ROUTLEDGE HANDBOOK OF SPORTS THERAPY, INJURY ASSESSMENT AND REHABILITATION

The work of a sports therapist is highly technical and requires a confident, responsible and professional approach. The *Routledge Handbook of Sports Therapy, Injury Assessment and Rehabilitation* is a comprehensive and authoritative reference for those studying or working in this field and is the first book to comprehensively cover all of the following areas:

- Sports injury aetiology
- Soft tissue injury healing
- Clinical assessment in sports therapy
- Clinical interventions in sports therapy
- Spinal and peripheral anatomy, injury assessment and management
- Pitch-side trauma care
- Professionalism and ethics in sports therapy.

The Handbook presents principles which form the foundation of the profession and incorporates a set of spinal and peripheral regional chapters which detail functional anatomy, the injuries common to those regions, and evidence-based assessment and management approaches. Its design incorporates numerous photographs, figures, tables, practitioner tips and detailed sample Patient Record Forms. This book is comprehensively referenced and multi-authored, and is essential to anyone involved in sports therapy, from their first year as an undergraduate, to those currently in professional practice.

Keith Ward has practised as a Sports Therapist since 1995. He has taught at a number of colleges and universities, and since 2009 has been a full-time lecturer on the BSc Sports Therapy programme at University College Birmingham (UCB), UK. He runs a small private practice in Cannock, Staffordshire. His first book, *Hands-On Sports Therapy*, proved popular with students of sports therapy and became a recommended text for many courses. Since 2012, he has been Managing Editor of the *Journal of Sports Therapy* (the 'JST'). He is a member of the Society of Sports Therapists (SST), a member of the Register of Exercise Professionals (REPS), a Fellow of the Royal Society of Public Health (RSPH), and a Fellow of the Higher Education Academy (HEA). Keith holds a biomedical BSc Rehabilitation Studies degree and Diplomas in Sports Therapy, Sports Massage, Exercise Referral, Naturopathy, and Acupuncture. He is currently completing an MA in Learning and Teaching.

ROUTLEDGE HANDBOOK OF SPORTS THERAPY, INJURY ASSESSMENT AND REHABILITATION

Edited by Keith Ward

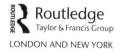

Routledge
Taylor & Francis Group

LONDON AND NEW YORK

First published in paperback 2018

First published 2016
by Routledge
2 Park Square, Milton Park, Abingdon, Oxon OX14 4RN

and by Routledge
711 Third Avenue, New York, NY 10017

Routledge is an imprint of the Taylor & Francis Group, an informa business

© 2016, 2018 K. Ward

British Library Cataloguing-in-Publication Data
A catalogue record for this book is available from the British Library

Library of Congress Cataloging in Publication Data
Routledge handbook of sports therapy, injury assessment, and
rehabilitation / edited by Keith Ward.
p. ; cm.
Handbook of sports therapy, injury assessment, and rehabilitation
Includes bibliographical references and index.
I. Ward, Keith (Keith D.), editor. II. Title: Handbook of sports
therapy, injury assessment, and rehabilitation.
[DNLM: 1. Athletic Injuries--therapy. 2. Athletic Injuries--diagnosis.
3. Sports Medicine. QT 261]
RD97
617.1'027--dc23
2015001364

ISBN: 978-0-415-59326-7 (hbk)
ISBN: 978-1-138-55906-6 (pbk)
ISBN: 978-0-203-80719-4 (ebk)

Typeset in Bembo
by Saxon Graphics Ltd, Derby

I dedicate this book with love to my wife Angela, our children Dennie and Arielle, and of course to my mom and dad (Peter and Nina). You have all given me so much love and support.

KW

CONTENTS

CONTRIBUTORS

Jo Baker BSc PG Cert MSc MSST, Lecturer in Sports Therapy, London Metropolitan University, UK.

Amy Bell BSc MSc MCSP BASRAT, Physiotherapist and Graduate Sports Rehabilitator, UK.

Hannah Boardman BSc PG Cert MSc MSST, Lecturer in Sports Therapy, University College Birmingham, UK.

Anthony Bosson BSc PG Cert MSST, Lecturer in Sports Therapy, Technological and Higher Education Institute of Hong Kong.

Aaron J. Caseley BOst MSc BOsC, Senior Lecturer in Sports Therapy, Faculty of Health and Social Sciences, Leeds Metropolitan University, UK.

Rob Di Leva BSc MSc, Sports Therapist, Australia.

Troy Douglin BSc PG Cert MSc MCSP, Lecturer in Sports Therapy, University College Birmingham, UK.

Kate Evans BSc PG Cert MSc MSST, Programme Director and Senior Lecturer in Sports Therapy, University of Wales Trinity David, UK.

Andrew Frampton BSc PG Cert MSST, Lecturer in Sports Therapy, University College Birmingham, UK

Nick Gardiner BSc PG Cert MSST, Lecturer in Sports Therapy, London Metropolitan University, UK.

Mike Grice BA BOst PG Cert BOsC, Lecturer in Sports Therapy, University College Birmingham, UK.

Adam Hawkey BSc MSc FBIS BASES REPS, Lecturer in Biomechanics, Abertay University (Dundee), UK.

Ian Horsley BSc MSc Phd MCSP MMACP MACPSM, English Institute of Sport (Regional Lead Physiotherapist, NW), UK.

Mark I. Johnson, Professor of Pain and Analgesia, Leeds Metropolitan University, Leeds Pallium Research Group, UK.

Jeanette Lewis BSc PG Cert MSST, Lecturer in Sports Therapy, University College Birmingham, UK.

Greg Littler BSc PG Cert MSc MCSP MSST, Senior Lecturer in Physiotherapy, University of Central Lancashire, UK.

Andrew Mitchell BSc PG Cert MSc Phd NSCA, Senior Lecturer, Sport and Exercise Science and Sports Therapy, University of Hertfordshire, UK.

Paul Robertson BSc PG Cert MSc BASES UKSCA, Senior Lecturer in Sports Therapy, University College Birmingham, UK.

Graham N. Smith, Chartered and HCPC Physiotherapist, Rehabilitation and Sports Injury Consultant, Glasgow, UK.

Philip Smith Grad Dip MSc MCSP, Senior Lecturer in Sports Therapy, Coventry University, UK.

Peter K. Thain BSc PhD MSST, Senior Lecturer in Sports Therapy, University of Bedfordshire, UK.

Tim Trevail BSc PG Dip SMA IRMA, Head of Academic Studies (Physical Health), Think Education Group, Australia.

Lee Young BSc PG Cert BASRAT, Lecturer in Sports Therapy, University College Birmingham, UK.

ACKNOWLEDGEMENTS

I would like to thank everyone who has helped us to get this thing together – it has certainly been a long, hard road to the destination of publication! I would like to express specific thanks to each of the following co-authors, subtle contributors, intelligent grafters, general supporters and jolly good friends:

- All colleagues from the Sports Therapy Department at University College Birmingham (UCB): Hannah Boardman; Glyn Curtis; Troy Douglin; Laura Ellery; Andy Frampton; Charlotte Gautrey; Mark Godwin; Mike Grice; Chris Holland; Tim Leary; Jeanette Lewis; Joe Matthews; Holly Mills; Marilena Nikolaidou; Paul Robertson; Steve Walker; Matt Willett; Marie Woodward; and Lee Young. There is a great sense of camaraderie at UCB and I have learnt so much from all of you …
- All past UCB sports therapy lecturing team alumni: Aaron Caseley; Sarah Catlow; Rob Di Leva; Ian Lahart; Greg Littler; Richard Morgan; Phil Smith; Tim Trevail.
- All UCB sports therapy students past and present (of course).
- All other significant people supporting the sports therapy team at UCB – Jane Abbey; Paul Barnes; David Bean; Andy Burston; Roland Hegarty; Matt Holmes; Adam Hubbard; Dianne Hudson; Kirendeep Jagdev; Dave Jenkins; Issy Johnson; Elaine Limond; Theresa Morris; Elaine Penn; Stephen Popple, Jo Reid; Andy Roberts; Ed Stanhope; Ruth Walton; Kat Whelan; Amy Williams.
- From the SST: Kate Cady; Sophie Drake; Colin Jackson; Jen Jones; Howard Piccaver; Graham Smith; Keith Waldon.
- John Annan; Jo Baker; Darryl Bagley (St John's Ambulance); Tom Baldwin (LWW); Amy Bell; Anthony Bosson (THEI, Hong Kong); Bob Bramah; Nick Dinsdale; Kate Evans; Susan Findlay; Lennard Funk (The Shoulder Doc); Nick Gardiner; Ann Gates (Exercise Works); Dom Gore; Kevin Hall; Lucy Hammond; Adam Hawkey (BASES); Ian Horsley (EIS); Jane Johnson; Mark Johnson (Leeds Pallium Research Group); Dean Madden (Aston Villa FC); Jason McCarthy (Wolverson Fitness); Andrew Mitchell; Alison Rushton (University of Birmingham); Keith Simmonds (Therapy World); Graham Taylor; Peter Thain.
- The publishing team at Routledge (especially Will Bailey, Ed Gibbons, Simon Whitmore and Joshua Wells).

- The copy-editor, Gary Smith.
- Dr Vicente Castells MB ChB MRCGP DA (UK) for his kind help in reviewing the 'Pitch-Side Trauma Care' chapter.

Many thanks to all the people involved in the photographs.

- The photographers included: Hannah Boardman, Anthony Bosson, Charlotte Gautrey, Jeanette Lewis, Keith Ward, Angela Ward, Arielle Ward and Angela Woodward.
- The models included: Aaron Caseley, Kieron Collins, Rob Di Leva, Greg Littler, Holly Mills, Marilena Nikolaidou, Dennie Rouse, Tim Trevail, Ruth Walton, Keith Ward and Angela Ward.
- The sports therapists included: Andrew Frampton, Paul Robertson, Tim Trevail, Keith Ward, Marie Woodward and Lee Young.

FOREWORD

Prior to 1990 there was no such thing as a sports therapist. This does not mean that anyone who participated in sport did not sustain injuries or receive primarily basic treatment from trainers, first aiders, physios and doctors. It does mean that, until that point, there was not a specific profession in the UK with its own clearly defined professional title, training, education and scope of practice, dedicated to sports and exercise therapy. However, a well-established and similar model did exist in the United States, which had been in existence since 1950; the model was that of the athletic trainer. This was also a practitioner who was playing an extremely vital role in sports medicine teams at all levels of the American sporting spectrum. Consequently, there was an urgent need for something comparable in the UK. Hence the birth of sports therapy and sports therapists.

Since 1990, sports therapist has become a firmly established occupational title. Similarly, sports therapy is now a respected profession that is firmly established within the sport and exercise medicine family in the UK. A significant reason for this was the development of graduate programmes which, through their validation and accreditation processes, set educational and professional benchmarks that are identifiable and applicable. Significantly, it is this graduate benchmark that is becoming increasingly used by governing bodies in sport and regulatory organizations as the minimum standard required for recognition and professional approval.

It is now acknowledged that sports therapists working in a multidisciplinary sport and exercise medicine team complement the other professionals and practitioners involved, which can only benefit the sports participant and potential patient/casualty. Sports therapists also have the ability to work as autonomous practitioners in an environment and industry that is extremely demanding and frequently unforgiving; hence the need for sports therapists who are appropriately educated and prepared.

A sports therapist requires knowledge, skills, expertise and competencies in five key areas. These are the prevention of injury; the recognition and evaluation of injury; management, treatment and, if appropriate, referral; rehabilitation; and education and professional practice issues. They are 'pillars of knowledge' that need to be built upon strong academic foundations.

In my opinion this *Handbook of Sports Therapy* has managed to establish these foundations. In doing so the editor and contributors have produced a publication that, I believe, will become a valuable asset to anyone studying sports therapy. The content has been carefully compiled to cover the concepts required in each of the five key competency areas by a cadre of contributors who, predominantly, work in higher education and within the subject area. Consequently, they understand the needs of the students they are responsible for educating and training. More importantly, sport and exercise therapy are linked between each contributor, which can only enhance the credibility of the material produced.

Another significant feature is that the editor has ensured that there is a consistency between each chapter, in both format and referencing, as well in the style of writing. This is extremely difficult to do but so important, especially when there are as many individuals contributing not only to the publication in its entirety, but to each specific chapter. For that achievement alone, the editor must be applauded and credited. I know that students of sports therapy will find this an extremely valuable handbook and one that they will refer to many times during their training and when they qualify. It is also a book that sets an academic benchmark for other specific sports therapy publications to follow. Therefore, I welcome this *Routledge Handbook of Sports Therapy, Injury Assessment and Rehabilitation*, and I will watch, with interest, to see how it evolves in the future alongside the exciting profession that it supports.

Professor Graham N. Smith
Chartered and HCPC Physiotherapist
Rehabilitation and Sports Injury Consultant
Glasgow (UK)

PREFACE

Even in a new age of information and technology, academic textbooks sit proudly and essentially as part of the base of the traditional hierarchical pyramid of research and information sources. Reputable academic textbooks (and handbooks) take a significant amount of time to develop and produce, and aim to provide evidence-based presentations of theoretical concepts and principles on often broad topic sets. I hope that the information in this book, which has been carefully gathered, appraised and presented, may almost inadvertently demonstrate a subtle tribute to all the therapists and scientists, academics and medics, researchers and writers, bloggers and tweeters, athletes and aspirant students who each effectively combine and contribute to an ever-evolving knowledge base.

This book is primarily aimed at *students* of sports therapy. While we have attempted to pitch some advanced concepts and develop a critically evaluative awareness, the main emphasis is on providing foundation and developmental information. The year 2015 is a fantastic time for sports therapists, given the growth and interest in all forms of sport and the clearly established public health need for widespread exercise participation. Not surprisingly, there has been a steady increase in the number of people choosing to study and practise in this exciting area. Since back in the day, athletes have been getting fitter and performing better because of the support they get from their team. The team today (at the higher levels) will be multidisciplinary, professionally organized, evidence-informed, progressive and technically advanced. Even in private practice, sports therapists are steadily gaining the increase in recognition that they deserve for helping their athletes and patients prepare for, and recover from, their chosen sports and physical activities. With increasing recognition and acceptance comes increasing demand and expectation.

The educational demands of graduate programmes in sports therapy obviously require appropriate, reliable and accessible reference resources; moreover, the standards of practice (the so-called 'competencies' of a sports therapist), which continuously undergo re-evaluation, must be achieved and evidenced by all who wish to achieve qualification. To demonstrate true competency in sports therapy is to be able to safely, effectively and autonomously demonstrate the ability to assess, manage and advise patients and athletes; this includes their fitness, their injuries, their needs and goals. Obviously, from the outset this is something much easier said than done, and clearly it takes time, effort and dedication to achieve such competency in such a specific area of health care.

This handbook is in no way any substitute for undertaking a comprehensive and recognized qualification, but along the way we hope that readers can better appreciate the remit of a sports therapist in any given situation, what constitutes our scope of practice, and importantly understand where sports therapists fit in alongside other health professionals.

To maintain focus, we have not attempted to discuss many of the more distinct specialities, methodologies, techniques and applications which are clearly essential component aspects in the wider delivery of sports therapy. Hence there is little mention, for example, of sports nutrition, sports psychology, advanced biomechanics, motor control or fitness assessment; nor are there expansive presentations of rehabilitation applications (whether regional, global or sports-specific) – other resources will provide all of this far more effectively. Simply, we have presented principles, overviews and discussions.

Most of us will recognize that the available 'evidence' (to support or refute anything) does not always equate to acceptable or transferrable validity or reliability – and this boils down to the very quality and type of research that is available, as well as how well it is accessed, translated and integrated. There will always be more questions, more proposals, hypotheses and anecdotes, and more debate. Sports therapists in this era are trained and expected to be relatively autonomous, and to be evidence-based. The concept of 'evidence-informed practice' is trichotomous and complementary and welcomes to the decision table, alongside the evidence-based and expert consensus guidelines, the contribution of individual practitioners' experience, expertise and clinical reasoning, as well as the utility of the 'patient culture' (i.e. the individual patient's or athlete's beliefs, values, situation and goals) which present in every single case.

This handbook has been an honest effort. We make no claim to perfection; and we accept in a critical world that almost any content can be legitimately challenged. We respect the progressive nature of contemporaneous information and enquiry. Whether student, experienced practitioner or lecturer, I think most of us should be able to appreciate that *the more we learn – the more we learn there is to learn*. I've certainly learnt a lot working on this handbook and I hope that you too can learn a little more, wherever you are on your own sports therapy journey.

Best regards to all.

Keith Ward
Cannock, Staffordshire, 2015

1

SPORTS INJURIES

Basic classifications, aetiology and pathophysiology

Keith Ward and Andrew Mitchell

This chapter aims to support a foundation understanding of sports-related injuries. It is expected that all professionals involved in the care of active exercising populations will view the topics of injury classification, injury aetiology and injury pathophysiology as fundamental to their knowledge base, and it is hoped that this chapter's overview can clarify some of the essential components of these core topics and explain the mechanisms occurring as the body attempts to repair tissue following injury.

Classifications of sports injuries

Sports injuries occur for innumerable reasons. They can be due to poor preparation for activities undertaken, to over-enthusiastic training, to inherent biomechanical problems or simply due to pure accident, such as a fall from a bike or horse, an unavoidable collision, slip or mistimed tackle. Table 1.1 provides some consideration for the various ways in which sports-related injuries may be presented or categorized, with important terms and concepts identified for the sports therapist to gain familiarity with. Any injury must go through a period of healing, and the resulting outcome will depend on a number of factors, such as: the type and severity of injury; the particular tissues involved in the injury and their capacity for resolution (repair or replacement); the early management provided; the age and general health of the individual; factors impeding the healing and rehabilitation process; and, crucially, how the injury is managed during the days, weeks and months that follow. One important aspect of broader injury assessment and management, especially in professional and team settings, is that of injury surveillance. The 'Orchard Sports Injury Classification System' (OSICS) is one established tool for providing audits and coding of injury diagnosis in sports injury surveillance systems. OSICS incorporates detailed lists of regional injuries and provides coding specific to sports medicine (Orchard, 2010; Rae and Orchard, 2007). The authors suggest that with efficient injury surveillance and documented identification of prevalence and incidence of specific injuries in specific sports, injury prevention strategies can be improved.

All sports have a collection of common injuries associated with them – whether the sport is recreational or professional, individual or team, contact or non-contact, agility, endurance or power-based. Injuries may also be regionally categorized; and by being knowledgeable of the causes and presentations of common injuries associated with each body region, the sports

Table 1.1 Classifying sports injuries

Stage of healing	Immediate / acute / reactive / sub-acute / post-acute / proliferative (repair) / dysrepair / remodelling (chronic) / degenerative / pathological
Severity	Minor, moderate and severe / I–III degree / type 1–4 (muscle disorders and injuries) / insignificant / ongoing / catastrophic / complicated
Tissue type	Skin / fascia / muscle / tendon / bursa / capsule / ligament / fibro-cartilage / hyaline cartilage / bone / blood vessel / nerve / viscera
Aetiology	Mechanism / primary / secondary / macrotrauma / repetitive microtrauma (overuse) / stress (tensile; compression; torsion; bending; shear) / intrinsic issue / extrinsic issue / direct / indirect / functional disorder / structural injury / instability (passive / dynamic) degenerative / insidious / sequelae / complications / predisposition / re-injury / preventable / accidental / compensatory / physiological / psychological
Age, gender, body type and performance level	Male / female / child / adolescent / adult / middle-aged / elderly / disabled / ectomorph / mesomorph / endomorph / novice / veteran / recreational / amateur / elite / professional
Body region	Head / facial / spinal / cervical / thoracic / lumbar / sacral / coccygeal / abdominal / pelvic / upper extremity / shoulder / elbow / wrist / hand / fingers / lower extremity / pelvic / hip / knee / ankle / foot / toes
Sports-related	Individual / team / contact / non-contact / high-risk / endurance-based / power-based / agility-based / linear / multidirectional / environment / terrain / level / position
Training, preparation and competition	Fitness: under-conditioned / over-trained / inadequate recovery, fatigue and physiological change (underperformance / overtraining syndrome) / sports-specific / nutritional deficiencies / dehydration / psychological factors / equipment factors / inadequate warm-up / cool-down / lifestyle factors / inadequate risk assessment or needs analyses / inadequate prehabilitation / access to medical and therapeutic support
Pain and symptoms	Types of pain (e.g. sharp; shooting; deep; throbbing; aching; stinging) / pain scales (e.g. VAS/NRS 0–10) / local pain / referred pain / radicular pain / somatic pain / peripheral neuropathic pain / myofascial pain / trigger point pain / DOMS / phantom pain / pain threshold / pain tolerance / pain syndromes (complex regional pain syndrome; fibromyalgia) / central sensitization / psychogenic pain / allodynia / hyperalgesia / hypoalgesia / causalgia / analgesia / nociception / noxious stimuli / nociceptive pain / dysaesthesia / fatigue / inhibition
Audit	Injury surveillance / statistical analyses – prospective / retrospective (i.e. numbers; percentages); populations (e.g. general; age; gender; sport; level; injury); prevalence (i.e. how common) / incidence (i.e. how often in a given timeframe); time out of action / games missed

therapist is able to clinically reason the differential diagnoses when undertaking assessment, as well as consider optimal prevention and rehabilitation strategies.

Alongside the most well-recognized sports-related injuries, the sports therapist must also be prepared and able to respond to the multitude of other medical conditions and concerns that may present in their work. These can include everything from known pre-existing conditions to acute infections, allergic reactions and the potentially more subtle psychosocial issues. With such a broad spectrum of conditions and the obvious potential for mismanagement and development of complications, the sports therapist must be efficient in screening and assessing their patients/athletes so as to be sure that individuals are managed as safely and effectively as possible and that medical advice is always sought whenever there is a lack of certainty or any doubt regarding the seriousness of the presenting condition. Conditions where the sports therapist must demonstrate cautiousness in their practice are extremely wide-ranging and not always obvious; they can range from contagious skin conditions (fungal; bacterial; viral) to complex injury presentations or suspicious clinical 'red flag' signs. If the practitioner has any doubt as to the suitability of the patient to receive sports therapy, then it is essential that medical advice is sought.

Functional regional anatomy and pathology are detailed elsewhere in this text, alongside the process and methods for efficient practical clinical assessment and strategies for management. Sports therapists will recognize that confident clinical reasoning strategies are central to being able to autonomously perform competent professional and ethical decision-making during both the assessment and the management of their patients/athletes.

Acute injuries and conditions

One single significantly traumatic episode can result in an acute injury, or aggravation of an existing injury, and the mechanism of that injury may be obvious. The classifications of contact injuries differ and are dependent on the type of tissue that suffers the damage. Acute bone injuries include fractures and periosteal contusions (bone bruising), while articular cartilage can experience osteochondral and chondral damage. Ligament injuries include sprains (graded I–III degree); joints can also suffer capsular irritations, dislocations, labral or meniscal damage. Acute *functional* muscular disorders include fatigue-related conditions, exercise-induced muscle disorders (EIMD) and exercise-associated muscle cramps (EAMC); and *structural* muscular problems include graded (mild, moderate or total) tears and contusions (Mueller-Wohlfahrt *et al.*, 2013). Cook and Purdam (2009) have documented the condition of an acute reactive tendinopathy. Acute skin injuries obviously include cuts, abrasions, lacerations and puncture wounds. Bursae can be subject to traumatic bursitis, which is most common at the hip (i.e. trochanteric), knee (pre-patellar and infra-patellar) and elbow (olecranon). Acute injuries to peripheral nerves can include transient neuropraxia (temporary paralysis ['conduction block'] resulting from direct impact or over-tensioning), axonotmesis (traumatic damage to the axon of the neuron) or neurotmesis (more severe neuronal and sheath damage); these have been traditionally classified by both Seddon (in 1943) and Sunderland (in 1951) (Faubel, 2010).

Traumatic head injuries are extremely common in sports. High-risk sports include combat sports, where the head is a legitimate target (boxing; martial arts); contact sports such as rugby and football; non-contact sports such as motor racing, equestrian, gymnastics and trampolining; and sports where head injury is rare but potentially severe (golf; cricket). Head and facial injuries include: skin wounds; contusions; eye gouging; perichondral haematoma (a blow to the ear causing subchondral haemorrhage [bleeding under the cartilage of the ear] which can separate tissues and restrict nutrient supply to the cartilage, leading to fibrosis and thickening – commonly known as 'cauliflower ear'); epistaxis (nose bleed); cranial or facial bone fractures; dental injury (dislodged teeth); temporomandibular joint (TMJ) dislocation; concussion and intracranial haemorrhage. Concussion is a common presentation and always a serious concern – its assessment and management are discussed in Chapter 4.

Contact injuries

Contact injuries occur as a result of an extrinsic force such as a collision with another player, or being struck by an object such as a hockey stick. Sporting examples of contact injuries include:

- Rugby: where the tackler hits the ball carrier on the anterior aspect of the knee causing a forced hyperextension, and sustains a posterior cruciate ligament sprain.
- Football: where two players go for a tackle and make shin-to-shin contact resulting in one player sustaining a fractured tibia and fibula.
- Basketball: where the player receiving a pass has a finger hyperextended by the ball, resulting in ligamentous sprain.

Non-contact injuries

Non-contact injuries occur as the body interacts with its environment. These may relate to individual predisposition (such as regional static and/or dynamic instability or previous injury), or simply to the combinations of forces and body positioning that occur during sport. Examples of non-contact injuries include:

- Rugby: where the player accelerates rapidly in order to chase or evade an opponent and sustains a hamstring tear.
- Football: where the player performs a change of direction or cutting manoeuvre resulting in forced inversion, and sustains a lateral ankle sprain.
- Basketball: where the player lands in full knee extension, or pivots on a flexed knee with the foot planted, and sustains an anterior cruciate ligament sprain.

Overuse injuries and chronic conditions

Whiting and Zernicke (1998) define use as 'normal functional loading' and overuse as 'repeated overload or force application'. Overuse injuries occur as a result of a repetitive overload or micro-trauma and therefore the mechanism of injury may be less obvious. Classification of overuse injury differs depending on the type of tissue that suffers the damage. Overuse bone injuries include stress fractures, apophysitis, osteitis, periostitis and bone strain. At synovial joints, capsulitis or synovitis can occur, articular cartilage can suffer from chondropathy and fragmentation; osteoarthritis is the most common degenerative musculoskeletal condition. The fibro-cartilaginous intervertebral discs and the meniscal cartilages of the knee are vulnerable to degenerative changes. While delayed onset muscle soreness (DOMS) may not be specifically categorized as an overuse muscle condition (as it can occur due to one single intense bout of unaccustomed exercise), it can present as a recurring problem; chronic exertional compartment syndrome (CECS) is recognized as an overuse condition. Tendinopathy, and in particular degenerative tendinopathy (tendinosis), is a highly prevalent overuse condition. Blisters, calluses and corns are examples of overuse conditions affecting the skin. Bursae are vulnerable to trauma from repeated impact or repetitive friction from tendon movement and can develop bursitis, which typically presents as visibly localized, extra-articular swelling and redness, and associated pain, tenderness and impaired function. Overuse nerve injuries may present as nerve irritations at their mechanical interfaces, which can be associated with adverse neural tension. A range of neural symptoms, such as distal paraesthesia, weakness in motor distribution and radicular pain can occur. Beyond this, peripheral neuropathy is the developmental dysfunction (abnormal firing and pain generation) from peripheral neural tissue (resulting from such situations as prolonged compression, local ischaemia and hypoxia, local neuroma or systemic demyelinating disease) (Butler and Tomberlin, 2007).

Sporting examples of overuse injuries include:

- Tennis: where the adolescent tennis player increases intensity of tennis play using the semi-Western or Western grip and sustains metacarpal stress fracture (Tagliafico *et al.*, 2009).
- Runners and cyclists: where the constant and repetitive flexion and extension of the knee causes the iliotibial band to rub against the lateral femoral epicondyle and the athlete suffers iliotibial band syndrome (ITBS).
- Swimming: where technical faults in conjunction with structural and functional imbalances can contribute to rotator cuff (sub-acromial) impingement.

Children and adolescents

There are a host of injuries and problems associated with younger age groups, for example the common adolescent growth spurt conditions, such as Osgood–Schlatter's lesion – a traction apophysitis, or micro-avulsion, of the patella tendon at the tibial tuberosity; Sinding–Larsen–Johansson lesion – a similar pathology which affects the attachment of the patella tendon at the inferior pole of the patella; and Sever's lesion – affecting the Achilles tendon insertion at the calcaneus. The majority of these conditions tend to settle within months and are generally recognized as being 'self-limiting' – that is they usually resolve within a predictable timeframe (months), and where intervention focuses upon symptom management (i.e. cryotherapy; taping), activity modification and progressive soft tissue and manual therapy. Occasionally, complications such as continued pain or fragmentation can occur (Gholve *et al.*, 2007).

There are several other common children's conditions with characteristic presentations simply attributed to musculoskeletal immaturity. Legg–Calve–Perthes disease is an idiopathic osteochondropathy of the hip, with characteristic flattening of the femoral head. It affects males more than females and is most commonly unilateral. The condition, which is associated with delayed skeletal maturity, typically begins with synovitis of the joint capsule, followed by an avascular (and necrotic) stage, which often leads to fragmentation and malformation. During this process, the child is likely to present with local aching and a painful limp. Once identified, ossification restarts and continues as activities are modified and the condition settles down, typically over a two-year period. Prognosis is generally good, but early onset osteoarthritis can be a concern (Placzek and Boyce, 2006).

Epiphyseal growth plate fractures are not uncommon. The growth plate is a cartilaginous centre of ossification at the metaphysis (between the diaphysis and epiphysis) in the long bones of adolescents. The growth plate can be considered as a vulnerable link – tendons and ligaments are relatively stronger than the growth plate and are also considerably more elastic, and as such the plate, being weaker, can give way when exposed to excessive stress. In adolescents, growth plate disruption is actually more common than ligamentous injury (Shanmugam and Maffulli, 2008). Once full skeletal maturity has occurred, the plate becomes a structurally stronger epiphyseal line (of mature bone) and is no longer active as an ossification centre. The condition can occur following a single trauma or from chronic stress. Certain individuals may have additional predisposing factors for epiphyseal growth plate fractures, such as being overweight, or underweight and tall, or simply sexually immature. Common sites for disruption are the: phalanges of the hand; distal radius; proximal and distal humerus; proximal and distal fibula; proximal and distal tibia; proximal and distal femur. Like many other types of fracture, there are established classification systems, the most recognized being the 'Salter–Harris' system (I–V), which categorizes different fractures according the degree of damage to the growth plate and the line of fracture or fragmentation (Peterson, 1994). A slipped capital femoral epiphysis (SCFE) occurs as the femoral shaft shifts proximally on the epiphysis. It occurs more in males than females and is frequently bilateral (McRae, 2006). The main complication associated with growth plate fractures is disruption to the normal process of bone lengthening and development and the possibility of deformity (Caine *et al.*, 2006). Growth plate fractures usually require cast immobilization and possibly operative fixation. Osteochondritis dissecans (OCD) is an adolescent idiopathic condition affecting subchondral bone and its adjacent articular cartilage, resulting in fragmentation of articular tissue. The intercondylar region of the femur at the knee, the talus at the talocrural joint and the capitulum at the elbow are the most commonly affected areas (Shanmugam and Maffulli, 2008). It is a condition that occurs more commonly in sporting males. Insidious onset of pain, swelling and restricted joint movements are characteristic symptoms, usually confirmed via plain radiographs or MRI (magnetic resonance imaging). Scheuermann's disease is a physeal osteochondropathy affecting the thoracic vertebral end growth plates. The condition, which is more common in active adolescents and young adults, typically leads to a 'wedging', usually of several adjacent vertebral bodies, and characteristically results in a kyphotic posture (MacAuley, 2007). The so called 'greenstick' fractures of long bones only occur in children and adolescents. These present as incomplete breaks on the convex side of the immature bone.

The sports therapist must also be vigilant to being able to recognize the possibility of symptoms that could be associated with underlying structural or developmental abnormality. Such conditions, although rare, include: lumbarization (abnormal separation and mobilization of S1 from S2); sacralization (abnormal fusion between L5 and S1); cervical rib (abnormal additional costal bone); pars defect (an abnormal neural arch, most commonly at L5); hooked acromion (abnormal inferior angulation of the acromion process – reducing the subacromial space); bipartite or multipartite patella (abnormal segmentation of the patella – usually unilateral and more common in males); discoid meniscus (abnormal discoid configuration of the meniscus); tarsal coalition (abnormal fibrous fusion of adjacent tarsal bones). Such presentations serve to remind us that all individuals are unique and every single patient's anatomy is different and has the potential to be the primary cause of their symptoms.

In addition to their developmental predisposition to particular kinds of injury, children and adolescents have some degree of increased vulnerability to injury simply because of limitations in their experience of situations and their awareness of their body and space (spatial awareness). Furthermore, younger athletes are sometimes 'pushed' inappropriately by parents or coaches. Brukner and Khan (2009) have presented the 'ugly parent syndrome', in which symptoms ranging from simple head, stomach and muscle aches to stress-related sleep and emotional disturbances may occur simply due to the excessive parental pressure to compete. Children should be encouraged but not forced and any participation in sport should be for the child's enjoyment (not the parent's) and healthy development at this stage of life. Additionally, in supervised sport, children should be matched appropriately, be provided with correct equipment and made aware of the rules and the reasoning behind them.

Males and females

MacAuley (2007) states that females may be more prone to sports injuries for anatomical reasons, and it is known that females are more vulnerable to specific types of sports injury when compared to males (for example, ACL injuries, patella dislocation and patellofemoral pain syndrome). The prevalence of males experiencing adolescent traction apophysitis or osteochondrosis is significantly higher. It has also been said that males are more prone to injury, experience more injuries and die more frequently from injuries simply because they are more likely to engage in risk-laden behaviour (Udry, 1998). Perhaps the issue of gender predisposition to injury becomes more apparent with inexperienced or recreational athletes, who are less likely to have access to the training methods and medical support that is normally available to elite athletes.

Males and females of the human species have many anatomical and physiological differences, but, as highlighted by Bennell and Alleyne (2009), they have far more similarities than males and females of many other species. A number of average and very generalized differences are recognized (Table 1.2), many of which are contentious for a number of reasons, not least the uniqueness of every individual and the potential for both anatomical and physiological development via training and nutrition. Hence such generalizations must be recognized as such;

Table 1.2 Average anatomical and physiological differences between males and females

Males	Females
Commence adolescent growth spurt around 13 years of age.	Commence adolescent growth spurt around 11 years of age.
No menarche, menstrual cycle, pregnancy or menopause.	Commence menarche between 12 and 14 years of age. Experience regular monthly menstrual cycles. May experience one or more pregnancies (period of 37–42 weeks, culminating in childbirth). Menopause (cessation of normal menstrual cycle) in middle age.
Reach maximal height around 20 years of age.	Reach maximal height around 16 or 17 years of age.
Generally are taller and heavier.	Generally are shorter and lighter.
Higher centre of gravity.	Lower centre of gravity.
Heavier and thicker bones.	Lighter and thinner bones.
Larger articulatory surfaces.	Smaller articulatory surfaces.
More distinct muscle attachment sites.	Less distinct muscle attachment sites.
Proportionally longer limbs.	Proportionally shorter limbs.
Proportionally wider biacromial width.	Proportionally narrower biacromial width.
Lesser elbow carrying angle.	Greater elbow carrying angle.
Proportionally larger thorax.	Proportionally smaller thorax.
Penis and testicles, small amount of breast tissue.	Vagina, ovaries and breasts.
Proportionally thicker waist.	Proportionally narrower waist.
Proportionally deeper pelvis and narrower hips.	Proportionally shallower pelvis and wider hips.
Lesser femoral angle of inclination.	Greater femoral angle of inclination.
Lesser genu valgus and Q angle.	Greater genu valgus and Q angle.
Lower average body fat composition (14%).	Higher average body fat composition (26%).
Greater subcutaneous body fat around abdomen and upper body.	Greater subcutaneous body fat around hips and thighs.
Higher lean body mass.	Lower lean body mass.
Greater muscle mass.	Lesser muscle mass.
Greater percentage of blood in body fluid.	Lesser percentage of blood in body fluid.
Larger heart and lungs.	Smaller heart and lungs.
Greater stroke volume and cardiac output.	Lesser stroke volume and cardiac output.
Lower resting heart rate.	Higher resting heart rate.
Lower blood pressure.	Higher blood pressure.
Greater respiratory rate and vital capacity.	Lesser respiratory rate and vital capacity.
Greater aerobic capacity and VO2 max.	Lesser aerobic capacity and VO2 max.

and clearly stereotypical classifications have their limitations. However, it is important for the sports therapist to recognize the definitive, apparent or potential characteristics of males and females; and in so doing, the aetiology of injuries may be more readily ascertained and the prevention and management of injuries improved.

Within sports medicine, females are frequently discussed as a special population, just as are children, older athletes and the disabled. The average or generalized differences highlighted in Table 1.2 will help the sports therapist appreciate some of the gender-unique issues that females may have to contend with. Clearly, any individual having less than ideal biomechanics for particular sports is at a disadvantage and offers an obvious increased vulnerability to injury. However, it must be recognized that many individuals do not conform to such generalizations; and also the majority of active individuals will choose to undertake sports and training to which they are best suited.

The hormonally regulated menstrual cycle, or monthly period, is a normal part of the female reproductive cycle. During the cycle, a woman bleeds from her uterus via the vagina for a period of three to seven days; this is known as menstruation – a process repeated every month until menopause – unless fertilization of her ovum occurs and she becomes pregnant. There are other normal reasons for absent periods (amenorrhea), such as taking the contraceptive pill. Some females experience occasional pre-menstrual syndrome, which has been defined as a collection of emotional and physical symptoms (for example: anxiety; depression; mood swings; headaches; fluid retention; abdominal and back pain; breast soreness) and which commonly occur prior to the monthly cycle. Interestingly, it has been identified that regular exercise may help to reduce such symptoms. Dysmenorrhea (painful menstrual cramps) can also occur early in the cycle due to transient ischaemia in the smooth muscular wall of the uterus. There are a number of menstrual irregularities which are associated with frequent and intense exercise, as explained by Bennell and Alleyne (2009). These include: delayed menarche (delayed commencement of menstrual bleeding); oligomenorrhea (irregular menstruation); amenorrhea (absent menstruation). Sports therapists, although not expected to be expert in such matters, should recognize, or at least aim to identify, when menstrual issues may be present.

Two main complications of menstrual cycle irregularities include reduced fertility and reduced bone mass. Particularly, amenorrheic female athletes have increased incidence of stress fractures; and osteoporosis is a concern for post-menopausal women with reduced bone mass, and therefore predisposition to pathological fractures (Sherry and Wilson, 1998).

The 'Female Athletic Triad' was first presented in 1992 by the ACSM (American College of Sports Medicine) as a term to describe a condition characterized by a combination of: (1) disordered eating (most commonly anorexia nervosa and bulimia nervosa); (2) delayed menarche or amenorrhoea (intense exercise related); and (3) (amenorrhoeic) osteoporosis or osteopenia.

However, a recent IOC consensus statement regarding 'Relative Energy Deficiency in Sport' and the acronym term 'RED-S' have been presented. RED-S has been defined and designed in an effort to supersede the term Female Athletic Triad (Mountjoy *et al.*, 2014). In presenting the RED-S condition, the aim was to emphasize the pathophysiological complexity and multisystem involvement, and the fact that, while aetiology can vary, the condition may affect both men and women. In RED-S the imbalance in energy availability and energy expenditure is evident; and as Swe Win and Thing (2014) explain, there also occurs a misbalance between training load and training recovery. However, it is important to appreciate the critical response to the IOC statement by De Souza *et al.* (2014a), who ascertained that it was '*ill-conceived and poorly defended*'. They argue that the progressing research platform and established practical management strategies for affected female athletes must continue, and that the 'Female Athletic Triad' concept and definition should not be subsumed under the umbrella of RED-S.

The signs and symptoms of this condition are not always easy to recognize, and indeed individuals can appear 'normal'. Pantano (2009) stated that *'physical therapists must be responsible for recognizing, treating and preventing the Female Athlete Triad'*. Disordered eating, or 'eating distress' may be due to psychological, biological or sociological factors (MacAuley, 2007) and can lead to a whole host of health problems, not least low energy availability. It is, however, more prevalent in sports where athletes are required to maintain a specific body weight and composition, such as gymnastics, synchronized swimming, ballet or distance running (Back and Smethurst, 2004). It is certain that affected individuals are likely to be discreet in their behaviour. Disordered eating results in calorific and nutritional deficiency and signs of such can include loss of muscle tone, skin problems, cold extremities, swollen face and ankles. Where there is imbalance in energy availability and energy expenditure, both short-term (performance deficits; stress fractures) and long-term (osteoporotic fractures; infertility) health consequences can manifest. Other consequences of insufficient energy availability include low immunity and risk of infection, and chronic fatigue. A recent Female Athletic Triad expert consensus statement (De Souza *et al.*, 2014b) recommended a set of pre-participation screening questions for vulnerable female athletes:

- Have you ever had a menstrual period?
- How old were you when you had your first menstrual period?
- When was your most recent menstrual period?
- How many periods have you had in the past 12 months?
- Are you presently taking any female hormones (oestrogen, progesterone, birth control pills)?
- Do you worry about your weight?
- Are you trying to or has anyone recommended that you gain or lose weight?
- Are you on a special diet or do you avoid certain types of foods or food groups?
- Have you ever had an eating disorder?
- Have you ever had a stress fracture?
- Have you ever been told you have low bone density (osteopenia or osteoporosis)?

Taking place over 37 to 42 weeks and involving three trimesters, pregnancy brings with it normal physical and physiological changes, a certain vulnerability to both mother and foetus and a collection of potential complications. Some of the more obvious changes occurring during pregnancy include: weight gain; breast enlargement; lung compression and diaphragm displacement; shift in centre of gravity with progressive lumbar lordosis; fluid retention; ligamentous laxity; increasing joint stress; and emotional changes. It is usual for active women to continue to exercise during pregnancy. Reasons not to exercise include: infection; fetal distress; placenta praevia; pregnancy-induced hypertension; pre-term rupture of membranes; persistent second or third trimester bleeding (Cowey, 2006; MacAuley, 2007). Particular signs of exercise being inappropriate include: dyspnoea; dizziness; chest pain; persistent headache; radicular pain; carpal tunnel syndrome; leakage of amniotic fluid; decreased fetal movement; calf pain or swelling (indicating the possibility of deep vein thrombosis [DVT]); and any other individual concerns. Furthermore, exercise is contraindicated in the first trimester where there is history of spontaneous abortion. Any concerns should be discussed with or referred to the individual's GP, midwife or gynecologist.

The female's breast is an apocrine mammary gland. Its primary function is to produce breast milk (lactation) for breastfeeding. Breasts overlie the pectoral region and are predominantly composed of connective fatty tissue (collagen, elastin and adipose tissue). The superficial

Cooper's ligaments suspend the breast's fascia to the overlying skin superiorly from the clavicular region and each breast contains a nipple, areolar, lactiferous (milk) lobes and ducts, blood vessels, nerve fibres and lymphatic channels. The majority of lymph from the breast region channels to the axillary lymph nodes. Females have to contend with the potential for direct traumatic injuries involving their breasts, which can lead to haematomas. Although males can suffer nipple problems, females have increased predisposition, particularly those undertaking distance running. 'Jogger's nipple' is where nipples are constantly irritated by the friction of clothing. Bleeding is common, and prevention is key. Excessive up and downward movement of breasts during exercise is also an issue and can easily lead to pain and reduced performance; correctly fitting sports bras should be recommended (Bennell and Alleyne, 2009). Finally, breast cancer, although far from being unique to females, is one of the most common cancers; regular self-examination for unusual lumps, skin dimpling or discolouration, nipple changes or bloody discharge must be encouraged.

Complications of injury

Not all sports or exercise-related injuries and problems follow a straightforward course of recovery. Injuries can become chronic, affecting ability to train or compete; secondary, or compensatory, injuries can develop; health problems can worsen; tissues can degenerate or fail to heal effectively; injuries can be recurrent; infection can occur (or reoccur). Recovery can be slow and problematic; setbacks are not uncommon. On return to full sporting action, if underlying aetiologies have not been attended to, or appropriate progressive and final stage rehabilitation undertaken, then re-injury or new injury can result. Comorbidities commonly exist which compound the injury's recovery process. Patients may not have been provided with a confirmative medical diagnosis, meaning increased potential for inappropriate management. Of course, patients may not even receive appropriate intervention or advice in the first instance. Furthermore, patients/athletes may not follow recommendations (for various reasons – intrinsic and extrinsic) which can have significant negative impacts on eventual outcomes. Non-adherence (more historically referred to as 'non-compliance') is a complex topic and involves a host of psychosocial factors (Magee *et al.*, 2008). Greenhalgh and Selfe (2006) present a summary of the psychosocial 'flag system': 'yellow flags' – emotional and behavioural factors; 'blue flags' – social and economic factors; 'black flags' – occupational factors; and 'orange flags' – psychiatric factors. Iatrogenic factors can also occasionally contribute to long-term problems; these relate to adverse effects of therapeutic or medical intervention. Therapists should aim to appreciate how long-term injuries can impact on the individual. Loss of self-esteem, financial implications and developing frustrations, fears and depression are all real concerns, particularly in professional sport. In an ideal setting these will be considered and managed carefully and responsibly.

Even when full and appropriate rehabilitation has taken place, the athlete could still be faced with a range of post-injury detriments, for example: reduced tissue strength; joint instability; excessive repair (scar) tissue; adverse stiffness; muscular weakness; motor control issues; persistant pain; restricted joint mobility; adverse neural tension; soft tissue calcification; early onset osteoarthritis; deformity; fear of use or apprehension. The sports therapist must aim to recognize when injuries are not responding as should be expected and they should be able to make autonomous decisions on appropriate recommendations, such as referral for second opinion, or for imaging or other investigation.

Injury aetiology

With Dr Andrew Mitchell

Forces acting upon the human body

The human body is remarkably resilient to the stresses and strains exerted upon it by not only activities of daily life, but also sports and exercise. In daily life, humans exert force on the ground and stairs while walking, in opening and closing doors and by lifting or carrying objects. During sports and exercise we exert often greater force on the ground, and more often while running than walking, and we also apply force against balls, clubs, racquets, water and wind. In contact sports such as rugby, force is applied against other human beings. On a daily basis the tissues of the body experience innumerable loads of varying intensities and suffer no ill effects. Injury only occurs when a force overloads the tissues' ability to withstand it, resulting in tissue failure and damage. Force may be defined as *'the mechanical action or effect applied to a body that tends to produce acceleration'* (Whiting and Zernicke, 1998).

There are a number of forces that athletes are subjected to that may cause injury. Gravity is the force that has the greatest influence on human movement (Mester and Macintosh, 2000) and is a downward force tending to accelerate objects at 9.8 m s^{-2} (Whiting and Zernicke, 1998). A ground reaction force (GRF) is a force that acts from the ground on any structure that is in contact with it (for example, the hands in a cartwheel, or the feet during gait). If any part of an athlete's body is in contact with the ground it will exert a force upon it, the ground in turn will then exert a force that is equal and opposite.

The impact force from an external source making contact with the body can cause injury (for example, being tackled in rugby or hyperextending a finger while catching a basketball). Compressive forces from structures within the body acting upon each other can cause injuries, for example, landing on one's feet from a high fall could result in compression of the femur, tibia, fibula, tarsals or any other weight-bearing bones, causing fracture. Intrinsic tensile forces, such as those at the musculotendinous junction or across a ligament acting over a joint can result in muscle tears, sprains or avulsion fractures.

Uniaxial forces

An axial force is a force that acts along the longitudinal axis of a structure. There are three forms of uniaxial loading: compression, tension and shearing (Figure 1.1).

Compressive forces cause a crushing or squeezing of the tissues. Compression of a high load can cause a single traumatic injury, for example, being struck on the forearm with a hockey stick, which may result in bruising of the forearm musculature or, more significantly, a fracture of the radius or ulna. Typical compression injuries include fractures, stress fractures, haematoma,

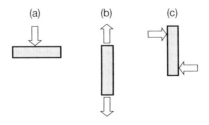

Figure 1.1 Uniaxial force of injury: (A) compression; (B) tension (C) shearing.

puncture wounds and, as a complication, myositis ossificans. Compressive forces can also be more subtle. Abnormal bony projections, for example, can cause repetitive compressive stress to local soft tissues (most commonly tendons) during joint movement. Also, where peripheral nerves pass through narrow anatomical tunnels (mechanical interfaces), compression can cause restriction to normal movement (adverse neural tension) and also restriction of normal blood flow to the nerve.

Tensile forces cause a pulling, longitudinal stretching of tissues. Tension of a high load can cause soft tissue tears and ruptures, whereas intermittent tension can strengthen muscle and tendon. Tensile injuries include ligamentous sprains, musculotendinous tears and avulsion fractures.

Shear forces cause a horizontal or oblique stress movement of one tissue over another, for example an excessive anterior tibial shear force acting on the anterior cruciate ligament can cause sprain or rupture. Shearing injuries include: sprains; meniscal and labral tears; long bone spiral fractures; isthmic spondylolistheses; and certain tendinopathies. Shear forces have been shown to increase within the knee joint if the supporting musculature is fatigued, which can put the knee at a greater risk of non-contact ACL injury (Chappell *et al.*, 2005). Equally, shear forces of a low load, with repetition, can lead to abnormal stress to tissues, such as with frictional foot blisters (Yavuz and Davis, 2010). Tendon and fascial tissues are particularly vulnerable to shear stress, for example the 'whipping' shear stress exposed to the Achilles tendon or the plantar fascia easily created in the presence of excessive foot pronation during running gait. Tendons are also vulnerable to the abusive overloading that can occur during episodes of rapidly repeated activity, especially where less than ideal biomechanics present (Sharma and Maffulli, 2006) – a common cause of acute reactive tendinopathy (Cook and Purdam, 2009).

Compression, tension and shearing stresses often combine and act on the same joint during sporting movements. For example, in the throwing athlete's elbow, tension is applied to the medial stabilizing structures, compression is applied to the lateral structures and a shearing force is exerted to the posterior structures (Cain *et al.*, 2003).

Multiaxial forces

Torque can be thought of as a rotational force and is the product of the magnitude of the force applied and length of the moment arm. When a muscle contracts it produces torque over the joint it crosses and this forms the basis for human movement. Torque caused by muscles rarely causes tissue damage; instead it is usually torque caused by an external source that is responsible for injury. There are two forms of multiaxial loading: bending and torsion (Figure 1.2).

A structure such as a long bone will bend if a force is applied to it, perpendicular to its longitudinal axis. During the bending situation, compression is applied to the concave surface and tension occurs at the convex surface. Bone is better at resisting compression rather than tension, and if the magnitude of force is great enough, fracture will occur on the side of the bone under tension.

A structure will experience torsion if a twisting force is applied to it along its longitudinal axis. A non-anatomical example of this is removing the cap from a bottle of water. A shear stress is created along the bone during a torsion injury. A typical torsional injury is a spiral fracture which is commonly seen in sports such as skiing and snowboarding, and as momentum is occurring and with the leg firmly fixed in the snow, the individual rotates around it during the fall, potentially resulting in excessive force to the lower limb bones. Obviously, such forces can lead to injury of any of the involved tissues (bone; muscle; tendon; ligament; cartilage; skin; nerve; blood vessel; viscera). Different tissues have differing properties and capacity to withstand different forces, and injury is usually sustained to the weakest tissues (or links) in the kinetic chain as these are the tissues that will fail first when put under stress and strain.

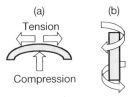

Figure 1.2 Multiaxial force of injury: (A) bending; (B) torsion.

There are a number of factors that determine the nature and severity of injury when force is applied to human tissues:

- **Area**: the risk of injury increases when force is applied to smaller areas.
- **Direction**: some tissues are more efficient at dissipating force in certain directions.
- **Duration**: acute injuries usually occur very quickly (30-50 ms), while overuse injuries occur over a much longer period of time.
- **Frequency**: acute injuries usually occur as a result of a single traumatic overload, while overuse injuries occur as a result of chronic repetitive loading.
- **Location**: where the force is applied to the structure will determine the tissues' ability to withstand it.
- **Magnitude**: injury occurs if the amount of force applied exceeds the tissues' ability to withstand it.
- **Rate**: if a force is applied quickly it may cause injury, but if that same force is applied gradually the tissues may well be able to withstand it.
- **Tissue type**: the large mass of the quadriceps muscles are less likely to suffer injury after a blow compared to the bony prominence of the olecranon process.
- **Variability**: whether the magnitude of the applied force is variable or constant will determine the extent of injury sustained.

Primary and secondary injury

A primary injury is one that occurs as an immediate and direct result of a trauma – for example, sustaining a haematoma on the thigh after being struck by a hockey ball. A primary injury is an acute catastrophic failure of the tissues. A secondary injury has a gradual onset and may appear some time after the initial trauma due to a disruption in blood flow, nerve supply or structural vulnerability. For example, degenerative change in the Achilles tendon (tendinosis) is associated with increased risk of spontaneous rupture (Kannus and Józsa, 1991). Another form of secondary injury is known as a compensatory injury, and can occur when an athlete consciously or unconsciously adjusts their biomechanics in order to accommodate for a primary injury. For example, a long-distance runner recovering from a lateral ankle sprain may subconsciously modify their gait, causing increased risk of stress fractures of the foot, or other problems through the kinetic chain.

Macrotrauma and microtrauma

Macrotrauma is an injury from a single acute force that causes immediate tissue damage such as a fracture, contusion, muscle tear, ligamentous sprain or neurotmesis. While microtrauma following appropriate loading is central to the process for progressive increases in strength and resilience in tissues (during either rehabilitation or fitness training), inappropriate microtrauma when repetitively or chronically overloading tissues at a microscopic level can lead to a breakdown in tissue structure. The forces involved in a single microtrauma will not cause injury; but it is the repeated inappropriate loading and resulting weakening of the tissue, due to insufficient recovery, that leads to degenerative conditions and in some cases subsequent macrotrauma. Taljanovic *et al.* (2011) present the example of repetitive microtrauma occurring from overhead hitting in female volleyball players, initially causing laxity of the inferior capsule which can lead to subsequent avulsion of the humeral attachment of the inferior glenohumeral ligament.

Stress, strain and deformation

The response of human tissue to progressive force application can be elastic or plastic in nature. Figure 1.3 shows how excessive force application can result in tissue deformation. If the load is applied at point A and released at point X, before reaching the elastic limit or yield point, the tissue will not suffer any long-term deformation and will return to its original shape and size. The response of the tissue to the stress is elastic. If, however, the load is applied at point A, but not released until point Y, which is beyond the elastic limit, the tissue will suffer long term deformation and will not return to its original shape and size. In such a case, the response of the tissue is plastic.

If the applied load exceeds the tissues' ultimate failure point then mechanical failure occurs. Figure 1.4 demonstrates how excessive force application can result in tissue failure. The tendon will cope with a high load applied at point A, before failure at point T. Muscle tissue will deform under low load, then respond stiffly before failure at point M. Bone responds stiffly to the load applied at point A, and undergoes minimal deformation prior to failure at point B (Whiting and Zernicke, 1998).

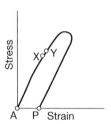

Figure 1.3   Stress–strain curve showing tissue deformation.

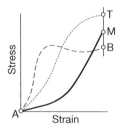

Figure 1.4   Stress–strain curve showing tissue failure (T = tendon; M = muscle; B = bone).

RISK FACTORS FOR INJURY

With Dr Andrew Mitchell

The sports therapist will appreciate that a major component of injury prevention is understanding and assessing the intrinsic and extrinsic risk factors. Leadbetter (1994), cited by Whiting and Zernicke (1998), identified a number of factors that can contribute to injury:

- contact or impact
- dynamic overload
- inflexibility
- muscle imbalance
- overuse
- structural vulnerability
- rapid growth.

Such factors are fundamentally interlinked and may act in unison to cause injury. For example, if an athlete has tightness in a hamstring muscle as a result of a history of previous strains, then inflexibility, muscle imbalance and subsequently dynamic overload may contribute to a new acute hamstring strain. In many cases, these factors may be identified by pre-participation screening, monitoring and evaluation of athletes. If a potential risk factor is observed then the sports therapist can implement prehabilitation techniques in order to reduce the chance of injury occurring. Meeuwisse (1994) presented an original multifactorial model of athletic injury aetiology, which aimed to demonstrate: the intrinsic risk factors predisposing the athlete to injury; the exposure to extrinsic risk factors during training or competition; the susceptible athlete; the inciting event; and the resultant injury. This model has been slightly modified in recent presentations, and remains relevant.

While there are numerous factors that contribute to an athlete sustaining an injury, these may be divided into two basic groups: intrinsic risk factors, which are individual, functional, anatomical, physiological, psychological and pathological and from within the body; and extrinsic risk factors, which are external, resulting from training and preparation errors, inappropriate equipment, environmental conditions and the very nature of competition.

Table 1.3 Intrinsic and extrinsic risk factors predisposing to injury

Intrinsic factors	*Extrinsic factors*
Structural and biomechanical abnormalities	Equipment
(e.g. excessive Q-angle; pes planus; leg	Footwear
length discrepancy)	Surface
Gait abnormality	Terrain
Muscle imbalance	Gradient
Age	Training errors
Excessive or limited flexibility	Coaching errors
Sex, size and body composition	Environmental conditions
Physiological issues	Nutritional issues
Previous injury	Sports officiating errors
Impaired proprioception and joint positional	Opposition players
sense	Inciting event
Sports-specific technique errors	
Psychological issues	

A thorough pre-participation/season screen can identify many intrinsic risk factors for an athlete and in some cases enable the sports therapist to intervene in order to mobilize, strengthen or enhance neuromuscular control where indicated. Formal profiling, particularly in professional settings, is utilized to establish a background picture of the individual athlete's health and injury status and functional ability performance. Profiling can include the individual's: previous medical history; injury history; body composition; blood pressure; blood constituents; nutritional status; lung function; heart function; basic cognitive functioning; balance and coordination; flexibility testing; functional movement screening (FMS); muscular strength and endurance assessment; VO2 max testing; agility testing; and sports-specific fitness assessment.

Structural and biomechanical abnormalities

The following common lower limb abnormalities are generally considered injury risk factors until proved otherwise because they alter biomechanics and may place excessive strain on involved structures during repetitive or excessive loading in sports or exercise. These may be unilateral or bilateral:

- excessive lateral, anterior or posterior pelvic tilt
- coxa valga and vara
- femoral anteversion and retroversion
- genu valgus and varus
- excessive Q-angle
- patella alta and baja
- 'frog-eyed' and 'squinting' patella
- genu recurvatus
- tibia varus and increased tibial external torsion
- ankle equinus
- valgus and varus heels
- rearfoot varus and rearfoot valgus
- plantarflexed first ray
- forefoot varus
- hallux valgus
- hallux rigidus
- pes cavus and planus
- excessive pronation or supination
- leg length discrepancy (true or apparent).

Average Q-angles are in the region of 10° for males and 15° for females; 20° is considered excessive (see Chapter 10 for Q-angle measurement technique). An excessive Q-angle has been shown to be a risk factor for patellofemoral pain syndrome (Haim *et al.*, 2006; Waryasz and McDermott, 2008) and lower limb stress fractures (Cowan *et al.*, 1996). Leg length inequality has been shown to be linked with lower extremity injury in runners (Fields *et al.*, 2010; Wen *et al.*, 1998) and specifically stress fractures (Korpelainen *et al.*, 2001) (see Chapter 9 for true and apparent leg length measurement techniques). Gait abnormalities are common and easily lead to injury problems. Runners with less pronation at heel or mid-foot strike, and those with laterally directed roll-off, may be at a greater risk of sustaining lower limb overuse injuries (Ghani Zadeh Hesar *et al.*, 2009). Equally, runners with excessive pronation and those exhibiting greater medial pressures are at risk of exercise-related lower leg pain (Willems *et al.*, 2006). Chapter 2 provides a detailed discussion of gait assessment.

Many upper limb injuries are caused by muscular imbalance caused by tightness or weakness, but a number of biomechanical factors may contribute to upper limb injury, including:

- abnormal shape and angulation of the acromion
- reduced subacromial space
- abnormal scapula shape and malpositioning
- excessive elbow carrying angle (>15°)
- cubitus recurvatus and other hypermobility.

Muscle imbalance

Clark (2001) suggested that muscle imbalance is caused by a number of factors such as overtraining, postural stress, poor neuromuscular or technical efficiency and pattern overload. In turn, predictable patterns of kinetic dysfunctions occur, such as those identified by Janda (1983).

Muscle tightness or weakness of one muscle (agonist) can cause inhibition in the antagonist, which in turn causes dysfunction in the kinetic chain. Therefore the tight or hyperactive muscle dominates against the weak or inhibited muscle and disrupts normal function over the joint. The athlete compensates for this dysfunction by making postural modifications and by placing greater emphasis on the synergistic muscles to those that are weak. Clark (2001) referred to this as synergistic dominance and suggested that these muscles are now required to do more work in contributing to acceleration and deceleration and as a result may be more at risk of injury. Janda (1983) divided the muscular system into two: those muscles prone to tightness (movement group) and those prone to weakness (stabilization group).

Movement group characteristics
- Prone to developing tightness or hyperactivity.
- More active during functional movement patterns.
- Dominate during fatigue situations.
- Dominate when performing new movement patterns.
- Usually cross two joints.

Stabilization group characteristics
- Prone to developing weakness or inhibition.
- Less active during functional movement patterns.
- Prone to myokinematic and arthrokinematic inhibition.
- Easily fatigued.
- Usually cross one joint.
- Janda (1983) identified the muscles that are commonly found in each group.

Movement group (prone to tightness)
- Gastrocnemius
- soleus
- hip adductors
- hamstrings
- rectus femoris

- iliopsoas
- tensor fascia lata
- piriformis
- erector spinae
- quadratus lumborum
- pectoralis major
- upper trapezius
- levator scapulae
- sternocleidomastoid
- scalenes
- flexors of the upper limb.

Stabilization group (prone to weakness)

- Peroneals
- anterior tibialis
- posterior tibialis
- gluteus maximus
- gluteus medius
- abdominals
- serratus anterior
- rhomboids
- lower trapezius
- deep cervical flexors
- extensors of the upper limb.

Athletes with a muscle strength imbalance between the ankle inverters and everters have been shown to have an increased risk of lateral ankle sprain, as did athletes with a low dorsiflexion-to-plantarflexion strength ratio (Baumhauer *et al.*, 1995). Weak dorsiflexors and delayed peroneal reaction time contribute to the risk of sustaining an ankle sprain (Willems *et al.*, 2006). Weak adductor muscles are a risk factor for sustaining new groin injury (Engebretsen *et al.*, 2010), while hip extensor muscle imbalance has been shown to be associated with the incidence of low back pain in female athletes (Nadler *et al.*, 2001). Similarly, athletes who sustain knee injury have been shown to have significantly weaker hip abductors and external rotators (Leetun *et al.*, 2004). Furthermore, a hamstring-to-quadriceps isokinetically assessed strength ratio (HQR) below the normal average (where hamstring strength is less than 50 per cent of quadriceps) has been shown to increase the risk of non-contact knee overuse injuries in female athletes (Devan *et al.*, 2004).

Motor control issues

Reduced ability of the athlete to optimally recruit musculature during physical activity, particularly in multidirectional sport, can predispose to injury. In the dynamic and rapidly changing sporting environment, efficient motor control requires at least multi-faceted instant responsiveness. This process is partly informed by trained and ingrained feedback and feed-forward neuromuscular proprioceptive signalling, in addition to all the other multisensory inputs from each concurrent situation (environmental inputs). The neuromuscular system is also further challenged to respond to the varying duration, repetition, intensity and adaptation associated with any movement. Pain, restriction, weakness, neural or circulatory deficits compound the process.

Excessive or limited flexibility

The effects of a limited range of motion at a joint are diverse and may contribute to acute or overuse injury. For example, limited dorsiflexion range of motion is a risk factor for ankle sprains (Willems *et al.*, 2006), while it is also a risk factor for Achilles tendinopathy in volleyball players (Malliaras *et al.*, 2006). Conversely, genu recurvatus (hyperextending knee) has been shown to increase the risk of overuse injuries in the knee in female athletes (Devan *et al.*, 2004).

Joint hypermobility syndrome

Joint hypermobility, when associated with symptoms, is termed joint hypermobility syndrome (JHS). JHS can be due to hereditary, congenital, developmental or acquired factors. Obviously, there is increased potential for decreased static stability following significant damage to joint stabilizing structures. A key component to the development of this condition is where poor recruitment of dynamic stabilizers is evident. JHS, when in its most severe form, presents as a multi-systemic, hereditary connective tissue disorder, which typically results in chronic disability. Recognized genetic connective tissue disorders showing such joint instability include Marfan's Syndrome and Ehler's Danlos Syndrome – these conditions, unfortunately, are likely to present with a host of other complications (including vascular problems, paraesthesias, chronic fatigue, faintness, malaise and even flu-like symptoms) (Simmonds and Keer, 2007).

The more general form of the condition is most prevalent in females. It presents with laxity and increased fragility of connective tissue; patients are also likely to demonstrate reduced proprioceptive functioning and altered (delayed) neuromuscular reflexes. JHS predisposes individuals to damage and injury because of the instability, altered biomechanics and proprioceptive deficits. Characteristic musculoskeletal features also include clicking and clunking, subluxations and dislocations. Such characteristics are normally observed during early development (Simmonds and Keer, 2007). For assessment, the original nine-point 'Beighton Score' (Beighton *et al.*, 1973) has more recently been incorporated into a more comprehensive and validated set of criteria termed the 'Brighton Criteria' (Grahame, 2000; Hakim and Grahame, 2003). The Beighton Score is a simple nine-point screening protocol. It incorporates assessing the patient's ability to: place their hands flat on the floor from standing without bending their knees; extend their elbows (left and right) beyond 10° hyperextension; extend their knees (left and right) beyond 10° of hyperextension; passively approximate their thumbs (left and right) to their forearm; and passively extend their fifth fingers (left and right) to 90°. The 'Brighton Criteria' (Grahame, 2000), categorizes patients with JHS when they are symptomatic and when they present with 'major criteria' (i.e. 4/9 or greater on the Beighton Score; and/or arthralgia for longer than three months in four or more joints); or where in addition to one of the 'major criteria' they also present with two or more 'minor criteria' (including: dislocation or subluxation in more than one joint, or in one joint on more than one occasion; soft tissue rheumatism with three or more lesions (such as epicondylalgia, tenosynovitis or bursitis); or an abnormal skin presentation (such as striae, hypermobility, thin skin or scarring).

JHS is a condition that may be under-recognized and poorly managed. Sports therapists should take care during any objective assessment, manual therapy, soft tissue therapy or exercise prescription so as not to exacerbate the condition or increase instability. While athletes during routine screening sessions should be easily identified with this condition, many patients attending for clinical assessment may be more likely to present with JHS simply as a comorbidity (i.e. as a background to their main complaint) rather than as the primary reason for attendance. Hence, the sports therapist should utilize strategies to improve stability as well as focus on supporting the management of the primary complaint. General recommendations include improving dynamic stability, proprioception, joint positional sense and muscular endurance (particularly in the core or spinal region and around all vulnerable joints).

Age

Greater age was identified as a risk factor that may contribute to running injuries in a systematic review by van Gent *et al.* (2007), but in contrast they also identified studies that suggest increasing age is in fact a protective factor. Runners with more than ten years of running experience have been shown to have an increased risk of Achilles tendinopathy (Knobloch *et al.*, 2008).

Body size and composition

Body mass index (BMI) is a simple (but limited) measure for identifying where individuals may be overweight – the individual's weight in kilograms is divided by their height in metres squared. Because factors such as individual fitness, muscle mass and ethnic origin are not taken into account with BMI, it is only a proxy indicator of obesity (NOO, 2009). However, a higher BMI has been shown to increase the risk of ankle sprains in high-school athletes (McHugh *et al.*, 2006) and elite athletes (Pefanis *et al.*, 2009). A higher BMI has also been shown to increase the risk of lower extremity injury in male recreational runners (Buist *et al.*, 2010). Heavier and shorter football players are also at a greater risk of thigh muscle injuries (Fousekis *et al.*, 2010); while taller and heavier military recruits, and those with a higher BMI, are at greater risk of ankle sprain (Waterman *et al.*, 2010).

Physiological issues

Cardiorespiratory endurance has been identified as a risk factor for ankle sprains in males (Willems *et al.*, 2006) and male and female military recruits (Waterman *et al.*, 2010). Genetic risk factors for musculoskeletal injuries have been found for the Achilles tendon, the tendons of the rotator cuff muscles and the anterior and posterior cruciate ligaments (Collins and Raleigh, 2009). Reduced dynamic knee stability caused by metabolic fatigue may increase the risk of knee injuries in women by reducing knee flexion angles in single-leg jump landings (Ortiz *et al.*, 2010), although similar results have been shown in both males and females (Brazen *et al.*, 2010).

An increase in non-contact ACL injuries during the ovulatory and pre-ovulatory phases of the menstrual cycle in female athletes has been shown (Adachi *et al.*, 2008; Hewett *et al.*, 2007). Oligomenorrhea, amenorrhea and low bone mineral density have been identified as injury risk factors in female high-school athletes (Rauh *et al.*, 2010).

Neuromuscular fatigue has been identified as a significant factor in functional muscle disorders such as EAMC. Fatigue also contributes to impaired performance and therefore predisposes to all manner of traumatic injuries.

Previous injury

Previous injury is widely identified as a significant risk factor for sustaining a subsequent injury. For example, a previous history of ankle sprain is a significant risk factor for re-injury (McHugh *et al.*, 2006); and previous history of musculotendinous groin injury is a risk factor for new groin injuries (Engebretsen *et al.*, 2010). A previous injury to the back has also been shown to be a risk factor for back pain in tennis players (Hjelm *et al.*, 2010). It is important to recognize that all significant musculoskeletal injuries undergo a repair process which involves replacement of original tissue with scar tissue (predominantly type 1 collagen), which does not have the same functional properties.

Impaired joint position sense

Athletes with functional ankle instability have been shown to have poor ankle joint positional sense and are more likely to exhibit a more inverted ankle joint position before, at and after heel strike (Delahunt *et al.*, 2006).

Sports-specific technique errors

Brukner and Khan (2009) identify a number of technique faults which may increase the athlete's risk of injury, such as poor lateral pelvic control contributing to iliotibial band syndrome, or too wide a grip in the bench press, leading to pectoralis major tendinopathy.

Psychological issues

A number of psychological factors may contribute to the incidence of injury in sport; these can include anxiety, fatigue, depression, excitation and fear, and can result in abnormal behaviours and impaired performance. It is important to evaluate the risk or threat, personality type and which coping strategies may be applicable (Whiting and Zernicke, 1998).

Nutritional issues

Nutritional status has a significant influence on the risk of injury while training and competing. A lack of protein will delay recovery and rehabilitation (Holmes, 2003), while nutritional deficiencies such as a lack of carbohydrates can cause fatigue. Disordered eating has been shown to be associated with increased risk of musculoskeletal injury in female athletes (Rauh *et al.*, 2010) and female athletes with disordered eating are twice as likely to sustain an injury (Thein-Nissenbaum *et al.*, 2011). Poor diet and hydration are obvious factors which can contribute to short-term poor performance. Persistently disordered eating (such as with anorexia nervosa or bulimia nervosa) and the associated malnutrition can lead to a range of systemic issues including osteoporosis, anaemia, hypotension, irregular cardiac rhythm, renal disease and neural and mental disorders.

Extrinsic risk factors

Extrinsic risk factors are external influences which may contribute to injury. These may be the athletes' immediate environment, such as the surface or terrain, the choice of equipment used or training errors. A simple risk assessment, regular checks of equipment and frequent monitoring and evaluation of the athlete's training programme can all help to reduce the risk of injury as a result of an extrinsic risk factor.

Equipment

Equipment can aid in the prevention of injuries but may also contribute to an athlete sustaining an injury. In the majority of cases protective equipment serves its purpose and protects the athlete from injury. It has been suggested that in a small minority of cases protective equipment such as the helmet and shoulder pads may, in fact, contribute to injury such as heat stress (Whiting and Zernicke, 1998). Sporting equipment has been implicated as an injury risk factor in a number of sports. A common issue is that, although it may be safe and functional, the equipment is often inappropriate for the athlete using it. For example, a tennis player using a tennis racket with too large or too small a grip will be at an increased risk of wrist and elbow injury. Equally, the string tension may be inappropriate or the racquet may be too stiff (Hennig, 2007). In a sport such as cycling there is a higher risk of injury if the bike is not correctly set up for the cyclist. Incorrect bike set-up has been shown to increase the risk of injury in triathletes and multisport athletes (Cipriani *et al.*, 1998). The factors that need to be considered are seat height, seat position, reach and cleat position (Brukner and Khan, 2009). Athletes should be discouraged from borrowing equipment which may be ill-fitting and therefore unsuitable.

Footwear

Although footwear could be classed as part of the athletes' equipment, it is presented separately here because of the diversity of the types of footwear worn by athletes and because footwear choice during the athletes' activities of daily living are equally important to consider. Running shoes are not only worn by runners and triathletes, but by any athlete using running as part of their training programme. More experienced runners are less prone to injury (Fredericson and Wolf, 2005) and it is the less experienced runners who are more inclined to wear ill-fitting or worn-out athletic running shoes. Equally, wearing shoes that are not tied up reduces the support offered by the shoe and increases the loading on the Achilles tendon (Rowson *et al.*, 2010). There is no one shoe that is the perfect running shoe for all athletes due to the diverse array of foot structures and lower limb biomechanics of the running population. Instead, the athlete should look to purchase the most appropriate shoe for their purpose and look to have a simple observational gait analysis and running shoe prescription, which are widely available at specialized running shops. In this way they purchase the most appropriate footwear for their foot structure and gait pattern. In the event that foot structure may be contributing to injury, orthotics or insoles may be required. If so, it is important to seek advice from a specialist sports podiatrist, who can carry out a lower limb biomechanical assessment and prescribe the athlete custom-built orthoses. Off-the-shelf orthotics are not designed individually for the athlete, may not fulfil their required purpose and can contribute to injury by inappropriately modifying the athlete's biomechanics. Athletes with prescribed orthotics may be required to wear them in their general everyday footwear as well as their athletic footwear.

Athletes wearing inappropriate footwear are a common sight: for example, a football player going out for a run while wearing artificial-turf football trainers or a netball player playing netball wearing running shoes. In these cases, they are putting themselves at an increased risk of injury because they are using a shoe for a purpose it was not designed for. Athletes may also wear inappropriate footwear for the type of training they are doing or for the surface they are training on. There is little in the way of evidence-based literature examining the effects of running spikes on the lower limb biomechanics of an athlete. These shoes have spikes over the forefoot and midfoot which strike the ground as the heel normally makes no contact with the ground while running at speed. The 'negative heel' is common in running spikes and observed when the shoe is placed on a flat surface – the heel is seen to be lower than the forefoot. This may increase eccentric load at the heel and predispose to Achilles tendinopathy and shin pain. Increasing heel lift in running spikes may reduce the risk of sustaining these injuries. Running flats are running shoes worn by athletes in races and at times in training. The use of these types of shoe have been shown to reduce the contact area between the shoe and the ground, increasing the maximum forces experienced by the athlete beneath the entire foot and specifically the lateral forefoot, which is an area of increased stress fracture risk in men (Queen *et al.*, 2010).

Wearing footwear that is too small for the athlete's foot size has been shown to cause injury (Morrison and Schöffl, 2007), while wearing footwear that is too large can cause imbalance, increase the risk of lower extremity injury and potentially induce falls (Paiva de Castro *et al.*, 2010). A study by Teyhen *et al.* (2010) examined the running shoes of 524 US soldiers and showed that poor shoe choices are very common. They showed that 35 per cent of individuals wore incorrectly sized shoes, 57 per cent wore running shoes that were inappropriate for their foot type, 35 per cent had excessively worn shoes and 63 per cent had no idea on the guidelines for running shoe replacement. Excessive shoe wear has also been implicated as an injury risk factor in triathletes (Cipriani *et al.*, 1998) and runners (Taunton *et al.*, 2003).

The type of ski or snowboard boot worn has a significant impact on the risk of injury the individual will be exposed to. Wearing soft boots in either sport puts the individual at a greater risk of injury compared to wearing rigid boots (Pino and Colville, 1989; Sacco *et al.*, 1998). The wearing of rigid boots has reduced the incidence of ankle injuries in skiing; however, in turn, the risk of knee injury has increased dramatically (Pujol *et al.*, 2007).

Surface

Training or competing on surfaces that are too hard or too soft may contribute to an overuse injury, while surfaces that are slippery, sticky, wet or uneven can contribute to acute injury. A number of studies show higher rates of injury sustained on first- and second-generation artificial turf compared to natural grass, while the current data suggest that the injury rate is similar on third-generation and natural grass surfaces. It has also been shown that playing tennis on clay is safer than playing on hard courts or grass (Dragoo and Braun, 2010). It has been suggested that clay causes fewer injuries because it has low frictional resistance and that surfaces with high frictional resistance are a significant risk factor (Nigg and Segesser, 1988).

Terrain

Athletes such as orienteers and hill runners, who predominantly run off-road on rough surfaces, are at an increased risk of injuries such as ankle sprain (Creagh and Reilly, 1998; Fordham *et al.*, 2004). Running on sand has been shown to increase the relative risk of sustaining mid-portion Achilles tendinopathy (Knobloch *et al.*, 2008). Running on a cambered surface has been shown to significantly alter the kinematics of the knee (Gehlsen *et al.*, 1989). This may contribute to lower extremity overuse injury in a similar way as a leg length discrepancy would. Equally, there may be an increased risk of a lateral ankle sprain on the outside (lower) foot as the ankle may be more inclined to invert on heel strike.

Gradient

Excessive uphill or downhill running have been shown to contribute to the risk of injury as the change in gradient significantly alters the biomechanics of the gait cycle. Uphill running has been shown to significantly increase hip flexion and knee extension torques in the rectus femoris compared to level running (Yokozawa *et al.*, 2007). This is due to the fact that there is greater forward lean of the trunk and less knee extension torque during uphill running. Excessive downhill running has been implicated as a risk factor for sustaining overuse injury (Fredericson and Wolf, 2005), with a −9° gradient causing impact force peaks to increase by 54 per cent and parallel braking force peaks to increase by 73 per cent (Gottschall and Kram, 2005).

Training errors

It has been shown that a significant correlation exists between number of training hours and incidence of injury (Almeida *et al.*, 1999; Fordham *et al.*, 2004; Wolf *et al.*, 2009). Rapid increases in training volume increases the risk of injury (Almeida *et al.*, 1999; Fredericson and Wolf, 2005), while lack of adequate rest has been shown to increase the incidence of overuse injuries. Running excessive distances in the same direction around a running track has been associated with the development of iliotibial band friction syndrome (Fredericson and Wolf, 2005). Once the athlete is running more than 40 miles per week there is a significant increase in the risk of lower extremity overuse injury (Fredericson and Misra, 2007) and runners with high weekly mileage are at risk of recurrent lower extremity stress fracture (Korpelainen *et al.*, 2001). The higher training loads and excessive intensity observed at the start of pre-season training corresponds to higher injury rates (Killen *et al.*, 2010). Running speed is a risk factor for acute injuries such as ankle sprains (Willems *et al.*, 2006). Poor technique while weight training has been shown to increase injury risk in the shoulder (Kolber *et al.*, 2010) and trunk (Quatman *et al.*, 2009).

Inappropriate cross-training can bring about any of the training errors listed above, but also expose the athlete to risk factors such as inappropriate footwear, equipment, surface, terrain or gradient. Cross-training is also a risk where athletes are exhibiting poor technique and are training unsupervised by qualified coaches. A high incidence of injury has been observed as a result of cross-training, with more than one-third of swimming injuries occurring out of the pool during activities such as strength training (Wolf *et al.*, 2009). Poor technique is a risk factor for many sports-specific overuse injuries such as medial epicondylalgia ('golfers elbow') (Bayes and Wadsworth, 2009) and lateral epicondylalgia ('tennis elbow') (Kelley *et al.*, 1994). Faults in sports-specific techniques which are not corrected may contribute to overuse injury, especially when the athlete trains for long periods of time.

Environmental conditions

Environmental conditions have a significant impact on athletes training and competing outdoors as they experience extremes of heat, cold and humidity, all of which may cause injury or illness. Adequate warm-up, cool-down, rest periods, nutrition and the replacement of fluid and salt are widely recommended for athletes training or competing under stressful environmental conditions. Guidelines on the prevention of environmental illness are published by a number of organizations such as the ACSM, the NSCA (National Strength and Conditioning Association) and NATA (National Athletic Training Association). Athletes exposed to cold, wet or windy conditions are at risk of cold injuries such as hypothermia, frostbite, chilblains and immersion ('trench') foot (Cappaert *et al.*, 2008). There are a number of events where athletes are at risk of cold injuries: those taking part in water, such as swimming and sailing; alpine sports; endurance events such as marathons and triathlons and basic military training. Hypothermia has been seen in open water swimming events (Castro *et al.*, 2009) and a higher BMI is associated with a decreased risk of hypothermia (Brannigan *et al.*, 2009). Extreme cold may cause hypothermia during endurance events and significantly more drop-outs (Agar *et al.*, 2009). It has also been shown that training seasons have an effect on the incidence of Achilles paratendinitis, with significantly more recruits sustaining the condition in winter months (Milgrom *et al.*, 2003). It is thought to be caused by the decreased temperature increasing the viscosity of the lubricant in the paratenon, which increases friction.

In endurance events such as marathon running, 4–15 °C is the most advantageous temperature range, while the risk of drop-outs and the numbers requiring medical attention increase dramatically as the temperature rises above 15.5 °C (Roberts, 2007). Heat stress increases the numbers of drop-outs due to heat stroke and hyponatraemia, while cold stress increases the numbers of drop-outs and when combined with rain increases the numbers of runners seeking medical attention (Roberts, 2007). Marathon performance slows as the temperature rises from 5 to 25 °C in both male and female runners and this affects the slower runners taking part (Ely *et al.*, 2007). As the temperature during the event rises, so does the risk of heat exhaustion and heatstroke in athletes. An athlete is suffering from heatstroke if their core (rectal) temperature is greater than 38 °C and they require immediate cooling until the rectal temperature drops below 38 °C (Armstrong *et al.*, 2007). A number of marathons with starting temperatures of >21 °C have ended with cancellation and mass casualty incident (Roberts, 2010).

Soft tissue repair process

The following section presents an overview of the soft tissue healing process. Generically, Watson (2012) has described four overlapping phases: bleeding, inflammation, proliferation and remodelling. Numerous authors have written extensively on this topic, including good early review articles by Barlow and Willoughby (1992) and Hardy (1989). Anderson *et al.* (2009), Houglum (2010), Knight and Draper (2008), Lieber (2002), Norris (2004) and Prentice (2011) each provide informative book chapters. In order to successfully assess and manage patients with soft tissue injury, sports therapists must understand basic pathophysiological theory, be able to recognize the signs and symptoms in their injured patients/athletes and appreciate the full sequence of events which typically occur during each phase. It is essential to appreciate that the following section describes a generic cascade of events which may typically occur in an average injury involving, for example, an injured ligament or area of skin; it is beyond the scope of this text to explore in detail the subtleties of healing processes involving specific injuries to specific tissues. There are numerous additional healing processes to understand, particularly when presented with injuries involving muscle, tendon, skin, bone, nerve or visceral damage. Readers are therefore directed towards key recent articles for detailed overviews of specific tissue pathophysiology and classification, such as those provided by: Cook and Purdam (2009), Kaeding and Best (2009) and Rees *et al.* (2013) (tendinopathy); Boage *et al.* (2012), Giamberardino *et al.* (2011), Mueller-Wolfahrt *et al.* (2013) and Valle *et al.* (2015) (functional and structural muscle conditions); Enoch and Leaper (2005) and Li *et al.* (2007) (skin healing); Bennell and Kannus (2003) (bone healing); and Butler and Tomberlin (2007) (nerve injuries).

The immediate (bleeding and haemostasis) phase

The immediate phase of a typical traumatic soft tissue injury is characterized first by bleeding and second by haemostasis. At the time of injury, bleeding from ruptured blood vessels in the affected tissues occurs to varying degrees. The amount of bleeding depends primarily on the severity and extent of the injury as well as the inherent vascularity of the involved tissue. The bleeding phase is normally short-lived (minutes) but may last for a few hours. As haemostasis (the inherent mechanisms involved in the cessation of bleeding) begins, the body is concomitantly initiating an inflammatory response. One of the body's first responses to bleeding is vasoconstriction, which is triggered initially by the release of noradrenaline from mast cells in the connective tissues local to the injury site. Further chemical stimulation for vasoconstriction is provided by serotonin, which is released by platelets. Vasoconstriction (vascular spasm) is the body's attempt to minimize blood loss, but will only last for a few minutes at most. Vasoconstriction also contributes to an additional aspect of the initial response to injury; a process known as secondary ischaemic (hypoxic) death, where local tissue cells on the periphery of the injury site – initially unaffected by the inciting event – begin to die due to an insufficient blood supply. The resulting cell necrosis is caused by a lack of oxygen, and hence hypoxia occurs (Knight, 1995). Digestive enzymes from the gathering phagocytic leucocytes can also spill over from the injury site and contribute further to the death of surrounding cells. Mast cells affected by secondary death release a number of chemical mediators, including histamine, which are essential to the ensuing inflammatory response. At the injury site, further mechanisms contribute to the coagulation cascade and resulting 'platelet plug'. Mediators such as the glycoprotein 'von Willebrand factor' (vWF) are released from the endothelial walls of affected blood vessels and contribute to the activation of circulating platelets (thrombocytes). The platelets proliferate, become sticky, and begin to adhere to the blood vessel walls and to each other (platelet aggregation). This process is further facilitated by the release of a prothrombotic lipid – thromboxane – from the platelets themselves. The process of platelet adherence is termed 'pavementing'. At the same time as platelet plug formation, the process of fibrinolysis occurs. There follows an ongoing series of chemical and enzymatic responses, particularly those involving plasma protein-based clotting factors. Platelet activation also stimulates the Hageman factor XII plasma enzyme to contribute to the coagulation cascade. Prothrombin is then converted to thrombin. Thrombin converts the soluble plasma protein fibrinogen into a more insoluble material called fibrin, which form into strands (Li *et al.*, 2007). The coagulation process results in the formation of a lattice-patterned fibrin mesh, which acts somewhat like a cement and binds together with the platelet plug and all other debris at the site (dead cells and metabolites). The plug and fibrin mesh form a temporary patch, and if bleeding is successfully stemmed, haemostasis is complete. During haemostasis, a careful equilibrium between coagulation and anti-coagulation (blood fluidity – mediated by such chemicals as heparin [also released by mast cells]) needs to be reached so as to achieve the desired state of haemostasis, while also providing necessary blood supply.

The acute inflammation phase

Acute inflammation is the vascularized tissues' initial reaction to any irritant or pathogenic agent or traumatic injury. Inflammation will result from any sufficiently damaging burn or chemical injury, infection, autoimmune disorder or mechanical trauma. In terms of tissue healing, this phase is sometimes referred to as the 'lag phase' because of the inherent weakness and insufficiency of the injury site. Watson (2012) presents a simplified overview of a recognized generic sequence of chemically mediated cellular and vascular responses to soft tissue damage which forms the normal, initial and essential inflammatory phase of healing. Vascular events essentially aim to provide a supply of specialized cellular effectors to the injury site, and the cellular events attempt to contend with pathogenic agents and clear (debride) the affected site of debris. Typically beginning within an hour of injury, peaking in magnitude of activity for two or three days, before gradually fading over two or three weeks, the acute inflammatory

Table 1.4 Five generic and cardinal signs of inflammation

Swelling (tumor)	Redness (rubor)	Heat (calor)	Pain (dolor)	Loss of function (functio laesa)
Due to damaged local vessels and the ensuing haemodynamic response (vasodilation, vasopermeability) Leaked plasma proteins increase extracellular osmotic pressure and draw more fluid from local capillaries Extravasated fluids and cells accumulate in the interstitial spaces. Lymphatic obstruction is a contributing factor Swelling is also known as oedema	Due to the haemodynamic response (increased blood flow) at the affected site, near to the skin's surface Reddening of skin is known as erythema Increased blood flow through a region is termed hyperaemia	Due to the haemodynamic response (increased blood flow) at the affected site, near to the skin's surface	Due to mechanical, thermal and chemical stimulation of nociceptors. With any pain experience, there is also a central (nervous system) component	Due to damaged structures, loss of tissue integrity (and reduced tensile strength), pain, swelling and/or muscular spasm

phase offers a defence against foreign substances, a disposal system for dead and dying (necrotic) tissue cells, a warning sign of damage and injury (pain), and attempts to immobilize and compartmentalize the affected area and set up a chain of events for the proliferative repair phase. The five classic, or cardinal, signs of inflammation, which are non-specific to the cause of damage, are: swelling (*tumor*); redness (*rubor*); heat (*calor*); pain (*dolor*); and loss of function (*functio laesa*) (Punchard *et al.*, 2004). The two essential chemically mediated haemodynamic events occurring as the inflammatory response are vasodilation and vasopermeability (Houglum, 2010). The process begins soon after the body has begun contending with the initial trauma and instigating the process of haemostasis. Vasodilation, which is autonomic relaxation and widening of blood vessel walls (arterioles and previously dormant capillaries) – leads to a decrease in vascular resistance and hence an increase in local blood flow (hyperaemia). Fluid leakage from the affected vessels into the interstitial spaces occurs as they become more permeable. Diapedesis is the term to describe the outward passage of blood cells (principally leucocytes), along with plasma proteins and other chemicals, through the vessel walls. The extravasated fluid is referred to as exudate. The increasing vascular hydrostatic pressure forces the fluid and particulate contents from the capillary outwards into the tissues. Gradually, local blood flow slows and a state of haemoconcentration occurs. Importantly, the exudate becomes more gel-like as it binds with hyaluronic acid (released from mast cells), and gradually, due to reducing stimuli, the haemodynamic response fades. The inflammatory exudate's gel-like consistency (sometimes described as the 'inflammatory soup') helps to contain the injury site and reduces the potential for inflammatory reactions occurring in surrounding tissues (Watson, 2012).

The hallmark characteristics of inflammation are the typically visibly obvious swelling (oedema), redness (erythema) and surface heat. Pain may occur due to stimulation of polymodal nociceptors (mainly involving the fast-conducting A-delta nerve fibres) during the initial trauma, and the resulting acute inflammatory response (with continuing stimulation of sensory nerves – involving slow-conducting unmyelinated C fibres – from the developing oedema and possible presence of muscular spasm); in addition there is chemical stimulation of nociceptors from locally released substances including prostaglandins, histamine and bradykinin. Nociceptors themselves also release the chemical neuropeptide 'substance P', which as well as stimulating further histamine release from local mast cells (to maintain the haemodynamic response), also contributes to the ongoing perpetuation of nociceptive messaging which is transmitted along afferent pathways towards the dorsal horn of the spinal cord; from here pain is modulated in numerous ways (via ascending and descending messaging in the central nervous system).

Substances such as histamine, leucotaxin, bradykinin, prostaglandins and the 'complement cascade' (numerous plasma-derived proteins) are among the main chemical mediators for the haemodynamic response. Leucocytes become chemically attracted to the site, and begin to marginate along blood vessel walls. They are able to pass through the permeable walls of the blood vessels (a process known as diapedesis) and via chemotaxis (chemical attraction) are drawn to the site of damage. The first leucocytes to gather in numbers are neutrophils (also known as polymorphonuclear leucocytes – PMNs). Neutrophils are chiefly responsible for early and aggressive phagocytosis, but may only provide around 7–10 hours of activity, and do not reproduce in the process. Their main phagocytic response is geared towards pathogenic agents, rather than larger cellular debris. As they die, neutrophils release chemical mediators which contribute to the chemotaxic attraction of larger, longer-lasting phagocytic leucocytes (monocytes) to the site (Knight and Draper, 2008). Other chemical mediators of phagocytosis include the complement cascade and a number of growth factors, which are the key substances able to chemically stimulate cell proliferation, differentiation and growth. The monocytes quickly differentiate into macrophages at the site, and continue to combat any ongoing infection and perform the main 'clean up' and debridement of the affected site. The basic process of phagocytosis is to engulf, digest and remove pathogens and tissue debris.

Many of the events occurring within the acute inflammatory phase occur simultaneously and will continuously interact. The acute stage response gradually fades and will normally last until damaged tissue has been contained, tissue debris removed, and new capillary networks have begun to be laid down. Towards the end of this phase, as the initial stimulations subside (chemical and mechanical), the hallmark haemodynamic and cellular responses also reduce.

Practitioner Tip Box 1.1

Chemical mediators are the plasma-derived or cell-derived chemical messengers that act directly on blood vessels, inflammatory cells or other cells. They are involved in propagating the complex cascade of events during all phases of tissue healing. During the bleeding and inflammatory phases they are variously released, mainly from the following:

- Blood plasma
- Endothelial cells (in blood vessel walls)
- Platelets (thrombocytes)
- White blood cells (WBC or leucocytes) including basophils, neutrophils, monocytes and
- macrophages
- Mast cells (in connective tissue)
- Damaged tissue cells

Practitioner Tip Box 1.2

Chemical mediators, which are involved in the complex cascade of events during the bleeding and inflammatory phases of tissue healing, include the following:

- Noradrenaline
- Histamine
- von Willebrand factor
- Thromboxane
- Prothrombin
- Thrombin
- Hageman factor VII
- Serotonin
- Prostaglandins
- Substance P
- Heparin
- Bradykinin
- Leucotaxin
- Nitric oxide
- Complement cascade
- Hyaluronic acid
- Growth factors
- Lactic acid

Table 1.5 The acute inflammatory phase

Duration	Within 1 hour to 2–3 weeks (gradual fade)
Signs and symptoms	Swelling, redness, heat, pain and impaired function
Key features	Chemically mediated vascular and cellular response
	Haemodynamic response:
	Vasodilation
	Vasopermeability
	Hyperaemia
	Haemoconcentration
	Increased hydrostatic pressure
	Production of exudate
	Cellular response:
	Chemotaxis
	Leucocyte margination and diapedesis
	Phagocytosis
	Chemical and mechanical/thermal irritation of nociceptors

Macrophages, which are activated later in the inflammatory phase than other phagocytes, work anaerobically, and as such release lactic acid as a metabolic by-product, as well as vascular endothelial growth factors (VEGF); these act as key stimulants for the next stage of healing – proliferation.

The well-documented 'pain–spasm–pain cycle' is a common characteristic feature of the sub-acute phase, where chemical stimulation of the free nerve endings contributes to the local pain experience, which then triggers a protective mechanism causing involuntary muscle spasm during static postures, leading to further pain. Concurrently, there may also be a reduction of muscle activity during movement (Roland, 1986). The fundamental combination of tissue structural damage, loss of tensile strength, localized swelling, protective muscular spasm and resulting mechanical and chemical perpetuation of pain leads to impaired functioning of the affected tissues in the injured individual. The severity and degree of impairment depends upon numerous factors.

The proliferative repair phase

As the inflammatory phase fades, so begins the proliferation, or early repair, phase. Typically lasting for approximately 3–4 weeks, it is characterized by the establishment of a new vascular network (neovascularization) in order to facilitate the process of delivering and supporting the cells (fibroblasts) involved in the repair of damaged tissue. The actual type of repair depends upon the type of tissue which is predominantly damaged. Knight and Draper (2008) explain that there are two basic types of initial repair process: reconstitution and replacement. Reconstitution may be 'perfect' or 'imperfect'. Perfect reconstitution is where the injured cells are replaced by identical cells – but this can only occur in those tissues which have a normally high rate of turnover and replacement – i.e. tissue cells which have a high regeneration capacity. Such cells are termed 'labile' and are found in such tissues as those forming the epidermis of the skin and in the linings of the respiratory, gastrointestinal and genitourinary tracts. Although dependent on severity of damage and individual capacity to heal, the resultant repair from perfect reconstitution is likely to be perfect! Imperfect reconstitution occurs with tissues formed from 'stabile' cells – such as those forming the liver, pancreas and kidneys. Imperfect reconstitution is where damaged cells are replaced by a combination of identical cells and connective tissue, which will be predominantly type-III collagen at this stage. Imperfect reconstitution can occur in response to skeletal muscle fibre damage, due to the presence of satellite cells, which contribute to a micro-regeneration of tissue, but regeneration capacity is still limited (Barlow and Willoughby, 1992). Replacement is the repair process for 'permanent' cells – cells which have limited or no regenerative capacity, such as those forming nerve tissue, cardiac muscle and ligamentous tissue. This type of repair replaces original cells with 'simpler' connective tissue cells. The replacement repair process also occurs whenever the soft tissue damage is sufficiently extensive to disrupt the basic cellular framework. Scar tissue (collagen) is laid down (synthesized) to replace the original tissue – a process referred to as 'collagenization'. The majority of soft tissue injury sites heal by imperfect reconstitution, with a repair (replacement) process rather than a complete regeneration (reconstitution). Garrett (1990) identified that repair with new collagen does not begin until around five days following injury; Norris (2004) also describes the 'lag phase' as the period of time from immediate injury to the beginning of collagen synthesis (i.e. the bleeding and inflammatory phases). During this period, pain and oedema are present and tensile strength is reduced.

Angiogenesis – the formation of a new vascular network – is an essential factor during this phase of healing. Stimulated by activating growth factors (such as VEGF, angiogenesis factor

[AF] and platelet-derived growth factor [PDGF]), fresh capillary buds (branches) begin to appear and are formed from the dividing endothelial cells from existing vessels in the injured area (Li *et al.*, 2007). As they develop, the new capillary buds migrate towards one another, eventually forming a series of capillary arches. Once fully formed, the capillary arches provide a new and effective and localized vascular supply throughout the damaged tissue. The network of capillary arches is referred to as the capillary arcade (Knight and Draper, 2008), and the neovascularization facilitates delivery of fibroblasts, myofibroblasts, oxygen and nutrients and also provides a drainage system for removal of metabolites and other tissue debris, all of which are essential for effective repair.

Table 1.6 The proliferative repair phase

Duration	3–4 days to 3–4 weeks
Signs and symptoms	Pain and impaired function (dependent on severity); localized swelling and reddening with superficial injury
Key features	Chemical mediation and chemotaxis via cytokines and growth factors
	Angiogenesis:
	Endothelial proliferation
	Neovascularization
	Capillary budding, arching and arcade formation
	Repair via reconstitution (regeneration) or replacement (scar tissue)
	Fibroplasia:
	Fibroblast and myofibroblast proliferation
	Granulation tissue
	Collagenization – type III collagen
	Degranulation
	Neoinnervation
	Devascularization
	Reduced tensile strength in affected tissue

Table 1.7 Main growth factors released in response to injury

Growth factor	Abbreviation	Function
Platelet-derived growth factor	PDGF	Early growth factor in healing; stimulates fibroblasts and angiogenesis; promotes remodelling; stimulates production of other growth factors
Transforming growth factor	TGF	Promotes ECM and cell replication
Vascular endothelial growth factor	VEGF	Stimulates angiogenesis
Insulin-like growth factor 1 (also known as mechano-growth factor)	IGF1	Promotes neurogenesis; stimulates myoblast proliferation
Fibroblast growth factor 2	FGF2	Promotes ECM; stimulates fibroblasts and endothelial cells; enhances number and diameter of regenerating muscle fibres
Tumor necrosis factor	TNF	Stimulates inflammatory and immune responses
Nerve growth factor	NGF	Stimulates neurogenesis

Source: adapted from Mangine *et al.*, 2012.

The stimulation for increased fibroblastic activity (fibroplasia) is also provided predominantly by cytokines and growth factors (such as Transforming Growth Factor [TGF], Tumor Necrosis Factor [TNF], Insulin-like Growth Factor [IGF] (also known as Mechanogrowth Factor [MGF]), Nerve Growth Factor [NGF] and basic Fibroblast Growth Factor [bFGF]). Growth factors are released from a range of cells, including platelets, mast cells and macrophages in the final stages of inflammation. Further release of growth factors occurs during the early proliferative phase from the extracellular matrix (ECM) of the injury site and also from the gathering fibroblasts themselves (Boage *et al.*, 2012). As fibroblasts proliferate, granulation tissue begins to form within the existing ECM and platelet plug/fibrin mesh. The tissue being produced is partly fibrous (i.e. collagen, elastin and reticulin) and partly non-fibrous (i.e. fluid and protein – water, mineral salts and glycosaminoglycans or 'GAGs'). The developing structure of the matrix strengthens and supports the tissues and provides a means for diffusion of tissue fluid and nutrients between capillaries and cells (Placzek and Boyce, 2006). Fibroblasts themselves produce collagen, proteoglycans and elastin, which are all essential components of scar tissue formation and maturation (Houglum, 2010). Fibroblasts lay down collagen (principally type III at this stage), which forms a far more significant seal over the injury site than that which was provided by the early fibrin patch and exudate gel during the initial stages of injury. Fibronectin, an adhesive glycoprotein, is plentiful at the site (within the gel) and improves the adhesion of fibroblasts to the fibrin patch. Hyaluronic acid (released from mast cells during inflammation) also assists in facilitating fibroblast and myofibroblast migration to the site due to its fluid-drawing properties. The collagen is laid down in a haphazard manner, essentially creating a quite random matrix. Myofibroblasts also begin to proliferate at the margins of the injury. These are then oriented towards the centre of the damaged tissue and have an actin filament content and resultant contractile properties (similar to that of smooth muscle cells), which means they are able to pull wound edges together. Type-III collagen is fundamentally thin, weak, soluble and lacks robust cross-linkages. It is vulnerable to re-injury, but tensile strength begins to increase after the first week. As the proliferation phase continues, the original fibrin patch is reabsorbed (in a process known as degranulation). In addition to its neovascularization, the replacement tissue also begins to develop a network of pressure- and tension-sensitive nerve cells (a process of localized neurogenesis or neo-innervation), which can lead to additional noxious stimulation when the area is externally compressed or stretched (Houglum, 2010). The area is also likely to remain visibly swollen and reddened, particularly if it is superficial, due to the increased water content, vascularity and significant amount of immature collagen at the site. As the repair tissue matures, typically by day 12, type-III collagen is gradually beginning to be replaced by type-I. A process of devascularization also begins, which involves obliteration of the newly formed capillary network (Watson, 2012).

The remodelling and maturation phase

The remodelling phase begins as the proliferation phase is fading and can last for a year or more. The number of capillaries, fibroblasts, myofibroblasts, macrophages and more all gradually diminish and the activity in the region returns to a near pre-injury state. During remodelling, the gradual organization of collagen takes place – this is termed 'collagen transition'. Type-III collagen is replaced by the stronger, more insoluble, more permanent, type-I collagen – with different tissues (muscle; tendon; ligament; fascia; skin) having different functional and structural requirements. Cross-linkages throughout the fibres occur more readily as fluid content in the area is reduced. Wound contraction via myofibroblast activity continues (Betz *et al.*, 1992) and is generally beneficial to the resulting quality of tissue, unless joint or tissue mobility is

Table 1.8 The remodelling and maturation phase

Duration	2–3 weeks to 1 year or more
Signs and symptoms	Improving function (dependent on severity and effectiveness of healing process)
Key features	Collagen transition:
	Type-III collagen gradually reinforced and replaced by type-I collagen
	Reduction in water content and numbers of capillaries, fibroblasts, myofibroblasts and macrophages
	Increasing scar tissue density, collagen cross-linkages and tensile stress

compromised. As maturation takes place, the collagen fibres model in response to the lines of mechanical stress applied to them – as in the concept of Davis' law of soft tissue and the long-established principle of 'specific adaptation to imposed demands' (SAID) (Stearns, 1940). Optimal scar tissue formation occurs when a physiological balance is maintained between its ongoing synthesis (production) and lysis (breakdown and reabsorption) during the remodelling phase (Hardy, 1989).

Chronic inflammation

In certain cases, the normal process of soft tissue healing does not take place. Chronic inflammation occurs when the healing does not progress successfully into the proliferation stage. Essentially a breakdown in the normal process of acute inflammation, chronic inflammation may persist for months or more and can result in an excess of scar tissue formation and associated functional deficits (Holey and Cook, 2011). Various reasons exist for this occurrence, including: presence of foreign bodies at the injury site; bacterial infection; invasion of microorganisms which are able to survive in large phagocytes; antigen–antibody adverse immune reactions; and perhaps most commonly, ongoing mechanical irritation. Whereas acute inflammation has a short onset and a relatively short duration, by definition, chronic inflammation typically has a long onset and a long duration. However, Watson (2008) explains that there are two forms of chronic inflammation: chronic supervention on an original acute reaction; or chronic inflammation in the absence of acute reaction ('ab initio').

Although the characteristic features of chronic inflammation differ according to type, there are likely to be low concentrations of normal chemical mediators, and neutrophils are replaced with prolonged presence and activity of larger phagocytes at the injury site, which produce harmful cytotoxins. There is continued production of exudate, but this does gradually reduce, albeit later than normal. Concentrations of essential growth factors at the site are reduced. Debridement (phagocytosis) is likely to be incomplete and a low-grade inflammatory response persists. Gathering fibroblasts produce a 'granuloma', or mass of weak type-III collagen, which begins to surround the injury site – this is the start of 'fibrosis' rather than the normal process of fibroplasia. There will be simultaneous tissue destruction, inflammation and attempted healing, and different tissues will respond differently to the process. Prentice (2011) states that there is no recognized timeframe in which acute inflammation transitions to chronic inflammation.

Factors affecting healing

A large number of factors can affect the overall quality of healing, both positively and negatively; these may be local or systemic. During the early phase, the quality of healing response will be directly influenced by the very nature (tissue involvement) and severity of injury, its initial management and the degree of post-injury mechanical aggravation (as opposed to appropriately graded therapeutic mechanical stress). Early presentations such as excessive oedema or bleeding, haematoma formation, or a large degree of tissue separation or muscle spasm can all impede the normal process. Enoch and Leaper (2005) explain how, in particular, growth factors and cytokines play an essential role in healing processes across each of the phases. Alterations in any of these components or disruption in their functional role can impair the healing response. Additional important factors to consider which have influence on healing (positively or negatively) include: the age of the individual; general health and presence of comorbidity; whether operative intervention was undertaken (repair or reconstruction); infection; immunosuppression; systemic vascular disease; obesity; diabetes; nutritional deficiency (malnutrition) (especially with regard to vitamin A and C, minerals zinc and copper and protein); use of supplementation (there is gathering evidence to warrant consideration of supplements such as arginine, leucine, HMB [hydoxy-beta methylbutyrate] and glutamine) (Williams *et al.*, 2002); and use of medications (especially regarding non-steroidal anti-inflammatories [NSAIDs], corticosteroids and anti-coagulants). Hypertrophic (excessive collagen deposited at the injury site) or keloid (excessive collagen deposited in the surrounding tissue) scarring can also lead to a less desirable local outcome. Placzek and Boyce (2006) explain that glucosamine, found within type-II collagen, has importance in the process of soft tissue repair, being a precursor for such compounds as chondroitin sulphate and hyaluronic acid. Glucosamine also increases proteoglycan production. However, evidence is limited with regard to its effects when taken as a dietary supplement. Bloch (2013) advocates supplemental vitamin C and E as antioxidants to combat the damaging free radicals produced by leukocytes during the early inflammatory phase.

Obviously, the sports therapist has a wide range of specialist interventions available to support the injured athlete back towards optimal function, and any management provided should be based on appropriate assessment and will be carefully and individually tailored to suit each particular phase of healing. Beyond this, an important issue surrounding therapeutic care is that of patient adherence, or non-adherence, to the therapeutic intervention and advice (Magee *et al.*, 2008). Even if the patient or athlete is adhering to the recommended advice, there is still potential for re-injury. The resulting tensile strength of tissue following minor injury is an indicator of outcome. When overviewing average healing timeframes and outcomes in different tissues, muscle tissue may have near normal tensile strength 7–11 days following minor damage, with a 90 per cent contraction ability following the remodelling phase (Houglum, 2010). Tendon strength is likely to be 85–95 per cent normal, and ligaments likely to be near to normal within a year. By comparison, articular cartilage is likely to be near normal within six months, and bone within 8–12 weeks following fracture (depending on type). It is important to recognize that although a functionally successful outcome is highly likely for an uncomplicated soft tissue injury following sports therapy intervention, it cannot be guaranteed!

This chapter has presented an introductory overview of topics fundamental to the understanding of sports injuries: classifications, aetiology and repair processes. It has been beyond the scope of this text to explore in greater detail specific tissue pathophysiology (i.e. the processes involved in the healing and repair of muscle, tendon, ligament, bone, skin, nerve and viscera) and also the relatively complex topic of pain. Obviously, it is an essential requirement that all practitioners involved in the prevention, assessment and management of sports injuries undertake appropriate, evidence-informed and continued professional development. The field of sports and exercise medicine is overtly and continuously re-evaluating its evidence-base, and cutting-edge research enables new light to be shone on all aspects of this specialized area, hence all aspiring sports therapists must be recommended to consolidate their foundational knowledge in each of the areas discussed, and to keep abreast of the latest and most current information.

References

Adachi, N., Nawata, K., Maeta, M. and Kurozawa, Y. (2008) Relationship of the menstrual cycle phase to anterior cruciate ligament injuries in teenaged female athletes. *Archives of Orthopaedic and Trauma Surgery*. 128 (5): 473–478

Agar, C., Pickard, L. and Bhangu, A. (2009) The tough guy pre-hospital experience: Patterns of injury at a major UK endurance event. *Emergency Medicine Journal*. 26 (11): 826–830

Almeida, S.A., Williams, K.M., Shaffer, R.A. and Brodine, S.K. (1999) Epidemiological patterns of musculoskeletal injuries and physical training. *Medicine and Science in Sports and Exercise*. 31 (8): 1176–1182

Anderson, M., Parr, G. and Hall, S (2009) *Foundations of athletic training: Prevention, assessment and management*, 4th edition. Lippincott, Williams and Wilkins. Philadelphia, PA

Armstrong, L.E., Casa, D.J., Millard-Stafford, M., Moran, D.S., Pyne, S.W., Roberts, W.O. and American College of Sports Medicine (2007) Exertional heat illness during training and competition. *Medicine and Science in Sports and Exercise*. 39 (3): 556–572

Back, D. and Smethurst, M. (2004) The female triad. *Sports Injury Bulletin*. 43: 9–10

Barlow, Y. and Willoughby, J. (1992) Pathophysiology of soft tissue repair. *British Medical Bulletin*. 48 (3): 698–711

Baumhauer, J.F., Alosa, D.M., Renström, P., Trevino, S. and Beynnon, B. (1995) A prospective-study of ankle injury risk-factors. *American Journal of Sports Medicine*. 23 (5): 564–570

Bayes, M.C. and Wadsworth, L.T. (2009) Upper extremity injuries in golf. *Physician and Sports Medicine*. 37 (1): 92–96

Beighton, P.H., Solomon, L. and Soskolne, C.L. (1973) Articular mobility in an African population. *Annals of the Rheumatic Diseases*. 32: 413–417

Bennell, K. and Alleyne, J. (2009) Women and activity-related issues across the lifespan. In Brukner, P. and Khan, K. *Clinical sports medicine*, revised 3rd edition. McGraw-Hill. NSW, Australia

Bennell, K. and Kannus, P. (2003) Bone. In Kolt, G. and Snyder-Mackler, L. (eds) *Physical therapies in sport and exercise*. Churchill Livingstone. Philadelphia, PA

Betz, P., Norlich, A., Wilske, J., Tubel, J., Penning, R. and Eisenmenger, W. (1992) Time-dependent appearance of myofibroblasts in granulation tissue of human skin wounds. *International Journal of Legal Medicine*. 150: 99–103

Bloch, W. (2013) Muscle healing: Physiology and adverse factors. In Mueller-Wohlfahrt, H.W., Ueblacker, P., Haensel, L. and Garrett, W.E. (eds) *Muscle injuries in sports*. Thieme. Stuttgart, Germany

Boage, L., Van Den Steen, E., Rimbaut, S., Phillips, N., Witvrouw, E., Almqvist, K.F., Vanderstraeten, G. and Vanden Bossche, L.C. (2012) Treatment of skeletal muscle injury: A review. *International Scholarly Research Network (ISRN) Orthopedics*. 2012: n.p.

Brannigan, D., Rogers, I.R., Jacobs, I., Montgomery, A., Williams, A. and Khangure, N. (2009) Hypothermia is a significant medical risk of mass participation long-distance open water swimming. *Wilderness and Environmental Medicine*. 20 (1): 14–18

Brazen, D.M., Todd, M.K., Ambegaonkar, J.P., Wunderlich, R. and Peterson, C. (2010) The effect of fatigue on landing biomechanics in single-leg drop landings. *Clinical Journal of Sports Medicine* 20 (4): 286–292

Brukner, P. and Khan, K. (2009) *Clinical sports medicine*, revised 3rd edition. McGraw-Hill. NSW, Australia

Buist, I., Bredeweg, S.W., Lemmink, K.A.P.M., van Mechelen, W. and Diercks, R.L. (2010) Predictors of running-related injuries in novice runners enrolled in a systematic training program: A prospective cohort study. *American Journal of Sports Medicine*. 38 (2): 273–280

Butler, D.S. and Tomberlin, J.P. (2007) Peripheral nerves: Structure, function and physiology. In Magee, D.J., Zachazewski, W.S. and Quillen, W.S. (eds) *Scientific foundations and principles of practice in musculoskeletal rehabilitation*. Saunders, Elsevier. St Louis, MO

Cain, E.L., Dugas, J.R., Wolf, R.S. and Andrews, J.R. (2003) Elbow injuries in throwing athletes: A current concepts review. *American Journal of Sports Medicine*. 31 (4): 621–635

Caine, E.L., DiFiori, J. and Maffulli, N. (2006) Physeal injuries in children's and youth sports: Reasons for concern? *British Journal of Sports Medicine*. 40: 749–760

Cappaert, T.A., Stone, J.A., Castellani, J.W., Krause, B.A., Smith, D. and Stephens, B.A. (2008) National athletic trainers' association position statement: Environmental cold injuries. *Journal of Athletic Training*. 43 (6): 640–658

Castro, R.R.T., Mendes, F. and Nobrega, A.C.L. (2009) Risk of hypothermia in a new Olympic event: the 10-km marathon swim. *Clinics*. 64 (4): 351–356

Chappell, J.D., Herman, D.C., Knight, B.S., Kirkendall, D.T., Garrett, W.E. and Yu, B. (2005) Effect of fatigue on knee kinetics and kinematics in stop-jump tasks. *American Journal of Sports Medicine*. 33 (7): 1022–1029

Cipriani, D.J., Swartz, J.D. and Hodgson, C.M. (1998) Triathlon and the multisport athlete. *Journal of Orthopaedic and Sports Physical Therapy*. 27 (1): 42–50

Clark, M. (2001) Muscle energy techniques in rehabilitation. In Prentice, W. and Voight, M. (eds) *Techniques in musculoskeletal rehabilitation*. McGraw-Hill. New York

Collins, M. and Raleigh, S.M. (2009) Genetic risk factors for musculoskeletal soft tissue injuries. *Genetics and Sports*. 54: 136–149

Cook, J.L. and Purdam, C.R. (2009) Is tendon pathology a continuum? A pathology model to explain the clinical presentation of load-induced tendinopathy. *British Journal of Sports Medicine*. 43: 409–416

Cowan, D.N., Jones, B.H., Frykman, P.N., Polly, D.W., Harman, E.A., Rosenstein, R.M. and Rosenstein, M.T. (1996) Lower limb morphology and risk of overuse injury among male infantry trainees. *Medicine and Science in Sports and Exercise*. 28 (8): 945–952

Cowey, C. (2006) Women in sport. In Higgins, R., Brukner, P. and English, B. (eds) *Essential sports medicine*. Blackwell Publishing. Oxford, UK

Creagh, U. and Reilly, T. (1998) Training and injuries amongst elite female orienteers. *Journal of Sports Medicine and Physical Fitness*. 38 (1): 75–79

Delahunt, E., Monaghan, K. and Caulfield, B. (2006) Altered neuromuscular control and ankle joint kinematics during walking in subjects with functional instability of the ankle joint. *American Journal of Sports Medicine*. 34 (12): 1970–1976

De Souza, M.J., Williams, N.I., Mallinson, R.J., Koehler, K., *et al.* (2014a) Misunderstanding the female athlete triad: Refuting the IOC consensus statement on relative energy deficiency in sport (RED-S). *British Journal of Sports Medicine*. 48 (20): 1461–1465

De Souza, M.J., Nattiv, A., Joy, E., Misra, M., Williams, N.I., Mallinson, R.J., Gibbs, J.C., Olmsted, M., Goolsby, M. and Matheson, G. (2014b) 2014 Female athlete triad coalition consensus statement on treatment and return to play of the female athlete triad: 1st International Conference held in San Francisco, California, May 2012 and 2nd International Conference held in Indianapolis, Indiana, May 2013. *British Journal of Sports Medicine*. 48: 289

Devan, M.R., Pescatello, L.S., Faghri, P. and Anderson, J. (2004) A prospective study of overuse knee injuries among female athletes with muscle imbalances and structural abnormalities. *Journal of Athletic Training*. 39 (3): 263–267

Dragoo, J.L. and Braun, H.J. (2010) The effect of playing surface on injury rate: A review of the current literature. *Sports Medicine*. 40 (11): 981–990

Ely, M.R., Cheuvront, S.N., Roberts, W.O. and Montain, S.J. (2007) Impact of weather on marathon-running performance. *Medicine and Science in Sports and Exercise*. 39 (3): 487–493

Engebretsen, A.H., Myklebust, G., Holme, I., Engebretsen, L. and Bahr, R. (2010) Intrinsic risk factors for groin injuries among male soccer players: A prospective cohort study. *American Journal of Sports Medicine*. 38 (10): 2051–2057

Enoch, S. and Leaper, D.J. (2005) Basic science of wound healing. *Surgery*. 23 (2): 37–42

Faubel, C. (2010) Nerve injury classifications – Seddon's and Sunderland's. *The Pain Source* http://thepainsource.com/2010/07/nerve-injury-classifications-seddons-and-sunderlands, accessed July 2011

Fields, K.B., Sykes, J.C., Walker, K.M. and Jackson, J.C. (2010) Prevention of running injuries. *Current Sports Medicine Reports*. 9 (3): 176–182

Fordham, S., Garbutt, G. and Lopes, P. (2004) Epidemiology of injuries in adventure racing athletes. *British Journal of Sports Medicine*. 38 (3): 300–303

Fousekis, K., Tsepis, E., Poulmedis, P., Athanasopolous, S. and Vagenas, G. (2010) Intrinsic risk factors of non–contact quadriceps and hamstring strains in soccer: A prospective study of 100 professional players. *British Journal of Sports Medicine*. 50 (4): 465–474

Fredericson, M. and Misra, A.K. (2007) Epidemiology and aetiology of marathon running injuries. *Sports Medicine*. 37 (4–5): 437–439

Fredericson, M. and Wolf, C. (2005) Iliotibial band syndrome in runners: Innovations in treatment. *Sports Medicine*. 35 (5): 451–459

Garrett, W.E. (1990) Muscle strain injuries: Clinical and basic aspects. *Medicine and Science in Sports and Exercise*. 22: 436–443

Gehlsen, G.M., Stewart, L.B., Vannelson, C. and Bratz, J.S. (1989) Knee kinematics: The effects of running on cambers. *Medicine and Science in Sports and Exercise*. 21 (4): 463–466

Ghani Zadeh Hesar, N., Van Ginckel, A., Cools, A., Peersman, W., Roosen, P., De Clercq, D. and Witvrouw, E. (2009) A prospective study on gait-related intrinsic risk factors for lower leg overuse injuries. *British Journal of Sports Medicine*. 43 (13): 1057–1061

Gholve, P.A., Scher, D.M., Khakharia, S. (2007) Osgood–Schlatter syndrome. *Current Opinion in Pediatrics*. 19 (1): 44–50

Giamberardino, M.A., Affaitati, G., Fabrizio, A. and Costantini, R. (2011) Myofascial pain syndromes and their evaluation. *Best Practice and Research Clinical Rheumatology*. 25: 185–198

Gottschall, J.S. and Kram, R. (2005) Ground reaction forces during downhill and uphill running. *Journal of Biomechanics*. 38 (3): 445–452

Grahame, R. (2000) Pain distress and joint hyperlaxity. *Joint Bone Spine*. 67: 157–163

Greenhalgh, S. and Selfe, J. (2006) *Red flags: A guide to serious pathology of the spine*. Churchill Livingstone, Elsevier. London, UK

Haim, A., Yaniv, M., Dekel, S. and Amir, H. (2006) Patellofemoral pain syndrome: Validity of clinical and radiological features: *Clinical Orthopaedics and Related Research*. 451: 223–228

Hakim, A. and Grahame, R. (2003) A simple questionnaire to detect hypermobility: An adjunct to the assessment of patients with diffuse musculoskeletal pain. *International Journal of Clinical Practice*. 57 (3):163–166

Hardy, M.A. (1989) The biology of scar formation. *Physical Therapy*. 69 (12): 1014–1024

Hennig, E.M. (2007) Influence of racket properties on injuries and performance in tennis. *Exercise and Sport Sciences Reviews*. 35 (2): 62–66

Hewett, T.E., Zazulak, B.T. and Myer, G.D. (2007) Effects of the menstrual cycle on anterior cruciate ligament injury risk: A systematic review. *American Journal of Sports Medicine*. 35 (4): 659–668

Hjelm, N., Werner, S. and Renström, P. (2010) Injury profile in junior tennis players: A prospective 2-year study. *Knee Surgery, Sports Traumatology, Arthroscopy*. 18 (6): 845–850

Holey, E. and Cook, E. (2011) *Evidence-based therapeutic massage: A practical guide for therapists*, 3rd edition. Churchill Livingstone, Elsevier. London, UK

Holmes, S. (2003) Undernutrition in hospital patients. *Nursing Standard*. 17 (19): 45–52

Houglum, P. (2010) *Therapeutic exercise for musculoskeletal injuries*, 3rd edition. Human Kinetics. Champaign, IL

Janda, V. (1983) *Muscle function testing*. Butterworth. London, UK

Kaeding, C. and Best, T.M. (2009) Tendinosis: Pathophysiology and non-operative treatment. *Sports Health: A Multidisciplinary Approach*. 1: 284

Kannus, P. and Józsa, L. (1991) Histopathological changes preceding spontaneous rupture of a tendon: A controlled study of 891 patients. *Journal of Bone and Joint Surgery (American Volume)*. 73A (10): 1507–1525

Kelley, J.D., Lombardo, S.J., Pink, M., Perry, J. and Giangarra, C.E. (1994) Electromyographic and cinematographic analysis of elbow function in tennis players with lateral epicondylitis. *American Journal of Sports Medicine*. 22 (3): 359–363

Killen, N.M., Gabbett, T.J. and Jenkins, D.G. (2010) Training loads and incidence of injury during the preseason in professional rugby league players. *Journal of Strength and Conditioning Research*. 24 (8): 2079–2084

Knight, K.L. (1995) *Cryotherapy in sports injury management*. Human Kinetics. Champaign, IL

Knight, K.L. and Draper, D.O. (2008) *Therapeutic modalities: The art and science*. Lippincott, Williams and Wilkins. Baltimore, MD

Knobloch, K., Yoon, U. and Vogt, P.M. (2008) Acute and overuse injuries correlated to hours of training in master running athletes. *Foot and Ankle International*. 29 (7): 671–676

Kolber, M.J., Beekhuizen, K.S., Cheng, M.S.S. and Hellman, M.A. (2010) Shoulder injuries attributed to resistance training: A brief review. *Journal of Strength and Conditioning Research*. 24 (6): 1696–1704

Korpelainen, R., Orava, S., Karpakka, J., Siira, P. and Hulkko, A. (2001) Risk factors for recurrent stress fractures in athletes. *American Journal of Sports Medicine.* 29 (3): 304–310

Leetun, D.T., Ireland, M.L., Willson, J.D., Ballantyne, B.T. and Davis, I.M. (2004) Core stability measures as risk factors for lower extremity injury in athletes. *Medicine and Science in Sports and Exercise.* 36 (6): 926–934

Li, J., Chen, J. and Kirsner, R. (2007) Pathophysiology of acute wound healing. *Clinics in Dermatology.* 25: 9–18

Lieber, R.L. (2002) *Skeletal muscle structure, function and plasticity: The physiological basis of rehabilitation,* 2nd edition. Lippincott, Williams and Wilkins. Philadelphia, PA

MacAuley, D. (2007) *Oxford handbook of sport and exercise medicine.* Oxford University Press. Oxford, UK.

Magee, D.J., Zachazewski, J.E. and Quillen, W.S. (2008) *Pathology and intervention in musculoskeletal rehabilitation.* Saunders, Elsevier. St. Louis, MO

Malliaras, P., Cook, J.L. and Kent, P. (2006) Reduced ankle dorsiflexion range may increase the risk of patellar tendon injury among volleyball players. *Journal of Science and Medicine in Sport.* 9 (4): 304–309

McHugh, M.P., Tyler, T.F., Tetro, D.T., Mullaney, M.J. and Nicholas, S.J. (2006) Risk factors for noncontact ankle sprains in high school athletes: The role of hip strength and balance ability. *American Journal of Sports Medicine.* 34 (3): 464–470

McRae, R. (2006) *Pocketbook of orthopaedics and fractures,* 2nd edition. Churchill Livingstone, Elsevier. London, UK

Meeuwisse, W.H. (1994) Assessing causation in sport injury: A multifactorial model. *Clinical Journal of Sports Medicine.* 4 (3): 166–170

Mester, J. and MacIntosh, B.R. (2000) Balance and control of movement summary. In Nigg, B.M., MacIntosh, B.R. and Mester, J. (eds) *Biomechanics and biology of movement.* Human Kinetics. Champaign, IL

Milgrom, C., Finestone, A., Zin, D., Mandel, D. and Novack, V. (2003) Cold weather training: A risk factor for Achilles paratendinitis among recruits. *Foot and Ankle International.* 24 (5): 398–401

Morrison, A.B. and Schöffl, V.R. (2007) Review of the physiological responses to rock climbing in young climbers. *British Journal of Sports Medicine.* 41: 852–861

Mountjoy, M., Sundgot-Borgen, J., Burke, L., Carter, S., Constantini, N., Lebrun, C., Meyer, N., Sherman, R., Steffen, K., Budgett, R. and Ljungqvist, R. (2014) The IOC consensus statement: Beyond the Female Athlete Triad – Relative Energy Deficiency in Sport (RED-S). *British Journal of Sports Medicine.* 48: 491–497

Mueller-Wohlfahrt, H.W., Haensel, L., Mithoefer, K., Ekstrand, J., English, B., McNally, S., Orchard, J., van Dijk, C.N., Kerkhoffs, G.M., Schamasch, P., Blottner, D., Swaerd, L., Goedhart, E. and Ueblacker, P. (2013) Terminology and classification of muscle injuries in sport: The Munich consensus statement. *British Journal of Sports Medicine.* 47: 342–350

Nadler, S.F., Malanga, G.A., Feinberg, J.H., Prybicien, M., Stitik, T.P. and DePrince, M. (2001) Relationship between hip muscle imbalance and occurrence of low back pain in collegiate athletes: A prospective study. *American Journal of Physical Medicine and Rehabilitation.* 80 (8): 572–577

Nigg, B.M. and Segesser, B. (1988) The influence of playing surfaces on the load on the locomotor system and on football and tennis injuries. *Sports Medicine.* 5 (6): 375–385

NOO (National Obesity Observatory) (2009) *Body Mass Index as a measure of obesity.* www.noo.org.uk/uploads/doc789_40_noo_BMI.pdf, accessed February 2014

Norris, C.M. (2004) *Sports injuries: Diagnosis and management,* 3rd edition. Butterworth Heinemann. London, UK

Orchard, J. (2010) *The Orchard Sports Injury Classification System (OSICS-10.1)* www.johnorchard.com/about-osics.html, accessed March 2014

Ortiz, A., Olson, S.L., Etnyre, B., Trudelle-Jackson, E.E., Bartlett, W. and Venegas-Rios, H.L. (2010) Fatigue effects on knee joint stability during two jumping tasks in women. *Journal of Strength and Conditioning Research.* 24 (4): 1019–1027

Paiva de Castro, A., Rebelatto, J.R. and Aurichio, T.R. (2010) The relationship between wearing incorrectly sized shoes and foot dimensions, foot pain, and diabetes. *Journal of Sports Rehabilitation.* 19 (2): 214–225

Pantano, K.J. (2009) Strategies used by physical therapists in the U.S. for treatment and prevention of the female athlete triad. *Physical Therapy in Sport.* 10: 3–11

Pefanis, N., Papaharalampous, X., Tsiganos, G., Papadakou, E. and Baltopoulos, P. (2009) The effect of Q angle on ankle sprain occurrence. *Foot Ankle Specialist.* 2 (1): 22–26

Peterson, H.A. (1994) Physeal fractures. Part 3: Classification. *Journal of Pediatric Orthopedics*. 14 (4): 439–448

Pino, E.C. and Colville, M.R. (1989) Snowboard injuries. *American Journal of Sports Medicine*. 17 (6): 778–781

Placzek, J.D. and Boyce, D.A. (2006) *Orthopaedic secrets*, 2nd edition. Mosby, Elsevier. Philadelphia, PA

Prentice, W.E. (2011) *Principles of athletic training: A competency-based approach*, 14th edition. McGraw-Hill. New York

Pujol, N., Blanchi, M.P.R. and Charnbat, P. (2007) The incidence of anterior cruciate ligament injuries among competitive alpine skiers: A 25-year investigation. *American Journal of Sports Medicine*. 35 (7): 1070–1074

Punchard, N.A., Whelan, C.J. and Adcock, I. (2004) Editorial: The Journal of Inflammation. *Journal of Inflammation*. 1: 1–4

Quatman, C.E., Myer, G.D., Khoury, J., Wall, E.J. and Hewett, T.E. (2009) Sex differences in weightlifting injuries presenting to United States' emergency rooms. *Journal of Strength and Conditioning Research*. 23 (7): 2061–2067

Queen, R.M., Abbey, A.N., Wiegerinck, J.I., Yoder, J.C. and Nunley, J.A. (2010) Effect of shoe type on plantar pressure: A gender comparison. *Gait and Posture*. 31 (1): 18–22

Rae, K. and Orchard, J. (2007) The Orchard Sports Injury Classification System (OSICS-10). *Clinical Journal of Sports Medicine*. 17 (3): 201–204

Rauh, M.J., Nichols, J.F. and Barrack, M.T. (2010) Relationships among injury and disordered eating, menstrual dysfunction, and low bone mineral density in high school athletes: A prospective study. *Journal of Athletic Training*. 45 (3): 243–252

Rees, J.D., Stride, M. and Scott, A. (2013) Tendons: Time to revisit inflammation. *British Journal of Sports Medicine*. http://dx.doi.org/10.1136/bjsports-2012-091957, accessed May 2013

Roberts, W.O. (2007) Heat and cold: What does the environment do to marathon injury? *Sports Medicine*. 37 (4–5): 400–403

Roberts, W.O. (2010) Determining a 'do not start' temperature for a marathon on the basis of adverse outcomes. *Medicine and Science in Sports and Exercise*. 42 (2): 226–232

Roland, M.O. (1986) A critical review of the evidence for a pain–spasm–pain cycle in spinal disorders. *Clinical Biomechanics*. 1 (2): 102–109

Rowson, S., McNally, C. and Duma, S.M. (2010) Can footwear affect Achilles tendon loading? *Clinical Journal of Sports Medicine*. 20 (5): 344–349

Sacco, D.E., Sartorelli, D.H. and Vane, D.W. (1998) Evaluation of Alpine skiing and snowboarding injury in a northeastern state. *Journal of Trauma-Injury Infection and Critical Care*. 44 (4): 654–659

Shanmugam, C. and Maffulli, N. (2008) Sports injuries in children. *British Medical Bulletin*. 86: 33–57

Sharma, P. and Maffulli, N. (2005) Current concepts review: Tendon injury and tendinopathy, healing and repair. *Journal of Bone and Joint Surgery*. 87 A (1): 187–196

Sharma, P. and Maffulli, N. (2006) Biology of tendon injury: Healing, modelling and remodelling. *Journal of Musculoskeletal Neuronal Interactions*. 6 (2): 181–190

Sherry, E. and Wilson, S.F. (1998) *Oxford handbook of sports medicine*. Oxford University Press. Oxford, UK

Simmonds, J.V. and Keer, R.J. (2007) Hypermobility and the hypermobility syndrome. *Manual Therapy*. 12: 298–309

Stearns, M.L. (1940) Studies on the development of connective tissue in transparent chambers in the rabbit's ear, part 2. *American Journal of Anatomy*. 67: 55–97

Swe Win, K. and Thing, J. (2014) 'The fatigued athlete' and RED-S: Lessons from the field and the BASEM spring conference. *British Journal of Sports Medicine Blog*. http://blogs.bmj.com/bjsm/2014/04/16/the-fatigued-athlete-and-red-s-lessons-from-the-field-and-the-basem-spring-conference-2, accessed April 2014

Tagliafico, A.S., Ameri, P., Michaud, J., Derchi, L.E., Sormani, M.P. and Martinoli, C. (2009) Wrist injuries in non-professional tennis players: Relationships with different grips. *American Journal of Sports Medicine*. 37 (4): 760–767

Taljanovic, M.S., Nisbet, J.K., Hunter, T.B., Cohen, R.P. and Rogers, L.F. (2011) Humeral avulsion of the inferior glenohumeral ligament in college female volleyball players caused by repetitive microtrauma. *American Journal of Sports Medicine*. 39 (5): 1067–1076

Taunton, J.E., Ryan, M.B., Clement, D.B., McKenzie, D.C., Lloyd-Smith, D.R. and Zumbo, B.D. (2003) A prospective study of running injuries: The Vancouver Sun Run 'In Training' clinics. *British Journal of Sports Medicine*. 37 (3): 239–244

Teyhen, D.S., Thomas, R.M., Roberts, C.C., Gray, B.E., Robbins, T., McPoil, T., Childs, J.D. and Molloy, J.M. (2010) Awareness and compliance with recommended running shoe guidelines among US army soldiers. *Military Medicine*. 175 (11): 847–854

Thein-Nissenbaum, J.M., Rauh, M.J., Carr, K.E., Loud, K.J. and McGuine, T.A. (2011) Associations between disordered eating, menstrual dysfunction, and musculoskeletal injury among high school athletes. *Journal of Orthopaedic and Sports Physical Therapy*. 41 (2): 60–69

Udry, J.R. (1998) Why are males injured more than females? *Injury Prevention*. 4: 94–95

Valle, X., Tol, H. and Hamilton, B. (2015) Muscle injury classification. In FC Barcelona, Aspetar and FIFA Medical Centres of Excellence. *Muscle Injuries Clinical Guide 3.0*. http://media3.fcbarcelona.com/media/asset_publics/resources/000/154/690/original/MUSCLE_INJURIES_CLINICAL_GUIDE_3.0_LAST_VERSION_pdf.v1428569103.pdf, accessed June 2015

van Gent, R.N., Siem, D., van Middelkoop, M., van Os, A.G., Bierma-Zeinstra, S.M.A., Koes, B.W. and Taunton, J.E. (2007) Incidence and determinants of lower extremity running injuries in long distance runners: A systematic review. *British Journal of Sports Medicine*. 41 (8): 469–480

Waryasz, G.R. and McDermott, A.Y. (2008) Patellofemoral pain syndrome (PFPS): A systematic review of anatomy and potential risk factors. *Dynamic Medicine*. 7: 9

Waterman, B.R., Belmont, P.J., Cameron, K.L., DeBerardino, T.M. and Owens, B.D. (2010) Epidemiology of ankle sprain at the US military academy. *American Journal of Sports Medicine*. 38 (4): 979–803

Watson, T. (2008) *Electrotherapy: Evidence-based practice*, 12th edition. Churchill Livingstone, Elsevier. London, UK

Watson T. (2012) Soft tissue repair and healing review. www.electrotherapy.org/assets/Downloads/tissue%20repair%202012.pdf, accessed June 2013

Wen, D.Y., Puffer, J.C. and Schmalzried, T.P. (1998) Injuries in runners: A prospective study of alignment. *Clinical Journal of Sports Medicine*. 8 (3): 187–194

Whiting, W.C. and Zernicke, R.F. (1998) *Biomechanics of musculoskeletal injury*. Human Kinetics. Champaign, IL

Willems, T.M., De Clercq, D., Delbaere, K., Vanderstraeten, G., De Cock, A. and Witvrouw, E. (2006) A prospective study of gait related risk factors for exercise-related lower leg pain. *Gait and Posture*. 23 (1): 91–98

Williams, J.Z., Abumrad, N. and Barbul, A. (2002) Effect of a specialized amino acid mixture on human collagen deposition. *Annals of Surgery*. 236 (3): 369–375

Wolf, B.R., Ebinger, A.E., Lawler, M.P. and Britton, C.L. (2009) Injury patterns in Division 1 collegiate swimming. *American Journal of Sports Medicine*. 37 (10): 2037–2042

Yavuz, M. and Davis, B.L. (2010) Plantar shear stress distribution in athletic individuals with frictional foot blisters. *Journal of the American Podiatric Medical Association*. 100 (2): 116–120

Yokozawa, T., Fujii, N. and Ae, M. (2007) Muscle activities of the lower limb during level and uphill running. *Journal of Biomechanics*. 40 (15): 3467–3475

2

CLINICAL ASSESSMENT IN SPORTS THERAPY

*Keith Ward, Mike Grice, Rob Di Leva, Kate Evans, Jo Baker
and Adam Hawkey*

This chapter will discuss methodology in clinical assessment for sports therapy. A number of strategies, models and approaches – drawn from the wider fields of clinical sports and exercise medicine, orthopaedics, physiotherapy, osteopathy, athletic training and sports science – are presented in context with a consideration for how these may be incorporated into sports therapy practice. The chapter will also present implications of using clinical reasoning to reach working hypotheses and differential diagnoses, alongside an appreciation of factors that can influence the selection of interventions, and how these may affect the overall patient/athlete management plan. The consultation process will be explained, including an exploration of theories of best practice and the subtleties of undertaking a reliable and efficient patient history, including the identification of important nuances which underpin the therapeutic relationship. Following this, the principles and components of objective physical assessment will be presented, including structuring the process of examination and appreciating reliability and validity. Regional assessment approaches and specific techniques are discussed in the regional chapters of this book.

Introduction to clinical assessment

When a patient presents with an injury or complaint, the sports therapist is responsible for carrying out a systematic assessment to identify the reason for the pain or dysfunction and to determine the best possible interventions to assist them back to full function. Magee (2008) identifies the importance of establishing a 'sequential method' so as to ensure that nothing is overlooked. The main components of the consultation process can be separated into four main areas, routinely presented in terms of the acronym 'SOAP' (Quinn and Gordon, 2003):

- **S**ubjective assessment (appropriate personal, lifestyle, medical and injury information provided by the patient).
- **O**bjective assessment (technical, measurable physical examination performed by the sports therapist).
- **A**ssessment (analysis of assessment findings and formation of a 'differential diagnosis').
- **P**lan (formation of a 'problem list' and set of short- and/or longer-term goals).

The information gained from assessment is instrumental in forming a differential diagnosis which, for efficacy, must employ a certain level of clinical reasoning, which in simple terms is the decision-making process based on professional judgement and interpretation of the presenting information. The subjective assessment is an investigatory interview between the therapist and patient/athlete. The therapist should work to find clues during this assessment, which lead to the determining cause of the presenting condition. The main method of data collection in the subjective assessment is through specific and targeted communication between the therapist and patient. The information gathered is mainly qualitative data, and the quality of the information is therefore dependent on such factors as the questions asked, how the patient/athlete recounts their story, and how the therapist interprets their responses.

Following on from the subjective assessment is the objective assessment; and this is focused on gathering measurable clinical data. Objective assessment aims to produce mainly quantitative data with numerical or other graded values (i.e. degrees of joint range of movement; leg length measurements; strength ratings; positive or negative special test results). On completion of the assessment, the sports therapist will evaluate documented data to develop a rationale for the working hypothesis, differential diagnosis and prognosis of the presenting complaint, and determine a plan for the treatment modalities that can be adopted. The prognosis is the predicted (considered and estimated) level of function that the patient may attain within a certain time frame; and this prediction of recovery will help to guide the intensity, duration and frequency of the selected intervention(s), and will also aid in their justification (Dutton, 2008). To enable the sports therapist to obtain the best possible information from both the subjective and objective assessment, it is important to recognize the importance of the developing therapist–patient relationship, and how effective methods of communication influence the whole process.

Communication skills

The consultation process is a major medium of communication between the sports therapist and patient, and it is essential to invest time to perfect the skills which underpin this crucial aspect of practice. The information extracted from the patient in the initial consultation provides the basis for a successful assessment and eventual outcome. Lipkin (1997) identifies three functions of the consultation:

1. information gathering;
2. development and maintenance of the therapeutic relationship;
3. communication of information.

These three functions are intrinsically linked. For instance, a patient who does not particularly trust (or like) a sports therapist is less likely to divulge all necessary information; similarly, a patient who is anxious may not comprehend information clearly. The consultation process can quite frequently present challenges to the novice therapist who must aim to be friendly and flexible but also professional, confident and authoritative. The sports therapist–patient relationship directly determines the quality and completeness of information elicited and understood (Lipkin, 1997).

The communication between the sports therapist and patient is the integral part of the consultation process (Travaline *et al.*, 2005). The role of good communication skills in medical and allied health professions is well documented (Ferrari, 2006). Patients who understand their therapist are far more likely to acknowledge health problems, understand their treatment options and positively modify their behaviours (Bogardus *et al.*, 1999). An effective sports

Table 2.1 Functions of the consultation process

- To determine and monitor the nature of the problem
- To develop, maintain and conclude the therapeutic relationship
- To carry out patient/athlete education and implementation of treatment plans

therapist–patient relationship should aim to give the patient a sense that they have been heard and feel allowed to express their concerns in a respectful, caring and empathetic environment. This should also allow the patient to reflect their feelings and convey their story in their own words.

The Good Back Consultation

The 'Good Back Consultation' was a product of a research study carried out to determine what patients with chronic low back pain perceived as good clinical communication (Laerum, 2006). The guidelines from this research can be applied to other clinical settings and patient presentations. The key findings were:

- Patients wanted to be taken seriously (i.e. be seen, heard and believed).
- Patients wanted to be given an understandable explanation of what is causing their problem (i.e. use of diagrams, models and analogies).
- Patients wanted to have patient-centred communication (i.e. where patient perspectives and preferences are sought).
- Patients wanted to be told what can be done to improve their condition (i.e. by the patient and by the therapist).

Verbal communication

Verbal communication in the context of sports therapy is not confined to face-to-face meetings. Involvement with sports teams can mean that telephone conversations are needed, and it is important that the therapist can articulate themselves in such a way that they can be understood without the need for face-to-face contact. It is important to understand that different patients/ athletes will prefer to receive information in different formats; as a therapist it is important to make sure the most effective communication methods are utilized (Laerum, 2006).

It is common in sporting environments to discuss the athlete's status with the medical team on a regular basis. While there are certain issues of informed consent with regard to the sharing of personal information, when appropriate the sports therapist must be able to present information about athletes in a format and language that is understandable to the people in attendance. The language used for the media or management will be different from the language used with the medical team, and may be different again when talking with the athlete. It is also important to consider appropriate use of language when dealing directly with the athlete, particularly when summarizing consultation findings. Adaptive skills are important for effective communication (Travaline *et al.*, 2005).

Developing a conducive and therefore effective patient–therapist relationship allows for a more accurate exchange of information. This dictates how information is delivered, and depending on how the patient/athlete interprets information, the sports therapist must be able to adapt their language terminology and use of jargon for different patients – the patient must at all times be able to understand what is being conveyed. Understanding the patient's belief systems and their interpretation of their problem, their expectations of how long recovery will take and the type of treatment they will receive, allows the therapist to map out a process of

Table 2.2 Adaptive communication skills

- Assess what the patient/athlete already knows
- Assess what the patient/athlete wants to know
- Be empathic
- Speak clearly
- Keep information simple
- Tell the truth
- Be hopeful
- Watch the patient's/athlete's body and face for non-verbal communication
- Be prepared for reactions

Source: adapted from Travaline *et al.*, 2005.

care. Such a process allows goals to be created to determine whether the initial hypothesis is materializing, or whether some confounding variables have materialized which might alter the prognosis (Matthews *et al.*, 1993). The sports therapist can be likened somewhat to a detective, seeking clues in the subjective and objective assessments so as to determine the likely pathology or dysfunction, as well as the aetiology. This is an essential component of clinical practice.

Personal contact

Palpation is a powerful non-verbal stimulus and communication medium (Willison and Masson, 1986). Sports therapists use palpation to ascertain anatomical and symptomatic information and to help provide a therapeutic intervention (Roger *et al.*, 2002). Contact is made with patients throughout the consultation process when examining and during treatment, whether instructing and positioning, facilitating movement or providing soft tissue therapy, mobilization techniques or other interventions. Contact and handling should be carefully explained to ensure that the patient is prepared and informed as to why it is necessary.

The sports therapist may sometimes work in unique settings; this can require that a working space needs to be created in a less than conventional setting. Such settings, where the boundaries between professional palpation and personal/intimate touch could become more easily blurred or obscured, must still be managed professionally. Sports therapists, as do all other health care professionals, require clear definitions and firm boundaries in order to maintain therapeutic efficacy and commitment (Schiff *et al.*, 2010). In best practice, the therapist makes an effort to explain what is likely to happen during the examination (CSP, 2012; SST, 2012). The patient will make assumptions of the therapist's clinical competency based on their handling skills – too vigorous (rough) handling will indicate insensitivity or a lack of empathy; too soft a handling technique may indicate a lack of confidence or inappropriate touch. Whether the handling is too vigorous or too soft, it will at the very least be ineffective.

Non-verbal communication

Alongside face-to-face and telephone communication, the sports therapist will also need to be able to deliver effective email and text communications. As always, the recommendation here must simply be to aim to be clear and professional. There is great potential to utilize electronic communication for confirming appointments and updates, but also for optimizing patient/athlete adherence to therapeutic programmes.

It is estimated that 60–65 per cent of interpersonal communication is conveyed via non-verbal behaviours (Burgoon *et al.*, 2009). Sports therapists should be aware of both their own and their patient's non-verbal behaviours and communication. Non-verbal behaviour ('body language') includes touch, eye contact, facial expressions, gestures, body positioning and movement, listening, observing and using silence (Duncan, 1969; Exline, 1971). It is important to appreciate how non-verbal behaviour can contribute to the patient–therapist relationship.

Facial expression is one of the more straightforward non-verbal behaviours to identify and interpret. Ekman and Friesen (1971) identified several facial expressions of emotion that are identifiable across cultures, and there are obvious benefits of smiling and presenting pleasant facial expressions during the consultation process. Quite simply, a smile can convey feelings of contentment, happiness and pleasure, and can be very welcoming. Other facial expressions to consider when undertaking a consultation are those that convey genuine interest and concern at the patient's injury or problem. Patients will interpret appropriate facial expressions as indicators of empathy and interest, and this will support the development of rapport and trust. Eye contact can also influence the rapport between the therapist and patient. Effective use of eye contact serves to regulate interaction between the therapist and patient as well as to exercise subliminal social control, and help to facilitate service and task goals (Kleinke, 1986). A therapist may communicate their respectful interest in the patient's story through eye contact and show that there is engagement and an understanding from what is being said. Gestures and postures are used naturally and also deliberately as adjuncts to verbal communication to amplify verbal cues. During the consultation process, the patient may exhibit gestures or postures that indicate pain or apprehension, which may not be conveyed so obviously during verbal or facial expressions. The patient's posture may also demonstrate their level of tension or relaxation. For example, an adopted position of shoulder elevation can be possibly indicative of guarding, or a form of pain apprehension and tension; a slumped shoulder position may indicate a low mood state. Frequency of postural changes may also indicate the patient's level of agitation or anxiety.

Active listening is an important tool in the consultation process. It implies not only listening to the content of what is being said, but also interpreting and understanding feelings from how things are said (Banville, 1978). Positive gestures should be used to show the patient that they are being heard. Nodding in agreement, making detailed notes about what they are saying and then being able to repeat back what they have said are key strategies to demonstrate interest and responsiveness. Inevitably during the consultation process, periods of silence can occur. Periods of silent reflection need to be protected, and the sports therapist should aim to (briefly) embrace such an atmosphere.

Picking up cues in the subjective assessment is a key element to determine the way the therapist reacts and uses the information immediately, or so as to develop the bigger picture and use the information constructively later on. Listening for cues can prompt the therapist to implement individualized processes to engage with the patient. It is usually a collaborative approach that will be favourable to develop effective rapport. Following the initial consultation, the development and fostering of an effective patient–therapist relationship is built on the ongoing communication systems (Travaline *et al.*, 2005); and both verbal and non-verbal (face-to-face and electronic) forms of communication (which must be two-way) constitute this essential feature of practice. All key communicated information and advice regarding patients must be documented on their records; this includes information delivered via telephone, email or text.

Subjective assessment

The first stage of any consultation process is the subjective assessment; this is the patient's opportunity to tell their story. The subjective assessment must aim to provide the sports therapist with all necessary personal details, including medical history, as well as a clear initial understanding of the patient's aetiology and source of symptoms, and their perspective on their condition. By the end of the subjective assessment the sports therapist should know about the patient's functional abilities and restrictions. This includes what they are able to do in terms of walking, lifting, sitting, training and specific sport activities, as well as work and home activities of daily living (ADL). The subjective assessment should also identify possible barriers, precautions or contraindications to further assessment, treatment or management. An efficient subjective assessment is fundamental to effective injury management (Refshauge and Gass, 2004). It is estimated that 80 per cent of the necessary information to explain the presenting problem can be provided by a thorough subjective assessment (Dutton, 2008). The subjective assessment lays the foundation for effective patient/athlete care. It is also important to note that by the end of the subjective assessment, the patient's interpretation of the severity, irritability and nature (SIN) of their symptoms should have been established. The SIN of symptoms influences which objective tests are to be selected, and also which treatment methods may be applicable. During

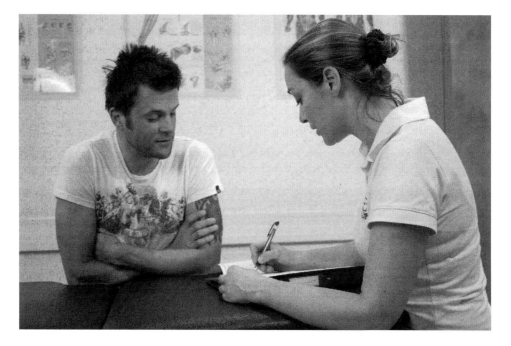

Photo 2.1 Undertaking subjective assessment.

Table 2.3 Key factors for effective subjective assessment

- Demonstrate professional appearance and behaviour at all times (overfamiliar, unprofessional behaviour does not inspire confidence).
- Wherever possible, provide a private, quiet and non-distracting environment (subjective assessments can contain highly confidential information and should be conducted in settings that maximize the patient/athlete's privacy).
- Always introduce yourself to new patients/athletes, and identify your role.
- Gain informed consent.
- Position yourself at the same level as the patient/athlete to avoid establishing dominance in the relationship.
- Know and respect the cultural norms and values of individual patients/athletes, and adjust interviewing techniques accordingly.

Table 2.4 Components of subjective assessment

Subjective assessment component	Reason for information
Presenting complaint	To determine the main reason for the visit. At this point, it is the patient's perception of their complaint.
Personal details (contact details; GP details; family history; occupation; social history)	To gather essential information, including age, gender, home and work situation, dependents and possible hereditary pathology.
Exercise and sports	To understand the patient's exercise and training routine (types; frequency; intensity) and sporting activity (types; level; position).
Past medical history (PMH)	To ascertain relevant medical history (investigations; interventions; trauma, illnesses), to review general health of body systems (e.g. digestive, respiratory systems) and identify any recent weight loss, dizziness or general malaise.
History of present complaint (mechanism of injury; onset; initial management)	It is important to record the circumstances of injury – both for clarification and for clues as to probable tissue involvement, and for medico-legal purposes.
Body chart (location of symptoms; genesis and any referral of pain)	Type and area of current symptoms, including pain and any paraesthesia (abnormal sensations).
Pain	Many cases of pain will be spontaneous in onset, or be related to perceived injury. The history of chronic pain must be fully explored. Pain of an insidious nature requires further investigation. Severity, irritability and nature (SIN) must be documented. Pain severity is recorded via visual analogue (or numerical rating) scale (VAS/NRS).
Frequency of symptoms	The subjective assessment should show how often the patient suffers pain. Frequency can help to identify the irritability of symptoms and highlight possible aggravating factors.
Duration	The duration of pain carries minimal diagnostic value. However, episodes of limited duration of pain suggest a lesser problem in terms of disability, but not necessarily lesser pathology.
Progression	If the symptoms are worsening, this may indicate an underlying pathological condition.
Precipitating factors	A patient who has pain-free intervals might identify activities that can bring on their pain. A record of precipitating factors provides a description of the patient and their problem.
Aggravating factors (AF)	Particular movements or activities will commonly aggravate a patient's pain. Listing aggravating factors provides a description of the patient and their problem, and foreshadows the assessment of disability. It provides some guidance as to which movements to undertake with care, or to possibly avoid, in objective assessment.
Relieving factors (RF)	Patients might identify factors that relieve their pain. These could include medications and interventions such as ice packs or hot baths. They may also include certain postures or activities. It is expectable that patients with a painful joint will feel better in postures that do not load that joint (e.g. lying down).
Associated features	Associated features suggestive of a more serious disorder may be more reliable than persistence of pain. Associated features can be explored during a systems review and during the general medical history.

the subjective assessment, the sports therapist should try not to ask questions or gather history that solely attempts to prove their hypothesis; it is important to keep an open mind as to what the reasons for the symptoms might be, and from this broad subjective assessment approach they can then begin to plan the objective assessment and start to rule out possible hypotheses. If the therapist starts from a narrow assessment base then the findings can also be narrow and the therapist may miss some vital clues as to the reason for the symptoms. It is important that the therapist develops a routine for the subjective assessment process but not be bound by that routine when they achieve additional clinical findings. The assessment order presented in this text is by no means definitive; however, it may be useful to break down the subjective assessment into a set of identifiable sections. It is worth noting that some of these categories will not be particularly relevant, nor will each question need to be asked for each patient. The subjective assessment must guide the objective assessment; but the temptation can sometimes be to put too much emphasis on the objective assessment and abbreviate the subjective assessment, whereas in reality, quite the opposite should be true.

Record keeping

During the consultation process, sports therapists must complete consultation and assessment forms for each patient. For the newly qualified therapist, the familiar structure and layout of the patient record form may serve as a memory prompt to ensure that all required information is obtained from the patient. It is essential from a legal and professional perspective that an accurate record of the consultation procedure and outcome is kept; importantly, it may be used to support the practitioner's actions should they be required to defend themselves against any claims of negligence or malpractice. It is also essential so that the therapist can revisit notes to compare clinical presentations and maintain clinical vigilance from one assessment to the next. (A sample 'Confidential Patient Record Form' is provided in the Appendix.)

Notation and legal requirements

Any assessment notes should be thorough but concise. It is expected that medical records are full, contemporaneous (up to date), legible and stored securely. All attendances and entries must be dated and initialled; this includes any advice given to the patient (even if provided over the telephone or via email or text). It is the duty of the sports therapist, as part of their professional standards of conduct, performance and ethics (SST, 2012), to ensure that full records are maintained. The use of standardized abbreviations assist note taking to reduce the amount of time required to produce and maintain athlete medical records. It is important that the sports therapist uses standardized abbreviations that facilitate information recording quickly and efficiently, and also so that patient data can be readily disseminated to colleagues and other medical professionals where appropriate. It is equally important that agreed standardized lists of abbreviations are used where a multidisciplinary team is responsible for the care of patients/athletes. The patient record form must be considered as a working legal document. Well-presented patient records safeguard both the practitioner and the patient, and provide a reference to previous treatments and advice. It is recommended that patient records are fully updated within 24 hours of seeing the patient. If in hard copy, all entries should be written in black ink, with any errors in the notes crossed through and initialled by the therapist who is making the correction (correction fluid should not be used). If electronic records are being held, these must be stored in a secure, password-protected system, and each update to the records should be saved as a separate file; robust back–up storage is also to be recommended. Patient records are confidential documents and must be stored in keeping with the Data Protection Act (1998) (ICO, 2013).

The record form must contain a section regarding 'informed consent'. There are two basic components to this; first, there is an information exchange – meaning that information from both sides is clearly and truthfully disclosed and understood. For this, the patient must understand that they need to provide all the necessary personal and medical information; and the therapist must provide the patient with a clear explanation of what is proposed during the assessment and treatment session. Second, consent signifies voluntariness on the part of the patient, i.e. they agree to what has been proposed (Sim, 1996). It is essential that this aspect of the process is effectively undertaken for a number of reasons, not least to offset the potential for accusations of malpractice or negligence from patients who may claim that they were not expecting to be physically examined, for example. There may be situations where informed consent is not so easily achieved, such as when there are language barriers or mental health issues; the sports therapist must in such instances still take steps to achieve informed consent – in the case of mental health issues, perhaps a partner, parent, carer or other chaperone can provide this. In the case of children, the parent or guardian must provide it. Beyond this, it is only for the optimal outcomes that informed consent to assessment and treatment is achieved; and so that the sports therapist can proceed safely. Informed consent must also be achieved prior to the sports therapist sharing any patient records with third parties (such as another health care professional, sports team or insurance company). The sports therapist must also recognize that the patient is entitled to access their records at any time.

It is recommended that if any assessment of 'intimate areas' is required, then this should be clearly noted on the record form and initialled by the patient after an explanation of the procedure. It is advisable that adults' consultation records be kept for eight years; in the case of children (under 18 in Wales and England, under 16 in Scotland) it is considered best practice for all records to be kept until the athlete is 21 years old, and a further eight years after that. After this time, all records should be destroyed as confidential waste.

The patient's personal details

The consultation process involves the initial stage of collecting administrative information. Essential details to be ascertained include: the patient's full name; date of birth; address; telephone number; email address; occupation(s); GP name; GP practice address and contact telephone number. Clarifying the patient's marital status and whether they have any dependents can be important features for clinical reasoning; such information may indicate the various external pressures the patient faces. It is efficient to consider a number of additional aspects of the patient's lifestyle and situation as they may have an effect on their ability to adhere to future advice and rehabilitation; for example: Have they recently moved house? Do they have new-born children? Do they care for elderly relatives? Do they have a long commute? Are they self-employed? It is essential that the physical components of the patient's lifestyle are effectively explored, especially with regard to their exercise and sporting regimes. The sports therapist must understand what exercise, training and recovery the patient/athlete incorporates into their normal routine. Their training history, current programme, fitness level and goals should be discussed, as should their sport(s) activities. If the patient is a competing athlete or belongs to a team, the sports therapist should ascertain to what level they compete, what their particular sport/position entails, whether they are under the care of a medical doctor or sports practitioner as part of the team environment, and, if they have a coach or manager, are they aware of their visit?

Practitioner Tip Box 2.1

Questions for the patient during subjective assessment

- Appropriate questions (e.g. What activities seem to aggravate your condition?)
- Short and clear questions (e.g. On a scale of 0–10, with 10 being the worst pain imaginable, how much pain are you in at this moment?)
- Closed questions (e.g. What sports do you do?)
- Open questions (e.g. Can you explain what happened?)
- Responsive questions (i.e. questions which are presented in response to the previous information provided by the patient)
- Special questions (*'to determine the nature of the patient's condition, differentiating between benign neuromusculoskeletal conditions which are suitable for manual therapy and systemic, neoplastic or other non-neuromusculoskeletal conditions which are not suitable for treatment'*) (Petty, 2011)

Previous medical history and general health

A general medical history needs to be obtained from the patient so that their health condition is understood, and to identify whether they have any congenital, hereditary, developmental or acquired comorbidities of significance. Further to this, are there any familial health issues of relevance (for example, history of cancer or heart disease)? It is important to clarify whether the patient is under the care of another health professional currently, such as their GP – if so, the reason for this must be discussed (and documented). It is essential to record what medications the patient is taking, ideally this will include either the brand (proprietary) name (the name given by the pharmaceutical company that produces it) or the generic (scientific) name (the name of the active ingredient in the medicine that is decided by an expert committee and is understood internationally) (NHS, 2012). The sports therapist needs to identify whether the medication is on prescription or non-prescription ('over the counter' – OTC), and should appreciate why the patient is taking the medication, what the dosage and frequency is, whether there are any adverse or side-effects and how long the patient has been taking them. A brief 'systems review' should also be undertaken. This means that the sports therapist should ascertain the patient's general health regarding their musculoskeletal, neurological, gastrointestinal, endocrine, cardiovascular, respiratory and renal systems. Furthermore, any medical investigations or interventions of significance (recent or major) must be documented; these can include blood tests, imaging, injection therapy or operative interventions. Other information that is important to ascertain can include confirming any history of allergic reactions, recent weight loss or gain, dizziness, malaise, nausea, depression or anxiety and, in females, menstrual problems or pregnancy (Petty, 2011). The sports therapist must be particularly vigilant to the details of any medical condition which may be relevant to the patient's main complaint and how it may be objectively assessed and managed. At this point in the subjective assessment, the therapist may have already gathered enough information to have identified precautions or contraindications to further assessment or treatment; clues to the possibility of serious underlying pathology ('red flag' signs and symptoms) may also be presented during subjective assessment. Sports therapists must be responsible for identifying and recommending or requesting medical assessment when signs, symptoms and history suggest the possibility of any serious pathology, and indeed whenever clarification of a medical condition or approval for sports therapy intervention is required.

Practitioner Tip Box 2.2

Example 'red flag' signs and symptoms

- History of malignancy
- Severe, unrelenting or worsening pain
- Severe pain with no apparent history of injury
- Night pain
- Pain unrelated to movement
- Severe spasm
- Loss of appetite
- Recent unexplained weight loss
- Significant neurological symptoms (e.g. cauda equine syndrome; drop attacks)
- Significant cardiorespiratory symptoms (e.g. shortness of breath; warm, discoloured, swollen limbs)
- Feeling generally unwell (malaise) (e.g. unexplainable fever or fatigue)
- Lesions which have failed to heal
- Unusual lumps or growths

* This list is not exhaustive. Any suspicion of serious underlying pathology requires urgent medical referral.

Questioning may also extend to any problems involving the rest of the kinetic chain; for example, has a patient with a current back problem sought treatment previously for any hip, knee, ankle or foot injuries, even if they are on the contralateral side of the body? Previous injuries may seem insignificant to the patient but they can be very important to the sports therapist who is attempting to put together a picture of the patient's intrinsic biomechanical history. It is also important to ascertain all other current or previous injuries or problems to ensure the therapist does not aggravate these while assessing and treating the main complaint.

Social history and family history

Information about the patient's living circumstances, marital status and details of lifestyle and leisure activities offers information about their social and family history. Certain psychosocial factors may be identified and recognized by the therapist as being 'yellow flag' signs. Throughout the assessment, the therapist should aim to identify predictors of chronicity, elements of risk behaviour, fears and fear avoidance, distorted belief patterns, low mood and possible external stressors, all of which can influence choice of treatment interventions, and can greatly influence the patient's prognosis (George *et al.*, 2008). Patients with underlying psychosocial issues may sometimes elect to withhold certain personal or medical information; such situations can also affect how pain and symptoms are reported (especially with persistant pain); patients may also be less likely to adhere to advice, even if this is unintentional. Certain patients can sometimes be involved in compensation claims with insurance companies following accidents and incidents, and therapists should recognize that this can be an influence in how they respond to assessment (Ferguson, 2009). Therefore there is an onus on detecting such underlining mechanisms. Exploring psychosocial factors forms the cornerstone for a strong patient–therapist relationship; it does, however, require an extremely sensitive, mature and confident approach, but it can be conducive to the delivery of effective care and optimal outcome, which may not have been otherwise assumed. The 'family history' considers the risk factors and potential for conditions which may have a genetic predisposition (such as ankylosing spondylitis; cancer; heart disease; hypertension; psoriasis; or rheumatoid arthritis); and hence the sports therapist will have increased awareness for suspicion of such conditions in their differential diagnosis. A careful consideration of the patient/athlete's situation and family history may also highlight such background issues as alcoholism, depression or drug dependency. Considering the family history of the patient can help to outline their relationships with others and their domestic situation. Awareness of such factors can help to influence management decisions and home care advice.

The history of the main complaint

In situations where the current injury appears to be a reoccurrence, previous assessment findings, treatment methods, functional outcomes and time frames should be established (this may include orthopaedic investigations and interventions, physiotherapy or even previous sports therapy). Whether the injury or condition is new or reoccurring, an understanding of how it first occurred is essential. The 'mechanism of injury' (MoI) may be simply viewed as a single traumatic event or as a result of repetitive microtrauma. Either way, the onset and history of the presenting complaint must be fully explored with careful questioning; and the therapist must provide full opportunity for the patient to recall and explain their experience. The sports therapist should use open-ended questions wherever possible to elicit information during subjective assessment. It is important that the patient has the opportunity to recount their story in their own words and understanding, particularly in explaining the history of their presenting condition. How and what the patient focuses on provides valuable insight into their perception of the relative importance of the symptoms being experienced.

Symptom assessment

Once the mechanism of the injury is established, the therapist should discuss the symptoms that the patient has experienced. It will be helpful to identify: what symptoms were experienced immediately at the time of injury; how severe they were; where these symptoms were felt; whether there were any abnormal sounds or sensations at the time of injury; how the area looked immediately after the injury; whether the symptoms altered from the time of the injury to present, and if so, how; whether the injury occurred during sport or exercise, and if so, whether they were able to play on.

It is important to establish if the athlete has acute, subacute or chronic symptoms, as the management options for each can be quite different. In the acute injury presentation, where the mechanism of injury is known, the potentially injured structures should be identified. Once the therapist has established the pain type, location, severity and number of pain problems (i.e. P1; P2), they may wish to question the patient on the behaviour (or pattern) of symptoms. The goal here is to establish whether pain is constant or intermittent in nature. True constant pain is unremitting, with no relief. It can be useful to ask someone who says they are in constant pain if it is hurting currently. Many patients will describe pain as constant, but it may not be painful when the question is asked during the subjective history. Constant pain that does not vary in intensity, or where no position of ease can be found, must be viewed as a red flag sign and referral considered. Constant pain that varies in intensity can be indicative of inflammatory or infective processes. Intermittent pain that comes and goes is often mechanically stimulated and is typical of many sports injury presentations. The therapist may also question the patient regarding their 24-hour behaviour of symptoms. This can help to establish how symptoms alter from morning to evening and night, as well as following activity or rest. In the morning, the therapist should establish the patient's symptoms on waking and on rising (i.e. getting out of bed). Prolonged morning pain and stiffness also suggests inflammation. Conversely, minimal or absent pain in the morning is associated with degenerative conditions such as osteoarthritis (Petty, 2011). Evening symptoms are often dictated by the patient's daytime activity levels and perhaps their occupation. Pain that is aggravated by movement is often worse at the end of the day. Night symptoms can indicate more serious pathology and must be explored fully. The sports therapist should establish if the patient has any difficulty sleeping due to their symptoms. If symptoms are relieved by lying down, this may represent the unloading of load-bearing symptom-producing structures. If the patient can only find comfort and relief and therefore sleep in one position, this can indicate the locality of a structural issue. It is important to note any positions of relief. If the patient is woken by symptoms, these should also be noted. It needs to be established if waking from sleep is associated with movement; for example, it is not uncommon for an injured medial collateral ligament of the knee to be aggravated by turning over onto the unaffected side while sleeping in bed, provoking enough pain to wake the patient. It is important to note the frequency of such painful events; how often per night, per week, and how long it takes for the pain to subside and for the patient to return to sleep. The therapist should also aim to identify any changes to the sleeping environment – this can include the type and number of pillows and the type of mattress, and how recently these may have been changed. These are particularly important with regard to spinal or back pain. Pain that prevents the patient from getting to sleep or, once woken, cannot be alleviated with a change of position or medication and prevents them from returning to sleep should be taken seriously, with referral to their GP. Information regarding the patient's symptoms must be compared on subsequent visits so that an objective view of their progress can take place.

Maitland *et al.* (2005) consider the patient's pain severity and irritability, as well as the nature of the disorder (SIN). These characteristics are important to guide the therapist's clinical impression of the problem. The severity of the injury is determined by the extent of injury, the type of pain and the intensity of pain. The 'visual (or verbal) analogue scale' (VAS) (or numerical rating scale – NRS) is helpful when determining both severity and irritability. The VAS is a numerical pain intensity scale of 0–10, where 0 indicates no pain at all and 10 represents the worst pain imaginable. The VAS is a subjective measurement instrument that is designed to measure the pain characteristic that is believed to range across a continuum of values. The patient identifies on the line the point that they feel represents their perception of their current state. The VAS score is determined by measuring (on a scale of 0–10 cm) from the left-hand end of the line to the point that the patient marks (Wewers and Lowe, 1990). The far left end indicates 'no pain' and the far right end indicates 'worst pain ever'. The score is out of 10 and may be recorded as 2/10 (little pain) or 7/10 (moderate pain) and so on. The VAS has most value when looking at change within individuals, and less value for comparing across a group of individuals at one time point.

A patient complaining of sharp, stabbing pain rated as 8/10 on a VAS can be categorized as having a high severity. A patient complaining of a dull ache which is no more than 3/10 may be deemed low to moderate severity. As a standalone characteristic, the severity of pain carries modest diagnostic weight. Patients may describe their pain as severe, but this does not necessarily suggest a serious or threatening condition. The severity and VAS score must be considered as part of all other clinical findings and in the context of other features. It is, however, helpful to record the severity of pain at baseline and on subsequent visits, using the quantitative measure of the VAS (Carlsson, 1983; Chapman *et al.*, 1985; Strong *et al.*, 1991), as this provides a measure of how the pain is changing. This should be more reliable than the patient's or

Visual Analogue Scale for Pain (VAS)

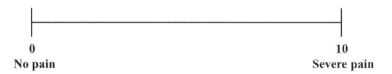

0   10
No pain   **Severe pain**

On the line provided, please mark where your 'pain status' is today.

For actual examination, the scale should measure from 0-10cm
(Magee, 2008; Wewers and Lowe, 1990)

Photo 2.2   The visual analogue scale.

therapist's memory of severity over time. Alongside the severity of pain, it is important to establish the irritability of pain symptoms. Pain irritability is assessed by how vigorous an activity is before symptoms appear, the severity of those symptoms and the time it takes for those symptoms to subside once aggravated (Koury and Scarpelli, 1994; Maitland *et al.*, 2005; Smart and Doody, 2007). Appreciating irritability helps the therapist determine how physically vigorous they can be throughout the objective assessment which follows, as well as the dosage of intervention. There is value in regulating how rigorous the assessment will be; this is chiefly to avoid exacerbating symptoms while still maximizing outcomes (Barakatt *et al.*, 2009).

As part of a full subjective review of the patient's complaint, the sports therapist must explore which factors appear to aggravate or ease the patient's condition, and also what they have done to help manage the condition. How was the injury initially managed? Did any assessment take place? Did the patient/athlete apply a PRICE (protection, rest, ice, compression and elevation) or other regime? Were there any referrals for further assessment such as an orthopaedic consultation or imaging? Were medications prescribed or taken?

Aggravating factors (AF) are particular movements, positions, activities or other things (such as heat applications) that might be responsible for reproducing or increasing the patient's symptoms. The exact movement or position, the delay in the onset of symptoms, intensity of symptoms and the duration of the increase in symptoms should be explored. Where more than one pain problem is established, aggravating factors can help establish the relationship between problems. If all symptoms are aggravated by the same factors it can be that the symptoms are related and are provoking the same structural dysfunction. Aggravating factors may be more functional in nature, so it may be necessary to consider questioning the patient on their ability to perform ADLs or sports-related movements, as well as establishing whether they are able to maintain a normal conditioning programme. Such restrictions can become objective markers of the efficacy of the rehabilitation programme.

Relieving factors (RF) are movements, positions or perhaps certain self-administered interventions (such as ice, heat, massage, strapping or OTC medications) that may help to alleviate symptoms. The sports therapist should establish exact movements or positions which appear to decrease the intensity or delay the onset of symptoms. This information can provide the therapist with insight as to how easily symptoms may be attenuated during treatment. It may also provide an insight into the structures that are implicated. As with aggravating factors, multiple pain problems eased by the same factors can indicate a relationship and a commonality of dysfunctional tissue.

Pain itself is a complex topic; it can be broadly categorized as being nociceptive, peripheral neuropathic and/or centrally sensitized. Symptoms that are brought on by physical movement and biomechanical loading, but resolve soon after the movement and loading has ceased, can usually be deemed mechanical in nature. Prolonged inflammatory injury pathologies such as bursitis, capsulitis and some tendinopathies can become chronic in nature and may also reflect an acute-on-chronic episode. The therapist can ask the patient to describe the type of pain they are experiencing and try to elicit the qualities this pain has. Newham and Mills (1999) identified general types of pain often associated with particular tissues. For instance, conditions involving bone pain may be associated with reports of deep, boring, nagging or dull pain. Post-acute muscle pain is associated with dull aching. Peripheral nerve root pain is associated with sharp, shooting, lightning-like pain. Sympathetic nerve pain is often reported as being a burning, stinging, pressure-like pain; damaged highly vascular structures can manifest pain as a throbbing and diffuse sensation. It is also interesting to note that Mense (1993) associated deep pain with muscles and superficial pain with joint injury. It is therefore beneficial to question the depth and characteristic of the patient's pain. Obviously, pain is often the primary complaint and reason for the initial sports therapy consultation. Understanding pain requires the sports therapist to appreciate the complexities that are involved in a patient's or athlete's pain. Pain is subjective and different for each individual. There are a host of factors that determine pain. It is particularly helpful for the therapist to aim to gather specific information so as to be able to understand the genesis of the patient's pain (the 'genics'). The general sources of pain, therefore, may be simply categorized as myogenic, arthrogenic, neurogenic, discogenic, viscerogenic or psychogenic, for example. Doubell *et al.* (2002) identified common characteristics of pain mechanisms. Nociceptive pain is generated due to noxious mechanical, thermal and/or chemical stimulation of peripheral receptors and is modulated in the brain. It is typically localized and predictable in its behaviour. Examples of nociceptive pain include that resulting from ligamentous sprains, fractures, impact trauma, inflammation and myofascial pain. Non-systemic peripheral neurogenic pain often follows neural distribution patterns, and can be characterized by burning, sharp or shooting type pain, and may be provoked by movement and positioning (i.e. nerve tensioning and/or compression). Persistent pain that stems from central sensitization can be widespread, more diffuse and likely to be challenging for the patient to explain or understand. Sports therapists will appreciate that, while the central sensitization of pain is very much associated with chronic pain situations, there is a central component (modulation) to all pain presentations. Centrally sensitized persisting pain is complex and multifaceted, but can involve dysfunctional neural processing associated with psychological components which can manifest in hyperalgesia (a heightened sense of pain in the periphery), allodynia (an abnormally painful response to innocuous stimuli) and altered behaviours (such as fear avoidance), which can contribute   to the situation.

Somatic referred pain is perceived in a region innervated by nerves or branches of nerves other than those which innervate the primary source of pain, where that source lies in one of the tissues or structures of the body wall (soma) or limbs (Merskey and Bogduk, 1994). A similar definition applies to referred viscerogenic pain, save that the primary source lies in one of the organs of the body. An example of this is the left arm and jaw pain that can occur during myocardial infarction. In both somatic and visceral pain the primary pain is produced by the stimulation of the peripheral endings of nociceptive afferent fibres. In contrast, neurogenic pain is pain produced by the stimulation of peripheral axons themselves, or their cell bodies (rather than their peripheral endings). Radicular pain is a subset of neurogenic pain, in which pain is evoked by stimulation of the nerve roots or dorsal root ganglion of a spinal nerve. In neurogenic pain, the pain is perceived in the region of the affected nerve. Neurogenic pain is a form of referred pain. It differs, however, from somatic and visceral referred pain in that it does not involve the stimulation of nerve endings, and does not involve convergence. Rather, it is perceived as arising from the periphery because the nerves from that region are artificially stimulated proximal to their peripheral distribution (Merskey and Bogduk, 1994). Centrally sensitized pain tends not to follow a pattern and is less predictable. The patient may also use emotional descriptions to describe their pain, such as it being unbearable or insufferable. This may indicate a habitual, psychosocial or behavioural element to their symptoms. A sclerotome is a region of bone that is innervated by a particular spinal segment (Grieve, 1988). Sclerotomal referred pain extends beyond its locality and is often overlooked for others of a more muscular origin.

When the patient presents with pain, one of the main objectives is to attempt to establish where the pain is coming from as accurately as possible. However, in some instances the patient may have pain arising from a region which may be greater than that initially indicated, such as with referred pain, or pain which only manifests when tissues are aggravated; or they may have more than one pain problem. If the patient has more than one pain, which are presumably separate in origin, a separate history should be taken for each. Each symptom may have a different cause and mechanism requiring different clinical investigation and management, or they may be linked due to the compensational biomechanical changes from the first injury. If the patient has multiple complaints related to one source, the separate histories should be combined.

Location of symptoms

Any relevant signs or symptoms should be recorded on the body charts on the patient record form. These show anterior, posterior and lateral views of the body, and it can be useful to ask the patient to complete this as they can more accurately locate the site of their symptoms. Obviously, the areas identified as painful or otherwise symptomatic by the patient are recorded. It is recommended that therapists label the identified areas of symptoms – making sure that symptoms have been clearly marked, and on the correct side of the body! Areas of scarring (such as surgical, atrophic, hypertrophic or keloid), bruising (contusion) and abnormal and unpleasant sensation (such as paraesthesia or dysaesthesia) should also be recorded. Simple abbreviations may be used to identify symptoms which have been labelled on the charts (i.e. P1 = pain 1; P2 = pain 2; C = constant; I/M = intermittent; P+Ns = pins and needles) (Petty, 2011). As a matter of clinical diligence, the therapist should check all other relevant anatomical areas for related symptoms such as stiffness or discomfort. Once these areas have been cleared a tick (✓) is placed on that area on the body charts. The information documented may not identify exact structures at fault, but the therapist can justify any relationships between symptoms, or decide whether each symptom is individual. Referred pain is the term given when the area of symptoms does not align directly with the structures at fault. Referred pain by definition is perceived in a region remote from the actual source of pain.

Patients will also present when they are not necessarily in pain or otherwise symptomatic. This can be challenging as it may be initially perceived that there is nothing specifically to assess or treat. However, sports therapists may advise completion of a functional movement or intrinsic biomechanical screen to assess the range and quality of movements at key areas, particularly those that are implicated in the patient/athlete's sport, and which may then be able to highlight possible dysfunctions at risk of becoming problematic.

The clinical impression and differential diagnosis

By the end of the subjective assessment the sports therapist should be aiming to have a differential diagnosis and justifiable clinical impression (working hypothesis) of the patient. Good verbal and non-verbal communication skills, along with appropriately selected questions, should enable the therapist to generate hypotheses based upon the MoI, the onset, the signs and symptoms and SIN, the VAS, the AF and RF and the body charts. The therapist should be aiming to link all key patient information so as to contextualize which structures and tissues may be injured and also what the root aetiology may be. The differential diagnosis is a set of named conditions that the sports therapist has clinically reasoned, based on the patient's history. The clinical impression incorporates a full and individualized appreciation of the underlying causes, including the patient's gender, age, general health, fitness, wellness and medical history, previous injuries, biomechanics, lifestyle factors (such as ergonomics, smoking, alcohol and diet), as well as psychosocial and environmental factors. It has been recommended that clinicians aim to generate up to five differential diagnoses (Elstein *et al.*, 1978). The considered differential diagnosis that the therapist establishes should then be prioritized, with the most serious condition being tested first in the objective assessment. It can be useful to categorize the differential diagnoses into the order 'life threatening', 'life changing' or 'treatable'. It may simply be that certain precautions or contraindications to objective assessment or treatment interventions have been identified by this point (Petty, 2011).

The objective assessment is then used to prove or disprove the hypothesis. The objective assessment should begin by attempting to identify any serious condition, and if positive, an immediate referral may be required. Once the therapist is convinced that there is no underlying serious pathology or referral concern, they can continue the objective testing to ascertain if the presenting condition is treatable. Objective testing and prioritizing can be a slow process when the therapist is training or newly qualified, but as more experience is gained these tests can be conducted more efficiently with a higher degree of confidence and competency.

Practitioner Tip Box 2.3

Optimizing the assessment process

- Demonstrate professional appearance, attitude and behaviour at all times.
- Inform and explain to the patient the process of assessment.
- Overfamiliar, unprofessional behaviour does not inspire confidence.
- Wherever possible, provide a quiet, non-distracting private environment. The patient history contains highly confidential information and should be undertaken in settings that show respect for this.
- Understand and respect cultural norms and values of individual patients and adjust consultation techniques accordingly.
- Inform the patient of the process of assessment and treatment and clarify that it is their responsibility to provide all required health information.
- Do not become overly fixated with taking notes at the expense of ignoring the patient.
- Give explanations in a language that the patient can comprehend.
- Be an attentive, non-judgmental, active listener, and an alert observer throughout the consultation process.

- Be mindful not to interrupt prematurely, and control any urges to fill every pause or silence with another question.
- Avoid the use of overly complex medical jargon.
- Give the patient enough time to reflect on their answers to questions.
- Engage patients to become partners in the rehabilitation process.
- Determine their health care goals and expectations about their care.
- Observe non-verbal behaviours throughout the consultation.
- Acknowledge the value of the patient's information through the use of supportive statements during and at the end of the consultation.
- Once all main personal details and general health questions have been completed, the sports therapist may then ask open-ended questions such as 'How can I help you today?' or 'What seems to be the problem?' to explore the history and background of the main complaint.
- The sports therapist should verbally summarize their understanding of the data and ask the patient if it is an accurate portrayal of the information that has been provided.
- If the consultation yields contradictory information, the therapist should revisit earlier areas of inquiry to check for consistency of response and/or ask the patient for clarification.
- Beware of prematurely cutting off a line of diagnostic inquiry.
- Although the patient's presenting symptoms may strongly suggest a particular diagnosis, failure to adequately explore alternative explanations may cause the therapist to falsely reject an important differential diagnosis.
- Provided the correct safeguards are in place, the therapist should ask the patient to email or telephone any additional information pertinent to their care that they may have forgotten to mention during the consultation.

Source: adapted from Lipkin, 1997.

Objective assessment

The adjective 'objective' is defined in the Longman Dictionary (1995) as *'existing independently of the mind'*. Objective assessment is based upon observable phenomena. In order to be objective in assessment, one must observe and be impartial to what is seen. The objective assessment aims to ensure that the therapist has assessed all probable causes of the patient's symptoms in a way that prioritizes risk. Sports therapists should aim to be able to associate the complaint with a specific region and, if appropriate, specific anatomical structures. The physical assessment process is the inspection, palpation and measurement of the body and its parts (Gross *et al.*, 2009). It is the step in the process that follows the subjective assessment, and it precedes the reaching of a clinical diagnosis. The purpose of the objective assessment is to establish the most likely (working) diagnosis using information generated from the clinical impression (hypothesis) formed in the subjective assessment. The process involves the gathering of evidence to support or disprove the differential diagnosis. With any applied test procedure, the therapist is seeking to reproduce symptoms of the primary complaint (these are known as comparable signs) and to compare the injured or problematic to the unaffected side (bilateral comparison). According to Maitland *et al.* (2005), two assumptions can be made when performing physical assessment; the first assumption is that if symptoms can be reproduced or eased, then the test has somehow affected the problematic structures. The assumption here is that all tests have the ability to isolate structures, be they anatomical or physiological. Any test conducted as part of an objective assessment is likely to stress a number of structures and can therefore implicate more than one locally or remotely (proximal or distal). The second assumption is that any abnormal response detected in a structure which could theoretically be responsible for the symptoms experienced is therefore suspected to be the source of the symptoms. The sports therapist needs to ensure that they have an appreciation of the wider pathological and biomechanical issues that can cause a structure to break down, not just identify which tissue has been damaged.

Table 2.5 Components of objective assessment

Objective assessment component	Principles
Observations	General observation of the patient in standing, seated or lying. Observing for skin presentations, muscle contours, asymmetries and other irregularities.
Static postural assessment	General impressions of the patient's musculoskeletal structure, spinal curves, shoulder and pelvic positioning and alignment of joints.
Active, passive and resisted physiological movements	Assessment of the patient's range of movement that includes active and passive ranges as well as active resisted strength, this may also include an analysis of the active and passive range of motion for the joints above and below the injured area (as in 'clearing').
Accessory movements	Movements that cannot be performed by the patient themselves but can be performed and assessed passively by the therapist.
Intrinsic biomechanical screen	A screening tool that takes a joint-by-joint approach to analyse movement dysfunctions.
Meaningful task analysis	The task that the patient functionally needs to be able to perform, but is unable due to symptoms.
Functional task analysis	Usually used as a screening tool to identify the patient's functional ability.
Muscle tests	The response and strength of muscles of the injured area using manual muscle testing. Muscle length tests aim to preferentially isolate and assess specific muscle flexibility.
Neurological tests	These include dermatomal, myotomal, reflex and neural tension testing. Cranial nerve testing may also be employed where applicable.
Palpation	A detailed assessment via touch and feel of the injured area. Involves palpation of the skin and subcutaneous tissues, anatomical landmarks, associated joint lines, ligaments, tendons and muscles.
Special tests	Used to try to confirm diagnosis of structures or the underlying condition that is causing symptoms.

While the sports therapist is guided to follow a reliable and sequential process of assessment, there is a certain clinical autonomy to the process. The patient whose subjective assessment leads the sports therapist to suspect (hypothesize) serious injury (such as a significant joint instability or stress fracture) may wish to prioritize certain stages of this objective assessment process. The prioritizing of stages during the objective assessment should help to confirm the hypothesis without unnecessarily aggravating the patient's symptoms.

The skilled therapist who has generated a comprehensive clinical impression from a detailed subjective assessment may also choose to prioritize the objective assessment in less severe injury presentations. This is a particularly useful skill in a team environment where the opportunity for a comprehensive initial consultation may not be available. The ability to quickly confirm the diagnosis hypothesis without discounting any serious injury or pathology allows the therapist to spend more time treating the patient and addressing the underlying causes.

Petty (2011) explains that prior to objective assessment, the therapist should have a firm plan for which tests to include, and also how they should be carried out. While many assessments will require the therapist to attempt to carefully reproduce patients' symptoms, an awareness of how severe and irritable symptoms are is crucial – in such cases it is important to not cause provocation. The sports therapist should also be mindful to perform fewer tests and to allow for rest periods between tests. Conversely, where symptoms are not so obviously severe or easily irritated, the therapist can consider utilizing combination movements, repetitive movements, and more functional or loaded movements to reproduce symptoms.

Observations

The first part of the objective assessment is the visual inspection; it is essential to conduct an efficient whole-body observational assessment, which then forms the basis of the overall evaluation of the patient. In the first instance, the body should be viewed as one entity as dysfunction at one segment can affect other parts through the biomechanical/kinetic chain. It is important that the sports therapist, possibly knowing prior to the visual inspection which body part is injured, does not isolate their inspection to that segment. The therapist may have formulated initial differential diagnoses from the subjective assessment, and the objective assessment will narrow these down, confirming or denying initial thoughts (Jones and Rivett, 2004). It is essential that the sports therapist remains open-minded at this stage. Observation can inform the therapist about certain specific factors which can then be further investigated throughout the physical assessment, including:

- information about the pathology itself;
- possible causes of the problem and therefore management options to correct it;
- information regarding symptom behaviour;
- information for selecting or requesting specific assessments/tests.

Following a whole-body (general) observational assessment (which should not normally take any longer than a minute or two), the injured area should be subjected to a more specific visual inspection, providing the therapist with a good initial insight into the problem in question. This is an inspection of the surface of the affected area observing for colour, contour and surface markings. It should be noted that aspects of this observation can be inadvertently or mistakenly influenced by the preceding history, leading to a less objective assessment than would be desired.

Observations begin from the moment the patient enters the clinical environment, and clues to problems can present, for example avoidance of certain movements when they are sitting in the waiting room, walking through the door, how they open the door, how they sit down or stand from a seated position, whether they cross their legs and whether they sit to one side, for example. This is an informal observation that can sometimes be the most valuable assessment as the patient will be acting most naturally, especially when compared to a more formal assessment when they are aware that the therapist is assessing them. However, a more detailed visual inspection will be conducted in the 'anatomical' and 'fundamental' positions. The importance of the anatomical position is that it provides a frame of reference with which to compare an 'ideal' body, whereas the fundamental position gives a reference specific to that individual. It could be argued that without a pre-injury image of the individual, the fundamental position is of little use. The patient may be standing, seated or lying for the initial inspection. The positioning for the observation is important. If the patient experiences their symptoms in a seated position and the therapist observes them in standing then the therapist will miss vital postural clues that may indicate why they are symptomatic.

There are a number of key features that the sports therapist should record during inspection. On inspection of the affected area, the therapist should know what bony landmarks are expected to be seen, and which landmarks are not expected to be seen (unless dysfunction is present). In addition to bony landmarks, the therapist should inspect muscle tone, size (hypertrophy; atrophy), surface tendons, and aim to notice any tremors or fasciculations.

Observations are obviously compared bilaterally. While this gives a good frame of reference for the patient as an individual, it is imperative that their dominant side is determined, recorded and considered, as this can have a significant impact on their structural composition. This is especially important in athletes, as their dominant side may be used more than in a non-athlete and may therefore exacerbate the difference. There may be evidence of 'handedness patterns'. Kendall *et al.* (2005) describe specific alterations to posture throughout the body, particularly at the shoulder and hip with muscular mal-adaptations. It must also be considered that the patient/ athlete's somatotype, body fat percentage, general stature and gender will affect the landmarks to be seen. For example, a male rugby prop would obviously have very different visual landmarks compared to a female gymnast. Other surface markings to pay attention to are scars. Although it is hoped that the patient will have disclosed any previous injuries or operations during the subjective assessment, the visual inspection is an opportunity to confirm this. If any scarring is seen which was not disclosed in the patient history, it should be discussed. It is worth remembering that scars can be as a result of minor abrasions, burns or lacerations, not always from operations, and this can explain why they may have not been noted previously. If scars are due to surgical procedures the therapist should explore further (if this was omitted in the subjective assessment). In such cases, the therapist needs to be clear as to whether it was arthroscopic or open surgery, if any metal fixtures were implanted, when the surgery was carried out and if there were any complications or infections. Such details can influence the therapist's clinical decision making when determining possible diagnosis and treatment plan.

Superficial evidence of traumatic injury can often be obvious to the therapist and the athlete themselves, and it goes without saying that if there is evidence of severe open wounds, structural deformity or protruding objects, the athlete must receive urgent medical attention. There may be evidence of deeper trauma. Observation of the surface skin can provide essential information as to the injury sustained. If the athlete has sustained a trauma to the surface which has not broken the skin, there may be haemorrhage under the skin surface which will appear as a haematoma (bruise). This area will usually appear blue or black in colour and may track down the limb with gravity over time. The bleeding may be a result of surface contact or may be due to damaged structures at a deeper level. If the athlete is seen soon after injury (within a few hours) the area may simply appear red from the initial impact. The blue–black colour normally

(a) Anterior

(b) Posterior

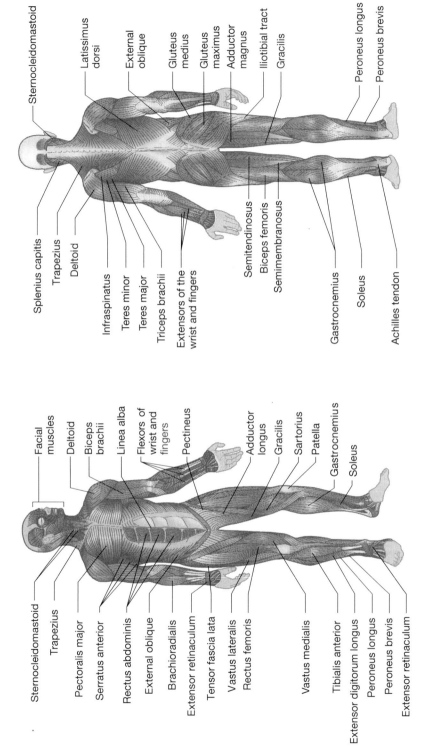

Facial muscles
Deltoid
Biceps brachii
Linea alba
Flexors of wrist and fingers
Pectineus

Sternocleidomastoid
Trapezius
Pectoralis major
Serratus anterior
Rectus abdominis
External oblique
Brachioradialis
Extensor retinaculum
Tensor fascia lata
Vastus lateralis
Rectus femoris

Adductor longus
Gracilis
Sartorius
Patella
Gastrocnemius
Soleus

Vastus medialis
Tibialis anterior
Extensor digitorum longus
Peroneus longus
Peroneus brevis
Extensor retinaculum

Sternocleidomastoid
Splenius capitis
Trapezius
Deltoid

Latissimus dorsi
External oblique
Gluteus medius
Gluteus maximus
Adductor magnus
Iliotibial tract
Gracilis
Peroneus longus
Peroneus brevis

Infraspinatus
Teres minor
Teres major
Triceps brachii
Extensors of the wrist and fingers

Semitendinosus
Biceps femoris
Semimembranosus

Gastrocnemius
Soleus

Achilles tendon

Figure 2.1 Superficial muscles (anterior and posterior) (source: adapted from Sewell *et al.*, 2013).

appears over the following days due to a reaction of blood with haemoglobin. After this, it can take up to two weeks for bruising to disappear, and in this time it will change from blue–black to green to yellow. The therapist can see approximately what area was injured and when it occurred, which may also support the subjective information. If the area appears warm and reddened it is also an indication that inflammation is present due to the vasodilation of local capillaries. Swelling can be caused by bleeding at the time of injury (tends to be rapid where more vascular tissue has been damaged); it may also be caused by damage to the joint capsule; or it may be due to the resulting vasodilation and vasopermeability occurring during early inflammation. Joint capsular damage and inflammatory reactions tend to have a more gradual onset. The gradual onset of inflammation typically peaks over a 48–72-hour period, but may persist for much longer; it involves the leaking of inflammatory exudate into the interstitial spaces. If the inspected area appears sweaty (confirmed by touch) this may indicate a sympathetic autonomic response. If such sympathetic activity is suspected, the sports therapist may also consider an investigation of the spinal segment relating to the autonomic innervation of that particular area. When inspecting any area, bilateral comparison must be undertaken, and if the therapist has any images or video of the patient then it may be useful to compare these also. Natural asymmetries due to the individual's structure or any functional imbalance or limb dominance are often seen and should be noted. It is, however, important to recognize that patients can have asymmetry without symptoms, and vice versa.

Postural assessment

Traditional posture analysis originates to some degree from the work of Braune (1877). Cadavers were frozen in a hanging position so they rested in the 'normalstellung' and the cadavers were then dissected along the frontal, sagittal and transverse planes to identify the centre of gravity (CoG). This was intended to be merely a reference point and not necessarily the 'ideal posture'; however, the 'plumb-line' measurements are still taught to assess posture to this day. Kendall *et al.* (2005) explain that ideal postural alignment centres the body's CoG over its base of support (BoS). It is essential when observing posture to consider the whole body entity, as dysfunction at one area can affect function in another. The relationship of body segments may be inherent, but there are many factors that affect posture (Magee, 2008). These include, but are not limited to, age, gender, emotional factors, muscle tone, neural control, fatigue and physical activity. IFOMPT (2010) defines posture as *'the alignment and positioning of the body in relation to gravity, centre of mass and base of support'*. Magee (2008) offers the following definition: *'Posture, which is the relative disposition of the body at any one moment, is a composite of the positions of the different joints of the body at that time… Correct posture is the position in which minimum stress is applied to each joint… Any static position that increases the stress to the joints may be called faulty posture.'* Kendall *et al.* (2005) present detailed discussions on posture (including 'ideal' posture, plumb-line assessments and regional postural presentations). The sports therapist will understand that what is 'normal' for one may be 'abnormal' for another; and that postural dysfunction does not automatically result in symptoms, or even predisposition. Lederman (2011) argues how evidence to support the 'postural–structural–biomechanical' (PSB) model of aetiology has been eroded in recent years. This argument implies that: postural asymmetries and imperfections are normal variations (i.e. not necessarily pathological); neuromuscular and motor control variations are also normal; there is individual capacity to tolerate such variations; and pathological biomechanics do not necessarily determine symptoms. However, while it is important to appreciate the potential pitfalls and limitations of the PSB model, principles for optimal posture must still be understood, these include:

- optimal loading on the musculoskeletal system;
- centre of mass over its base of support;
- optimal efficiency for movement;
- muscular balance between agonistic pairs;
- optimal positioning for organ activity.

Fryer (2011), Lee (2011) and McGill (2011) each recognize the value of undertaking postural assessment as a component of the full subjective and objective patient assessment. During *et al.* (1985) supported the need for assessment of posture, finding that there was a significant difference in posture between healthy subjects and those with spondylolisis. Brence (2012), however, does identify a number of limitations associated with the static postural assessment, not least the issues associated with both inter and intra-rater reliability. Valid and reliable posture or joint analysis (without the use of X-ray) depends on a number of factors including operator experience (Picciano, 1993), how the patient is standing and whether measuring instruments are used. Posture can be assessed in a number of positions and from a variety of angles; all combinations can provide useful information. The 'anatomical' position and the 'fundamental' position can both be used to assess the patient's posture statically. While the anatomical position is central as a baseline, where patients can be compared against recognizable norms and against one another; the fundamental position is the relaxed, natural stance which is unique to each person. In each of these positions the patient should be assessed anteriorly, posteriorly and laterally, left and right.

The static postural assessment can be undertaken using a weighted piece of string (the 'plumb-line') hanging vertically – or simply via use of an imaginary vertical line. From the anterior view, it is obvious that for symmetrical assessment the line should bisect the centre of the body via the sternum, umbilicus and midpoint between the knees and feet. Similarly, in the posterior view the line will pass through the occipital protuberance, all spinous processes, the midline of the sacrum and pelvis, and down equidistantly between the knees and feet. However, from the lateral view it is perhaps most useful as guidelines have been suggested for 'normal' alignment (Kendall *et al.*, 2005). In the 'ideal' lateral posture the plumb-line passes through the following: the earlobe; the centre of the glenohumeral joint; the greater trochanter; slightly anterior to the midline of the knee joint; and slightly anterior to the lateral malleolus. Within the body, from the lateral aspect, the imaginary plumb-line would pass through the odontoid process (the 'dens'), cervical and lumbar vertebral bodies and slightly posterior to the hip joint (Kendall *et al.*, 2005; Petty, 2011). In a clinical environment, the use of a 'postural grid' (large graph pattern on a wall) can assist the therapist in more accurately recording asymmetries in the anterior and posterior views (Fruth, 2014).

It is also essential, especially when assessing athletes, that they are observed in functional positions and during movements. During any individual standing or sitting positions, or walking or running, it is necessary to consider which sport-specific movements may have different requirements and considerations. These observed movements are likely to relate to the aggravating and easing factors stipulated during the subjective assessment.

As mentioned previously, in addition to the arguably limited information that static postural assessment may provide, for a long time it has been acknowledged that visual inspection of posture only has poor to fair reliability (Fedorak *et al.*, 2003). This has led to the development of a range of sophisticated assessment tools – although clinicians continue to use visual postural assessment due to its zero-cost and ease of use. However, advanced equipment is becoming more commonly utilized in clinical studies, alongside the use of still photographic images or visual assessment (Rillardon, 2003). Some therapists have been concerned about repeated

Table 2.6 Postural assessment checklist

Anterior view	Lateral view	Posterior view
Plumb-line (anterior view skeletal landmark coordinates)	Plumb-line (lateral view skeletal landmark coordinates – L&R)	Plumb-line (posterior view skeletal landmark coordinates)
Eye levels	Head positioning	Head positioning
Ear to shoulder distance	Curve of C spine	Ear to shoulder distance
Head positioning	Curve of T spine	Shoulder levels
Shoulder levels	Curve of L spine	Scapula position (angle/height/retracted/protracted)
Clavicle symmetry	Pelvic positioning (ASIS-PSIS comparison/ant tilt/ post tilt [unilateral/bilateral]/sway/L&R)	Curvature of spine (scoliosis/shift)
Sternal line	Knee positioning (genu flexus/recurvatus)	Pelvic position (PSIS levels/lateral pelvic tilt)
Nipple line	Muscle (bulk/symmetry):	Arm distance from body
Linea alba	*trapezius / deltoids / biceps / triceps / pectorals /*	Elbow/arm positioning
Curves of waist	*abdominals / quadriceps / ITB / hamstrings / tibialis*	Knee positioning (genu valgus/varus)
Arm distance from body	*anterior / gastrocnemius / soleus / Achilles tendon*	Ankle/foot (Achilles/calcaneus/valgus/varus heels)
Rib movement on respiration	Skin creases/fat folds	Muscle (bulk/symmetry):
Pelvis levels (ASIS/iliac crest scoliosis/lateral pelvic tilt)	Skin scars/bruises/conditions	*trapezius / deltoids / erector spinae / latissimus /*
Knee positioning (genu valgus/varus)	Other	*rhomboids / triceps / gluteals / hamstrings / gastrocnemius*
Patella positioning (normal/alta/baja)		*/ soleus / Achilles tendon*
Ankle/foot (arches/toes)		Skin creases/fat folds
Muscle (bulk/symmetry):		Skin scars/bruises/conditions
upper trapezius / deltoids / pectorals / abdominals /		Other
obliques / biceps / forearm / quadriceps / tibialis anterior		
Skin creases/fat folds		
Skin scars/bruising/conditions		
Other		

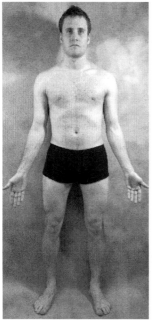 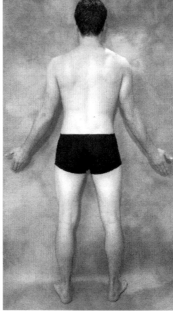 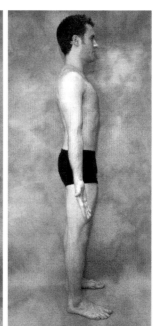

Photo 2.3 Anterior view postural assessment.

Photo 2.4 Posterior view postural assessment.

Photo 2.5 Lateral view postural assessment.

radiographic exposure on the spine during imaging (such as may take place in certain orthopaedic, chiropractic or other physical therapy settings), which has led to the development of skin surface assessment methods (Mannion *et al.*, 2004). In addition, video analysis and computer programs are becoming more widely utilized to assess posture, although due to the cost and time taken to set up equipment and to analyse information, it is not often used in clinical environments. There are also issues with confidentiality and ethical permission to video a patient. Kuo *et al.* (2009) acknowledged problems with skin markers used in video analysis and developed a new marker placement model suggesting that their model may have preferred clinical applications. Such development happens to highlight one of the key issues associated with video analysis in postural assessment. Another issue is the complex nature of technical approaches. Taylor (2010) in his review of the 'SpineDMS' ('Spinal Mouse') found it to be not only portable, but also fairly straightforward in application. The 'Rapid Entire Body Assessment' ('REBA') has been developed to assess working postures (Hignett and McAtamney, 2000), although its application to assess an injured population is not clear. 'Postural Assessment Software' ('PAS') has proved to be a reliable method of assessment, although Ferreira *et al.* (2010) concluded that the further developed the user's computer skills the more superior the reliability. In the majority of clinical settings, however, there is yet to be widespread use of advanced methods for postural assessment.

The sports therapist has to ensure that they understand the origin of any of the patient's main or recent postural changes. An example may be that the pelvis may appear anteriorly tilted when observing the body as a whole, but when the femur position is identified the position of the femur within the acetabulum may be 'normal' and the appearance of the anterior pelvis may be due to a genu recurvatus (hyperextending knee) which has altered the position of the femur and given the impression of an anterior pelvis. This 'body reading' approach has been widely taught by Myers (2009). One consideration when assessing posture using bony landmarks are the anomalies of the landmarks themselves. Preece *et al.* (2008) found numerous variations in pelvis morphology that could prevent the identification of a true anterior pelvic tilt.

Common postural conditions

There are numerous postural conditions that can present; these may be hereditary, congenital, developmental, acquired, structural and/or functional. An underlying mal-alignment, which may be congenital, can result in abnormal postural adaptations which may then lead to musculoskeletal changes which are less than optimal. Conditions such as Scheuermann's disease (an osteochondrosis of the thoracic and/or lumbar vertebrae in adolescents characterized by an anterior 'wedging' of vertebral bodies) can restrict thoracic movements, but may in the early stages seem like a normal postural kyphosis. Occasionally, dysfunction is caused by the activity undertaken by the athlete because their sport requires them to adopt unique body positions that the body's optimal posture is not designed for, such as with dancers and gymnasts.

There will always be muscular involvement (whether symptomatic or not) in any postural presentation. Muscles have a specific purpose based on their type and location. While postural muscles prevent the collapse of the skeleton, phasic muscles generate movement. Postural muscles do not fatigue as easily when compared to phasic muscles, which can generate greater forces, but fatigue more quickly. These muscles are also known as slow twitch (postural) and fast twitch (phasic) muscle fibres. When exposed to overuse or disuse, postural muscles have a tendency to become upregulated, leading to greater muscle tone with associated adaptive shortening. Muscles that are held in a shortened position for six weeks or more can lose up to 40 per cent of the sarcomeres due to the adaptation to that shortened position. It is essential that the sports therapist identifies any muscle shortening because this can have significant impact on the athlete's biomechanics and performance (Tarbary *et al.*, 1972). When postural muscles are overactive, the phasic muscles can become inhibited which can then lead to adaptive weakening and possible lengthening. When muscles are upregulated they can become overactive and held in a chronically shortened or lengthened position. Common postural patterns classically result in the 'upper cross' and 'lower cross' syndromes, as outlined by Janda (1980). Upper cross syndrome (UCS) is evidenced by:

- tight (short) pectoralis major and minor;
- tight (short) upper trapezius and levator scapulae;
- weak (long) lower trapezius, serratus anterior and rhomboids;
- weak (long) deep cervical flexors.

(Chaitow and DeLany, 2008; Liebenson, 2006)

The characteristics of UCS are often synchronous with rounded (protracted and medially rotated) shoulders and an exaggerated thoracic kyphosis. UCS is often seen in sedentary individuals, and also in very tall adolescents who habitually attempt to conceal their height. Complications associated with UCS can include headaches and thoracic outlet syndrome (neurovascular compression) (Moore, 2004).

Lower cross syndrome (LCS) (sometimes referred to as 'pelvic crossed syndrome') is evidenced by:

- tight (short) hip flexors;
- tight (short) lower spinal extensors;

- weak (long) rectus abdominus;
- weak (long) gluteus maximus.

(Chaitow and DeLany, 2008; Liebenson, 2006)

The characteristics of LCS are often synchronous with anterior pelvic tilt, increased lumbar lordosis and associated lower back pain (Chaitow and DeLany, 2008; Petty, 2011).

The 'ideal' spine as described by Kendall *et al.* (2005) presents (in the lateral view) with lordotic curvatures in the cervical and lumbar regions and kyphotic curvatures in the thoracic and sacral regions. Where these curvatures are reduced or exaggerated, descriptors may be attributed to them, such as 'flat back' (reduced lumbar lordosis). Both structural (fixed) and functional (adapted soft tissue) postural conditions relate to the individual's musculoskeletal architecture, imbalances and anomalies; their aetiology may be genetic (hereditary), congenital (simply present from birth), acquired (caused by events occurring after birth), developmental (occurring during early development), pathological (caused by disease), idiopathic (of unknown cause) or traumatic (caused by injury). While there are innumerable postural conditions, there now follows a brief overview of six broad categories of posture.

Kyphotic postures

The normal curvature of the thoracic region can be exaggerated, leading to local pain and functional muscular maladaptations. In severe cases the patient can present with neurological dysfunction or lung dysfunction (McMaster, 2007). The common presentation is with a hyperkyphosis through the thoracic region as a whole, or at its upper or lower segments, where the kyphosis can show as a more segmental and angular presentation. A forward head position, rounding of the shoulders (girdle protraction and possible medial rotation of the glenohumeral joint) and abducted scapulae are also common features, as in UCS. Muscles of the thorax (including pectoralis major and minor and the intercostals) are usually adaptively shortened, and the antagonistic thoracic erector spinae, rhomboid major and minor, serratus anterior, trapezius and erector spinae group are often adaptively lengthened and weakened (Houglum, 2010). There are three main types: postural kyphosis; congenital kyphosis; and Scheuermann's disease. Postural kyphosis is the most common type overall, where thoracic mobility is usually retained; its prevalence increases with age due to vertebral fractures, which may be related to osteoporosis or muscular atrophy (Ball *et al.*, 2009; Kado, 2007). Congenital kyphosis is uncommon, although it is often more severe than other forms; it is characterized by a failure of segmentation and can involve neural compression (McMaster and Singh, 1999). Scheuermann's kyphosis becomes apparent during adolescence, and more commonly in males, and affects around 10 per cent of the population (Magee, 2008). Its aetiology is unclear, with hereditary, developmental and environmental factors having been suggested (Draper, 2011; Lowe and Line, 2007). Finally, there is also a 'kypholordotic' postural presentation, which is a common compensatory increase in thoracic kyphosis due to exaggerated lumbar lordosis.

Lordotic postures

The normal curvatures of the cervical and lumbar sections of the spine can be exaggerated, leading to regional pain and functional muscular maladaptations. As with LCS, this posture is often identified in patients with anterior pelvic tilt. With a lordotic posture, patients often have hypomobile vertebral segments adjacent to hypermobile segments, which can exacerbate the condition and also make diagnosis and treatment difficult. Lumbar lordosis can be measured as an angle, where normal is 20–45°, which often increases with age (Lin, 1992). Fernand and Fox (1985) have previously suggested that less than 23° represents hypolordosis, and more than 68°

represents hyperlordosis. Hyperlordosis is of particular relevance to some dancers and gymnasts who require increased lumbar lordosis for aesthetic and performance reasons. However, this puts them at an increased risk of LCS, spondylolisthesis and facet joint stress, as well as a reduction in intervertebral foramen (Solomon, 2005). Increased shear forces on lumbar vertebrae, secondary to adaptive psoas tightness, may also occur, and lordosis can also lead to a 'swayback' presentation through compensation.

Swayback syndrome

Swayback posture is a combination of postural adaptations often rooted from an anteriorly shifted pelvis (in the sagittal plane). Although variants exist, swayback commonly presents with a posteriorly tilted pelvis, a reduced lumbar lordosis and most notably a compensation at the thoracic spine and cavity (the thorax) which is elongated and moves posteriorly, and the entire pelvis shifts anteriorly. The swayback posture is best observed in the lateral view, where the long kyphosis and posterior pelvic tilt are identifiable, and the greater trochanter can be assessed for being positioned anterior to the plumb-line (Kendall *et al.*, 2005). Although with a small sample size (*n* = 22), Mulhearn and George (1999) found that gymnasts with swayback posture were more likely to present with low back pain. Keer and Grahame (2003) noted that hypermobile individuals were at more risk of swayback syndrome, which may be due to excessive lumbar lordosis. A common feature is increased reliance on ligaments for postural stability. Although it has been acknowledged that these two postures are often used interchangeably, Kendall *et al.* (2005) provided guidelines for their differences: the lordotic posture is characterized by an increased lordosis in the lumbar spine and pain in the low back; the swayback posture is characterized by an increased kyphosis in the thoracic spine and thoracolumbar area, with possible pain reported at the thoracolumbar junction. It should be noted that with the swayback posture there may be a compensatory increase in lordosis. Corrections for swayback posture may include lower thoracic erector spinae, lower abdominals, external oblique and hip flexor conditioning and lengthening and down-regulating hamstrings and gluteals (Kendall *et al.*, 2005). In athletic populations with increased lordosis, where the hip flexors may be upregulated, rehabilitation may need to focus on retraining motor recruitment of rectus abdominus and external obliques, and downregulating the hip flexors through muscle energy techniques (MET) and other neuromuscular and stretching techniques.

Scoliosis

Scoliosis may be described as a curvature of the spine, observed in the frontal plane, and often with associated rotation of the spinal column. The posture is characterized by either a 'C' or 'S' shape when viewed posteriorly. Depending on the cause, severity and location of the curvature, patient presentations vary considerably. Four main categories of scoliosis have been presented: idiopathic; syndromic; neuromuscular/neuropathic; and congenital (Janicki and Alman, 2007). It has been estimated that approximately 80 per cent of scolioses are idiopathic (from no known cause) (Abul-Kasim and Ohlin, 2010). A syndromic scoliosis will most commonly present in childhood and is secondary to a recognized underlying disease (for example: Marfan's syndrome; Rett syndrome; or Beals syndrome) (SAUK, 2013). Differences in curve location, curve form and number of vertebrae affected can differ between scoliosis types. For example, Abul-Kasim and Ohlin (2010) suggested that a curve length involving more than eight vertebrae, with the furthest caudad vertebrae at L4 or L5, and a non 'S' shape curve indicates neuromuscular/neuropathic aetiology (which may result from such conditions as: cerebral palsy; spina bifida; muscular dystrophy; or spinal cord injury).

When examining patients with scoliosis, it is important to assess shoulder, scapulae and pelvic positioning (Janicki and Alman, 2007); leg length (true and apparent) should be also evaluated. Movements and palpation later in the objective assessment will provide further essential information. The traditional test for assessing scoliosis is ('Adam's') 'forward bend test', which assesses for asymmetry as the standing patient performs spinal flexion from the hips, with feet together and knees extended (Morrissey and Weinstein, 2006). For the scoliosis to be considered 'structural' the patient will retain the spinal curvature and show a 'rib hump' (unilateral costal protrusion) as they bend forward. If the spine shows a normal curve when forward bending (i.e. the scoliosis appears to normalize), they are considered to be less likely to have a structural scoliosis, and more likely to have a 'functional' scoliosis. When a scoliosis is identified, the sports therapist should consider the functional effect this deviation may have on the mechanics of the shoulder girdle, pelvic girdle, upper and lower extremity.

Flat back postures

The typical flat back posture commonly manifests in the lumbar spine, with either a reduced lordosis or even kyphosis. A lumbar spine angle of less than 20° is considered to be a flat back, although the caudad vertebrae level for measurement is debated (either L5 or S1), with the cephalad level being L1 (Szpalski and Gunzburg, 2004). The specific causes of flat back include degenerative intervertebral disc disease, spondylolisthesis or ankylosing spondylitis, and spinal fusion surgery (such as following corrective surgery for scoliosis) (Szpalski and Gunzburg, 2004). Aside from the post-operative aetiology, both genetics and muscular imbalance may increase flat back syndrome. For example, if the patient has long, weak hip flexors and shortened hip extensors, this may lead to a posteriorly tilted pelvis which, as a functional compensation, results in a flat back. A reduced lumbar lordotic curvature will generally result in reduced shock absorption through the spine and increased compressive loading through the discs and facet joints. Patients with flat back postures often experience chronic lower back pain (CLBP), find it difficult to maintain erect postures as the day progresses and may tend to flex at the hips or knees to compensate. In the thoracic region, a flatback may also be referred to as a 'military back', as it presents as a loss of normal kyphosis and an upright posture.

Leg length discrepancy

A leg length discrepancy (LLD) (or inequality – LLI) is where there is a measurable true or apparent difference between the lengths of the lower extremities; differences can exist due to structural or functional issues. A congenital cause is where the individual is born with abnormality affecting one (or both) limbs (and any of its skeletal components). There are also developmental conditions which have childhood onset and which can lead to deficient growth in a limb, for example a localized dysplasia (such as a tumour) causing restricted blood flow to a bone, which in turn can lead to avascular necrosis (AVN) (Morrisey and Weinstein, 2006). Trauma (such as a fracture) or operative intervention (such as a total knee or hip replacement – TKR/THR) are other common causes of LLD. Where actual shortening of skeletal structure is present, this is termed a 'true' (or anatomical) LLD. An 'apparent' (or physiological) LLD may give the impression of a structural imbalance, but is so categorized because the reason for the apparent shortening relates to soft tissue adaptation, which may be due to a myriad of neuromuscular conditions, dysfunctional patterns of use or occasionally it can be idiopathic. Contractures of soft tissues around arthritic joints can also lead to alterations in posture which may manifest in LLD (Sabharwal and Kumar, 2008). Discrepancies may not become evident until the patient/ athlete experiences problems with ambulation, or gradually worsening discomfort or movement restrictions involving, in particular, the lower extremities, but also the spine. Due to the spinal kinetic chain through to the pelvis, it is also possible that postural deficiencies (previously discussed) may also affect leg length. For example, scoliosis can alter pelvic alignment which can present as an apparent LLD (Morrisey and Weinstein, 2006). It is worth noting that Hoikka (1989) found poor correlation between LLD and lumbar scoliosis, but good correlation between pelvic tilt and LLD. McWilliams *et al.* (2011) discuss the management of LLI following THR; they suggest that following THR inequalities of 3 cm or more are likely to require re-operation, but those of 3 cm or less may not. Even in athletic populations, an LLD of 1 cm or less is usually considered as acceptably normal, unless identified as a cause of symptoms or compensatory movement dysfunction.

Assessment of LLD can range from simple observation – in standing (inspecting levels of bilateral pelvic landmarks), supine-lying (inspecting left and right medial malleolar positioning) and using a tape measure, or standing blocks, to radiographic imaging (Sabberwal and Kumar, 2008). To assess for true LLD, most authors recommend measuring unilaterally from the anterior superior iliac spine (ASIS) to the medial malleolus, and then comparing contralaterally (Magee, 2008). The patient should be supine-lying, and asked to 'square' their pelvis first by lifting up into a 'bridge' position and back down; legs should be 15–20 cm apart. In this method, however, the bony landmarks used may be significantly different due to the length of the ASIS differing from right to left (Preece *et al.* 2008) and this may falsely identify a true LLD. Furthermore, this measurement does not incorporate assessment of foot arch height, which the vigilant sports therapist will recognize. There is also potential for inaccurate measurement if not careful. The sports therapist may also decide to use a tape measure to assess the actual lengths of the tibia or fibula. Magee (2008), highlights how left and right limbs may be visually compared for discrepancies: femoral shortening can be assessed in a supine position, with the patient's hips and knees flexed to 90°, with feet off the couch supported by the therapist; tibial shortening may be observed in a prone position, with the patient's knees flexed to 90°. Apparent LLD may be assessed by taking a tape measurement from a central reference point (either the xiphoid process of the sternum or the umbilicus) to the medial malleolus. Inaccuracies associated with using a tape measure approach for true LLD include the possible lack of consideration for overlying soft tissue structures which may produce a functional discrepancy, but on imaging may show no bony differences. Morrisey and Weinstein (2006) note that positional angularities and subject movement, especially with younger patients, can flaw radiographic examination. These assessments should be conducted in parallel for optimal diagnosis. Practitioners may also use standing blocks as an 'indirect' measure of LLD, using the level of the pelvis as a guide. In a literature review conducted by Sabberwal and Kumar (2008) they found that standing block assessment tended to have lower reliability than a tape measure method. Consideration when using any method of LLD assessment should be given to the potential morphological differences between individuals.

Clearing tests

Clearing tests involve the assessment of key physiological movements at an associated joint to the affected region which may be the primary cause of the patient's main complaint, but as such may not be immediately obvious as it is not the main symptomatic region. Clearing will usually involve assessment of joints or regions above and below the affected joint. In simple terms, the sports therapist should understand that there can be a referral of pain or other symptoms from one region to another, and that clearing tests aim to identify this or rule it out (i.e. clear the associated region of primary involvement). For simplicity, referred symptoms are often categorized as being radicular (i.e. neurogenic, or of neural origin) or mechanical. Where the patient's symptoms are reproduced during any clearing test, the joint being tested cannot be considered 'normal' and will require further investigation (Petty, 2011).

Recommended regional clearing approaches

Each joint has its own set of physiological movements that can be applied during the clearing test to assess its integrity and any possible reproduction of symptoms. While clinical reasoning will support decision making on the process, the sports therapist is likely to clear the cervical and thoracic regions for upper extremity symptoms, and lumbar and sacroiliac regions for lower extremity symptoms. In addition, the therapist will normally clear the peripheral regions above and below the affected area. For an example, when there is elbow pain, the therapist will usually clear the cervical, thoracic, shoulder and wrist regions before proceeding to assess the elbow area. Some examples of movements to assess in clearing are presented below:

- The cervical, thoracic and lumbar regions can be assessed (cleared) by asking the patient to perform all main active ranges of movement (ARoM) (flexion, extension, lateral flexion left and right and rotation left and right), and then offering overpressure (OP) if asymptomatic. In addition, or alternatively, the sports therapist may elect to assess combination movements, such as 'quadrant' positions (for example, assessing lateral flexion in combination with rotation, and then adding a flexion or extension movement); OP may also be added. With spinal movements, the therapist must aim to recognize which movements and structures are compressing or tensioning, gapping or closing.
- The shoulder can be assessed (cleared) by asking the patient to perform all main ARoMs (flexion, extension, abduction, adduction, lateral and medial rotation), and then offering OP if asymptomatic. Protraction, retraction, elevation or depression can be used to clear the shoulder girdle. Alternatively, or in addition, combination movements can be used, such as hand behind back (HBB) (involving extension, adduction and medial rotation) and hand behind neck (HBN) (involving flexion, abduction and lateral rotation). The acromioclavicular joint can also be cleared by performing horizontal adduction, with or without medial rotation.
- The hip joint can be cleared by assessing the patient's response to standard ARoM (flexion, extension, abduction, adduction, medial rotation and lateral rotation), and then offering OP if asymptomatic. In addition, or alternatively, the sports therapist may elect to assess combination movements, such as 'quadrant' positions.
- The knee is usually cleared by assessment of flexion and extension, with OP if appropriate.
- The talocrural joint is usually cleared with dorsiflexion and plantarflexion, with OP if appropriate. The subtalar joint can be cleared with inversion and eversion, plus OP if asymptomatic.

Active movement assessment

Active range of movement assessment aims to examine the following: the quality of movement (observing for smoothness, control, deviation from requested pattern, compensation, clunking or crepitus); the production of pain during movement (locally or referred); the actual RoM (assessed in degrees, or possibly centimetres); any other symptoms (such as paraesthesia or anaesthesia), tension (sense and location of restricted motion due to soft tissue tension); and the willingness (or apprehension) of the patient to perform the particular movement. These aspects may be summarized as 'QPRSTW' (quality, pain, range, symptoms, tension and willingness). Essentially, ARoM involves assessing physiological movements plus OP when the patient's full active range is shown to be asymptomatic. OP is used to ascertain patient (and symptom) response at the end of available range and incorporates an appreciation of 'end-feel' at each joint. ARoM assesses contractile tissue (the musculotendinous tissue involved in producing the movement), hence if there is any damage or dysfunction in these tissues, the movement may provoke symptoms – however, as ARoM does not challenge the musculature against external resistance beyond gravity, the patient's symptoms may not actually be reproduced – hence, resisted movement, and more functional movement, testing may be required to elicit the symptom response. The sports therapist will appreciate that in addition to the contractile tissues, inert issues are also involved in the process of producing an ARoM, including neural tissue, articular surfaces and capsules, ligaments and fascial tissue. Prior to assessing ARoM, the sports therapist must demonstrate and explain what is required of the patient. They should note which movements (if any) cause pain or other symptoms, and question the patient on the specific onset of symptoms during range and the location, intensity and quality of any symptoms produced. If the subjective assessment leads the therapist to suspect fracture or dislocation as the primary complaint, then they must be cautious with any movement that may result in loading, translation or relocation of the affected bone or joint. If the patient's pain or other symptom reports are intense, severe, acute or highly irritable it may not be possible for the therapist to assess all movement ranges. Where an assessment of active range is possible, in addition to pain, the therapist should establish the quality of the movement produced. An abnormal movement may present as a 'jolting, jerky or bumpy' movement as opposed to smooth and coordinated. Certain joints require specific movement coordination, referred to as a rhythm. An example of this is the scapula–humeral rhythm (SHR) required for ideal glenohumeral movement and function. The therapist should instruct the patient to perform the required movements at a slow and controlled speed while making a note of the prime movers, synergists, joint rhythm and the muscle recruitment pattern, where appropriate. The therapist should also consider the functional role of muscles and not just the agonistic or concentric role presented in many textbooks. Compensatory movement patterns should also be noted. An example of a compensatory pattern is the patient who elevates their shoulder girdle before abducting or flexing their shoulder as a compensatory pattern for a possibly weak, inhibited or injured supraspinatus. The patient's facial expressions should also be observed for any signs of pain, discomfort or apprehension. Each movement is typically performed two or three times to ensure the therapist has the opportunity to make all the necessary observations. However, if the patient describes an increase in symptoms with repetition of movement, two or three repetitions may not be possible.

The assessment of ARoM is typically performed qualitatively, with the therapist subjectively estimating range. The result is then compared bilaterally and also to normative data. Where the therapist is unable to accurately estimate range or where the gains in range will be small, as in the case of the long-term injured athlete, the therapist may decide a quantitative approach is necessary. A goniometer or inclinometer (flexometer) can be used to measure angles and joint range more accurately than purely by eye. The most common 'universal' (plastic or stainless steel) goniometer is essentially a protractor which comes in a number of sizes suitable for measuring different joints; these have a 'stationary' arm and a 'moving' arm, which rotates about an axis on the protractor with a dial showing the degrees of movement. There are a number of inclinometers, including the original 'Leighton' type, which straps to the patient's body or limb, and consists of a circular 360° scale, with a weighted dial and a weighted pointer needle (Leighton, 1966). As the dial of the flexometer locks into one position, gravity draws the weighted end of the needle downwards to record the range achieved. Digital and bubble (fluid-filled, 'spirit-level' type) inclinometers are more commonly used currently. The most commonly used measurement method is the 0–180° system. Therapists should recognize the 'anatomic zero position'. This is where the start position for measurement is set at 0° and where the assessed joint is taken from a neutral position to its

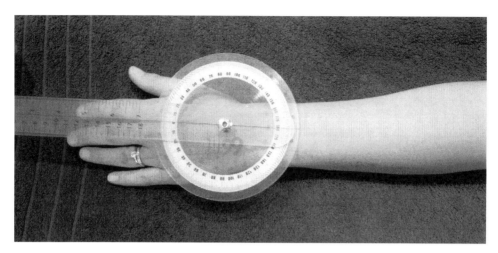

Photo 2.6   Assessing radial and ulnar deviation (start position – anatomical zero).

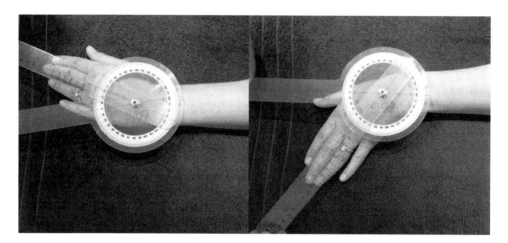

Photo 2.7   Assessing radial and ulnar deviation.

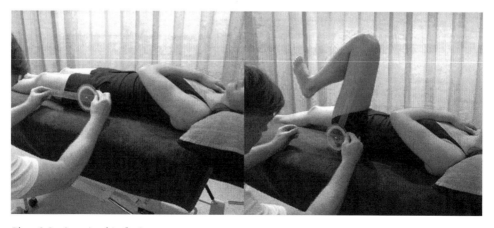

Photo 2.8   Assessing hip flexion.

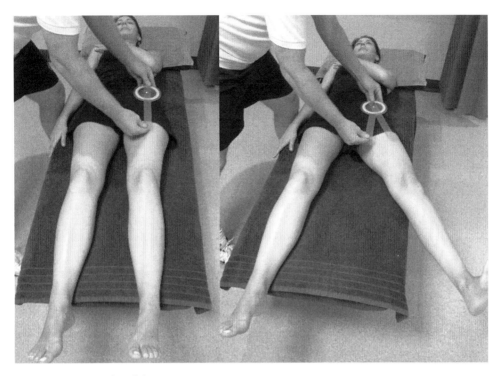

Photo 2.9   Assessing hip abduction.

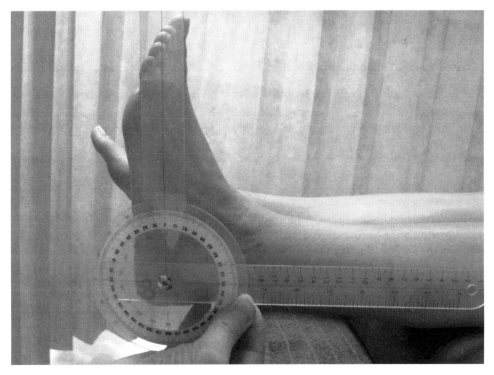

Photo 2.10   Assessing ankle dorsiflexion and plantarflexion (start position – anatomical zero).

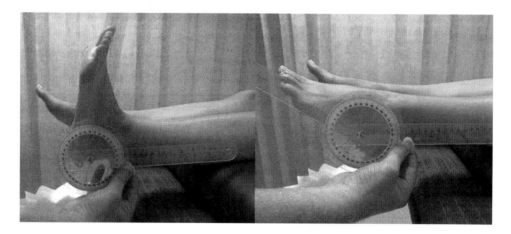

Photo 2.11 Assessing dorsiflexion and plantarflexion.

available outer range. Swann and Harrelson (2012) highlight that exceptions to this start position include medial and lateral rotation of the shoulder and hip, and forearm pronation and supination, where the start position will begin in mid-range. Ankle plantar and dorsiflexion is also measured from a mid-range anatomical zero position (the 'plantigrade' 90° position). The accuracy of the measurement is dependent upon the therapist's training, experience and their attention to detail. Houglum (2010) estimates accuracy of the experienced therapist to be within 3–5° of the true values (i.e. around 5° would be considered as the standard error of measurement).

The therapist should aim to relate any adverse findings of hyper- or hypomobility to the patient's age, gender, occupation, sport and past injuries and problems. It is not uncommon for a swimmer, or any athlete participating in repetitive overhead activities, to show some patterns of hypermobility; however, older patients/athletes more commonly present with patterns of hypomobility. Sporting contexts are essential to appreciate – consider the scrum-half in rugby union who has reduced shoulder horizontal adduction; this will significantly affect their ability to pass the ball.

Passive physiological movement assessment

Once the active ranges of movement have been conducted, the therapist should move on to the passive RoM (ProM) assessment. This requires the therapist to position the patient appropriately, instruct them to relax, take the weight of the limb and carefully move the target joint through its full available range. The non-affected side is normally tested first for baseline appreciation. The patient's response to movement must be appreciated (verbal and visual); and the sports therapist must utilize correct and repeatable handling skills and aim to interpret movement findings reliably. The PRoM can be measured in the same way as the active assessment using goniometric assessment (although it can be challenging to do this passively without assistance); a visually estimated assessment of range can also be used. Discrepancies in PRoM may be caused by such conditions as myofascial tension, contraction or spasm, soft tissue contractures, adverse neural tension, intra- or extra-capsular swelling, bursitis, tendinopathy, intra-articular joint restriction, mechanical derangement or patient pain and apprehension. In addition to assessing available RoM and quality, the PRoM assessment also allows the therapist to assess the 'end-feel'. The end-feel is a description of the sensation felt by the therapist as the joint is taken to

Table 2.7 Average regional active ranges of movement

Region and movement	Average RoM
Cervical flexion	45–50°
Cervical extension	70–85°
Cervical rotation	75–90°
Cervical lateral flexion	35–45°
Thoracic flexion	30–50°
Thoracic extension	25–45°
Thoracic rotation	35–50°
Thoracic lateral flexion	20–40°
Lumbar flexion	40–60°
Lumbar extension	30–42°
Lumbar rotation	3–18°
Lumbar lateral flexion	19–35°
Shoulder flexion	160–180°
Shoulder extension	50–65°
Shoulder abduction	170–185°
Shoulder adduction	50–75°
Shoulder medial rotation	60–90°
Shoulder lateral rotation	80–105°
Elbow flexion	140–150°
Elbow extension	0–10°
Elbow pronation	80–90°
Elbow supination	80–90°
Wrist flexion	70–80°
Wrist extension	60–80°
Wrist radial deviation	15–20°
Wrist ulnar deviation	30–40°
Hip flexion	110–125°
Hip extension	10–30°
Hip abduction	30–50°
Hip adduction	20–30°
Hip medial rotation	25–40°
Hip lateral rotation	40–60°
Knee flexion	130–145°
Knee extension	0–10°
Knee medial rotation	20–30°
Knee lateral rotation	30–40°
Ankle dorsiflexion	13–20°
Ankle plantarflexion	50–60°
Ankle inversion	30–40°
Ankle eversion	15–23°

Source: adapted from Cipriano, 2010; Kenyon and Kenyon, 2009; Magee, 2008.

Notes

The average ranges presented are for active movements. The sports therapist will recognize that ranges will vary according to positioning of the patient/athlete, and among populations. Factors including age, gender, body type, genetics, work, sports and training, injury, pain, weakness, general health, soft tissue tension, joint hypomobility or hypermobility, as well as fear or apprehension all influence the available active range of movement.

its actual end of range. It is achieved by the application of OP by the therapist. OP is the careful application of force into the joint's end range position. Occasionally in the pathological joint, pain or resistance may be felt during the application of OP. The therapist should record which of the following, if either, is present, and in which order they present: pain before resistance (typically noted as P > R); or resistance before pain (R > P). These findings can inform management options. *Normal* end-feels of joints may be simply classified as one of the following palpable presentations (Cyriax, 1996):

- Bone to bone end-feel: a hard, distinct, unyielding sensation that is painless. An example is elbow extension, where the range cannot exceed the closing of the olecranon process of the ulna into the olecranon fossa of the humerus, and the therapist feels an abrupt, hard restriction to further movement.
- Soft tissue approximation: a soft, painless end-feel represents a movement that is halted due to the compression of approximating soft tissue. The movement feels 'mushy', where often the muscles compress against each other and it is this that prevents further movement. An example is knee flexion, where passive compression of the posterior thigh against the posterior calf prevents further movement of the joint. The end-feel is gradual and soft.
- Tissue stretch end-feel: a firm, tensile, painless sensation of restriction represents movement that is prevented by ligamentous or capsular tension. Ligamentous tension can produce a more elastic end-feel; and capsular tension tends to produce a harder end-feel. Examples of more ligamentous end-feels are wrist flexion and extension; an example of a capsular end-feel is knee extension.

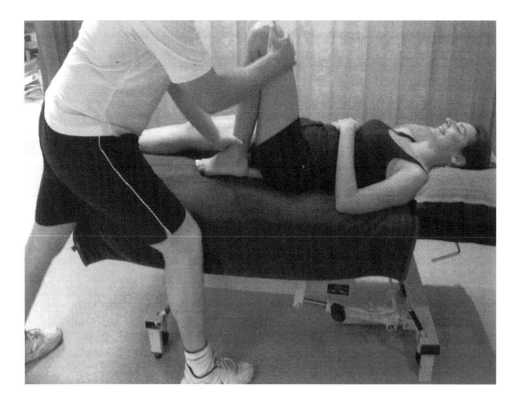

Photo 2.12   Assessing knee flexion end-feel.

A number of recognizable *abnormal* end-feels have also been presented (Cyriax, 1996; Magee, 2008). These include:

- Bone to bone end-feel: a hard, restricted and possibly painful end-feel; this can present in joints where a bone to bone end-feel is not normal. An arthritic joint, with cartilage degeneration, and osteophytic projections at the joint margins will typically show this type of end-feel.
- Springy end-feel: an abrupt, restricted, possibly painful, rebounding response to overpressure. This can occur when there is an internal mechanical derangement; the most common example of this is a meniscal tear in the knee.
- Capsular end-feel: a local, often painful, restricted, soft tissue tension where such an end-feel is not expected, such as with adhesive capsulitis of the shoulder, or in arthritic joints where the capsule is affected (Fruth, 2014; Petty, 2011).
- Empty end-feel: a lack of normal end-feel due to soft tissue damage (such as ligamentous sprain or tendon tear); or lack of normal end-feel due to pain being the limiting feature.
- Muscular spasm end-feel: a sudden, firm, tensioning end-feel due to involuntary muscular spasm; typically, either as a protective pain response, or as a feature of a neurological condition.

Where ligamentous rupture has occurred, there is likely to be a lack of restriction to excessive movement (i.e. gross instability) and the joint is permitted to exceed normal physiological movement. Where a springy end-feel is felt, often a hard end-feel on opposite structures will be observed. For example, a complete rupture of the calcaneofibular ligament of the talocrural joint will allow full, unhindered inversion (in neutral). This movement will continue until the medial ankle structures, such as the talus, medial malleolus and possibly even the calcaneous compress together to restrict range. It is always useful to ask the patient where they feel restriction during movement: in this instance, if the patient points to the medial aspect of the ankle, an abnormal end-feel may be considered. Where muscle spasm is present, it can be provoked during PRoM assessment; this may occur at the beginning, middle or end of range, and is often accompanied by the sharp sudden onset of pain. It is easily identified by asking the patient, again, to point to the cause of the restriction. For example, a lack of talocrural dorsiflexion early in range may be caused by spasm of the gastrocnemius. A premature 'springy' block to movement usually indicates an internal derangement in the joint itself, and may be accompanied by a clicking or locking sensation if articular cartilage, meniscal or labral structures are involved. An abnormal hard end-feel manifests as a bone-to-bone restriction on range of movement early within the joint's range. Unlike the springy block, the abnormal hard end-feel does not offer any spring-back to a comfortable range. The abnormal hard end-feel found early in range may be indicative of arthritic osteophyte formation. Each synovial joint movement also has the potential to be restricted by its joint capsule. Where the capsular pattern of restriction occurs prematurely, the therapist may consider a capsular pathology. Cyriax (1996), Magee (2008) and others have presented the movements most likely to be affected (restricted) with a capsular pathology; these are termed 'capsular patterns' and when understood, the sports therapist will be more able to suspect such conditions. As Magee (2008) states: *'If the capsule of the joint is affected, the pattern of limitation is the feature that indicates the presence of a capsular pattern in the joint… this pattern is the result of a total joint reaction.'*

Table 2.8 Regional capsular patterns

Joint/region	Movement restriction (in order of restriction)
Cervical spine	Lateral flexion and rotation equally limited, extension
Glenohumeral	Lateral rotation, abduction, medial rotation
Sternoclavicular	Pain at extreme end of range
Acromioclavicular	Pain at extreme end of range
Humeroulnar	Flexion, extension
Radiohumeral	Flexion, extension, supination, pronation
Proximal radioulnar	Supination, pronation
Distal radioulnar	Pain at extreme end of range
Radiocarpal	Flexion and extension equally limited
Thoracic spine	Lateral flexion and rotation equally limited, extension
Lumbar spine	Lateral flexion and rotation equally limited, extension
Sacroiliac	Pain when joint is stressed
Pubic symphysis	Pain when joint is stressed
Femoracetabular	Flexion, abduction, medial rotation (medial rotation may be first)
Tibiofemoral	Flexion, extension
Tibiofibular	Pain when joint is stressed
Talocrural	Plantarflexion, dorsiflexion
Subtalar	Inversion

Source: adapted from Cyriax, 1996; Magee, 2008; Petty, 2011.

Passive accessory movement assessment

Accessory movements are defined as those movements which a person cannot isolate and perform actively but which can be performed on the person by the therapist (Petty, 2011); accessory movement has also been referred to as 'joint play' (Mennell, 1960). Accessory movements should normally occur so as to facilitate smooth physiological movements. Restrictions in accessory movements can cause aberrant motion or pain (or both) in the physiological range. Simply; accessory movement involves a translation, compression or distraction of articular surfaces; the translator movements are described as glide, roll and spin. Gliding accessory movements have been described as when the same area of one articular surface meets new areas on the opposing articular surface; spin movements involve accessory rotation around a stationary axis; and roll movements are where one articular surface rolls on another and new areas of one articular surface will meet new areas of the opposing articular surface. Examples of such accessory movements, which clarify their direction, include: posteroanterior glide (PA); anteroposterior glide (AP); medial glide (MG); lateral glide (LG); and transverse glide (TG). When spinal accessory movements are performed, these are referred to as passive accessory intervertebral movements (PAIVMs); examples of these include central passive accessory movement (CPAM) and unilateral passive accessory movement (UPAM). When a compression movement is applied longitudinally to a peripheral joint and involves movement proximally towards the head it is termed 'cephalad' (from Greek – *kephale* meaning 'head'); when a distraction movement is applied longitudinally to take the target limb away from the body and separate joint surfaces it is termed 'caudad' (from Latin – *cauda* meaning 'tail').

Key to the effectiveness of passive accessory joint movement assessment is the therapist's handling, delivery and interpretation. Inter-rater reliability has been questioned (Schneider *et al.*, 2008; Snodgrass *et al.* 2007) and issues of reliability can relate to the specificity of the therapist's palpatory contact points, the amount of force used (such as with compression, distraction or gliding) and their ability to interpret findings. If any of the accessory movements associated with a particular joint are deemed to be restricted (hypomobile), then it follows that normal full-range physiological movements are likely to be adversely affected; additional factors contribute to the quality of movement, including hypermobility, pain and restricted soft tissue mobility. With such conditions, dyskinesia (gross abnormal movement pattern) will normally be observed. Accessory movements must be performed with the patient in a supported, relaxed position, and with the target joint in a 'loose-packed' position. The 'close-packed' (synarthrodial) position is where the associated articular joint surfaces are in maximal contact with each other, where primary static stabilizers are typically on tension and where a position of maximal congruency is present (Magee, 2008); this is an unfavourable position to test accessory movement. The loose-packed position is where the joint surfaces are not in maximal contact with each other, and where the primary static stabilizers are not on full tension – the joint is less than maximally congruent.

When assessing accessory movements the therapist has to be extremely focused on localizing their movements to the target joint. A firm understanding of the joint surfaces and directions of movement is essential. Unless the accessory movement is a compression or distraction, the delivery has to be applied close to the joint line, and the area should be as stable as possible so that the therapist can direct their forces appropriately. When assessing the movement available the therapist should move slowly and carefully, and aim to palpate and sense the range and quality of movement of the joint and surrounding tissue, which must include the detection of any pain or muscle spasm.

The shape of the articulating joint surfaces and direction of associated movements is defined to some degree by the so-called 'convex–concave rule'. This describes the directions of movement which are associated with a joint as being dependent upon the shape of the moving bone's surfaces (Schomacher, 2009). Kessler and Hertling (1983) distinguish that as a concave surface moves on a convex surface (where the convex surface is fixed), then the accessory movements (such as roll and glide) will occur in the same direction to the angular physiological movement. Conversely, if the convex joint surface moves on a fixed concave surface, then the accessory movement will be in the opposite direction to the angular physiological movement. The clinical relevance of the convex–concave rule has been questioned, however, and certainly its universal application. Banks and Hengeveld (2010) place lesser credence on the model for planning manual therapy, particularly with regard to pain; they suggest the use of the least painful accessory movement(s) as the starting point for joint mobilizations. When the involved accessory movements have been assessed, the sports therapist will record which movements were restricted, lax or otherwise symptomatic. This information will then contribute to decisions regarding hypothesis generation and resulting patient management.

Even after assessment has taken place and therapy is being delivered, the sports therapist must continuously monitor the patient response (for any improvement or possible aggravation). As Cook (2012) explains, effective delivery of manual therapy must involve assessing for *'within-session changes'*, and refers to it as a *'patient response-based method'*. The use of 'clinical indicators' should be incorporated into this approach. Clinical indicators are those movements which have been identified during assessment as being problematic (i.e. painful, restricted or the source of other symptoms); these movements should be re-tested 'within-session' following the delivery of manual therapy techniques. This will usually take the form of re-testing problematic active or functional movements.

Resisted movement assessment

Resisted movements are typically the last movements to be assessed in this section of the objective assessment. The primary purpose is to test the ability of the joint's surrounding contractile structures to protect the joint from excessive movement. In essence, the joint is actively taken to a mid-range. The therapist then applies their contact (firm, confident and specific handling is required) and instructs the patient to resist the movement. In so doing, the therapist is assessing the voluntary isometric contraction of the movement agonists (isotonic resistance can also be used). Where these contractile elements or the nerve supplying the contractile structures are at fault, pain and weakness will be observed. The resistance should be applied initially gently, with an instruction such as *'Don't let me move you'* or *'Just meet and match my resistance'* so that the patient knows not to resist the force with too much effort. This approach should be protective against aggravating symptoms, but allows for incremental increases in intensity; the contractions should be held for 3–5 seconds, and contralateral comparison must be made.

Manual muscle tests

The therapist may also undertake assessment of more specific muscle strength. This is where the therapist attempts to target specified muscle(s) rather than general group synergy. This is also usually done initially as an isometric contraction. The therapist should know the position, attachments and actions of the muscles to be tested. They should ask the patient to actively move the muscle into its action. For example, iliacus is a hip flexor and so the therapist positions the patient in supine-lying with the hip flexed, bringing the knee in towards the chest. The therapist instructs the patient to resist and then applies a force opposite to the muscle action. The patient should match the force of the therapist to produce an isometric contraction in which no movement occurs. This 'matching of force' approach allows a therapist of any size to administer a manual muscle test to a patient/athlete of any size. Pain, discomfort, weakness or any other symptoms provoked should be noted. The optimal muscle length for generating muscle tension is slightly greater than the resting length (Hamill and Knutzen, 2009). Manual muscle testing should be performed in this range. However, if adaptive shortening/lengthening of the muscle being tested has taken place then the length tension relationship may be altered.

Muscle strength throughout the range of movement can also be tested. In this test the muscle is again placed into its action with the therapist applying an opposing force, which attempts to take the muscle out of its action. The patient/athlete is instructed to resist the movement, but also to allow the movement to happen; it is testing the lengthening contraction. This enables the therapist to assess eccentric strength through a full range. The therapist should use an established strength-grading scale, such as the 'Oxford Grading Scale' (OGS). The OGS rates a patient's strength on a scale of 0–5. Strength is graded at 0 if no contraction is produced and no resistance is applied. A grade of 1 out of 5 (noted as 1/5) is characterized by slight contractile activity but no joint motion. A grade of 2/5 reflects the patient's ability to move the joint through its full range when gravity is eliminated by the patient's positioning; 3/5 is associated with the ability to move the joint through its full range against gravity; at 4/5, the patient is able to produce joint movement through the full range, against gravity and against moderate resistance; 5/5 is exemplified by maximal resistance applied through a full range and against gravity. Florence (1992) conducted research into the inter-rater reliability of manual muscle testing and found that a modified scale had good repeatability. Manual muscle testing can serve to indicate musculotendinous injury (pain and/or weakness) and neurological deficits (weakness). The sports therapist must also be able to interpret the possibility of 'emotional sensitivity' – where all resisted movements may be apparently painful (or weak); or 'intermittent claudication'– where discomfort results during sustained or repetitive contractions (Cyriax, 1996).

Table 2.9 Oxford Grading Scale (OGS) (for muscle testing)

Grade	Definition
0/5	No contraction
1/5	Visible/palpable muscle contraction but no movement
2/5	Movement with gravity eliminated
3/5	Movement against gravity only
4/5	Movement against gravity with some resistance
5/5	Movement against gravity with full resistance

Table 2.10 Modified Medical Research Council Scale (for muscle testing)

Grade	Definition
5	Normal strength
5–	Barely detectable weakness
4+	Same as grade 4, but muscle holds the joint against moderate to maximal resistance
4	Muscle holds the joint against a combination of gravity and moderate resistance
4–	Same as grade 4, but the muscle holds the joint only against minimal resistance
3+	Muscle moves the joint fully against gravity and is capable of transient resistance, but collapses abruptly
3	Muscle cannot hold the joint against resistance, but moves the joint fully against gravity
3–	Muscle moves the joint against gravity, but not through full mechanical range of motion
2	Muscle moves the joint when gravity is eliminated
1	A flicker of movement is seen or felt in the muscle
0	No movement

Source: adapted from Florence, 1992.

In certain cases it may be necessary to assess an athlete's strength isokinetically. Isokinetic strength reflects the ability of the contractile elements to produce a contraction at a constant speed through a full range of movement. This requires the use of specialized equipment; two of the most recognized isokinetic machine manufacturers include *Biodex* (Biodex Corporation, New York) and *Cybex* (Cybex Medical Division, Texas). Isokinetic machines can be used both diagnostically and in a rehabilitation context, and can be useful when muscle imbalances, dysfunction or altered recruitment patterns are the cause of the athlete's problem.

Muscle length tests

Muscle length tests are used to identify if the length of a muscle (and associated myofascia) is relatively normal, excessive or restricted as these will alter the length–tension relationships (Hamill and Knutzen, 2009). This is useful as the muscle that is too short will restrict joint range, whereas the muscle that is stretched or lengthened may allow excessive range of movement. Kendall *et al.* (2005) state that a muscle's length impacts on its strength capabilities. Muscles that are functionally lengthened may be weak or inhibited/downregulated; adaptive shortening may also have occurred in the opposing muscles. Muscles that are functionally shortened may be strong, or in spasm/upregulated and may be maintaining opposing muscles in a lengthened/downregulated position and state. In either case the function may be impaired due to the imbalance. The aim of muscle length testing is to move the attachments of the myofascia further apart, elongating the tissues so as to assess for potential contributions to functional impairments.

Typically, the proximal attachment(s) of the myofascia are fixed and the distal attachment(s) (via trunk or limb/appendage) are moved to produce the lengthening of tissue. A muscle that is hypomobile and lacking in strength may be referred to as having 'passive insufficiency'. At the point when a shortened muscle or restricted movement is identified, it may not be necessarily clear if the muscle is held in contracture or spasm, as both present as shortened. The type of treatment that may be required for each of these states is very different. If a muscle is held in a shortened position for more than six weeks the sarcomeres of the muscle can reduce by 40 per cent (Tarbary *et al.*, 1972). This suggests that the functional capacity of the muscle is reduced after this time. A muscle that is in contracture has become fibrosed and is unlikely to be detected on EMG (electromyography); a muscle that is in spasm is held in spasm neurologically and therefore is detectable on EMG. The issue in both presentations is that the tissues appear shortened in a clinical setting where EMG is not often available. One possible way to help identify the type of shortening, other than via EMG, is by using muscle energy techniques (MET). It has been proposed that a muscle that is in spasm, with a high level of EMG activity, may respond to MET and demonstrate decreased EMG activity following a low-level isometric contraction (Ribot–Ciscar, 1991). A muscle that is fibrosed and in contracture is unlikely to change with MET alone, and may require a more vigorous approach to affect the fibrosis (such as joint mobilization, specific soft tissue mobilization or myofascial release techniques). This is an important distinction to make in the assessment stage because it will inform treatment.

Neurological assessment

Neurological assessment within a sports therapy setting will in most cases seek to establish the integrity of the nervous system in particular context to the presenting complaint. When neural tissue is under sustained or frequent mechanical compression and irritation, the effects can include reduced peripheral sensory inputs, reduced motor outputs, reflex changes, weakness that may be in a myotomal pattern, pain that may be in a dermatomal pattern and also disturbances to the autonomic nervous system. In order to assess the integrity of the nervous system relative to the condition, usually when the subjective history indicates, the sports therapist will assess skin sensation (dermatomes), motor function (muscle strength and recruitment) (myotomes), deep tendon reflexes and neurodynamic testing. In special circumstances, a cranial nerve assessment may be required.

Dermatomal assessment

A dermatome is an area of the skin that is supplied by nerve fibres that originate from a single nerve root. The afferent nerve fibres are responsible for transmitting information regarding skin sensation to the central nervous system. Although there is a great variability in individual dermatomal distributions, generic 'dermatomal maps' are widely available and enable therapists to appreciate the approximate distribution of sensory nerve supply to all areas of skin (Downs and Laporte, 2011). When assessing neural integrity and areas of abnormal sensitivity, the sports therapist should correctly identify the dermatome and apply light touch, sharp touch and vibration to the various limb segments. This should be done slowly and bilaterally, starting with the unaffected side first; the patient should be asked to identify and describe any changes in sensation when comparing the unaffected to the affected side. For limbs, the therapist should carefully stroke circumferentially (first using cotton wool) around the limb, one stroke at a time, comparing left with right at the same level. It has been recommended that the patient is positioned comfortably and appropriately for upper or lower limb dermatomal assessment, and that they have their eyes closed to reduce visual input. The therapist applies a contact that is

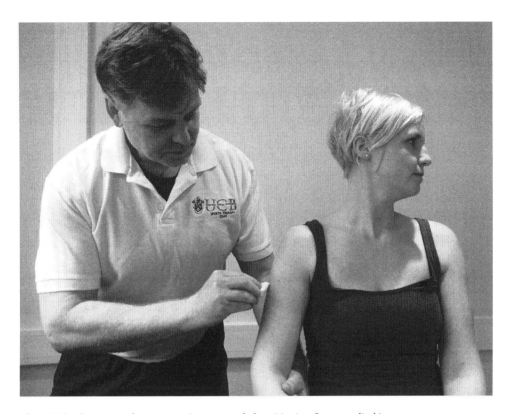

Photo 2.13   Dermatomal assessment (recommended positioning for upper limb).

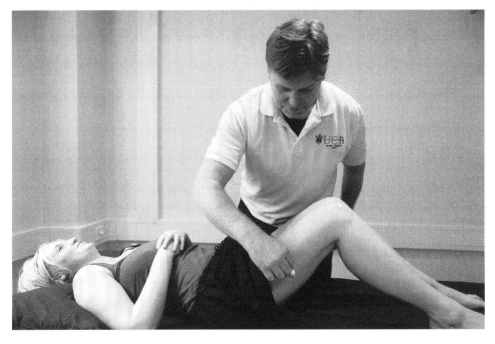

Photo 2.14   Dermatomal assessment (recommended positioning for lower limb).

Table 2.11 Dermatomes and myotomes

Spinal level	Dermatome area	Myotome
C3	Lateral neck	Cervical lateral flexors
C4	Above clavicle	Shoulder elevators
C5	Radial antecubital fossa	Shoulder abductors and elbow flexors
C6	Thumb	Elbow flexors and wrist extensors
C7	Middle Finger	Elbow extensors and wrist flexors
C8	Little Finger	Thumb extensors and finger flexors
T1	Ulnar antecubital fossa	Finger abductors and adductors
L2	Mid-Anterior thigh	Hip flexors
L3	Medial femoral condyle	Knee extensors
L4	Medial malleolus	Ankle dorsiflexors and inverters
L5	Dorsal 2nd/3rd toe web space	First toe extensors
S1	Lateral heel	Ankle plantarflexors and everters; hip extensors; knee flexors

Source: adapted from Fruth, 2014; Fuller, 2008; Magee, 2008.

light enough to affect the epidermis, but not so heavy that indentation occurs (Fruth, 2014). Any areas that the patient reports as being abnormal should be further evaluated with sharp touch (such as with the end of a reflex hammer) unilaterally to clarify the type and extent of abnormal sensation. Ability to differentiate temperatures can also be assessed. The therapist should then refer to a reliable dermatome map to identify the related spinal nerve root. The patient may experience one or more of the following abnormal sensations in the dermatome: dysaesthesia; paraesthesia; anaesthesia; hypoaesthesia; hyperaesthesia; hyperalgesia; or allodynia.

Myotomal assessment

Myotome is the term used to describe the group of muscles innervated by a single nerve root and is the motor equivalent of the dermatome. If a peripheral nerve lesion, nerve root compression or structural spinal defect is suspected, the sports therapist may test the strength of the individual muscles supplied by the suspected spinal segment to assist in confirming the diagnosis hypothesis. To do this, Magee (2008) emphasizes that the isometric resistance applied in myotomal testing should be held for a minimum of five seconds. An example of an affected myotome would be where a patient, complaining of weakness in biceps brachii, is suffering from a C6 nerve root compression which is causing symptoms such as loss of muscle power to the elbow flexor region.

Deep tendon reflex testing

A reflex is an involuntary, almost instantaneous movement performed in reaction to a stimulus. Deep tendon reflex testing involves the therapist tapping a specified tendon with a reflex hammer to ascertain the integrity of the reflex arc in question. A normal reflex arc involves sensory and motor components, and it is the integrity and functioning of these components which are being assessed. The principal sensory component being assessed is a response to a stretch stimulus via activation of the muscle spindles (intrafusal fibres) as the targeted tendon is momentarily stretched by the therapist's reflex hammer. The motor component involves a reflex contraction (initiated at the level of the spinal cord) of the associated muscle; such a response is also known as a stretch (myotatic) or spinal reflex. While many tendon reflexes may be assessed, the most commonly tested are the biceps (C5–6) and triceps brachii (C7–8) in the upper limb, and the patellar (L2–4) and Achilles (S1–2) in the lower limb.

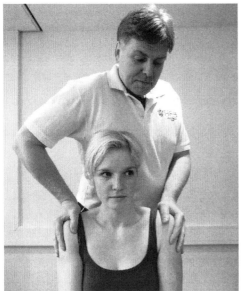

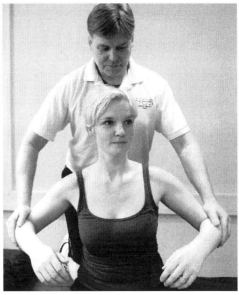

Photo 2.15 Upper limb myotomal assessment (C4: shoulder elevation).

Photo 2.16 Upper limb myotomal assessment (C5: shoulder abduction).

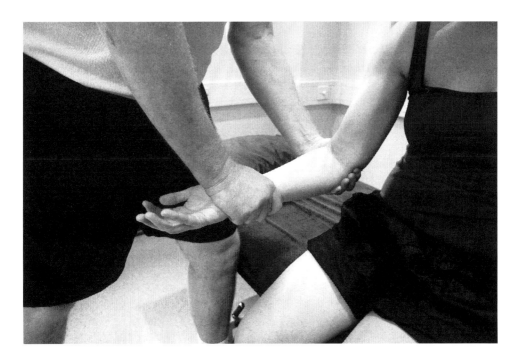

Photo 2.17 Upper limb myotomal assessment (C6: elbow flexion).

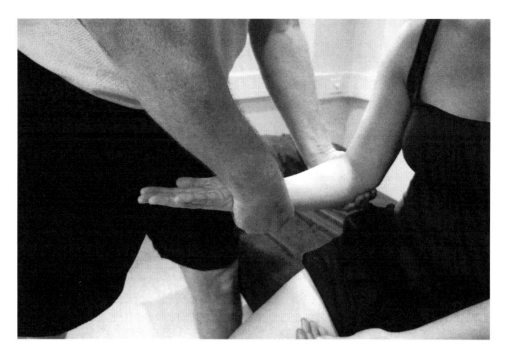

Photo 2.18   Upper limb myotomal assessment (C7: elbow extension).

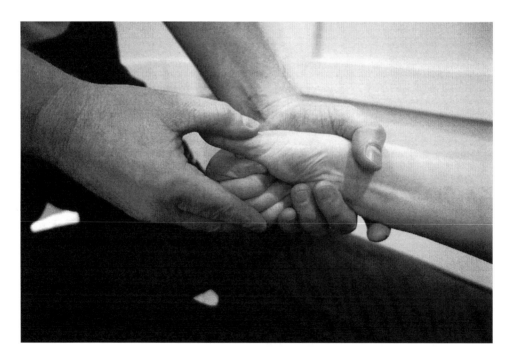

Photo 2.19   Upper limb myotomal assessment (C8: thumb extension).

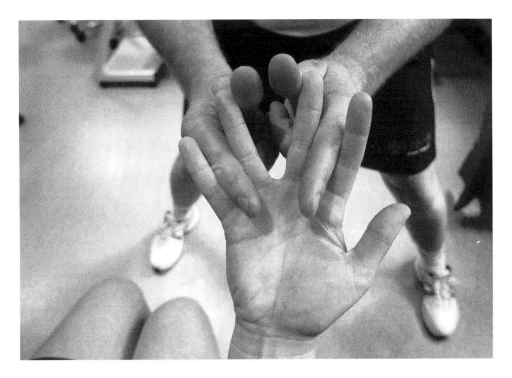

Photo 2.20   Upper limb myotomal assessment (T1: finger abduction/adduction).

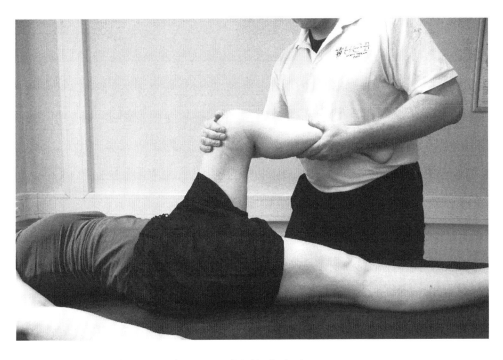

Photo 2.21   Lower limb myotomal assessment (L2: hip flexion).

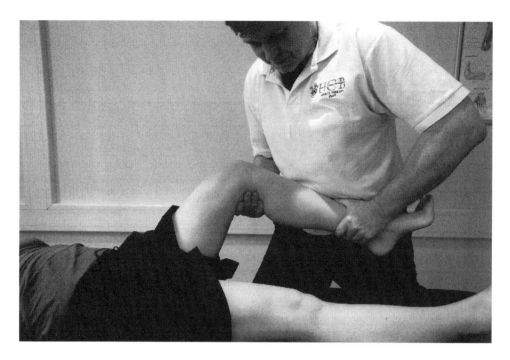

Photo 2.22 Lower limb myotomal assessment (L3: knee extension).

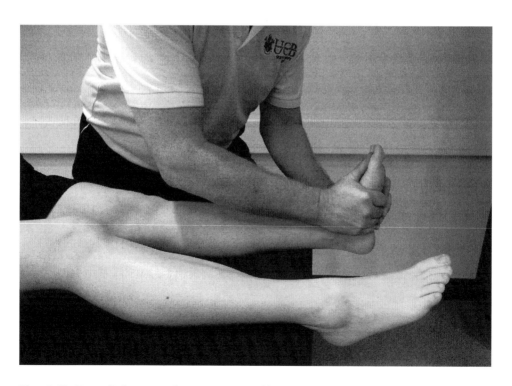

Photo 2.23 Lower limb myotomal assessment (L4: ankle dorsiflexion).

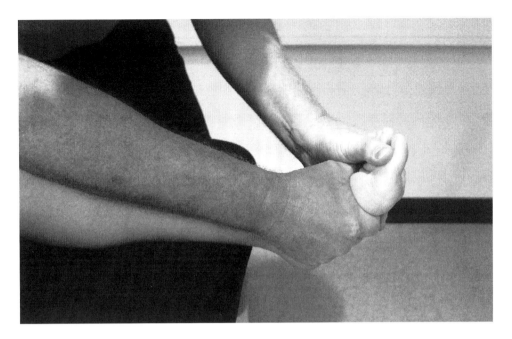

Photo 2.24   Lower limb myotomal assessment (L5: hallux extension).

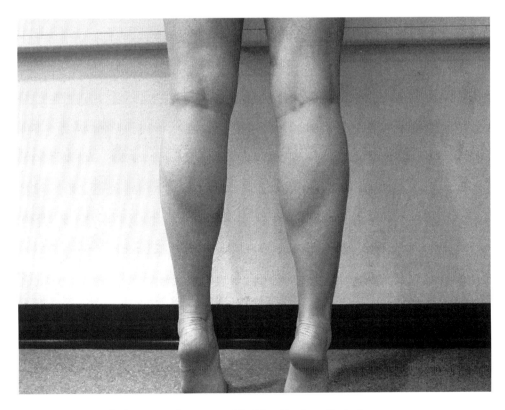

Photo 2.25   Lower limb myotomal assessment (S1–S2: ankle plantarflexion).

The sports therapist must aim to deliver an effective test (which involves correct positioning and explanation to the patient) and be able to reliably interpret the test response. The patient must be relaxed and positioned appropriately for the reflex test in question (there are usually options for each reflex test). The therapist should assess the non-affected side first. It is important that the therapist has the target muscle/tendon supported in a state of slight stretch, and that they hold the reflex hammer with a relaxed grip and produce a 'flicking' type movement with sufficient force to cause a stretch stimulus. It is recommended to tap the tendon five or six times; the reason for this is twofold – the therapist may not accurately tap the tendon, but also a repetition of tapping may evoke an exaggerated or clonus response.

An absent or diminished reflex response may present naturally without any underlying pathology (for example, deep tendon reflexes typically reduce with advancing age). There is also high potential for error in eliciting reflexes, although this will usually improve with practice. If there is a lesion involving the peripheral sensory or motor pathways, the reflex response will usually be diminished or absent. This is termed a 'lower motor neuron lesion' (LMNL), and is a common presentation due to such conditions as intervertebral disc herniations or any other interruption (compression or injury) of peripheral neural tissue (Fruth, 2014).

An exaggerated, heightened, brisk or clonus reflex response may indicate the need to assess for possible 'upper motor neuron lesion' (UMNL). Where this occurs, the therapist may first use the 'Babinski' test. This test involves stroking the plantar aspect of the patient's foot with the pointed end of a reflex hammer (from the heel, up along the lateral aspect of the sole, and across to the medial ball of the foot). A normal response to this is demonstrated by either no movement of the toes, or a 'down-going' response, where the toes curl into flexion. An abnormal (positive) response shows as an 'up-going' movement, where the toes 'fan out' and the hallux extends (Petty, 2011). The therapist may also assess for a clonus response. A clonus is an exaggerated reflex response associated with UMNL, and typically consists of involuntary intermittent muscle contractions produced by a fairly quick and sustained passive stretching of

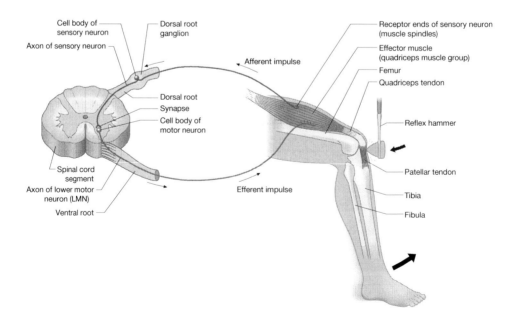

Figure 2.2 Deep tendon reflex testing (patellar reflex arc) (source: adapted from Sewell *et al.*, 2013).

a specific muscle; hence testing for such a reflex response does not involve tapping with a reflex hammer – this response is elicited by way of passive stretch (most commonly at the ankle where three or more rhythmic contractions of the plantar flexors occurs in response to sudden passive dorsiflexion). A positive Babinski test or clonus response is associated with possible UMNL disorders involving the brain and spinal cord and the patient should be referred for further medical assessment.

It is important to note that reflex changes alone do not indicate neural involvement and may not be considered a clinical finding. The therapist must also consider that apprehension and anxiety can increase the reflex response of the tendon reflex or make it difficult to elicit, hence the patient must be encouraged to relax. If the sports therapist is still struggling to elicit an effective reflex response, then the 'Jendrassik' manoeuvre may be used – for the lower limb this involves asking the patient to contract muscles in their upper body as a distraction technique (ask the patient to clasp their hands and to gently pull them apart in an isometric contraction) (Fruth, 2014). For the upper limb reflexes, the patient could be asked to push their legs together.

Table 2.12 Grading deep tendon reflexes

0	*Absent (areflexia)*
1+	Diminished (hyporeflexia)
2+	Average (normal)
3+	Exaggerated (brisk)
4+	Clonus (hyperreflexia)

Source: adapted from Bickley, 2013; Magee, 2008.

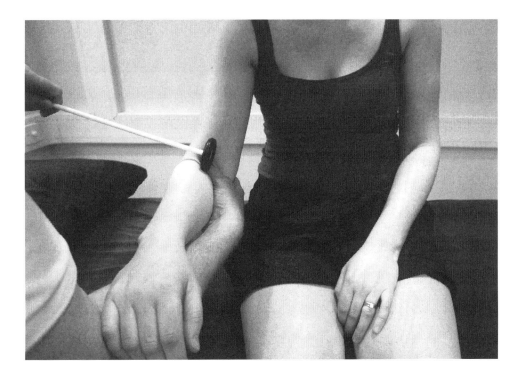

Photo 2.26 Deep tendon reflex testing (biceps C5–C6).

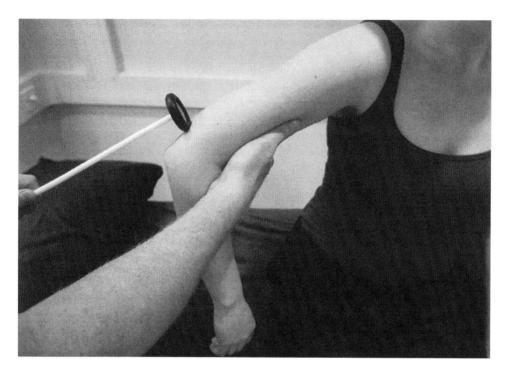

Photo 2.27 Deep tendon reflex testing (triceps C7–C8).

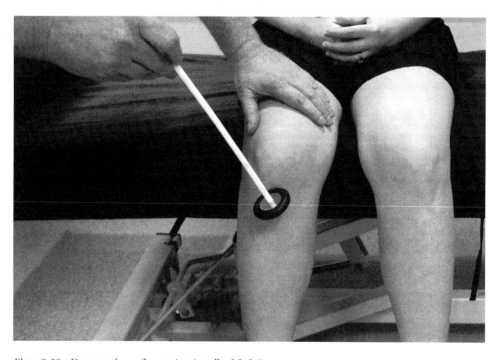

Photo 2.28 Deep tendon reflex testing (patellar L2–L4).

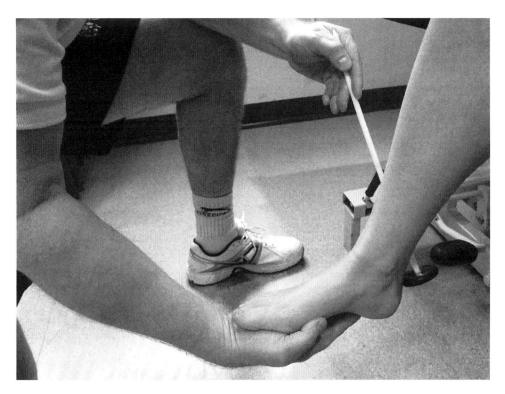

Photo 2.29   Deep tendon reflex testing (Achilles S1–S2).

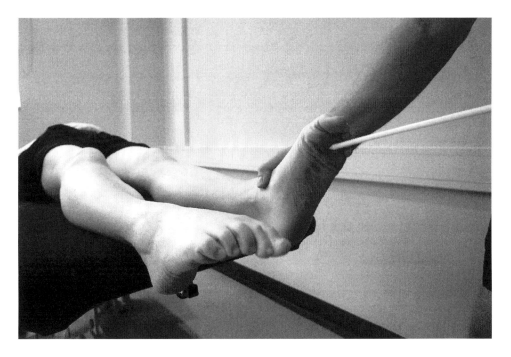

Photo 2.30   Babinski test.

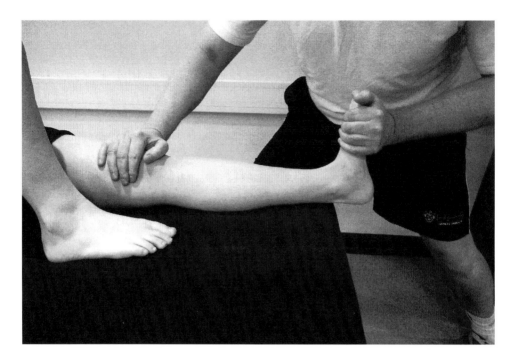

Photo 2.31 Clonus test.

Neurodynamic tests

Neurodynamic testing (also known as neural tension testing) is an established part of neuromusculoskeletal assessment, and involves carefully and selectively increasing the tension in a specific peripheral nerve in an attempt to elicit neural signs and reproduce the patient's symptoms. The specific major nerve is identified and isolated, and a tensile load is carefully applied by passively taking the patient's limb through a sequential set of multi-joint movements. If symptoms are generated via initial tensioning, the usual protocol, to help confirm neural involvement, is to desensitize (reducing the position of tension until symptoms subside) then adding a different sensitizing movement (such as neck flexion) to observe for reproduction of symptoms. Positive signs during such tests which may suggest adverse neural tension include: increasing or shooting pain (i.e. 'stretching' type pain or radicular pain); anaesthesia; paraesthesia; dysaesthesia; or simply reduced RoM.

The term 'neurodynamics' implies functional movement of the nervous system, and more explicitly, neurodynamics is the interaction between physiological and mechanical functions of the nervous system (Shacklock, 2005). Clinically, neurodynamic assessment should be undertaken in conjunction with assessment of other component functioning of the nervous system (sensory and motor), including palpation of peripheral nerves. Sports therapists must understand the five peripheral nerve plexuses (cervical – C1–4; brachial – C5–T1; lumbar – L1–4; lumbosacral – L4–S3; and sacral – S3–5) and the main peripheral nerves of the upper and lower limb, as well as appreciating the relationships and connectedness of the central and peripheral nervous systems.

The main upper limb neurodynamic tests (ULNTs) are principally for the median (C6–T1), radial (C5–T1) and ulnar (C7–T1) nerves, and their nerve roots and tributaries. These tests are used to identify any adverse limitations in neural tissue length, or for any apparent irritation at mechanical interfaces. Adverse neural tension, or mechanical irritation, affecting the upper extremity may be the cause of symptoms in any of the areas of the peripheral nerve distribution into the arm or hand. The cause of symptoms may originate at the spinal cord or meningeal level (as a result of intervertebral disc lesion, for example), at segmental nerve roots or anywhere along the length of either of the peripheral nerves. Potentially irritating mechanical interfaces include intervertebral foramen, myofascial tissue and bony grooves and tunnels. Positive signs from neurodynamic tests are present when neurological symptoms occur, or are reproduced, and ULNTs should be performed whenever there are indicators in the patient's history or from other objective test findings that adverse neurodynamics could be a factor in their symptoms. Conditions such as thoracic outlet syndrome (TOS), cubital tunnel syndrome and carpal tunnel syndrome (CTS) are classic upper extremity peripheral nerve conditions.

In the lower limb, the obturator and femoral nerves originate from the lumbar plexus (L2–4). The superior and inferior gluteal nerves and the sciatic nerve and its branches (tibial, common, superficial and deep peroneal, medial and lateral plantar nerves) all originate from the lumbosacral plexus (L4–S3). The main neurodynamic tests for the lower extremity are the 'slump' test, the straight leg raise (SLR) test and femoral nerve test; conditions such as sciatica, piriformis syndrome and tarsal tunnel syndrome (TTS) may be identified and assessed for irritability during

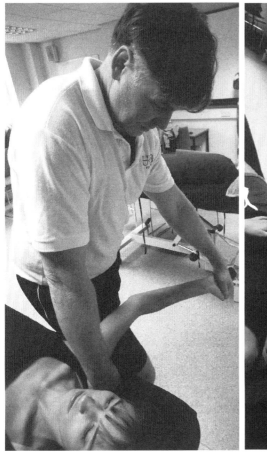
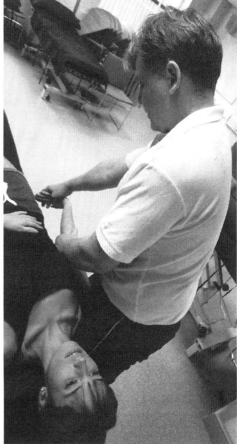

Photo 2.32   ULNT 1 (median nerve bias).   *Photo 2.33*   ULNT 2a (median nerve bias).

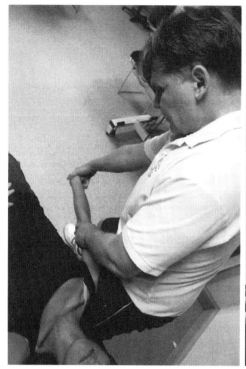 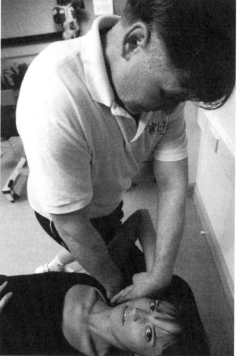

Photo 2.34   ULNT 2b (radial nerve bias).   *Photo 2.35*   ULNT 3 (ulnar nerve bias).

such testing procedures. There are variant approaches to ascertaining the presence of any adverse neural tension or symptom reproduction; the sports therapist will utilize their ability to carefully sensitize and desensitize the tissues. Butler (1991), Cook and Hegedus (2013), Magee (2008), Petty (2011) and others each provide detailed presentations on neurodynamic testing. Where appropriate, the manoeuvres of neurodynamic testing may be adapted as part of a neural mobilization strategy to ease symptoms and improve function (see Chapter 3).

Cranial nerve screening

There are 12 pairs of cranial nerves arising from the brain and brainstem as part of the peripheral nervous system (PNS). They have sensory, motor or mixed functions, and supply predominantly the face, head and neck. Each cranial nerve has a designated number (I–XII) and name (Cipriano, 2010). Cranial nerve testing is not necessarily a primary skill for sports therapists, but screening should be considered for patients/athletes that have recently suffered a head or neck injury (such as concussion or whiplash), and who are experiencing symptoms such as headaches, dizziness, diplopia (blurred vision), facial weakness or paraesthesia and postural sway (unsteadiness). The sports therapist should understand that, in addition to trauma, cranial nerve dysfunction can also be caused by infection, tumour, vascular lesion (such as a cerebrovascular accident – CVA or 'stroke'); alcohol and drug misuse; or by progressive degenerative conditions such as multiple sclerosis (MS), diabetes or Guillain–Barre syndrome (Fruth, 2014). Cranial nerves serve to facilitate olfaction (sense of smell), vision, gustation (sense of taste), audition (hearing), vestibular function (balance) and the motor control of muscles of mastication and the mouth (Fuller, 2008). It is particularly common for whiplash patients to demonstrate sensorimotor disturbance in addition to the more obvious musculoskeletal symptoms of neck pain and reduced RoM. Sensorimotor disturbance may result in the patient demonstrating joint positional errors (such as the inability to correctly repeat simple joint movements when eyes are closed), impaired oculomotor control (eye movement) or postural instability. There are a number of tests of balance and postural stability, including 'Romberg's test', in which the patient stands with feet together and their arms by their sides, first with their eyes open, then with their eyes closed. The therapist observes for any postural sway or tendency to fall (Khasnis and Gokula, 2003). Another assessment is the 'Balance Error Scoring System' (BESS), which is also incorporated into the latest Sports Concussion Assessment Tool (SCAT3) (Concussion in Sport Group, 2013). The modified BESS assesses the athlete's number of observed errors during performance of a series of three 20-second balance tests with closed eyes, hands-on iliac crests and, sequentially, double-leg stance, single-leg stance and tandem stance. Potential errors include opening eyes or moving out of position (Bell *et al.*, 2011; Guskiewicz, 2003). Where the sports therapist suspects cranial nerve dysfunction, unless trained to manage such presentations, referral should be considered.

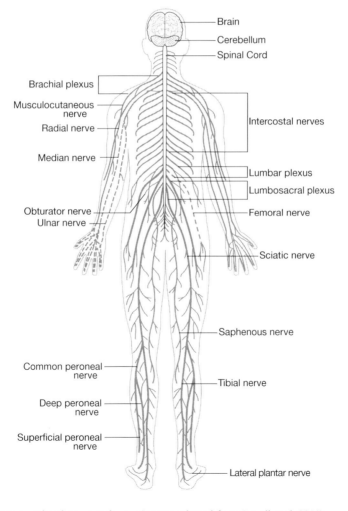

Figure 2.3 Main peripheral nerve pathways (source: adapted from Sewell *et al.* 2013).

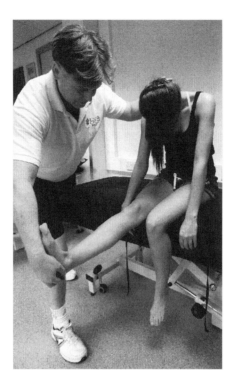

Photo 2.36　Slump test.

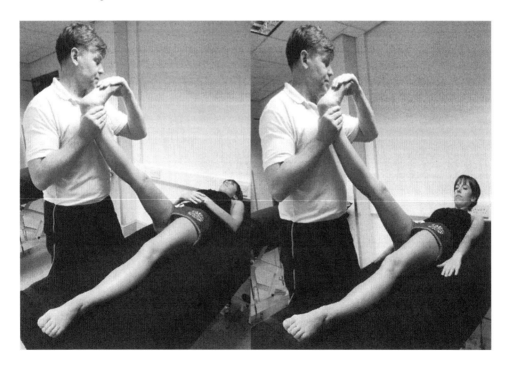

Photo 2.37　Straight leg raise test.

Special tests

Most usually comprising the final part of the assessment is the delivery of one or more special tests. These are used to attempt to confirm or deny probable/differential diagnoses. Most special tests are used in clinical orthopaedic assessment, and as the evidence-base evolves, their ranking in terms of reliability may be adjusted and also they may sometimes become modified. Due to this, and the fact that they are used in clinical environments by numerous therapists, there is frequently variability in terms of technique protocol (including positioning, handling, manoeuvres and interpretation) as presented in academic literature or as taught or performed by different therapists. There is, however, a certain universal terminology which is used when discussing special tests.

Special tests may be single or multi-planar, and they may aim to incriminate a specific structure or simply confirm a (dys)functional condition. Depending on the test concerned, positive findings may include: pain exacerbation and apprehension; pain reduction; crepitus (grating sensation); clunking (where one or more structural components move inappropriately or suddenly during the test); laxity (excessive joint movement; hypermobility); soft tissue tension; joint stiffness or restriction (reduced movement; hypomobility); weakness or loss of muscle recruitment (due to motor nerve interruption; flaccid paresis); abnormal end-feel (such as 'spongy' – indicative of capsular swelling; or an 'empty' end-feel); or other obvious joint or tissue abnormality. The uninjured limb should always be assessed prior to the affected limb so as to provide a comparison specific to the patient.

Cook and Hegedus (2013) explain reliability as the extent to which a test is free from error. Special tests should be repeatable for reassessment, and test findings should be reproducible. Reliability should relate to inter-tester (between more than one tester) and intra-tester (between

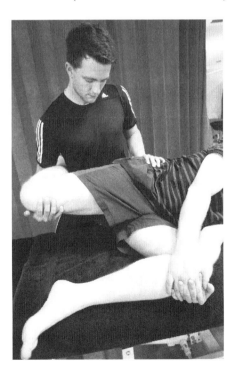

Photo 2.38   Femoral nerve test.

Table 2.13 Cranial nerve testing

Nerve	Normal function	Test
I Olfactory (sensory)	Smell	Assess patient's ability to detect distinctive aromas (e.g. coffee; essential oils)
II Optic (sensory)	Visual acuity	Use a 'Snellen Eye Chart' (progressively smaller letters) to assess acuity
III Oculomotor (motor and autonomic)	Eyelid movement; eye movement	Assess ability to open eyelids; assess eye movement using the 'H' test (eyes follow the therapist's finger in an 'H' pattern) – testing for 'smooth pursuit'
IV Trochlear (motor)	Eye movement	Assess eye movement using the 'H' test; and 'Convergence' test (therapist observes for downward and inward movement of eyes as they follow therapist's finger towards patient's nose)
V Trigeminal (sensory)	Face sensation; muscles of mastication	Assess resisted jaw deviation (lateral movements) and masseter strength (clenching); corneal reflex; and sensation of the face
VI Abducens (motor)	Eye movement	Use the 'H' test
VII Facial (sensory, motor and autonomic)	Taste on anterior 2/3 of tongue; eyelid movement; muscles of facial expression; saliva, tear and nasal mucosa secretion	Assess facial expressions (e.g. smile; frown; elevate and depress eyebrows; 'puff out' cheeks); taste (i.e. therapist puts something sweet on the patient's anterior tongue and asks them to identify it)
VIII Vestibulocochlear (sensory)	Hearing; balance	Perform a hearing test (e.g. with patient's eyes closed, the therapist rubs their thumb and finger pads together close to each ear and asks patient to identify when this is heard). Balance and postural stability can be tested with Romberg's test (assesses the patient's ability to stand unsupported, with eyes closed, for 30 seconds)
IX Glossopharyngeal (sensory and motor)	Gag reflex; taste on posterior 1/3 of tongue; saliva production	Assess for 'gag' reflex (tongue depressor carefully moved posteriorly towards the back of the throat until the gag reflex – laryngeal spasm – occurs)
X Vagus (sensory, motor and autonomic)	Muscles of the palate; thoracic and abdominal viscera	Observe for (palatine) uvula deviation at the back of the throat when saying 'Ahhh' (no lateral movement should be present)
XI Accessory (motor)	Sternocleidomastoid and trapezius movement	Ask patient to shrug (elevate) their shoulders and apply resistance; cervical flexion and rotation may also be tested. Observe for atrophy in sternocleidomastoid or trapezius
XII Hypoglossal (motor)	Tongue movement	Ask the patient to stick their tongue out – there should be no lateral deviation or atrophy

Source: adapted from Bickley, 2013; Fruth, 2014; Fuller, 2008.

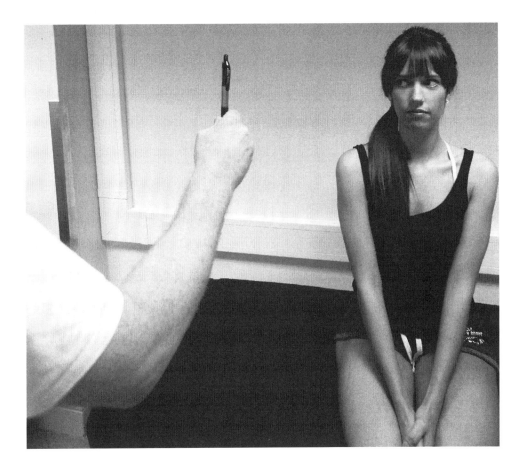

Photo 2.39   The H 'smooth pursuit' test.

the same tester on repeated application) performances. The sensitivity (Sn) and specificity (Sp) of special tests are evidence-based numerical values of reliability, and are expressed as a percentile. They are determined by data including true positives, true negatives, false positives and false negatives (Cipriano, 2010). Sensitivity has been described as the probability of a positive test result in someone *with* the pathology; and specificity as the probability of a negative test result in someone *without* the pathology. For a test to be deemed highly sensitive, it will have demonstrated an ability to identify when patients have the condition that the test is attempting to confirm (true positive), and additionally, it will reveal any false negative. For a test to be highly specific, it will have demonstrated an ability to exclude the tested condition, and will reveal any false positive. Glynn and Weisbach (2011) explain that sensitivity and specificity are

> statistical parameters that describe the measurement validity of a diagnostic test with regard to the relationship between the findings on the test compared to the findings on the reference standard. In this context, the diagnostic test is usually the clinical test under investigation and the reference standard (sometimes called the gold standard) is what is used to determine the true diagnosis.

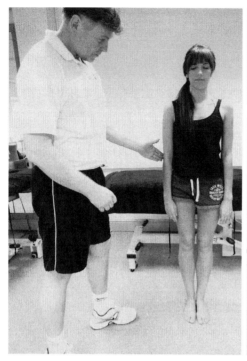 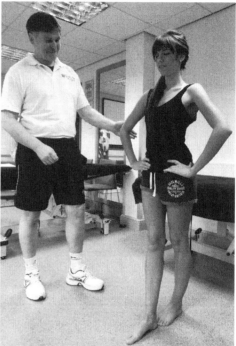

Photo 2.40 Romberg's test.   *Photo 2.41* Tandem stance balance test.

Hattam and Smeatham (2010) explain that a test with a 98 per cent sensitivity rating, for example, should therefore be recognized as being a fairly reliable test to clinically suspect the condition – but this opinion should only be reached in conjunction with other assessment findings.

As an example of special test sensitivity and specificity, a brief scenario is presented. One test for ACL (anterior cruciate ligament) rupture is the 'anterior drawer test' which involves the therapist pulling the tibia forward on the femur (the main movement that the ACL works to prevent). A positive test here would be excessive anterior movement of the tibia, with no discernable end-feel, and/or pain. The specificity of the test is the likelihood of someone with no rupture having a negative result – which is why the specificity of the test will ideally be high. The sensitivity of this test is the likelihood of someone with a rupture having a positive result. This information, however, is dependent on many factors, most commonly noted as false positives and false negatives. A false negative is when a negative result is displayed when the person does have the pathology being tested. In the example, a false positive would be that the tibia is translating – but the athlete has no ACL rupture. One possible explanation for this could be that the athlete has hypermobility syndrome and is lax at all ligaments. A false negative would be the tibia not translating but the athlete actually has an ACL rupture. A possible reason for this could be swelling in the joint preventing movement, or protective contraction of the hamstrings preventing the anterior translation. Interestingly, the 'anterior drawer test' for the ACL has been shown to have a fairly high sensitivity (Jackson *et al.*, 2003), but limited specificity.

Another issue is the topic of normative values for special tests. The important thing to recognize is that, while for some tests, sport-specific norms are necessary, norms are most commonly presented for average populations – they are 'normal' in a very general sense. Further to this, many special tests have little in the way of rigorous evidence to support their reliability or applicability. It is also essential to appreciate the uniqueness of every individual, not least their anatomy and function, but also their responses to injury and testing procedures – such variability can present during assessment, for example: articular surfaces, sizes and shapes; neural and vascular pathways; tendon positioning and attachments; structural deficiencies; and hypermobility). Certainly, sports therapists should understand that there are a host of potential flaws when delivering and interpreting special tests. Other factors which can sometimes adversely affect the reliability of special tests include:

- The timing of the test – certain special tests are more reliable either at the time of injury, before symptoms (such as oedema, spasm and increasing pain have manifest) or post-acutely. As such, it is usual after the initial event to wait for such limiting factors to have subsided. Magee (2008) suggests that special tests 'can be more accurately performed right after injury (during the period of tissue shock – five to ten minutes after injury), under anaesthesia, or in chronic conditions'.
- The protocol of the chosen test (i.e. positioning of the patient; the start position; the direction, angle, speed and range of the manoeuvre; the end position; stabilization of body areas).
- The sports therapist's handling technique (i.e. the positioning, support and direction of movement).
- The response and behaviour of the patient during testing (i.e. inability to relax – especially where pain or fear of aggravation is an issue; apprehension).
- Regional tissue involvement (i.e. swelling of a joint; comorbidities).
- The delivery of too many tests (can be provocative to irritable conditions; can cause confusion in diagnosis).

Finally, Magee (2008) summarizes that:

> special tests should be done with caution and may be contraindicated in the presence of severe pain, acute and irritable conditions of the joints, instability, osteoporosis, pathological bone diseases, active disease process, unusual signs and symptoms, major neurological signs, and patient apprehension.

Palpation

Palpation is the careful and specific identification and assessment of accessible tissue and structure through educated feel and touch. The skill of palpation is key to distinguishing between normal and abnormal (accessible) tissue. It is a psychomotor skill that can be taken for granted, and requires strong underpinning anatomical knowledge, clear communication and significant practice to perfect. The reliability of palpation (particularly inter-rater), however, has been questioned (Gerwin *et al.*, 1997; Lew *et al.*, 1997; Schneider *et al.*, 2008). Perhaps palpation is most useful for identifying and assessing abnormalities in more superficial anatomical structures, for identifying possible superficial soft tissue restrictions, and for identifying (and helping to therefore subjectively grade) localized pain and tenderness. Palpation is not to be confused with 'quick touch'. A quick touch of the area may be performed early on in the objective assessment to assess for changes in temperature and texture when compared bilaterally. A quick touch utilizes the back of the hand as the sensitive tool and will monitor for warmth or coolness as indicators of inflammation or circulation loss, respectively. A quick touch will check for asymmetries in skin texture, such as clamminess or sweating as indicators of sympathetic changes. A quick touch may also be used to gauge initial impressions of muscle tonicity or superficial sensitivity.

The main palpatory assessment, therefore, is normally undertaken later in the objective assessment, once the therapist has begun to formulate a hypothesis surrounding the damaged or involved tissue. The reason for the delay in palpation is that structures may be uncomfortable or painful to palpate. As such, palpating without a hypothetical foundation may lead the therapist to incorrectly diagnose an unrelated problem as being the origin of the patient's primary complaint. Palpation is most commonly performed using the pads and tips of the fingers and thumbs. These are the most sensitive parts of the hand for identifying texture, consistency and size. The back of the hand is the most appropriate part of the hand for sensing temperature and moisture differences. The amount of pressure applied for palpation is also important to note. Pressing too firmly can cause discomfort, and too much pressure lessens tactile sensitivity (Biel, 2005). Pressing too lightly may not allow for identification of underlying structures, and it can be ticklish and uncomfortable for the patient. An appropriate pressure would be deliberate and direct (i.e. performed with intent); its application should be slow and even. Sports therapists should attempt to gauge the 'pressure provocation threshold' (PPT) of the patient in relation to the local symptomatic response and the amount of pressure applied. It is recommended that palpation of an injured area should begin both distally and proximally to the area, and also initially superficially, before progressively more deeply. Sports therapists will also recognize that when, for example, spinal accessory movements are being assessed (for hyper- or hypomobility, pain or other symptomatic response) that these are utilizing palpatory assessment. Similarly, whenever soft tissue therapy is performed, palpation provides constant feedback so as to influence the delivery. The therapist should aim to carefully and systematically identify the structures underneath their fingers. The patient should be positioned so that they are as relaxed and comfortable as possible, and the body area to be palpated should be supported. The therapist may need to alter their own or their patient's positioning so as to effectively assess certain structures. When the sports therapist is required to palpate intimate areas of the patient, such as the pelvic region, or the chest region of the female, permission must first be gained, and they must avoid direct contact with genitalia or female breast tissue. Towels, alternate patient positioning and even the use of the patient's own hands to palpate through (therapist's hand on top of the patient's hand) can be utilized to overcome this sensitive issue.

The proficient therapist should aim to be able to discriminate between differences in tissue tension, muscle tone and texture. For example, is the muscle hypertonic, hypotonic or normal when compared bilaterally? Does the tissue texture reflect its original structure? Are there any fibrous bands of collagen – as with scar tissue healing – or possibly calcification, in the case of myositis ossificans? If the therapist can identify the shape, structure and tissue type, they should also be able to identify, or at least suspect, any abnormalities. The therapist should also aim to identify the thickness of the tissue. An abnormal enlargement may be as a result of bone thickening, synovial membrane thickening, cyst formation, fluid or swelling that may be intracellular or extracellular, intra or extracapsular. 'Effusion' may be defined as increased fluid accumulation within a joint capsule; and 'oedema' as a generic term describing increased fluid outside of a joint (Fruth, 2014). Additionally, the swelling may be extra-articular and localized, such as in the case of bursitis. Magee (2008) explains that the quality and characteristics of a swollen area can provide clues to the source of the fluid accumulation:

- Swelling which occurs soon after injury, and feels firm, thick, gel-like and warm is likely to be due to internal haemorrhage.
- Synovial joint swelling typically accumulates 8–24 hours post-injury. Synovial swelling will usually present with a boggy, spongy feeling.

- Infected swellings may involve pus, which may feel thick to the touch and does not fluctuate or vary. It is usually associated with other signs of inflammation such as heat and redness.
- Thickenings of the joint capsule feel firm and broad and are not malleable upon palpation. The thickness and firmness of the tissue often reflect the chronicity of the symptoms. Softer thickenings of the capsule are often more acute in nature and are associated with a recent onset.
- Bony or hard swelling within muscle tissue that is not pliable and does not fluctuate is often associated with new bone formation (calcification or ossification), and these may be associated with a recent trauma.
- Pitting oedema is an abnormal fluid accumulation that is thick and slow moving. It is characterized by the indentation left in the superficial tissues after the pressure of palpation has been removed. This longer-lasting swelling can be caused by circulatory stasis, such as with peripheral arterial disease, and may also result in reflex inhibition of surrounding muscles.

Palpation can reveal pulses, rhythms, tremors, fasciculation's, tensions, adhesions, thickenings, tender areas and tumours. Tumours may be benign (i.e. a harmless mass of cells), such as an epidermal or sebaceous cyst or lipoma (soft, localized fatty mass); but obviously, the sports therapist must be vigilant for detecting or suspecting the possibility of a malignant tumour (unregulated cancerous cell growth), such as carcinoma (involving epithelial cells) or sarcoma (involving connective tissue cells). While palpating any area, the therapist should also pay close attention to the patient's physical reactions, including compensatory muscle contraction and facial expressions, along with any reports of accompanying abnormal sensation. For example, palpation of a painful biceps femoris tendon may result in a compensatory contraction of gluteus maximus, and a grimacing expression. Generally, if the patient complains of pain and winces, the tenderness of palpation is graded more severely than the reporting of pain alone. Also, the patient who reports pain, grimaces and withdraws the joint may be graded as less severe than a patient who refuses palpation of the area completely. As with all elements of the objective assessment, the uninvolved side or limb should be palpated first to establish a baseline or an appreciation of the patient's 'norm'. Each objective assessment should include the palpation of bony landmarks and the attachments and body of all associated ligaments, muscles and tendons. Joint lines may be palpated as an indicator of disruption to intracapsular structures, such as the menisci of the knee. Any reports of pain should be noted, detailing the intensity and type of pain. Magee (2008) presented a tenderness grading scale (see Practitioner Tip Box 2.4). Direct bony tenderness that is sharp, severe and (where appropriate) aggravated with weight-bearing should be treated more cautiously, and the sports therapist should consider referral for X-ray. Guidelines for X-ray investigation relative to the risk of fracture are available. One notable example are the 'Ottawa Ankle Rules' (OAR) (Stiell *et al.*, 1992; 1994). The OAR state that, in addition to an inability to weight-bear, distinct tenderness found on palpation of the medial or lateral malleolus (or 6 cm proximally), tuberosity of navicular, base of the fifth metatarsal or head of fibula warrant further investigation based upon the likelihood of fracture. The 'Ottawa Knee Rules' (OKR) are guidelines for patients aged 55 or over who present with tenderness on the patella or head of the fibula, who have an inability to flex their knee to 90° or to weight-bear (Stiell *et al.*, 1996). In addition to skin, neuromusculoskeletal and vascular tissues, the sports therapist may also be required to palpate visceral tissue (such as abdominal, respiratory and pelvic organs) when there is the possibility that pain, injury, infection or other abnormality is present. Hence, an appreciation of anatomical positioning and palpatory approaches and findings relating to such must be developed so that any suspicious findings may be ascertained and appropriate medical assessment sought (Fruth, 2014).

Practitioner Tip Box 2.4

Palpation tenderness grading scale

Grade	Response
1	Patient complains of pain
2	Patient complains of pain and winces
3	Patient winces and withdraws the joint
4	Patient will not allow palpation of the joint

Source: adapted from Magee, 2008.

Functional tests

Basic functional testing may take place in the later stages of objective assessment – however, clinical reasoning may influence the inclusion of a more comprehensive functional testing process earlier in the assessment. Functional assessment should incorporate movements identified by the patient/athlete; the movements they cannot do and movements they wish or need to do for their sport or job. Up to this point the therapist may have only considered the injured area in relative isolation; hence this is the opportunity to examine the functional kinetic chain. Goldstein (1995) identified four areas of functional human movement that could be examined in the objective assessment. First, the therapist should identify the basic ADLs that are problematic for the patient, such as personal hygiene activities, eating, dressing and walking. If these pose no problem the therapist may then look to analyse the patient's ability to perform more challenging ADLs such as negotiating stairs and the movements required for cooking, cleaning, shopping and driving. Once these have been examined and deemed problem-free, the therapist may move on to functional work activities such as lifting, carrying, reaching, climbing, pushing and pulling activities. Finally, once the previous three have been cleared, the therapist can examine sporting movements such as jogging, sprinting, throwing, catching, hopping, jumping, striking, cutting and explosive power. It is important that the tasks the patient is being asked to perform are meaningful to them, especially if they feel that they cannot produce a pain-free movement that is essential to their job or sport.

The assessment of functional movements will often have a regional or sports-specific focus. For an ankle injury, the sports therapist may choose to examine the athlete's proprioceptive ability by asking them to hold a single leg balance with their eyes closed for 30 seconds (as with Romberg's test or the BESS); they may also progress to assess dynamic proprioception and strength and power by assessing their ability to double-leg calf raise, single-leg calf raise, double-leg jump and single-leg hop. The therapist may assess functional training movements such as the squat, lunge, dead lift or other Olympic lifts if applicable. Assessment of the athlete's ability to straight line run at varying percentages of their maximum speed can be useful for athletes whose sports require such function; agility may also be assessed via weave runs or by the performance of 90° and 180° turns at speed. Any further functional movements should be gathered from the understanding of the athlete's sporting requirements: do they kick, pass, hit, strike, throw or tackle, for example? The sports therapist must have a good understanding of the sporting requirements of their athletes. Without an understanding of the physiological and technical demands of the sport, the functional assessment will be too generalized.

Functional Movement Screening

Interestingly, Hoogenboom *et al.* (2012) provide a clear differentiation between screening, testing and assessment (see Practitioner Tip Box 2.5). Functional Movement Screening (FMS) can be classified as an extrinsic biomechanical approach; traditional FMS assesses how the body moves as a whole to identify aberrant movement patterns (Cook *et al.*, 2003; 2010). Visual assessment can be supported by video analysis. A number of functional assessment systems have been introduced with the aim of assessing kinetic chains as a whole in an attempt to identify faulty movement and motor control patterns which may lead to injury (Comerford and Mottram, 2012; Cook *et al.*, 2010). Following a standard functional assessment, patients/athletes may be categorized into one of three groups: 'acceptable screen' (i.e. cleared for activity); 'unacceptable screen' (i.e. at risk of injury unless movement patterns are improved); or 'pain with screen' (i.e. currently injured and requiring further assessment) (Cook *et al.*, 2010). Once any faulty movement patterns have been identified, a 'prehabilitation' or corrective programme is introduced. Cook *et al.* (2010) have also developed a Selective Functional Movement Assessment (SFMA) system which is designed for patients/athletes who are presenting with movement dysfunction (i.e. limitations or restrictions in mobility, stability or symmetry during specified movements) and/or pain. Arguably the main functional movements to be assessed are the overhead squat, the in-line lunge and the hurdle step over.

Overhead squat

The overhead (or deep) squat is a functional assessment of mobility and alignment. The athlete is asked to stand with feet hip-distance apart, feet facing forward. The athlete is handed a light bar (a broom handle is ideal). The athlete grips the bar with hands placed shoulder width apart and presses the bar directly overhead. The athlete then squats as deep as is possible for three repetitions, with the therapist observing body alignments from the anterior, posterior and lateral views. An ideal functional pattern will allow the athlete to squat to at least 90° knee flexion while maintaining the bar pressed overhead and within the base of support from the feet. In the anterior view, the foot, knee and hip remain aligned. Common faults for this movement include: a 'dropping in' or valgus movement pattern at the knee, which can be indicative of gluteus medius weakness or overpronation; limited knee flexion – and thus reduced squatting depth, which can be indicative of limited ankle dorsiflexion; or an inability to keep the bar over the feet, which indicates poor trunk mobility and stability.

Practitioner Tip Box 2.5

Differentiating between screening, testing and assessment

Term	Definition	Meaning
Screening	A system for selecting suitable people; to protect people from harm	To create grouping and classification; to check risk
Testing	The undertaking of questions and tests to gauge knowledge, information, experience and ability; measurement with little in way of interpretation	To gauge ability
Assessment	The examination or evaluation of something; the calculation of a value based on a number of factors	To estimate inability

Source: adapted from Hoogenboom *et al.*, 2012.

In-line lunge

The 'in-line lunge' is an assessment of dynamic balance and functional flexibility. It requires the use of an unweighted bar which is held in-line with the spine posteriorly and in contact with the back of the head, the mid-thoracic spine and the top of the sacrum. The athlete stands in a split stance, with the distance between the back foot's lead toe and the front foot's heel being equal to the length of the tibia. The feet are in-line as if standing on a balance beam. The athlete is then instructed to lunge forward on to the front leg without losing contact with the bar, losing balance, or the front foot's heel losing contact with the floor. This test assesses trunk, hip and ankle movement, and also lower limb balance and control.

Hurdle step-over

The 'hurdle step-over' (or 'walking lunge') is a functional assessment of hip stability and mimics the stride position found in the sprint gait. The athlete begins by positioning themselves in front of a hurdle. The toes are touching the base of the hurdle, and the hurdle height is set to the height of the athlete's tibial tuberosity. The athlete is given an unweighted bar that is held in a back squat position across the posterior shoulders. The athlete is then instructed to step one leg over the hurdle and touch the floor with the heel of the foot before returning to the start position. Common errors in this test include: an inability to keep the trunk upright; an inability to clear the hurdle with the test leg; an inability to keep the bar level across the shoulders; and a loss of balance.

Intrinsic biomechanics screening

Intrinsic biomechanical issues can be a root cause of a patient/athlete's dysfunction, and an understanding of the effects of poor intrinsic biomechanics is important. Hoogenboom *et al.* (2012) describe two subcategories of mobility dysfunction: those involving tissue extensibility restrictions (i.e. extra-articular limitations, such as active or passive muscle insufficiencies, adverse neural tension or myofascial restrictions); and those involving articular structures (such as with osteoarthritis or capsular adhesions). Stability dysfunction may also be viewed as having two subcategories – dynamic instability occurs when muscle recruitment is less than adequate; and passive (or static) instability is where joint laxity or hypermobility is present. However, both of these subcategories may have underlying motor control impairments. Building on the work of others (including Cook, 2001; Cook *et al.*, 2003; 2010; Krabak and Kennedy, 2008; Sahrmann, 2002) an intrinsic biomechanics model has been developed by Haines (2008) and has been used as a preparation for any movement programme. The programme is split into three key phases: 'normalize', 'stabilize' and 'functionalize'. The 'normalize' phase is designed to assess pelvic function, nerve and spinal mobility and muscle spasm; where dysfunction in these areas is identified treatment and/or exercises are used before progressing to the next phase. The 'stabilize' phase assesses motor control and strength of the trunk, and then provides progressive exercises to improve the motor control and strength before progression to the final phase. The 'functionalize' phase aims to address gross movement pattern dysfunctions within the kinetic chain. While requiring further research, the rationale for intrinsic screening is based on the premise that an athlete may be able to pass a standard FMS with no obvious extrinsic biomechanical faults, but in so doing, there can be underlying intrinsic biomechanical compensation which may go unnoticed unless specifically screened.

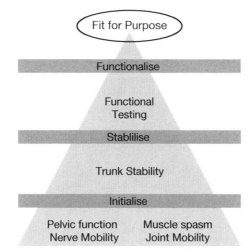

Adapted from Cook (2003), Haines (2008) and Krabak and Kennedy (2008)

Figure 2.4 Intrinsic biomechanics screening.

Gait assessment

When sports therapists undertake a gait analysis it is essential that they understand the basic phases and components of normal gait, and that they consider the possible reasons for any gait dysfunction. These could be biomechanical, due to pain ('antalgic gait') or because of central neurological disturbance – any of which may require referral. Gait is the term used to describe human locomotion. While the term is used interchangeably to distinguish between walking and running, it is more accurately defined as the way, or manner, in which humans walk or run. Gait analysis, therefore, is the systematic study of human motion via observation, augmented by instrumentation for measuring body movements, body mechanics and the activity of the muscles (Whittle, 2007). While basic and initial gait analysis can be undertaken in the clinic, or on a treadmill, gait analysis commonly involves measurement of the body's movement in time and space (kinematics) and the forces involved in producing these movements (kinetics). Kinematics can be recorded using a variety of systems, principally cine film or digital video, using footage from single or multiple cameras (in 2D or 3D), with passive or active reflective markers. To calculate movement kinetics, most gait analysis laboratories have floor-mounted load transducers, also known as force platforms, which measure ground reaction forces (GRF). Forces are normally plotted in three perpendicular directions against time, these being the vertical, anterioposterior (front–back) and mediolateral (inside–outside) forces (Parker, 2001). To detect the activity and contribution of individual muscles to movement, it is necessary to investigate their electrical activity. This is achieved via EMG, which uses surface electrodes attached to the skin to detect the electrical activity of muscles (Hawkey, 2005a). In this way it is possible to investigate the activation times of muscles and, to some degree, the magnitude of their activation, thereby assessing their contribution to gait. Deviations from normal kinematic, kinetic or EMG patterns are used to diagnose specific conditions, predict the outcome of treatments or determine the effectiveness of training programmes. Gait analysis, therefore, can be used to assess, plan and treat individuals with conditions affecting their ability to walk. It is also used in sports biomechanical assessment to help athletes run more efficiently, and also to identify posture- and movement-related issues in people with injuries. Strong foundational insight into normal walking patterns can help the sports therapist improve the efficiency of a patient/athlete's gait-related pathology. Such knowledge can assist the therapist in the patient management process, improving treatment and referral decisions and also the selection of orthotics or prosthetics, alignment parameters and identification of other variants that may enhance performance. Familiarity with gait terminology and function enables the sports therapist to communicate effectively with other members of the medical team and contributes to the development of a comprehensive treatment plan. When undertaking a basic and initial gait assessment in the clinical environment, perhaps as part of a functional movement assessment, the sports therapist must prepare appropriately:

- The patient should be sufficiently functional to be able to undertake gait assessment.
- The patient should be wearing shorts.
- The patient should be observed both with and without their shoes.
- There should be sufficient space to enable the patient to walk up and down the room two or three times, and also at varying speeds if appropriate.
- The therapist should observe the patient bilaterally, anteriorly and posteriorly (thereby attempting to appreciate what is occurring in each of the three cardinal planes – sagittal, frontal and transverse).
- The therapist should observe the patient's ability to walk slowly and, if appropriate, quickly.
- The therapist should observe what occurs during stance and swing phases bilaterally.
- The therapist should observe base of gait and foot width, foot angle, step length, stride length, vertical and lateral movements, reciprocal arm swing and general rhythm and quality of gait.
- The therapist should observe for what is occurring at the foot, ankle, knee, hip, pelvis, spine, shoulder and elbow left and right (this will include regional ranges of movement, patterns of movement and asymmetry).
- All key findings should be recorded.

Defining walking and running

Adult humans generally employ two primary methods of locomotion: walking and running. Although children may 'skip', adults do not tend to perform this method of locomotion (Minetti, 1998). Adults tend to walk at low speeds and run at higher speeds, and as walking and running are markedly different methods of locomotion, transitioning from a walk to a run is not necessarily a smooth and continuous process. Consequently, there are distinct changes from one mode to the other, evident from the use of motion analysis, force recordings and EMG (Hawkey, 2005b). During normal walking at least one foot remains in contact with the ground at all times, and both feet make contact with the ground during the mid-phase of a stride ('double stance'). The centre of mass (CoM) is highest at mid-step, when the hip of the stance leg is directly over the ankle. Running differs from walking in that there is foot contact with the ground before and after an aerial flight phase, and that both feet are never in contact with the ground at the same time (sometimes referred to as the 'double float phase') (Dugan and Bhat, 2005). The CoM is lowest at mid-step during foot contact, rather than at its highest as in walking. These differences lead to substantially higher magnitudes – approximately 50 per cent higher – in the vertical component of the GRF for running as compared to walking, and a decrease of approximately 35 per cent in the time of foot–ground contact (Hawkey, 2005b). The motor control required for normal gait is dynamic and multidimensional. A rapid processing of afferent inputs, integrative messaging within the brain and spinal cord and motor outputs occurs simultaneously. This involves multi-regional somatic mechanoreceptive and proprioceptive functioning, in conjunction with special sense information (mainly visual and vestibular reception). Due to the continuously repetitive, but adaptively responsive nature of gait, the process requires both 'feedback' mechanisms (where the body senses the stimulus of mechanical, visual, and kinaesthetic perturbation of the body in relation to its environment) and responds with required muscle activation accordingly; and 'feed-forward' mechanisms (i.e. the process of anticipating and responding to future or potential perturbations).

Gait cycle

The gait cycle is the period of time between any two identical events in the walking cycle. As the various events follow each other continuously, potentially any event could be selected as the onset of the gait cycle. However, the initial contact is generally selected as the starting and completing event. The gait cycle is divided into two phases: the stance phase and the swing phase. The stance phase is defined as the interval in which the foot is on the ground (approximately 60 per cent of the gait cycle), while the swing phase refers to the interval in which the foot is not in contact with the ground (approximately 40 per cent of the gait cycle) (Ounpuu, 1994). During evaluation of the walking gait cycle, the sports therapist can further assess each portion of these two phases. The stance can be subdivided into four phases:

1. heel strike to foot flat;
2. foot flat to mid-stance;
3. mid-stance to heel off;
4. heel off to toe off.

The swing phase can also be subdivided into three phases:

1. acceleration to mid-swing;
2. mid-swing;
3. mid-swing to deceleration.

Practitioner Tip Box 2.6

Walking gait cycle

Stance phase	Swing phase
• 60 per cent of total gait at normal walking speed	• 40 per cent of total gait, at normal walking speed
• Contact (heel strike)	• Acceleration (initial swing)
• Initial contact with the ground and loading response	• The limb begins to advance, free of the ground
• Double-leg support	• Swing through (mid-swing)
• Mid-stance (foot flat to heel off)	• The non-weight-bearing limb is advanced to where it passes directly underneath the body
• Single-leg support, with body directly over weight-bearing leg	
• Terminal stance and pre-swing (propulsion from heel off to toe off)	• Deceleration (terminal swing)
• Double-leg support	• Controlled slowing of swing in preparation for next heel strike
• Pushing off from the ground	

Source: adapted from Dugan and Bhat, 2005; Ounpuu, 1994; Whittle, 2007.

By evaluating each individual component of the walking gait cycle, the sports therapist obtains clues into specific gait problems and muscular weaknesses. Addressing these issues in a rehabilitation programme will lead to a more efficient gait pattern, resulting in decreased risk of injury, less energy expenditure, greater functional independence and improved muscular balance.

Practitioner Tip Box 2.7

Basic considerations in walking gait assessment

Consideration	Explanation
Ability, willingness or apprehension of patient	General, initial observations of the patient may reveal information indicating that gait assessment is inappropriate
Stance and swing phase components	These two phases of the gait cycle should be carefully observed and compared bilaterally
Quality of gait	General impressions relating to smoothness, range, responsiveness, stability and endurance
Cadence	Steps per moment of time (usually steps per minute). Average walking cadence is between 70–120 steps/min. 90 steps is approximately 2.5 mph As cadence increases, so does the percentage swing phase per limb. As cadence reduces, percentage stance phase increases
Regional issues	Locally restricted or excessive movement due to neurogenic or joint conditions, or myofascial tension or weakness
Regional ranges of movement	Important regional ranges of movement to assess during both stance and swing phases of gait particularly include hip, knee, ankle and first metatarsophalangeal joints (bilaterally)
Step	The advancement of a single leg
Step length	The distance from initial heel strike of one foot to the initial heel strike of the opposite foot
Stride	The advancement of both feet (one step from each foot)
Stride length	The full sequence from heel strike to heel strike on the same limb (one single stance to swing cycle)
Foot angle	The degree of out-turning (or in-turning) of the foot. Influenced by femoral and tibial torsion angles, orientation of the talocrural, subtalar and mid-tarsal joints, arch presentation and myofascial tension. Average foot angle is approximately 20–25°
Double support	Both feet in contact with the ground during initial contact and terminal stance
Base of gait (step width)	The distance between the mid-point of each heel during each of their contact phases. The average base of gait is approximately 7 cm, and rarely exceeds 10 cm. Tends to be wider in slow gait, and in ataxic gait, and narrower in faster gait
Reciprocal arm swing	In normal walking gait, the opposite hip and shoulder move in a similar and harmonious range of forward and backward motion during each step (i.e. the right arm swings forward at the same time as the left leg). This provides a dynamic counterbalance to the shifting CoG

Consideration	Explanation
Centre of gravity (CoG)	In standing, the average CoG is approximately 5 cm anterior to S2. During gait, with VD and LD occurring with each step, the CoG will normally produce a 'figure of 8' pattern within a 5 cm space within the pelvis
Vertical displacement (VD) of the CoG	During each step, the CoG moves rhythmically up and down. Its highest point is during mid-stance; its lowest point is in double-leg support. The total range of VD is normally 4–5 cm
Lateral displacement (LD) of the CoG	During each step, as weight transfers from one stance leg to the other, a lateral shifting in pelvic position, and CoG, occurs. Maximal LD occurs during mid-stance. The total range of LD is normally 4–5 cm
Muscular holding patterns	Some patients will demonstrate a tendency to hold certain muscle groups in a state of tension, thus restricting certain joint movements. This may be due to an underlying neurological condition, localized injury or pain and associated compensatory mechanisms, or simply because of habit

Practitioner Tip Box 2.8

Average regional biomechanical components of walking gait in relative sequence

Phase of gait	Key positions and movements
Stance phase	
• Contact/heel strike	Hip flexed to approximately 25–30°
	Knee slightly flexed (5–10°)
	Ankle slightly dorsiflexed (0–10°)
	Subtalar joint initially supinated (followed by rapid pronation)
• Mid-stance (foot flat to heel off)	Hip close to neutral
	Knee slightly flexed (5–10°)
	Ankle slightly dorsiflexed (5–15°)
	Subtalar joint moves from pronation to supination
• Terminal stance (heel off to toe off)	Hip extends to approximately 20°
	Knee slightly flexed to approximately 10°
	Ankle moves from dorsiflexion to plantarflexion (approximately 20°)
	Subtalar joint fully supinated
	Metatarsophalangeal joints fully extended
Swing phase	
• Acceleration (initial swing)	Hip extended to approximately 20°
	Knee flexes to approximately 40°
	Ankle plantarflexed to approximately 25°
• Swing through (mid-swing)	Hip moves towards neutral
	Knee remains in flexion (approximately 40–60°)
	Ankle moves towards neutral

Phase of gait	Key positions and movements
Deceleration (terminal swing)	Hip flexes to approximately (25–30°) Knee extends to approximately 5–10° Ankle remains in neutral/slightly dorsiflexed Subtalar joint moves to supination

Common gait problems

Practitioner Tip Box 2.9

Categories of gait dysfunction

Descriptor	Description	Reason
Antalgic gait	Short stance phase on affected limb, with gentle, tentative heel-strike	Secondary to injury or pain (for pain avoidance)
Arthrogenic gait	A compensatory gait typically showing increased flexion of the compensating joint or circumduction of the hip to provide sufficient foot clearance. Varies according to which joint(s) are affected	Secondary to joint stiffness (e.g. arthritis; arthrodesis; prosthesis), laxity, deformity or pain
Ataxic gait	Characterized by a wider base, slower, lurching, unsteady, staggering, and irregular gait	Secondary to underlying neurological conditions with sensorimotor disturbance
Circumduction gait	A compensatory gait, characterized by abductory circumduction to advance the affected limb	Secondary to joint stiffness (hip, knee or ankle), muscular weakness (e.g. weak hip flexors) or foot drop
Contracture gait	A compensatory gait pattern, whereby the patient compensates for restriction in one region with increased movement in another	Soft tissue contractures can occur following chronic joint changes or prolonged immobility. Most common at the hip and knee, but also the ankle
Equinus gait	A compensatory gait pattern to offset equinus deformity and reduced dorsiflexion. Typically presents as a more bouncy gait; the patient will walk more on their toes, with early heel off	Secondary to an ankle equinus deformity, where the Achilles tendon is shorter than normal. May be due to neurological disease (e.g. cerebral palsy) or a congenital or acquired condition
Foot drop ('steppage') gait	Characterized by an involuntary plantarflexed foot position. Compensatory increased hip flexion or circumduction occurs	Secondary to neurologically weakened ankle dorsiflexors

Descriptor	Description	Reason
Forward lean gait	Characterized by forward lean of the head and trunk	Secondary to such conditions as exaggerated kyphosis, osteoporosis, ankylosing spondylitis and Parkinson's disease
Hemiplegic/ hemiparetic/ flaccid gait	Characterized by a swinging, circumduction of the affected hemiplegic leg	Secondary to stroke (cerebrovascular event), spinal cord or other injury or illness. Flaccid hemiplegia is an ipsilateral motor impaired paralysis of the upper and lower extremities and trunk
Leg length discrepancy gait	Characterized by repeated dropping down onto the short leg during each step with the affected limb; will show increased movement of the trunk in the frontal plane towards the affected side. The longer leg may show increased flexion of the hip or knee during its swing phase to facilitate improved ground clearance	Secondary to leg length discrepancy
Parkinsonian ('festination') gait	Characterized by short, often quick but inefficient, shuffling steps, with minimal foot clearance during swing phase. Initial contact tends to be foot flat. The neck, trunk and knees tend to be flexed forward. The patient will usually show slowness of postural adjustment (bradykinesia)	Secondary to Parkinson's disease
Plantarflexor gait	Characterized by reduced or absent power in terminal stance and toe off, reduced stance phase and shorter step length on the unaffected limb	Secondary to neurologically weakened ankle plantarflexors
Psoatic limp gait	Characterized by an impaired swing phase. There may be a limp with circumduction (especially with hip lateral rotation, flexion and abduction) as well as exaggerated trunk and pelvic movement	Secondary to hip pathology (such as Legg–Calve–Perthes disease) which can result in a weakened or inhibited psoas major muscle
Scissors gait	Characterized by involuntary hip adduction tension causing knees to be drawn together and difficulty during the swing phase. This may be accompanied by stiff foot-dragging	Secondary to neurological disease, such as cerebral palsy, where spastic paralysis occurs. Diplegia is where the lower extremities are involved more than the upper. Paraplegia is typically defined as complete paralysis of the lower extremity

Descriptor	Description	Reason
Trendelenberg gait	Characterized by a downward pelvic tilt away from the affected side during the affected leg's stance phase. The trunk will typically shift laterally to the stance side to maintain CoG. Bilateral presentations will show exaggerated side to side movements in the frontal plane	Secondary to weakness or inhibition of the hip abductors (principally gluteus medius), which stabilize the pelvis during single leg stance

Source: adapted from Fruth, 2014; Houglum, 2010; Magee, 2008.

Some of the most common causes of gait problems are associated with overpronation or oversupination of the foot. Pronation, the movement that occurs as weight moves from the lateral aspect of the heel to the medial aspect of the forefoot, is necessary for normal gait; although too much or too little has the potential to cause injury. When overpronated, the three major joints are not in optimal alignment and can result in a structurally unstable foot, meaning the muscles, tendons and ligaments of the lower leg are forced to work harder to facilitate stabilization. Overpronators, therefore, are vulnerable to a range of conditions including plantar fasciitis, medial tibial stress syndrome (MTSS, or 'shin splints'), Achilles tendinopathy, iliotibial band syndrome (ITBS), patellofemoral pain syndrome (PFPS) and other overuse injuries. A supinated foot is sometimes referred to as a 'rigid lever' because it provides a firm base as weight shifts to the forefoot in the toe off phase of gait. Again, a certain amount of supination is necessary to generate the force needed to walk and run, but too much can decrease the foot's ability to absorb impact and, therefore, can lead to impact-related injuries. Those with high arches tend to over-supinate or under-pronate. Those with a supinated foot type, and especially runners, may be vulnerable to back, hip and knee problems. The most severe over-supinators also tend to experience recurrent ankle sprains and/or stress fractures. Runners who supinate excessively usually require the highest level of cushioning in their running shoes and should avoid shoes with stability features.

Although pain does not inhibit normal motion directly, deformity and weakness may result from an individual's attempts to attenuate pain through modifying their gait. Generally, joint reaction forces are magnified due to an increase in muscle forces crossing the joint. It is this increased joint contact force which is associated with increased discomfort. One mechanism for reduction of joint pain is to limit the muscle force output at the painful joint. This protective response can, in severe cases, lead to muscle atrophy and weakness. Muscle force requirements are trivial in normal individuals, with less than 25 per cent of normal strength generally needed for locomotion. However, in the case of certain diseases, which show decreased maximum muscle force, functional reserve is lost, endurance is compromised and normal ambulation may not be possible. In these cases orthotic management may be prescribed in order to prevent excessive and undesirable motion. Uncompensated calf weakness can result in diminished mid-stance control, while the increased rate and amount of dorsiflexion increases the functional demands on the quadriceps to maintain limb stability. More serious weakness in ankle dorsiflexion can show toe dragging and foot dropping during the swing phase of walking.

Quadriceps weakness diminishes knee control, leading to pronounced deficits in stance being observed. The knee also tends to over-flex, and a variety of other compensations are employed to preserve stability during weight-bearing. Compensations begin prior to weight acceptance (also known as late swing) and continue through support activity. Late swing hip flexion leads to passive knee extension through momentum transfer. Stance phase increased knee flexion is attenuated by hip extension and premature plantarflexion. Alternatively, external rotation of the affected limb orients the external force vector medial to the joint axis, minimizing the tendency toward knee flexion. Impaired proprioception can also inhibit walking due to diminished information about the position of the limb segment in time and space. This can result in decrements in walking velocity and stability.

Normal bipedal gait is achieved through a complex combination of automatic and volitional postural components. Normal walking requires stability to provide support of an individual's body weight, mobility of body segments and motor control to sequence those segments, while transferring body weight from one limb to another. Gait is, therefore, influenced by muscle strength, dynamic RoM, the shape, position and function of the numerous neuromusculoskeletal structures, including the ligamentous and capsular constraints of joints. The primary goal is that of being able to perform energy-efficient forward progression using a stable kinetic chain of joints and limb segments that work congruently and are not exposed to abusive biomechanical overload.

Clinical reasoning in sports therapy

In an open market, competition increases patients' expectations of an effective and efficient management approach (Noll, 2001). Clinical reasoning is the decision-making, or problem-solving, process used to determine the diagnosis and management of patients' problems (Jones *et al.*, 2008; Terry and Higgs, 1993). It has been defined as the *'thinking and decision-making associated with clinical practice that enables therapists to take the best-judged action for individual patients'* (Jones and Rivett, 2004). There are several recognized models of clinical reasoning, including: hypothetico-deductive or diagnostic reasoning, pattern recognition (experiential, inductive) and narrative reasoning (based on the patient's story) (Edwards and Jones, 2007; Elstein *et al.*, 1978; Jones, 1992; Jones and Rivett, 2004; Terry and Higgs, 1993). In hypothetico-deductive reasoning, the therapist generates a hypothesis based on data from the patient or athlete, which is then tested, and further hypotheses are generated until a management pathway is defined clearly. In pattern recognition, the therapist associates problems of the current patient with previously seen clinical problems and adopts a previously successful management strategy. The ability to deduce a clinical impression and generate a diagnosis hypothesis are fundamental skills in clinical reasoning. According to Wiener (1996), clinical reasoning is a major component of clinical competence and is a dynamic process that occurs before, during and after the collection of data through subjective assessment, objective assessment and (where appropriate) imaging, endoscopic or laboratory tests. Although a number of clinical reasoning models have been presented, therapists most commonly use one of the three methods presented, or a combination of methods, to produce a diagnosis.

Probably the most common clinical reasoning method is the hypothetico–deductive approach. In the hypothetico–deductive approach the initial hypothesis, or hypotheses, are generated early during the initial presentation of the problem. These are generated from the therapist's existing knowledge, associations and experience. Where more than one possible diagnosis is generated, the primary diagnosis is based upon probability of occurrence or prevalence and the therapist's experiences. The remaining theoretical explanations of the patient's symptoms are deemed differential diagnoses. Further questions or assessment are then oriented towards supporting or refuting the hypothesized diagnoses. If a hypothesis is discarded, the next likely diagnosis is considered and treated in the same way. Several hypotheses can be actively considered at any

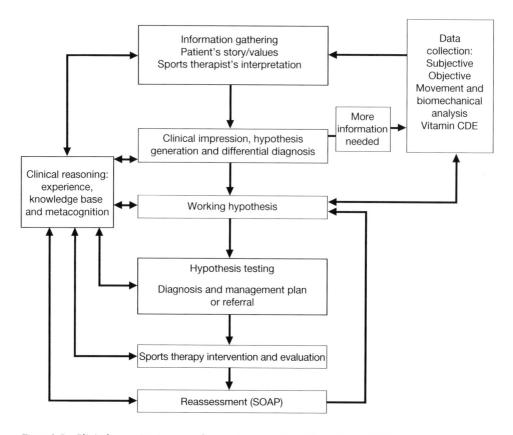

Figure 2.5　Clinical reasoning in sports therapy (source: adapted from Jones, 1992).

one time. Both awareness of probabilities (and prevalence) of injury and knowledge of causal pathways are important.

In clinical reasoning based on pattern recognition, a particular combination of symptoms, or even certain phrases used to describe a symptom, can very strongly suggest a diagnosis to the experienced practitioner. With experience, therapists will build their own internal library of patterns on the basis of their experience and existing knowledge. A simple example of this could be an athlete who presents with knee pain associated with 'clicking' or 'locking', who will often be hypothesized as having damaged their meniscus.

A third possible method of clinical reasoning involves the therapist looking for a single sign or symptom that is strongly indicative of a diagnosis. Pathognomonic signs and symptoms exist where a particular finding almost guarantees a certain diagnosis. This sign or symptom may not be unique to this diagnosis and may not directly imply a single specific diagnosis, but upon presentation the identified sign or symptom markedly intensifies the therapist's suspicion. For example, most sports therapists are taught that a 'pop' sound during a knee injury is indicative of an anterior cruciate ligament rupture, therefore any athlete with knee pain that describes such a sensation will generate such a hypothesis.

Clinical reasoning in subjective assessment
It is important that the sports therapist does not overlook the cues (or clues) that are presented by the patient in the subjective history. Challenges, however, do occur; the patient may, for

example, be a biased storyteller and the sports therapist's interpretation of their story may not be useful because the patient is not neutral in their view (Edwards, 2004). The sports therapist may also inadvertently play a biased role during subjective history taking – particularly if they have seen the presenting symptoms many times previously, and they may jump to conclusions regarding the condition. Accountability suffers when therapists follow assessment routines without considering and exploring alternatives (Jones, 1992). A useful prompt during this stage of history taking is the mnemonic 'VITAMIN CDE' for a 'systemic sieve' (see Table 2.14). The sports therapist must always consider body systems and possible presentations of conditions which may masquerade as neuromusculoskeletal symptoms. Jones (1992) proposed a five-stage model for structuring clinical reasoning for physical therapy (see Table 2.15).

Clinical reasoning in objective assessment

Subjective history taking should lead the objective assessment. During history taking, the patient may be fully clothed, so it can be difficult to notice any external evidence of injury or illness. As the sports therapist will have conducted an in-depth analysis of the injury/symptoms, including the possibility of systemic indicators, this information must influence first observational priorities. The main focus of the objective assessment is to test the established hypotheses and produce a working, clinical diagnosis, problem list and management plan.

Clinical reasoning in patient management

The clinical reasoning process continues throughout the ongoing patient management. Reassessment either provides support for hypotheses an the chosen course of action, or signals

Table 2.14 Systemic sieve

V	Vascular
I	Infective/inflammatory
T	Traumatic/toxic
A	Autoimmune
M	Metabolic
I	Iatrogenic
N	Neurological
C	Cancer
D	Degenerative
E	Endocrine

Table 2.15 Five-stage clinical reasoning model

Stage	*Considerations*
Source of the symptoms	The actual structure affected causing the symptoms
Contributing factors	Predisposing or associated factors (i.e. environmental, behavioural, emotional, physical and biomechanical factors)
Precautions and contraindications	Testing the various tissues to establish a symptom area (taking into consideration systemic factors)
Management	Technique selection. Treat the source or the symptoms?
Prognosis	Based on subjective and objective information gathered, the therapist should be able to make an informed prognosis

Source: adapted from Jones, 1992.

the need for hypothesis modification (Higgs *et al.*, 2008). The sports therapist must not forget their patient's beliefs and expectations nor their personal situation and potential for adherence to a rehabilitation plan. The patient may have actually presented with a previous or preconceived diagnosis, treatment and action plan in mind, and any deviation from this may hinder progress. Where clinical reasoning decisions are informed, shared and collaborated upon directly with the patient, the management plan and resulting outcomes are far more likely to be favourable (Higgs *et al.*, 2008).

Clinical Prediction Rules

Cook (2013), citing Glynn and Weisbach (2011), discusses the emergence of 'clinical prediction rules' (CPR) in physical therapy settings: *'clinical prediction rules are algorithmic decision tools (that use parsimonious clinical findings) designed to aid clinicians in determining a diagnosis, prognosis, or likely response to an intervention'*. In recent years CPRs have been developed for many patient presentations, and sports therapists are recommended to investigate and develop their appreciation of such prediction tools within their clinical reasoning strategy; but as with all areas of practice, an awareness of their methods of derivation, accuracy, validity and impact must be considered, as issues in these areas have been highlighted (particularly regarding the sample sizes in their derivation, the usefulness of generalization in prediction, and inter-rater reliability). Hence, for effective utilization, a process for efficient critical appraisal must be undertaken.

Potential errors in clinical reasoning

Clinical reasoning is only as good as the information on which it is based (Jones, 1992). There is significant potential for errors in clinical reasoning; these may include, variously: making assumptions; considering too few hypotheses; gathering limited data; confirmation bias; confusing inductive and deductive logic; having an over-emphasis on positive findings; and misinterpreting negative findings (Jones, 1992; Rushton, 2013).

It is essential that sports therapists do not assume descriptions from patients are accurate. Failure to recognize this can lead the therapist to assume incorrectly; for example, the patient may describe pain emanating from the piriformis muscle as 'hip pain' (as a pragmatic inference) unless questioned to a greater degree and more specifically. Similarly, patients will often describe their perception of a previous diagnosis which does not in actuality reflect what was diagnosed. If the sports therapist considers too few hypotheses the (real) reasoning for the symptoms may be missed. This type of narrow investigation and questioning may come about when the sports therapist is focused purely on the symptom area. A failure to sample sufficient patient information (data) is especially relevant for newly qualified therapists. In such a situation, the sports therapist's experience of previous patient presentations is limited, hence they may default to the memory of a patient that they have treated in the past with similar symptoms and assume that the new patient has the same condition if the history is similar. Sometimes these memories can be limiting because, through lack of experience, the sports therapist does not effectively explore other potential issues. Confirmation bias can occur when the therapist only obtains the information that they are looking for. If the therapist thoroughly believes that a patient has a certain condition and, upon testing, they present with some positive tests to confirm such a hypothesis, then the sports therapist may choose to ignore other tests for that condition that are negative because they do not support their hypothesis. Errors in detecting covariance can also occur. If the patient has two symptoms that appear to be linked it is important to clarify everything about their covariance. For example, knowing that a patient's knee pain and foot pain occur simultaneously is insufficient knowledge, and is not useful. The sports therapist would need to know more; for example, if the knee pain occurs on its own; if the foot pain occurs on its own; or if at some point both the knee and foot pain are asymptomatic. Covariance can also be confused with causality. If two symptoms do occur together it is important not to immediately link the two. Both symptoms may be affected by an area that is asymptomatic. In the knee and foot example above, the real cause may be a control issue at the hip that is causing pain at both the knee and foot. There can sometimes also exist confusion between deductive and inductive logic. Deductive reasoning involves pure logic. If, for example, an athlete has an AC (acromioclavicular) joint injury, then horizontal flexion is likely to be symptomatic (i.e. if the athlete has A, it is likely to be B). However, this does not work in reverse. If the athlete is symptomatic on horizontal flexion it does not mean that it is the AC joint problem.

Clinical reasoning in sports therapy is not always straightforward. As Kassirer *et al.* (2010) explain *'the principles of diagnosis and therapy are inextricably intertwined'*. Clinical reasoning requires a thorough, reflective and developmental approach which is underpinned by embedding into one's own practice an analytical processual methodology. It requires an engagement with best evidence and associated emerging concepts and paradigms.

Follow-up sessions, re-assessment approaches, and return-to-play decisions

Sports therapists are routinely involved in follow-up re-assessment of their patients/athletes. It is often unnecessary for the patient to undergo a full subjective and objective assessment for a primary complaint when a clinical diagnosis has been made and a treatment plan set, unless there are issues regarding progress or worsening, or if a new primary complaint is presented. Hence, follow-up appointments normally follow a SOAP format and begin with a short review of the patient's explanation and perception of their condition. The sports therapist should review the initial (and/or subsequent) subjective assessment notes, specifically focusing on the patient's symptoms and primary complaint. The patient should be questioned on any changes to the primary complaint, including pain type and quality, pain intensity, the painful area, pain referral patterns, 24-hour pain patterns, aggravating and easing factors (including medication) and any other abnormal symptoms the patient initially presented with. The therapist must also establish any effect of the treatment administered in the previous appointment or any issues with the home care advice, especially considering any rehabilitation exercise. The therapist should then review any comparable signs generated by the initial (and/or subsequent) objective assessment. Where positive tests or responses were provoked, these should be revisited. Where any bilateral comparisons were made, these too should be reviewed. Any relevant clinical findings should be set as objective markers (or clinical indicators) for treatment efficacy. Where the patient's subjective and objective findings have altered – whether improvement or a change or worsening of symptoms, the therapist may wish to consider undertaking a full assessment to assist with clinical reasoning and the formation of new diagnosis hypotheses. This is also true of the patient whose treatment and progression has reached a plateau. It is important to share any progression changes with the patient so that they can see the differences that have been made following treatment and rehabilitation. The patient/athlete can often lose sight during the rehabilitation process, of how far they have come when they are injured, especially if they are still experiencing symptoms and are not yet ready for a return to full training or competition.

Following completion of the subjective and physical examinations of a patient, the sports therapist must aim to have a clear appreciation of the source of symptoms or dysfunction, including involved anatomical structures. All relevant assessment findings should then be summarized in the form of a 'problem list' and, with the patient/athlete's background information very much in mind, a set of short term management goals and plan of therapeutic intervention can then be prepared. It is rare for one piece of information from either the subjective assessment, or one test from the objective assessment, to fully develop into one hypothesis (Petty, 2011). More commonly, it is the weight of evidence, and the interpretation of gathered data, from the whole assessment and reasoning process which facilitates the reliable hypothesis. Further to this, the sports therapist will recognize the importance of continuously appraising the effect of any clinical treatment or exercise during treatment or rehabilitation sessions.

Finally, return-to-play decisions are to be made by the sports therapist on a daily basis – in clinical, rehabilitation, training and competitive situations when assessing, guiding and advising athletes on when they are fit, conditioned, prepared, recovered and ready for a full return to competitive training or action. In a team environment, such decisions are usually made in conjunction with the medical, conditioning and coaching staff. Return-to-play decisions must also be made 'in the moment' in pitch-side situations where athletes have suffered injury. While this chapter has focused on clinical assessment, readers are directed towards the three-stage 'decision-based model' of return-to-play in sport as presented by Creighton and colleagues (2010) which incorporates: evaluation of medical factors (i.e. signs and symptoms; test findings; psychological state; and assessment of seriousness); participation risk (i.e. type of sport, position; limb dominance; level; and ability to protect); and final decision modification (i.e. time in season; pressure from the athlete; external pressures; conflicts of interest; and potential issues of litigation). The evidence-base for effective and specific return to play decision making is still in development; the current paradigm revolves around strong appreciation of background subjective and objective information, effective communication and recognition of ethical responsibilities.

Table 2.16 Using the SOAP approach in assessment and management

Subjective assessment	• In a first session, this will incorporate the full history of the patient/athlete and their condition
	• In follow-up sessions, this is a review and update (aiming to confirm any subjective improvement or worsening)
	• What is the main complaint?
	• Are there any other complaints or health concerns?
	• How and why has the main complaint come about?
	• Has a confirmative diagnosis been ascertained?
	• Does the condition appear straightforward – or more complex?
	• How has the condition been managed to date?
	• What is the extent of pain and other symptoms? (Severity / Irritability / Nature?)
	• What body regions are contributing to this condition?
	• What other factors are contributing to this condition (equipment; training; work; attitude; lifestyle; comorbidities)?
	• What are the aggravating and relieving factors?
	• What are the apparent functional limitations?
	• What are the patient/athlete's hopes and expectations? (Are these realistic or unrealistic?)
	• Is the patient/athlete likely to adhere to advice? (If so, what level of adherence can be expected?)
	• What is the clinically reasoned differential diagnosis and primary working hypothesis?
	• What is the plan for objective assessment (priorities; adaptations)?
	• Is there any need for a referral?
	• Has informed consent been obtained?

Objective assessment	<ul><li>In a first session, this will typically incorporate a full physical examination of the patient/athlete's main complaint and associated factors</li><li>In follow-up sessions, this is a review of main clinical indicators (aiming to confirm any objective improvement or worsening)</li><li>A review of patient/athlete exercises is important in follow-up sessions</li><li>What is apparent in observation (local and global)?</li><li>What can be gleaned from static postural assessment?</li><li>What functional tests might be appropriate for this patient?</li><li>Prioritizing – what are the most important movement tests to perform with this patient/athlete?</li><li>Consider the proximal, distal and local contributions to any condition</li><li>Is clearing required?</li><li>Do the active/passive/resisted movement tests all need to be bilaterally compared?</li><li>Which special tests will be most appropriate to confirm the hypothesis?</li><li>Does the physical assessment need to be more functional or intensive to test function or reproduce symptoms?</li><li>Which objective measures should be recorded?</li><li>What will be the best patient/athlete positioning / therapist positioning / handling techniques for each selected test?</li><li>Is there any need for a referral?</li></ul>
Assessment of findings	<ul><li>This is analysis of subjective and objective findings</li><li>The aim is to produce a clinical impression, diagnosis or other decision on the patient/athlete's main complaint or health status</li><li>What could this condition be?</li><li>Again, why has it occurred?</li><li>Specifically, what tissues/structures/regions are involved?</li><li>Is this a new injury/reoccurrence/result of other underlying weakness or instability/result of inappropriate training or sports technique or equipment?</li><li>Are there any comorbidities or complexities to this case?</li><li>If this is a new or reoccurring injury – what stage of healing is evident?</li><li>Are there any red or yellow flags?</li><li>Is there a need for a second opinion?</li><li>Is there a need for a referral for imaging, blood tests or other investigation?</li><li>Is there a need for a referral for other form of management?</li><li>Is the patient/athlete a suitable candidate for sports therapy?</li></ul>
Plan of management	<ul><li>This is the sports therapist's (or medical team's) decision on management which is discussed and agreed with the patient/athlete</li><li>This may include referral</li><li>This will certainly involve advice</li><li>A problem list and set of short-term SMART goals should be formulated and strategy for management prepared</li><li>Can the management plan be reliably justified?</li><li>Where therapeutic interventions are planned:</li><li>Are there any absolute or local contraindications or precautions?</li><li>Will management involve active as well as passive interventions?</li><li>Is treatment indicated today?</li><li>Will an assessment and advisory mind-set be maintained whilst providing treatment?</li><li>Has the treatment strategy been clinically reasoned (in terms of prioritizing and combining methods and techniques)?</li></ul>

- Can the sports therapist confidently explain why, where, when, how and how much of any proposed modality?
- Is there opportunity to assess the short-term effectiveness of any intervention (i.e. 'within session' clinical indicators)?
- For exercise rehabilitation, has positioning/technique/intensity/repetitions/sets/frequency been confirmed with the patient/athlete?
- Is there any need to document exercise rehabilitation for the patient?
- Is there any additional advice regarding exercise at home?
- Is there any additional advice regarding managing their condition generally?
- Has a follow-up session been arranged?

References

Abul-Kasim, K. and Ohlin, A. (2010) Radiological and clinical outcome of screw placement in adolescent idiopathic scoliosis: Evaluation with low-dose computed tomography. *European Spine Journal.* 19 (1): 96–104

Ball, J.M., Cagle, P., Johnson, B.E., Lucasey, C. and Lukert, B.P. (2009) Spinal extension exercises prevent natural progression of kyphosis. *Osteoporosis International.* 20: 481–489

Banks, K. and Hengeveld, E. (2010) *Maitland's clinical companion: An essential guide for students.* Churchill Livingstone, Elsevier. London, UK

Banville, T.G. (1978) *How to listen: How to be heard.* Nelson Hall. Chicago, IL

Barakatt E.T., Romano, P.S., le Ridd, D.L. and Beckett, L.A. (2009) The reliability of Maitland's irritability judgments in athletes with low back pain. *Journal of Manual and Manipulative Therapy.* 17: (3) 135–141

Bell, D.R., Guskiewicz, K.M., Clark, M.A. and Padua, D.A. (2011) Systematic review of the balance error scoring system. *Sports Health: A Multidisciplinary Approach.* 3 (3): 287–295

Bickley, L. (2013) *Bates' guide to physical examination and history-taking,* 11th edition. Lippincott, Williams and Wilkins, Philadelphia, PA

Biel, A. (2005) *Trail guide to the body: How to locate muscles, bones and more,* 3rd edition. Books of Discovery. Boulder, CO

Bogardus, S.T., Holmboe, E. and Jekel, J.F. (1999) Pitfalls and possibilities in talking about medical risk. *Journal of the American Medical Association.* 281 (11): 1037–1041

Braune, W. (1877) *An atlas of topographical anatomy after plane sections of frozen bodies.* Churchill. https://archive.org/details/atlastopographi00braugoog, accessed January 2014

Brence, J. (2012) *Drop the plumb-line ... static posture assessments were so last decade.* http://forwardthinkingpt.com/2012/10/02/drop-the-plumb-line-static-posture-assessments-were-so-last-decade, accessed February 2013

Burgoon, J.K., Guerrero, L.K. and Floyd, K. (2009) *Non-verbal communication.* Allyn and Bacon. Boston, MA

Butler, D. (1991) *Mobilisation of the nervous system.* Churchill Livingstone. Melbourne, Australia

Carlsson, A.M. (1983) Assessment of chronic pain: Aspects of the reliability and validity of the visual analogue scale. *Pain.* 16: 87–101

Chaitow, L. and DeLany, J. (2008) *Clinical application of neuromuscular techniques, Volume 1: The upper body,* 2nd edition. Churchill Livingstone. London, UK

Chapman, C.R., Casey, K.L., Dubner, R. and Foley, K.M. (1985) Pain measurement: An overview. *Pain.* 22: 1–31

Cipriano, J.J. (2010) *Photographic manual of regional orthopaedic and neurological tests,* 5th edition. Lippincott, Williams and Wilkins. Philadelphia, PA

Clarkson, H.M. (2013) *Musculoskeletal assessment: Joint motion and muscle testing,* 3rd edition. Lippincott, Williams and Wilkins. Philadelphia, PA

Comerford, M. and Mottram, S (2012) *Kinetic control: The management of uncontrolled movement.* Churchill Livingstone. Chatswood, NSW

Concussion in Sport Group (2013) Sports Concussion Tool (3) (SCAT3). *British Journal of Sports Medicine.* 47: 259

Cook, C.E. (2012) *Orthopedic manual therapy: An evidence-based approach*, 2nd edition. Pearson Health Science. Upper Saddle River, NJ

Cook, C.E. (2013) *A critical appraisal of clinical prediction rules*. Presentation from the 33rd IAOPT and Kaiser Hayward PT Fellowship Anniversary Symposium. www.iaopt.org/PDF/Part_5_Kaiser_Presentation_Cook.pdf, accessed January 2014

Cook, C.E. and Hegedus, E. (2013) *Orthopaedic physical examination tests*, 2nd edition. Prentice Hall. London, UK

Cook, G. (2001) Baseline sports-fitness testing. In Foran, B (ed.) *High performance sports conditioning*. Human Kinetics. Champaign, IL

Cook, G., Burton, L. and Fields, K. (2003) *Functional movement systems: The functional movement screen and exercise progressions manual*. Functional Movement. Danville, VA

Cook, G., Burton, L., Kiesel, K., Rose, G. and Bryant, M.F. (2010) *Movement: Functional movement systems. Screening, assessment and corrective strategies*. On Target Publications, Apos, CA

Creighton, D.W., Shrier, I., Shultz, R., Meeuwisse, W.H. and Matheson, G.O. (2010) Return-to-play in sport: A decision-based model. *Clinical Journal of Sports Medicine*. 20 (5): 379–385

CSP (Chartered Society of Physiotherapy) (2012) *Quality Assurance Standards*. www.csp.org.uk/professional-union/professionalism/csp-expectations-members/quality-assurance-standards, accessed December 2013

Cyriax, J. (1996) *Illustrated manual of orthopaedic medicine*, 3rd edition. Butterworth-Heinemann. Oxford, UK

Doubell, T.P., Mannion, R.J. and Woolf, C.J. (2002) The dorsal horn: State dependent sensory processing, plasticity and the generation of pain. In Melzack, R. and Wall, P. (eds) *Textbook of pain*. Churchill Livingstone. Edinburgh, UK

Downs, M.B. and Laporte, C. (2011) Conflicting dermatome maps: Educational and clinical implications. *Journal of Orthopaedic and Sports Physical Therapy*. 41 (6): 427–434

Draper, R. (2011) *Scheuermann's disease*. www.patient.co.uk/doctor/Scheuermann's-Disease.htm, accessed January 2014

Dugan, S.A. and Bhat, K.P. (2005) Biomechanics and analysis of running gait. *Physical Medicine and Rehabilitation Clinics of North America*. 16: 603–621

Duncan, S. (1969) Non-verbal communication. *Psychological Bulletin*. 72 (2): 118–137

During, J. (1985) Towards standards for posture: Postural characteristics of the lower back system in normal and pathological conditions. *Spine*. 10 (1): 83–87

Dutton, M. (2008) *Orthopaedic examination, evaluation, and intervention*, 2nd edition. McGraw-Hill. New York

Edwards, I. (2004) Clinical reasoning strategies in physical therapy. *Physical Therapy*. 84: 312–330

Edwards, I. and Jones, M. (2007) Clinical reasoning and expertise. In Jensen, G.M., Gwyer, J., Hack, L.M. and Shephard, K.F. (eds) *Expertise in Physical Therapy Practice*, 2nd edition. Elsevier. Boston, MA

Ekman, P. and Friesen, W.V. (1971) Constants across cultures in the face and emotion. *Journal of Personal and Social Psychology*. 17 (2): 124–129

Elstein, A.S., Shulman, L.S. and Sprafka, S.S. (1978) *Medical problem solving: An analysis of clinical reasoning*. Harvard University Press. Cambridge, MA

Exline, R.W. (1971) Visual interaction, the glances of power and preference. In Weitz, S. (ed.) *Non-verbal communication*. Oxford University Press. New York

Fedorak, C., Ashworth, N., Marshall, J. and Paull, H. (2003) Reliability of the visual assessment of cervical and lumbar lordosis: How good are we? *Spine*. 28 (16): 1857–1859

Ferguson, F. (2009) *A pocketbook of managing lower back pain*. Churchill Livingstone, Elsevier. Philadelphia, PA

Fernand, R. and Fox, D. (1985) Evaluation of lumbar lordosis: A prospective and retrospective study. *Spine*. 10 (9): 779–803

Ferrari, E. (2006) Academic education's contribution to the nurse–athlete relationship. *Nursing Standard*. 10: 35–40

Ferreira, E.A.G. (2010) Postural Assessment Software (PAS/SAPO): Validation and reliability. *Clinical Science*. 65 (7): 675–681

Florence, J.M. (1992) Inter-rater reliability of manual muscle test grades in Duchenne Muscular Dystrophy. *Physical Therapy*. 7: 115–122

Fruth, S.J. (2014) *Fundamentals of the physical therapy examination: Patient interview and tests and measures*. Jones and Bartlett Learning. Burlington, MA

Fryer, G. (2011) Invited response. *Journal of Bodywork and Movement Therapies.* 15: 38–40

Fuller, G. (2008) *Neurological testing made easy*, 4th edition. Churchill Livingstone. Gloucester, UK

George, S.Z., Fritz, J.M. and Childs, J.D. (2008) Investigation of elevated fear-avoidance beliefs for athletes with low back pain: A secondary analysis involving athletes enrolled in physical therapy clinical trials. *Journal of Orthopedic Sports Physical Therapy.* 38 (2): 50–58

Gerwin, R.D., Shannon, S., Hong, C.Z., Hubbard, D. and Gevirtz, R. (1997) Inter-rater reliability in myofascial trigger point examination. *Pain.* 69: 65–73

Glynn, P.E. and Weisbach, P.C. (2011) *Clinical prediction rules: A physical therapy reference manual.* Jones and Bartlett Publishers. Sudbury, MA

Goldstein, T.S. (1995). *Functional rehabilitation in orthopaedics.* Aspen Publishers. Gaithersburg, MD

Grieve, G. (1988) *Common vertebral joint problems*, 2nd edition. Churchill Livingstone. Edinburgh, UK

Gross, J.M., Fetto, J. and Rosen, E. (2009) *Musculoskeletal examination*, 3rd edition. John Wiley and Sons. Chichester, UK

Guskiewicz, K.M. (2003) Assessment of postural stability following sport-related concussion. *Current Sports Medicine Reports.* 2: 24–30

Haines, M. (2008) Module 1: Biomechanics coach. Unpublished course manual, Intelligent Training Systems. UK

Hamill, J. and Knutzen, K. (2009) *Biomechanical basis of human movement*, 3rd edition. Lippincott, Williams and Wilkins. London, UK

Hattam, P. and Smeatham, A. (2010) *Special tests in musculoskeletal examination: An evidence-based guide for clinicians.* Churchill Livingston. Edinburgh, UK

Hawkey, A. (2005a) Biomechanical alterations in gait on the Earth, Moon and Mars. *Spaceflight.* 47: 354–357

Hawkey, A. (2005b) Mechanics and energetics of human locomotion on the Earth, Moon and Mars. *Proceedings of the 5th Annual European Mars Conference.* Swindon, UK

Higgs, J., Jones, M.A., Loftus, S. and Christensen, N. (2008) *Clinical reasoning in the health professions*, 3rd edition. Butterworth Heinemann, Elsevier. UK

Hignett, S. and McAtamney, L. (2000) Rapid Entire Body Assessment (REBA). *Applied Ergonomics.* 31 (2): 201–205

Hoikka, V. (1989) Leg length inequality has poor correlation with lumbar scoliosis: A radiological study of 100 patients with chronic low back pain. *Archives of Orthopaedic Trauma Surgery.* 108 (3): 173–175

Hoogenboom, B., Voight, M.L. and Cook, G. (2012) Functional movement assessment. In Andrews, J.R., Harrelson, G.L. and Wilk, K.E. (eds) *Physical rehabilitation of the injured athlete*, 4th edition. Saunders, Elsevier. Philadelphia, PA

Houglum, P. (2010) *Therapeutic exercise for musculoskeletal injuries*, 3rd edition. Human Kinetics. Champaign, IL

ICO (Information Commissioners Office) (2013) *The guide to Data Protection.* www.ico.org.uk/Global/~/media/documents/library/Data_Protection/Practical_application/THE_GUIDE_TO_DATA_PROTECTION.ashx, accessed December 2013

IFOMPT (International Federation of Orthopaedic Manipulative Physical Therapists) (2010) *Glossary of terminology.* www.ifompt.com/Standards/SC+Glossary.html, accessed January 2014

Jackson, J.L., O'Malley, P.G., Kroenke, K., (2003) Evaluation of acute knee pain in primary care. *Annals of Internal Medicine.* 139: 575–588

Janda, V. (1980) Muscles as a pathogenic factor in back pain. *Proceedings of International Federation of Orthopaedic Manipulative Physical Therapists (IFOMPT) Conference.* Christchurch, New Zealand.

Janicki, J. and Alman, B. (2007) Scoliosis: Review of diagnosis and treatment. *Paediatrics and Child Health.* 12 (9): 771–776

Jones, M.A. (1992) Clinical reasoning in manual therapy. *Physical Therapy.* 72: 875–884

Jones, M.A. and Rivett, D.A. (2004) Introduction to clinical reasoning. In Jones, M.A. and Rivett, D.A. (eds) *Clinical reasoning for manual therapists.* Butterworth Heinemann. London, UK

Jones, M.A., Jensen, G. and Edwards, I. (2008) Clinical reasoning in physiotherapy. In: Higgs, J., Jones, M.A., Loftus, S. and Christensen, N. (eds) *Clinical reasoning in the health professions*, 3rd edition. Elsevier. Edinburgh, UK

Kado, D.M. (2007) Narrative review: Hyperkyphosis in older persons. *Annals of Internal Medicine.* 147 (5): 330–338

Kassirer, J., Wong, J. and Kopelman, R. (2010) *Learning clinical reasoning*, 2nd edition. Lippincott, Williams and Wilkins. Philadelphia, PA

Keer, R. and Grahame, R. (2003) *Hypermobility syndrome: Recognition and management for physiotherapists.* Butterworth Heinemann. London, UK

Kendall, F.P., McCreary, E.K., Provance, P.G., Rodgers, M.M. and Romani, W.A. (2005) *Muscles, testing and function with posture and pain*, 5th edition. Lippincott, Williams and Wilkins. Baltimore, MD

Kenyon, K. and Kenyon, J. (2009) *The physiotherapist's pocketbook: Essential facts at your fingertips*, 2nd edition. Churchill Livingstone, Elsevier. London, UK

Kessler, R.M. and Hertling, D. (1983) *Management of common musculoskeletal disorders: Physical therapy, principles and methods.* Harper and Row, Publishers Inc. Philadelphia, PA

Khasnis, A. and Gokula, R.M. (2003) Romberg's test. *Journal of Postgraduate Medicine.* 49 (2): 169–172

Kleinke, C.L (1986) Gaze and eye contact: A research review. *Psychological Bulletin.* 100 (1): 78–100

Koury, M.J. and Scarpelli, E. (1994) A manual therapy approach to evaluation and treatment of an athlete with a chronic lumbar nerve root irritation. *Physical Therapy.* 74: 549–560

Krabak, B. and Kennedy, D.J. (2008) Functional rehabilitation of lumbar spine injuries in the athlete. *Sports Medicine and Arthroscopy Review.* 16 (1): 47–54

Kuo, Y., Tully, E.A. and Galea, M.P. (2009) Video analysis of sagittal posture in healthy young and older adults. *Journal of Manipulative and Physiological Therapeutics.* 32 (3): 210–215

Laerum, E. (2006) What is 'the good back-consultation'? A combined qualitative and quantitative study of chronic low back pain athletes' interaction with and perceptions of consultations with specialists. *Journal of Rehabilitation Medicine.* 38 (4): 255–262

Lederman, E. (2011) The fall of the postural–structural–biomechanical model in manual and physical therapies: Exemplified by lower back pain. *Journal of Bodywork and Movement Therapies.* 15: 131–138

Lee, D. (2011) Invited response (evidence and clinical experience: The challenge when they conflict). *Journal of Bodywork and Movement Therapies.* 15: 148–150

Leighton, J.R. (1966) The Leighton flexometer and flexibility test. *Journal of the Association for Physical and Mental Rehabilitation.* 20 (3): 86–93

Lew, P.C., Lewis, J. and Story, I. (1997) Inter-therapist reliability in locating latent myofascial trigger points using palpation. *Manual Therapy.* 2 (2): 87–90

Liebenson, C. (2006) *Rehabilitation of the spine: A practitioner's manual*, 2nd edition. Lippincott, Williams and Wilkins. London, UK

Lin, R.M. (1992) Lumbar lordosis: Normal adults. *Journal of the Formosan Medical Association.* 91 (3): 329–333

Lipkin, Jr. M. (1997) The medical interview. In: Feldman, M., Phil, M. and Christensen, J. (eds) *Behavioral medicine in primary care: A practical guide.* Appleton-Lange. Stamford, CN

Longman Dictionary (1995) *Longman Dictionary of Contemporary English*, 3rd edition. Pearson. London, UK

Lowe, T.G. and Line, B.G. (2007) Evidence-based medicine: Analysis of Scheuermann kyphosis. *Spine.* 32 (19): 115–119

Magee, D. (2008) *Orthopedic physical assessment*, 5th edition. Saunders. London, UK

Maitland, G.D., Hengeveld, E., Banks, K. and English, K. (2005) *Maitland's vertebral manipulation*, 7th edition. Elsevier, Butterworth Heinemann. London, UK

Mannion, A.F. (2004) A new skin-surface device for measuring the curvature and global and segmental ranges of motion of the spine: Reliability of measurements and comparison with data reviewed from the literature. *European Spine Journal.* 13 (2): 122–136

Matthews, D.A., Suchman, A.L. and Branch, W.T. (1993) Making 'connexions': Enhancing the therapeutic potential of athlete–clinician relationships. *Annals of Internal Medicine.* 118 (12): 973–977

McGill, S. (2011) Invited response. *Journal of Bodywork and Movement Therapies.* 15: 150–152

McMaster, M. (2007) Lung function in congenital kyphosis and kyphoscoliosis. *Journal of Spinal Disorders and Techniques.* 20 (3): 203–208

McMaster, M. and Singh, H. (1999) Natural history of congenital kyphosis and kyphoscoliosis: A study of one hundred and twelve patients. *Journal of Bone and Joint Surgery.* 81 (10): 1367–1383

McWilliams, A.B., Grainger, A.J., O'Connor, P.J., Redmond, A.C., Stewart, T.D. and Stone, M.H. (2011) A review of symptomatic leg length inequality following total hip arthroplasty. *Hip International.* 23 (1): 6–14

Mennell, J. (1960) *Back pain: Diagnosis and treatment using manipulative techniques.* Little, Brown. Boston, MA

Mense, S. (1993) Nociception from skeletal muscle in relation to clinical muscle pain. *Pain.* 54 (3): 241–289

Merskey, H. and Bogduk, N. (1994) *Classification of chronic pain: Descriptions of chronic pain syndromes and definitions of pain terms*, 2nd edition. International Association for the Study of Pain Press. Seattle, WA

Minetti, A.E. (1998) The biomechanics of skipping gaits: A third locomotion paradigm? *Proceedings of the Royal Society, London.* 265: 1227–1235

Moore, M. (2004) Upper cross syndrome and its relationship to cervicogenic headache. *Journal of Manipulative and Physiological Therapeutics.* 27 (6): 414–420

Morrisey, R.T. and Weinstein, S.L. (2006) *Lovell and Winter's paediatric orthopaedics*, 6th edition. Lippincott, Williams and Wilkins. Philadelphia, PA

Mulhearn, S. and George, K. (1999) Abdominal muscle endurance and its association with posture and low back pain. *Physiotherapy.* 85: 210–216

Myers, T. (2009) *Anatomy trains*, 2nd edition. Elsevier. London, UK

Newham, D.J. and Mills, K.R. (1999) Muscles, tendons and ligaments. In Melzack, R. and Wall, P. (eds.). *Textbook of pain.* Churchill Livingstone. Edinburgh, UK

NHS (UK National Health Service) (2012) *Why do medications have brand names and generic names?* www.nhs.uk/chq/pages/1003.aspx?categoryid=73&subcategoryid=108, accessed December 2013

Noll, E. (2001) Clinical reasoning of an experienced physiotherapist: Insight into clinician decision making regarding low back pain. *Physiotherapy Research International.* 6 (1): 40–51

Ounpuu, S. (1994) The biomechanics of walking and running. *Clinics in Sports Medicine.* 13 (4): 843–863

Parker, K. (2001) Use of force platforms in physics and sport. *Physics Education.* 31: 18–22

Petty, N. (2011) *Neuromusculoskeletal examination and assessment*, 4th edition. Churchill Livingstone, Elsevier. Edinburgh, UK

Picciano, A. (1993) Reliability of open and closed kinetic chain subtalar neutral positions and navicular drop test. *Journal of Orthopaedic and Sports Physical Therapy.* 18 (4): 553–558

Preece, S., Willan, P., Nester, C.J., Graham-Smith, P., Herrington, L. and Bowker, P. (2008) Variation in pelvic morphology may prevent the identification of anterior pelvic tilt. *Journal of Manual and Manipulative Therapy.* 16 (2): 113–117

Quinn, L. and Gordon, J. (2003) *Functional outcomes: Documentation for rehabilitation.* Saunders. St. Louis, MO

Refshauge, K. and Gass, E. (2004) *Musculoskeletal physiotherapy: Clinical science and evidence-based practice*, 2nd edition. Butterworth Heinemann. London, UK

Ribot-Ciscar, E. (1991) Post-contraction changes in human muscle spindle resting discharge and stretch sensitivity. *Experimental Brain Research.* 86: 673–678

Rillardon, L. (2003) Validation of a tool to measure pelvic and spinal parameters of sagittal balance. *Revue de Chirurgie Orthopedique et Reparatrice de L'appareil Moteur.* 89 (3): 218–227

Roger, J., Darfour, D., Dham, A., Hickman, O., Shaubach, L. and Shepard, K. (2002) Physiotherapists' use of touch in inpatient settings. *Physiotherapy Research International.* 7 (3): 170–186

Rushton, A. (2013) Clinical reasoning in neuromusculoskeletal practice: To critically explore the application of clinical reasoning theory and literature to neuromusculoskeletal practice (sports therapy). Unpublished guest lecture. University of Birmingham, UK

Sabharwal, S. and Kumar, A. (2008) Methods of assessing leg length discrepancy. *Clinical Orthopaedics and Related Research.* 466 (12): 2910–2922

Sahrmann, S.A. (2002) *Diagnosis and treatment of movement impairment syndromes.* Mosby. St. Louis, MO

SAUK (Scoliosis UK) (2013) *Syndromic scoliosis.* www.sauk.org.uk/uploads/Syndromic%20scoliosis%20 08.13.pdf, accessed January 2014

Schiff, E., Ben-Ayre, E., Shilo, M., Levy, M., Schachter, L., Weitchner, N., Golan, O. and Stone, J. (2010) Development of ethical rules for boundaries of touch in complementary medicine: Outcomes of a Delphi process. *Complementary Therapies in Clinical Practice.* 16(4): 194–197

Schneider, M., Erhard, R., Brach, J., Tellin, W., Imbarlina, F. and Delitto, A. (2008) Spinal palpation for lumbar segmental mobility and pain provocation: An inter-examiner reliability study. *Journal of Manipulative and Physiological Therapeutics.* 31 (6): 465–473

Schomacher, J (2009) The convex–concave rule and the lever law. *Manual Therapy.* 14 (5) 579–582

Sewell, D., Watkins, P. and Griffin, M. (2013) *Sport and exercise science: An introduction*, 2nd edition. Routledge. Abingdon, UK

Shacklock, M. (2005) *Clinical neurodynamics: A new system of musculoskeletal treatment.* Butterworth Heinemann, Elsevier. Edinburgh, UK

Sim, J. (1996) The elements of informed consent. *Manual Therapy.* 1(2): 104–106

Smart, K. and Doody, C. (2007) The clinical reasoning of pain by experienced musculoskeletal physiotherapists. *Manual Therapy*. 12: 40–49

Snodgrass, S.J., Rivett, D.A. and Robertson, V.J. (2007) Manual forces applied during cervical mobilization. *Journal of Manipulative and Physiological Therapeutics*. 30 (1): 17–25

Solomon, L. (2005) *Apley's concise system of orthopaedics and fractures*, 3rd edition. Hodder Arnold. London, UK

SST (Society of Sports Therapists) (2012) *Standards of conduct performance and ethics*. www.society-of-sports-therapists.org/flipbooks/Standards%20of%20conduct%20performance%20and%20ethics/index.html, accessed December 2013

Stiell, I.G., Greenburg, G.H., McKnight, R.D., Nair, R.C., McDowell, I. and Worthington, J.R. (1992) The study to develop clinical decision rules for the use of radiography in acute ankle injuries. *Annals of Emergency Medicine*. 21: 381–390

Stiell, I.G., Greenburg, G.H., McKnight, R.D. Nair, R.C., McDowell, I., Reardon, M., Stewart, J.P. and Maloney, J. (1994) Decision making rules for the use of radiography in acute ankle injuries: Refinements and prospective validation. *Journal of the American Medical Association*. 271: 827–832

Stiell, I.G., Greenberg, G.H., Wells, G.A., McDowell, I., Cwinn, A.A., Smith, N.A., Cacciotti, T.F. and Sivilotti, M.L.A. (1996) Prospective validation of a decision rule for use of radiography in acute knee injury. *Journal of the American Medical Association*. 275: 611–615

Strong, J., Ashton, R. and Chant, D. (1991) Pain intensity measurement in chronic low back pain. *Clinical Journal of Pain*. 7: 209–218

Swann, E. and Harrelson, G.L. (2012) Measurement in rehabilitation. In Andrews, J.R., Harrelson, G.L. and Wilk, K.E. (eds). *Physical rehabilitation of the injured athlete*, 4th edition. Elsevier, Saunders. Philadelphia, PA

Szpalski, M. and Gunzburg, R. (2004) Spine arthroplasty: A historical review. In Gunzburg, R., Mayer, H.M. and Szpalski, M. *Arthoplasty of the spine*. Springer-Verlag. Berlin, Germany

Tarbary, J.C., Tarbary, C., Tardieu, C., Tardieu, G. and Goldspink, G. (1972) Physiological and structural changes in the cat's soleus muscle due to immobilization at different lengths by plaster casts. *Journal of Physiology*. 224: 231–244

Taylor, W.R. (2010) A novel system for the dynamic assessment of back shape. *Medical Engineering and Physics*. 32 (9): 1080–1083

Terry, W. and Higgs, J. (1993) Educational programs to develop clinical reasoning skills. *Australian Journal of Physiotherapy*. 39: 47–51

Travaline, J., Ruchinskas, R. and D'Alonzo, G.E. (2005) Athlete–physician communication: Why and how. *Journal of the American Osteopathic Association*. 105 (1): 13–18

Wewers, M.E. and Lowe, N.K. (1990) A critical review of visual analogue scales in the measurement of clinical phenomena. *Research in Nursing and Health*. 13: 227–236

Whittle, M.E. (2007). *Gait analysis: An introduction*, 4th edition. Butterworth Heinemann. Oxford, UK

Wiener, S. (1996). Clinical reasoning in health professions. *Annals of Internal Medicine*. 124 (5): 537

Willison, G.B. and Masson, L.R. (1986) The role of touch in therapy: An adjunct to communication. *Journal of Counselling and Development*. 64 (8): 497–500

3

CLINICAL INTERVENTIONS IN SPORTS THERAPY

Keith Ward, Rob Di Leva, Peter K. Thain and Nick Gardiner

This chapter explores and reflects upon the principles and applications of contemporary treatment interventions in clinical sports therapy. Specifically, it examines evidence-based practice (EBP), soft tissue therapy, manual therapy, cryotherapy, heat therapy, electrotherapy and taping and strapping. Sports therapists will recognize that treatment interventions are the most suitable techniques to be delivered once the athlete or patient has been appropriately assessed and therapeutic goals identified; such interventions must be employed in conjunction with progressive exercise rehabilitation. With the delivery of any therapeutic intervention, there must be full consideration of the following: therapeutic objectives; effective communication with the patient; the positioning of the patient; the therapist's working posture and their handling of the patient; treatment technique applications (including location, intensity, frequency and duration); and patient re-assessment. Obviously, there are times when the intervention will simply be the delivery of expert advice, which may be in the form of referral for medical assessment. An essential part of the intervention process in sports therapy is to consider how to best address any apparent causative (aetiological) factors to the patient's condition so as to reduce potential for re-occurrence. Interventions such as sports nutrition, sports psychology and exercise rehabilitation have not been included in this chapter.

Evidence-based practice

This chapter aims to explore the evidence-base to support sports therapy interventions, and additionally provide guidance for best practice. While the utilization of an evidence-base for all interventions is idealistic, it is the recommended approach in which health care professionals formulate clinical decisions, and is based upon the latest and best scientific evidence available for individual patients (Sackett *et al.*, 1996). Effective consideration and employment of EBP is processual. It is founded on clinical questioning, critique and appraisal of available evidence, appropriate integration and evaluation of clinical outcomes. The expert practitioner will apply 'evidence-informed practice' (EIP). True EIP is triadic and incorporates the essential evidence-based guidelines, the autonomy of the individual practitioner's experience and expertise (and their 'craft knowledge'), and the individual 'patient's culture'. Sackett *et al.* (1996) defined EBP as *'integration of the best research evidence with clinical expertise and patient values and circumstances to make clinical decisions'*. The process is also encapsulated by the term 'clinical reasoning'. According to Haynes *et al.* (2002), EBP must always incorporate: clinical expertise; reliable research evidence; and, crucially, patient preferences and actions. Efficient EBP is a seamless combination of factors which play a role in achieving one goal – the best possible advice and treatment for the patient. For practitioners, the process for delivery of EBP must embrace the ability to both critically appraise and integrate the research into practice. Critical appraisal involves the efficient selection, analysis and synthesis of research information; it also involves the ability to evaluate the usefulness of any adaptations incorporated into practice. Scott *et al.* (2013) state that *'It is imperative that a concerted effort is undertaken to ensure that research is pertinent to, meaningful to, and feasible for easy uptake into the clinical setting.'* Clinical experience alone does not substantiate up-to-date clinical research, and the sports therapist must strive, through reflection, to explicitly identify gaps in their knowledge and areas for development. Scott *et al.* (2013) present a selection of barriers to achieving EBP:

- insufficient time to search for evidence;
- too much evidence available (information overload);
- insufficient relevant and applicable evidence;
- lack of collation of related evidence;
- inadequate access to evidence;
- insufficient training in how to access evidence;
- poor presentation of evidence;
- limited confidence and competence in appraising the quality of evidence (epistemological issues);
- limited applicability of evidence for, or from, heterogeneous populations;
- bias in research (bias in publication; bias in population selection, allocation, performance or outcome);
- restrictions in practitioner autonomy;
- limitations in practitioner incentives or motivations;
- the influence of patient expectations.

Irrespective of the professional experience of a therapist, formulating a sound and critically reasoned rationale for the care of the patient is the underpinning reason for adopting EBP. Although operating within an EBP framework is a formal requirement for sports therapists, it must be acknowledged that all areas of contemporary sports therapy practice require ongoing development for optimizing the evidence-base; and this is the case for all areas of health care. Although anecdotally practitioners may find certain methods and techniques consistently effective, and patients may indeed request or expect them, the evidence-base may not be so strong as to be scientifically justifiable. Within the process of ongoing research, sports therapists, their organizations and educational institutions, must aim to advance their position via the generation of reliable and progressively valid practice-based evidence, which must especially be focused upon all specified areas of expertise currently being utilized effectively in clinical and sporting settings. Dinsdale (2012) presents a case for sports therapists in private practice to undertake their own clinical auditing (i.e. systematically monitoring and evaluating their own performance). Clinical auditing may incorporate the formal documentation of: patient assessment methodologies; baseline assessment findings and clinical indicators; intervention strategies, types and dosages; and outcome measures). A number of evidence-based outcome measures and disability indexes have been produced in recent years, including: DASH (Disability of Arm, Shoulder and Hand); SPADI (Shoulder Pain and Disability Index); MFPDI (Manchester Foot Pain and Disability Index); and ODI (Oswestry Disability Index – also known as the

Oswestry Low Back Pain Disability Questionnaire). Such disability indexes offer regionally focused baseline and outcome subjective assessments, which can support appraisal of therapeutic performance (Manske and Lehecka, 2012); they are also useful when conducting case study research.

Greenhalgh and colleagues (2014) have presented a fresh consideration for EBP as they describe its movement towards a renaissance and refocusing. EBP has, following its formal introduction over 20 years ago, established into a solid and energetic intellectual community of health researchers, educationalists and practitioners; but, as with any emergent approach, lessons must be learnt from its implementation, delivery, measured outcomes and analysis. Greenhalgh (2012), Greenhalgh *et al.* (2014) and Ioannidis (2005) have all highlighted issues associated with EBP, including: the misappropriation of the evidence-based 'quality mark'; the sheer volume of evidence (including clinical guidelines) and challenges associated with the implementation of such; the marginal statistical significance of benefits; the challenges associated with incorporating patient-centred care; and the challenges of mapping EBP to patients with multiple morbidity. In their appraisal, Greenhalgh *et al.* (2014) request a progressive shift towards 'real evidence-based medicine' (REBM) which:

- makes the ethical care of the patient its top priority;
- demands individualized evidence in a format that clinicians and patients can understand;
- is characterized by expert judgement rather than mechanical rule following;
- shares decisions with patients through meaningful conversations;
- builds on a strong clinician–patient relationship and the human aspects of care;
- applies these principles at community level for evidence-based public health.

Once qualified and in practice, mandatory continuous professional development (CPD) is the essential, ongoing process for practitioners. CPD should be multifaceted, formally organized, and designed to advance individual professional knowledge, understanding and practice. CPD is an absolute hallmark characteristic for all health care professionals. CPD aims to ensure that practitioners incorporate the most current and reliable approaches to their work. Straus *et al.* (2005), cited in Manske and Lehecka (2012), present questions that practitioners should ask of themselves:

- Am I asking any well-informed questions?
- Am I becoming more efficient in my searching?
- Am I critically appraising evidence?
- Am I integrating critical appraisals into my practice?
- Have I done any audits of my diagnostic, therapeutic or other performances, including measures of patient satisfaction?

Databases applicable to sports therapy

Contemporary research and information sources for best practice are readily available via 'open-access' or subscription-based online databases. One essential component for the successful employment of EBP is being able to critique the evidence for any particular strategy, methodology or technique for its validity or clinical usefulness. It is extremely important for all sports therapists to be able to develop their own appreciation of what constitutes 'reliable and valid' literature, and to be able to critique and appraise said literature – whether a paper discussing a multi-centre, double-blinded randomized control trial (RCT), a small-scale pilot study, or a case study or case series; or whether it is a systematic review or meta-analysis of a specified body of literature. According to Law and MacDermid (2008), there is a corresponding relationship between the quality of a study and the confidence of a clinical decision. The potential for bias is something the sports therapist must be able to identify, and this is a key component in the appraisal of the quality of any evidence. Bias may be considered as the tendency or disposition of researchers, authors, publishers or clinicians to present information and findings which may in some way not be a true representation. The concept of ranking levels of evidence is based on the principle that certain study types have more rigour; and higher-quality study designs provide more confidence to associated clinical decision making (Belsey and Snell, 2009). The International Centre for Allied Health Evidence (ICAHE, 2014) clarify that while there is not one standard hierarchy of evidence, there is a recognizable consensus of hierarchy pertaining to different types of research. Reliably constructed systematic reviews and meta-analyses rank highest because, by definition, they rigorously analyse data from multiple primary studies. Well-constructed primary experimental studies rank above observational studies because these will attempt to control for bias in their design (the highest ranking studies of this type are RCTs). Lowest in the ranking of research hierarchy is evidence-based opinion, such as that seen in narrative reviews, sometimes in editorial commentaries and in some textbooks. Table 3.1 presents a summary of hierarchical levels of research evidence; Table 3.2 presents a summarized hierarchy of information sources; and Table 3.3 presents the American Academy of Family Physicians' (AAFP) Strength of Recommendation Taxonomy (SORT).

Databases applicable to sports therapy

Below is a selection of online databases which are useful for accessing contemporary and archived research information relevant to sports therapy:

- AMED (Allied and Complementary Medicine)
- CINAHL (Cumulative Index to Nursing and Allied Health Literature)
- Cochrane Collaboration
- DARE (Database of Abstracts of Reviews of Effects)
- EMBASE
- HRC Academic (Health Reference Center Academic)

Table 3.1 Hierarchical levels of research evidence

Methodology	Relative ranking
Systematic reviews and meta-analyses	1
Randomized control double-blind trials (RCT)	2
Cohort studies	3
Case controlled studies	4
Cross-sectional studies	5
Case reports	6
Expert opinion, commentaries, ideas, editorials	7
Anecdotal (experiential, unpublished) opinion	8
Animal research	9
In-vitro research	10

Source: adapted from Cook, 2012; Dinsdale, 2008; Greenhalgh, 1997; Sackett *et al.*, 1996.

Table 3.2 Hierarchy of information sources

Information source	Relevance	Validity	Cost	Usefulness
Evidence-based textbook	High	High	High	High
Systematic review	High	High	High	High
Journal of Family Practice POEMs (patient-oriented evidence that matters)	High	High	Mod	High
Colleagues	High	High	Low	High–moderate
Practice guidelines (evidence-based)	Mod	High	Low	High–moderate
Cochrane Database	Moderate–high	High	Low	High–moderate
Standard textbook	High	Low	Mod	Mod
Standard journal review	High	Mod	Low	Mod
Practice guidelines (consensus)	Mod	Mod	Low	Mod
Internet (general)	Low–moderate	Low–moderate	Low	Low–moderate
Mass media	Low	Low	Low	Low

Source: adapted from Sackett *et al.*, 2000; Smith, 2005; Straus *et al.*, 2005; Vizniak, 2012.

Table 3.3 Strength of recommendation taxonomy (SORT)

Strength of recommendation	Definition
A	Recommendation based on consistent and good-quality patient-oriented evidence
B	Recommendation based on inconsistent or limited-quality patient-oriented evidence
C	Recommendation based on consensus, usual practice, opinion, disease-oriented evidence, or case series for studies of diagnosis, treatment, prevention or screening

Source: adapted from the Strength of Recommendation Taxonomy (SORT): A patient-centered approach to grading evidence in the medical literature from the *American Academy of Family Physicians* by Ebell *et al.*, 2004.

- MEDLINE
- NHS Evidence
- NICE (National Institute for Health and Care Excellence)
- PEDro (Physiotherapy Evidence Database)
- PubMed
- SciVerse SCOPUS
- SPORTDiscus
- Trip
- Zetoc.

Obviously, when searching such databases, sports therapists should aim to appreciate the difference between peer-reviewed, evidence-based journal articles, edited textbooks and conference proceedings, and those which are not. Introductory (summary) abstracts on such databases are especially useful, and are usually freely available. The sports therapist should also aim to use search terms which are most likely to provide the most applicable results (i.e. 'MeSH' terms: medical subject headings – which are a vocabulary of indexed terms used in some databases). Furthermore, such approaches as 'Boolean logic' may also be used. This is a simple method for specifically linking or separating two or more search terms for optimizing results, for example, using *'and'* between terms retrieves articles containing both terms; using *'or'* between terms retrieves articles containing either or all of the terms; and using *'not'* between terms excludes the retrieval of articles which contain the terms preceded with *'not'* in the search. Search term methodology may also employ use of truncation or 'wildcards' where, for example, a root word – plus a designated symbol (applicable to the database in question), such as ★ ? or @ – may be used to retrieve a wider range of results.

The sports therapist is advised to gain familiarity with the wide range of research that is undertaken in the field so that they can appreciate which methodology has been employed – or could be employed – and essentially, the reliability and validity of such. There are a number of simple, initial methods which may be used to either assist in the appraisal of study design (by identifying the key features of a study), or to help develop a viable literature review format (ICAHE, 2014; Sackett *et al.*, 1996); these include:

- 'PICO' (Problem/sample Population/Patient; Intervention/exposure/test; Comparators/Controls; and Outcomes/results);
- 'PIPOH' (Population; Intervention; Profession; Outcome; and Healthcare setting);
- 'PECOT' (Population; Exposure; Comparator; Outcome; and Time period);
- 'SPICE' (Setting; Perspective; Intervention; Comparison; and Evaluation);
- 'ECLIPSE' (Expectations; Client group; Location; Impact; Profession; and Service).

The sports therapist must also aim to be critical in their reading of research. Ioannidis (2005) presented a stirring article suggesting that much of the published research is false, and stated that *'claimed research findings may often be simply accurate measures of the prevailing bias'*. Certainly it can be observed that newer evidence frequently refutes previous evidence. Hence, sports therapists must aim to identify and note the research question, the study design, the ethical issues, the specified inclusion and exclusion criteria of the study, the method of data gathering and analysis, the time frame, the significance of results, the conclusions, the recommendations and the possibility of methodological flaws, confounders or bias. A number of established and straightforward critical appraisal tools have been produced to assist practitioners in their assessment of published research, such as;

- The Psysiotherapy Evidence Database 'PEDro scale' for measuring the methodological quality in clinical trials.
- The 'QUADAS' tool for assessing systematic reviews of diagnostic accuracy studies.
- The Critical Appraisal Skills Programme (CASP, 2014) tools for systematic reviews, randomised controlled trials, cohort studies, case control studies, economic evaluations, diagnostic studies, qualitative studies and clinical prediction rules.
- Organizations such as the UK-based Medical Research Council (MRC) and Centre for Evidence-Based Medicine (CEBM) provide comprehensive online resources for research educators, researchers, clinicians and students on areas such as critical appraisal, research design, research ethics, research funding and the implementation of EBP.

Practitioner Tip Box 3.1

Considerations in the critical evaluation of research

- Research title, aim and objectives
- Rationale
- Context
- Relevance
- Conceptual framework
- Theoretical framework
- Methodological design (e.g. primary; secondary; systematic approach)
- Research hierarchy (e.g. CEBM; SORT)
- Search and review strategies
- Critical appraisal tools (e.g. PEDro; QUADAS)
- Credibility
- Ethical issues
- Objectivity
- Precision of experimental delivery
- Cumulative weighting
- Outcome measure(s)
- Data collection
- Data analysis
- Confounding variables (uncontrolled factors)
- Interpretation
- Confirmability
- Statistical significance (e.g. the level of acceptable error ['alpha level']; the probability that the results are due to chance ['*p* value'])
- Correlation (measure of the relationship between variables)
- Triangulation (use of multiple data sources to confirm or refute findings)
- Trustworthiness
- Reliability
- Internal validity (e.g. historical issues; maturation or loss of participants; data issues)
- External validity (e.g. the 'Hawthorne effect', where participants' performance alters simply because they are being observed; multiple treatment interference)
- Bias (e.g. selection bias; conflicts of interest)
- PICO (patient/population/problem; intervention/exposure/test; controls/comparators; outcomes)
- Inclusion–exclusion criteria
- Recognition of design or conclusion limitations
- Conclusions
- Epistemology (analysis of the justified knowledge)
- Directions for future research
- Transferability potential
- Replication potential (repeatability/reproducibility)
- Synthesis potential
- Implications for practice
- Applicability to practice
- Contribution to the field

Table 3.4 Types of research

- Literature reviews (e.g. systematic reviews; meta-analyses; narrative reviews; document analyses)
- Qualitative studies (examination and analysis of beliefs, attitude, behaviour and interactions, and generation of non-numerical data; e.g. passive observation studies; participant observation studies; questionnaires; interviews; focus groups)
- Quantitative studies (generation of numerical data; e.g. case cohort studies; randomized control trials [RCTs])
- Mixed methods research (studies involving collection of both numerical and non-numerical data)
- Descriptive (non-experimental) research (studies which aim to describe characteristics of an individual or population group, e.g. unobtrusive job analysis)
- Experimental interventional studies (e.g. prevention strategies; diagnostic testing; acute interventions; training interventions; educational strategies; case studies; crossover studies)
- Case study (descriptive research involving a single individual, group, intervention or setting)
- Longitudinal studies (following a population over a time period, e.g. experiential; passive observational; prospective; retrospective; cohort; case-control)
- Cross-sectional studies (descriptive analyses of population groups, commonly for prevalences at a specific point in time)
- Time series studies (analyses of defined data obtained through repeated measurements during a designated time period)
- Grounded theory studies (theory derived from the analysis of participant responses)
- Ethnographic studies (interpretation of the activity of sub-cultural populations)
- Phenomenological studies (interpretation of specific aspects of population groups' perceptions of lived experiences)
- Epidemiological studies (quantitative analysis of prevalence and incidence of conditions and injuries)
- Questionnaires (e.g. Delphi survey method; Likert-coded; mixed methods)
- Interviews (e.g. structured; semi-structured)
- Focus groups (qualitative research involving small participant groups, assembled to engage in structured discussion)
- Translational research (e.g. where findings from animal studies are first tested in humans)
- *In-vitro* ('in-glass') studies (i.e. in a test-tube or petri-dish) and animal-based (a form of *in-vivo* – 'in the live') studies – both of these typically form early foundations to an area of investigation; they are relatively lower-level evidence due to the obvious limitations in relevance and transferability)

Source: adapted from Andrade and Clifford, 2012; Cook, 2012; Gratton and Jones, 2010; Hall and Getchell, 2014; Thomas *et al.*, 2005).

Therapeutic interventions

Obviously, prior to the delivery of any clinical intervention, the sports therapist must undertake an appropriate patient assessment. Aside from exploring all aspects of the patient's background, health status and main complaint(s), the therapist must aim, as a priority, to identify any reasons for proceeding with caution. Contraindications can range from straightforward locally avoidable conditions, such as an open wound or fungal infection, to more suspicious and concerning presentations such as 'clinical red flag' signs warranting immediate referral for medical assessment. It is beyond the scope of this chapter to review all contraindications to clinical sports therapy interventions, and reasons for using caution in practice, but sports therapists must become extremely confident with this fundamental aspect. Additionally, it is a professional and legal requirement to gain the patient's informed consent prior to delivery of any intervention and that all patient records are produced clearly and correctly, are completed and updated after each session and that they are stored in keeping with Data Protection legislations to ensure safety and confidentiality.

Soft tissue therapy

Manual techniques for affecting soft tissues have perhaps been more commonly recognized as being forms of massage therapy (including such variants as 'therapeutic', 'sports', 'remedial', 'corrective' and 'orthopaedic' massage); however, the authors of this text favour the use of the generic term 'soft tissue therapy' (STT), mainly to promote an appreciation of the technical components of the various approaches and applications to treating soft tissues, and to differentiate from any less professional forms. STT in general is an extremely popular component of sports and physical therapy, and is favoured by patients and therapists alike. Broadly, the field of STT incorporates a wide range of methodologies, approaches and techniques for an equally wide-ranging set of (purported) therapeutic objectives. Such objectives may include:

- generation of mental and physical relaxation;
- release of unwanted local muscular tension (mechanical or reflexive);
- promotion of local neuromuscular excitability (muscular stimulation);
- stretching of tight and shortened soft tissues (muscle and fascia);
- mobilization of restricted or painful joints;
- optimization of soft tissue adhesions, fibrosis or scar tissue formation;
- increase of circulatory flow (arterial, venous and lymphatic);
- enhancement of warm-up and preparation for physical activity (pre-event massage);
- improved recovery from training and competition (post-event massage; maintenance massage);
- recovery from fatigue;
- promotion and support of injury healing mechanisms;
- relief from pain;
- reduction of dyspnea and expulsion of unwanted secretions in respiratory conditions;
- support for the use of other therapeutic interventions;
- promotion of general health and well-being.

Clearly this is an extremely broad set of therapeutic objectives and the evidence to support the efficacy of STT in all of its forms and applications is limited, if not largely speculative; indeed, Weerapong *et al.* (2005) highlight how the widespread utility of massage in athletic settings is due more to coaches and athletes holding firm beliefs of its potential benefits, based on observation and experience, rather than because of a body of hard scientific, empirical data. Nevertheless, the therapy is consistently requested and offers the patient/athlete an extremely personalized and focused intervention. Among the most well-recognized STT techniques and approaches are: effleurage; petrissage; tapotement; vibrations and shaking; friction techniques; stretching techniques; soft tissue release techniques; myofascial release techniques; instrument-assisted soft tissue mobilization; manual lymphatic drainage; neuromuscular techniques; muscle energy techniques; and positional release techniques. It is usual for the sports therapist to use a combination of soft tissue techniques. Technique selection must be based upon a thorough patient assessment and identification of the intended therapeutic objectives, but also it is imperative that the sports therapist understands the likely mechanisms of effect and most reliable applications. STT for both athletic and general populations has been popular for decades, and there are a multitude of high-profile advocates. Evidence suggests that, when employed, STT may take up nearly half the total treatment time during physical therapy treatments (Hemmings, 2001; Weerapong *et al.*, 2005). STT is considered to be relevant to sports performance through a range of physiological effects (Hemmings, 2001). The main claims for STT relate to its ability to:

- increase local blood circulation (Goats 1994a; 1994b; Rinder and Sutherland 1995);
- enhance elimination of metabolic waste, including lactate clearance (Hemmings, 2001; Rinder and Sutherland, 1995);
- decrease sympathetic nerve activity (Callaghan 1993; Goldberg *et al.*, 1992; Sullivan *et al.*, 1991; Tiidus 2000; Weerapong *et al.*, 2005);
- contribute positively to the inflammatory process (Callaghan 1993; Goats 1994a; 1994b; Moraska 2005; Rinder and Sutherland 1995);
- reduce delayed-onset muscle soreness (DOMS) (Hilbert *et al.*, 2003; Zainuddin *et al.*, 2005);
- address restrictions, adhesions and fibrosis in soft tissues (Donaldson, 2012; Hunter, 2006; Myers and Frederick, 2012);
- inhibit muscle hypertonicity (Chaitow, 2007; Chaitow and DeLany, 2002);
- reduce perceived post-exercise fatigue (Robertson *et al.*, 2004);
- offset the negative aspects of stress (Field *et al.*, 2005; Moyer *et al.*, 2011).

Despite its popularity, the evidence of the effectiveness of STT as a general intervention is limited. Hyde *et al.* (2011) suggest that any soft tissue technique will have local mechanical and cellular effects, as well as associated neurological (indirect or reflexive) responses, which is a key aspect for practitioners to recognize. With regard to the effects of specific soft tissue mobilization (SSTM), Hunter (2006) describes: the local effects regarding blood and lymphatic flow, peripheral neural reception and the mechanical structural changes; the central effects which influence the general interpretation and regulation of nociception and threshold for neural

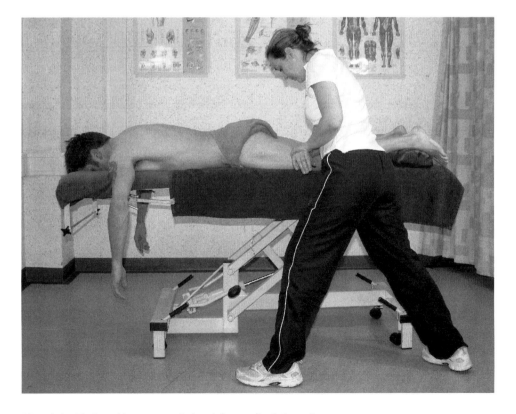

Photo 3.1   Ideal working posture during delivery of soft tissue therapy.

firing, which in turn may facilitate improved scope for motor patterning in rehabilitation; and the cognitive effects, which may include the generation of positive emotional responses (such as the reduced sense of fear or frustration or the improved sense of pleasure, safety and comfort),which can lead to improvements in decision making and behaviours. Such effects, it must be considered, relate not just to the treatment itself, but also to the therapeutic relationship and the setting. Galloway *et al.* (2012) provide a contemporary review of evidence to support massage therapy for athletic populations, and importantly highlight the need for practitioners to engage more effectively with the development of the evidence-base. Similarly, Brummitt (2008) reviewed the evidence for massage in aiding sports performance and rehabilitation. While numerous positive outcomes with regard to physical, physiological and psychological effect were identified in the literature, issues of flaws in study design were highlighted. Notwithstanding the evidence, the art, skill and specificity of the delivery and application of tissue palpation, pressure, depth, movement, stretch and proprioception, together with the time frame, duration, repetition and the response to the patient's reported levels of comfort or discomfort are each equally important to achieving the therapeutic objectives. The recognizable physical, physiological, psychological and cumulative effects of STT have certainly reasoned this modality to be suitable as a treatment within athletic and general populations, but developing the evidence-base to support the whole spectrum of applications and indications must be seen as a priority of the profession; in so doing, practitioners and researchers must look to find ways to reliably prepare studies, recruit participants, standardize interventions and measure outcomes. Future research in this area must appreciate the findings and recommendations of previous research and the critical analysis that it has faced. Provided below is an overview of the main methods and techniques utilized within the fields of STT.

Effleurage

Effleurage is a technique using rhythmic stroking movements. Effleurage is frequently used as a technique to commence, link and conclude STT sessions (Callaghan, 1993; Watt, 2008). When oil or lotion is being used, effleurage is the technique which is employed to apply it. The purported benefits of effleurage include promoting circulation, warming of tissue, the generation of relaxation, and through the effect of stretching muscle and fascia can help to ease painful and restricted areas (Briggs, 2001; Goats, 1994b; Watt, 2008). Deeper effleurage stroking techniques during treatment can be applied using a smaller and reinforced contact surface, and is applied in both longitudinal and transverse directions using the tip or pad of the thumb or fingers, the heel of the hand (hypothenar eminence), the knuckles, the flesh of the forearm, the ulnar border and more specifically the olecranon process. As a basic rule, whenever the practitioner is choosing to work more deeply they must work more carefully and slowly. There is a great advantage for deep transverse stroking over, for example, longitudinal stretching because it can target specific restrictions and work across the direction of the affected fibres ('across the grain'). Longitudinal stretching lengthens tissue, but it is limited in the fact that it preferentially affects (lengthens) the most elastic components of tissues, and in so doing will also actually bring tissue fibres closer together.

Petrissage

Petrissage describes a variety of techniques that rhythmically lift, compress, stretch and knead soft tissues. Techniques include wringing, picking-up and rolling, and may be delivered with a lifting, gripping and grasping type approach, or more compressively via the use of the palms of the hand.

The technique may be delivered in an alternating manner using both hands, or simply with a single hand. Petrissage can be slow, rhythmical and restful, but also energetic and invigorating. With a gentle, but firm grasp, the tissues are raised and stretched away from the underlying bone with alternate squeezing and relaxing of the tissues. Petrissage techniques collectively may promote reflex vasodilation and hyperaemia that can lead to a decrease in tissue swelling. Vigorous kneading may cause a decrease in muscle spasm and stretch tissues shortened by injury.

Tapotement

Tapotement consists of percussive movements which involve rhythmic tapping or controlled striking (Lewis and Johnson, 2006). Tapotement is purported to: cause erythema (reddening of the skin due to local hyperaemia); stimulate muscle fibres (potentially invoking the myotatic stretch reflex to raise tone); increase cellular activity; increase airway clearance and decrease dyspnea; mobilize respiratory secretions; cause systematic and sensory arousal and enhanced alertness; and cause pain reduction through counterirritant analgesia (Andrade and Clifford, 2008). Tapotement most commonly uses both hands alternatively and quickly. Techniques include: hacking; flicking; cupping (or clapping); pounding; tapping; beating; and pincement. Pincement is a technique performed at speed without aggressive pinching of the skin (Benjamin and Lamp, 2005); fingers and thumbs are used to lightly pluck and pick up superficial tissues.

Vibrations and shaking

Vibration and shaking techniques may be applied locally to specific soft tissues, or more generally to a muscle group. A brisk trembling type motion of the hands or fingers is employed. This technique is often used pre-competition with a view to 'excite' the muscles (Goats 1994a).

Friction techniques

The friction technique aims to separate tissue fibres and restore mobility where restriction, adhesions, fibrosis and degeneration are present (Cyriax and Coldham, 1984). Frictions provide localized movement to a specifically identified site (lesion) in the muscle, tendon, fascia or ligament, while also inducing hyperaemia. Donaldson (2012) explains that reparative cells (fibroblasts), which lay down collagen, are mechanosensitive; hence, friction massage may facilitate matrix production and are aimed to restore the tissues' mechanical properties during repair. Transverse friction techniques typically use reinforced thumb or finger tips, or the olecranon process (Cyriax and Coldham, 1984; Goats, 1994b; Watt, 2008). The technique may be delivered in a small circular motion (Goats, 1994b), or longitudinally, or perpendicular (transversely) to the orientation of the affected tissue fibres; and the technique should only be performed at the exact site of lesion (Donaldson, 2012). When the therapist applies friction to tendons and ligaments, it has been recommended that these tissues should be in a stretched position. In contrast, it is suggested that friction to muscle tissue is performed in a relaxed, shortened position (Cyriax and Coldham, 1984; Goats, 1994b). Donaldson (2012) highlights that much of the published evidence to support friction techniques has involved small sample sizes.

Therapeutic stretching

Whether deemed to be active, passive, static, ballistic, dynamic, maintenance, developmental or corrective, stretching involves a force application to lengthen tissue. Lederman (2014) proposes that 'functional range of movement' may be effectively maintained by forces generated during normal daily activity (or perhaps more explicitly, guided therapeutic daily activity) and that *'overloading is a training condition for adaptation in which physical challenges are raised above functional levels … and forces below the overloading threshold will be ineffective at inducing long-term range of movement change'*. Lederman (2014) also suggests that functional activities may be able to provide the required adaptations in restricted soft tissue movement, and that some manual stretching approaches may fail to provide this.

Indications for therapeutic stretching may include: mechanical lengthening for improving soft tissue and segmental length and alignment, and normalizing range of joint movement; improving circulatory flow to dehydrated connective tissues; reducing low-grade interstitial oedema; improving movement control; stimulation of tissue cells during repair (fibroblasts; myofibroblasts) via a process of mechanotransduction; and reducing nociceptive firing caused by structural compression, joint malalignment, low-grade oedema and restricted myofascia.

Mechanotransduction is simply the process whereby tissue cells respond to mechanical loads (Khan and Scott, 2009). Therapists will appreciate the difference between active and passive ranges of movement, and also how tension imbalances between antagonistic muscle groups can affect and restrict movement. Stretching techniques rely on neural, structural (musculoskeletal), elastic and potential plastic effects to alter the available ranges of motion. As Myers and Frederick (2012) explain, the effects of stretching will relate to the variable components of delivery (the 'task parameters') (i.e. force type, intensity, amplitude, duration, speed, direction, repetition and frequency). Lederman (2014) explains how any of these task parameters may be carefully 'amplified' during rehabilitation progressions. While mechanoreception is not limited to the following, neural effects of stretching rely on three main reflexes: stretch reflex (invoked via stimulation of the intrafusal muscle spindles); inverse stretch reflex (invoked via stimulation of golgi tendon organs); and the perception and control of pain via nociceptive and central mechanisms (Vujnovich and Dawson, 1994). The three neural reflexes together respond to and contribute to the regulation of muscular flexibility during stretching. Another important consideration is that it is never just muscle tissue which is being stretched. The non-contractile tissues may be more resistant to stretch compared to muscle tissue due to their different structural constituents and associated viscoelastic properties; it is also important to remember that scar tissue and fibrous adhesions also comprise connective tissue (Sapega *et al.*, 1981). With passive (assisted) stretching delivered by the therapist, the patient is positioned appropriately and remains as relaxed as possible. For optimal effects, the therapist must work with an understanding of where the stretching is to be focused. Some applications will involve attempting to fix and stabilize body areas which should not be moving during the stretch so as to localize the effect to the target area; other applications will incorporate a more global approach. As Myers and Frederick (2012) ascertain, *'the use of the word "isolated" in conjunction with the word "stretching" is difficult to justify when a straight leg lift test produces 240% of the strain in the iliotibial tract that it does in the hamstrings'*. The fact that motor control and task-specific muscle recruitment (to retrain functional movement patterns) are not being utilized during passive stretching shows another limiting aspect to its usefulness (Lederman, 2014). However, as part of a comprehensive strategy, the sports therapist will clinically reason their optimal approach. Debate continues regarding the optimal duration of stretching techniques to achieve lasting adaptation in soft tissue. Many authors recommend a gradual lengthening into the desired stretch position (aiming to inhibit the myotatic stretch reflex), with the stretch position held for 15–30 seconds (McAtee, 2013). Where there are fascial restrictions, stretches will need to be held for longer, but practitioners must recognize the highly individualized variants in regional tissue structure and composition, which means that there is not one single recipe for stretching restricted tissue. Jelveus (2011) has highlighted the plethora of evidence that indicates static stretching prior to athletic activity can reduce power output and speed, and moreover may even contribute to the potential for injury.

All stretching techniques must be performed within a physiological range, as overstretching causes damage (Alter, 2004). Such damage may occur in muscular, fascial, tendon, ligamentous, capsular or neural tissue. While peripheral nerves are able to withstand moderate stretching force, and indeed neural tensioning is a recognized therapeutic intervention, structural damage can occur when a nerve is stretched to 10 per cent of its physiological length, and tearing (neurotmesis) can occur at 30 per cent (Ylinen, 2008). Dynamic stretching has been part of the pre-event warm-up strategy which has been universally recommended in recent years due to its efficacy in aiding increased body temperature, joint mobility and neuromuscular firing, as well as offering some contribution to the increased strength, power, endurance, anaerobic capacity and agility which is promoted during thorough dynamic warm-up.

As discussed later in this section, soft tissues are anisotrophic, and there is an order-effect relating to the movements of joints; the therapist should keep these aspects in mind when attempting to perform passive tissue lengthening techniques (Hunter, 2006). It must also be recognized that soft tissue flexibility incorporates the tension (or 'tone') as held by the nervous system – which is why stretching in itself will not address such a component effectively – as well as the mechanical, elastic and plastic limitations to its end of range. Beyond this, there are other tissues which influence the range of movement available, not least all main peripheral nerves and all associated joint capsules. It is important to note that patients with hypermobility require special consideration so as not to develop further instability. Ylinen (2008) provides a comprehensive, practical guide to passive stretching techniques.

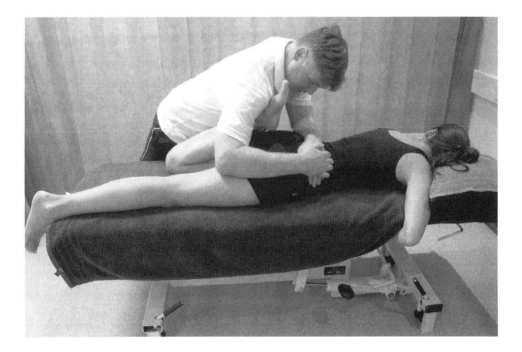

Photo 3.2   Passive stretching for the quadriceps group.

Soft tissue release

Soft tissue release (STR) requires the therapist to apply pressure into an area of restriction while it is being stretched. Basic STR strategies employ a procedure of first positioning the patient appropriately; shortening (slackening) the target tissues; applying a specific pressure into the area of soft tissue requiring release; and then, as the associated joint is slowly passively or actively mobilized, stretching of the tissues directly below the fixed point (Sanderson, 2012). The analogy of a 'key into a lock' has been used (Cash, 2012), where the therapist applies a 'key' (the pressure) into a 'lock' (the shortened restricted tissue) and then 'opens the door' (stretches the tissue); this may also be explained as 'pin and stretch'. Active STR involves the patient having to perform the joint movement and does mean that the therapist may be able exert a stronger reinforced pressure as they will have two hands available; passive STR has the therapist moving the patient with one hand and applying the pressure with the other.

Myofascial release

Fascia is a thoroughly integrated membrane of connective, viscoelastic tissue which covers and invests all structures of the body; fascia provides support and protection, and creates a structural unit. Fascia both separates and connects layers of muscle, compartments and cavities, as well as forming sheaths for nerves. Fascia thickens ligaments and joint capsules, and creates a continuous matrix that interconnects all structures of the body. Fascia is akin to a web that covers and interacts within the entire body. In order to appreciate how myofascial release (MFR) (may) work, it is essential to appreciate the main functional characteristics of fascia; such terms as viscoelasticity, thixotropy, creep and hysteresis require brief explanation. According to Schleip

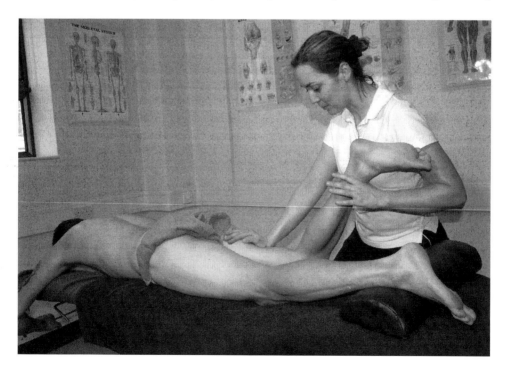

Photo 3.3   Soft tissue release for the hamstring group.

(2003), much of the work in myofascial therapy has been influenced by Rolf (1977), who was an early advocate of the requirement to therapeutically affect the ground substance of fascia with mechanical or thermal energy, and hence attempt to convert the substance aggregates from a dense gel-like state to a more fluid state, a process known as thixotropy, which itself is said to be due to the hydrophilic (water attracting) and viscoelastic (fluid-based elastic) properties of the fascial connective tissues. The fluid component of the ground substance (generated by the hydrophilic glycosaminoglycans) is essential to facilitate lubrication and synthesis of the collagen fibres it separates; and numerous factors can transpire to cause reduction in this fluid constituency (Chaitow and DeLany, 2002). The response of fascia to mechanical (tensile, shear and torsion forces) and thermal energy, in terms of its resultant plasticity (and potential for long-lasting deformation) is apparently time and force-dependent (Schleip, 2003). As such, fascia has been traditionally described as having 'creep' properties, which implies a relationship between time and stress on this connective tissue; a potential gradual conversion from 'gel' to 'sol' (fluid) state; a potential resulting effect on tissue length and freedom of movement; and further, an influence or effect on all related areas of the body. Barnes (1990) suggested that the time frame for thixotropic effect is 90–120 seconds. Hysteresis is the gradual resumption of viscoelastic structures to a resting length following deformation; the difference between pre- and post-loading strain is termed the 'set' (Atkins *et al.*, 2010; Bogduk and Twomey, 1987). Andrade and Clifford (2008) recommend that the best method for achieving longer-lasting plastic deformation of myofascial tissue, importantly without compromising its structural integrity, is to perform sustained, low-intensity forces. It is important to recognize that the purported effects of MFR are not universally accepted. Ingraham (2013) presents an eloquent analysis and argues against the inherent potential of fascia to 'release'; even Schleip (2003) has stated that plastic adaptation to moderate loading is *'impossible to conceive'*. Although advocates enthuse about the benefits of MFR, convincing evidence is still required for what exactly may be occurring during and after such intervention. Kidd (2009) builds an argument that MFR technique cannot be effectively evidenced, simply because of the inherent involvement and unique nature of each therapist's delivery. It is often implied that effective MFR is a therapeutic art relying on experience, skill and intuition; and while therapeutic outcomes can be readily evaluated, can the therapist be excluded from the process?

MFR consists of the focused releasing of both obvious and subtle restrictions evident within the myofascial network. Aside from the obvious limitations in soft tissue flexibility and ranges of movement, such restrictions can also cause entrapment of neural and vascular structures which are embedded within the tissue, potentially leading to neurological and ischaemic conditions (Fritz, 2005). Myofascial release technique involves either gross or local application, depending on the desired clinical outcome. Gross myofascial release concentrates on groups of muscles or sections of the body and is performed by a hand or one or two fingers fixing the affected tissue, while the other hand or finger(s) applies the stretch in parallel to the long axis of the tissues away from the fixing hand. Reinforced fingers or the elbow can be used to deliver slow and responsive techniques to fascia. The practitioner must hone their sense of how the fascia yields in response to the mechanical and thermal energy and the resulting thixotropic effect. Using the palms in a 'crossed-hands' technique allows gradual lengthening of fascial tissue in opposing directions following an initially static and sustained contact. Other foundational MFR techniques include arm and leg pulls, which offer subtle distraction as limbs are taken steadily through a range as the therapist senses yield. MFR is very much a process employing constant assessment and observation of effect and the patient must be encouraged to fully relax. Once tightness or restriction is identified and met, the tissue stretches are held until the therapist senses that tension has subsided, and are then progressed carefully (Andrade and Clifford, 2008; Manheim, 2008). Practitioners must aim to appreciate what effect the technique is having

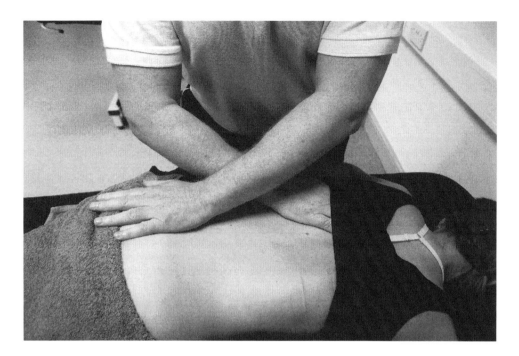

Photo 3.4   Myofascial release ('cross hands' technique) to thoracolumbar region.

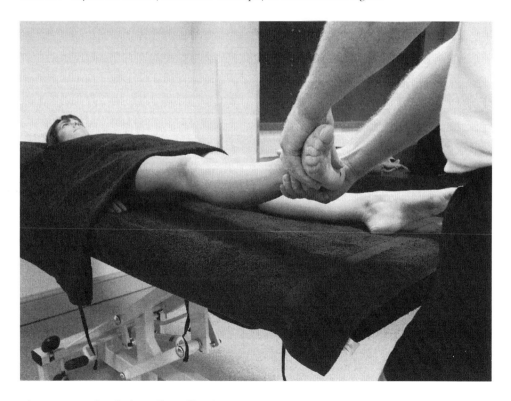

Photo 3.5   Myofascial release ('leg pull' technique).

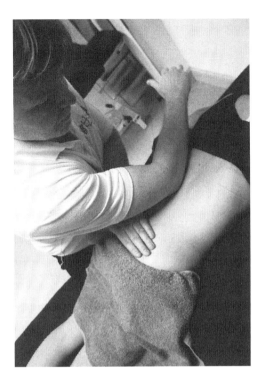

Photo 3.6   Myofascial release ('vertical stroking' technique).

during its application; constant palpatory monitoring is required. Furthermore, it is important to appreciate that, just as with joints and muscles, the presentation of fascia varies from patient to patient; it may be regular or irregular, dense or loose, bound or hypermobile (Earls and Myers, 2010). A systematic review of MFR interventions for a range of musculoskeletal conditions by McKenney *et al.* (2013) found that the majority of studies had positive outcomes, but due to the mixed quality (higher-quality experimental to lower-quality case studies), few conclusions could be drawn, and further randomized controlled trials are required.

Instrument-assisted soft tissue mobilization

Massage tools and instruments may offer the therapist assistance with corrective and deeper work, making remedial work more specific to areas of fibrosis, and may also reduce manual stress to thumbs, fingers, hands and the upper extremity (Hammer, 2012). Instruments to assist in the treatment of soft tissue dysfunction and other problems have been in use for many years in traditional Chinese Gua Sha therapy (Nielsen, 1995). Wooden, hard plastic, stone (such as jade) and high-grade stainless steel instruments ('tools') have become more commonplace in recent years to assist practitioners in the delivery of corrective soft tissue techniques, both for protecting thumbs and fingers and for facilitating increased precision. The concept of instrument-assisted soft tissue mobilization (IASTM) has been developed, and although evidence is in its infancy, Loghmani and Warden (2009) are among those who are demonstrating the potential for enhanced soft tissue therapy using stainless steel instruments. Looney *et al.* (2011), in a case series, presented evidence to support the use of 'Graston' instrument mobilization of the plantar fascia. Other recognized protagonists include Hammer (2008; 2012) and Hyde *et al.* (2011). It is proposed that specialized stainless steel instruments can be used as part of the palpatory assessment of tissues, and will 'amplify' the tactile and auditory senses. Orton (2013), in his brief review, described the versatility of such instruments, where multifaceted edges (blades) on a tool can facilitate improved precision and provide access to a host of usually challenging anatomical structures. Hence, this method can be extremely useful for attending to specific soft tissue problems associated with muscles, tendons, fascia, ligaments and scar tissue. By appreciating the need to assess the locality of any soft tissue lesion, the sports therapist will also understand the potential for unnecessarily aggravating tissue (and causing undue pain) if delivering IASTM treatment without due care. An emollient salve, typically with a base of beeswax and petroleum jelly, is the preferred medium for allowing smooth movement on tissue. Recognized methodology for IASTM incorporates the following:

- Selecting the appropriate tool and blade for the targeted tissue.
- Applying an initial 'scanning' assessment technique using an angle of approximately 30° to the skin (scanning techniques allow for superficial fascial and deeper soft tissue restrictions to be identified using the tool).
- Treatment methods include localized, short cross-fibre and 'J-stroke' techniques.
- Increased angles of application with maintained or increased pressure will increase depth and specificity of application.
- Blade size and contact area may be reduced to increase depth and specificity of application.
- Depth and specificity can also be achieved by altering the positioning of the body region (i.e. placing tissues on stretch or into shortened relaxation; or by guiding the patient to perform movement – active or resisted – during treatment).
- Both applied heat and warm-up exercises have been recommended for tissue preparation.
- Ice applications have been recommended pre- and/or post-treatment.

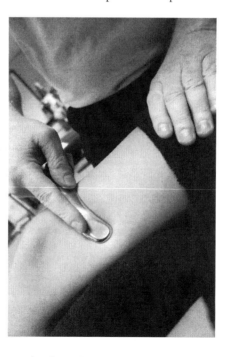

Photo 3.7   The 'i-assist' ('scanning' technique).

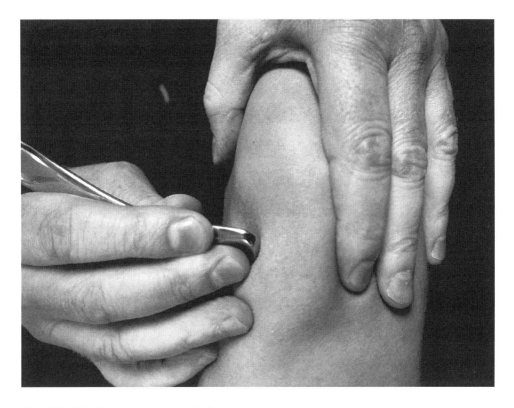

Photo 3.8 The 'i–assist' (treatment technique).

Manual lymphatic drainage

Manual lymphatic drainage (MLD) is a gentle advanced soft tissue technique which uses low-intensity pressures, strokes and joint movements, with the aim of manipulating skin and associated connective tissues to assist the function of the lymphatic system (French, 2011). As a secondary circulatory system, the lymphatic system comprises lymphatic vessels, lymph nodes and lymphatic ducts, which eventually drain into the left and right subclavian veins and return their fluid constituents to the general circulation. There are two primary functions of the lymphatic system; first, the collection and transportation of interstitial fluid, as lymph; and second, the production, storage and distribution of lymphocytes (specialized leucocytes – white blood cells), which are essential components of the immune system. The sports therapist may utilize aspects of MLD technique in acute stages of injury when oedema is present. Knowledge of location and direction of the main lymphatic vessels and nodes is central to this application (Andrade and Clifford, 2008). Instructing deep breathing, passive joint movements, elevation of limbs, physically encouraging circulatory flow in proximal vessels and pathways (including alternating gentle compressions over the anterior upper chest and shoulder area) are all potentially useful approaches. The lymph nodes that are proximal to the injury can be lightly massaged using circular, 'figure of eight' or 'J-shape' motions (French, 2011). These movements can be performed in conjunction with light effleurage techniques which follow the lymphatic pathway from the affected region towards the nearest set of proximal nodes, and followed with light stokes proximally away from these.

Myofascial trigger point therapy

Within neuromuscular therapy (NMT) there are a range of approaches and techniques. As Dejung *et al.* (2013) explain: *'In folk medicine it has always been known that finger pressure on a painful spot can reduce the pain'*. While the true aetiology of trigger points is still to be determined, trigger point therapy is a recognized soft tissue approach incorporating pressures, which are applied by the thumb, fingers, elbow or an applicator tool (such as a 'Jacknobber') to tissues deemed to be containing myofascial trigger points (MTrPs); this may also be known as ischaemic compression, or simply neuromuscular technique. Longitudinal or local stretching of the affected tissues, muscle energy techniques, positional release and myofascial release techniques are all commonly integrated into therapy designed to 'deactivate' the MTrPs. Ultrasound, laser, heat and cold (including 'spray and stretch') therapy have also been historically advocated. Invasive procedures such as dry needling, local anaesthetic and combination corticosteroid injections, as well as botulinum toxin ('botox') injections have also been advocated by some practitioners in resistant cases, although evidence is lacking. A combined NMT approach aims to eliminate MTrP activity and produce modifications in dysfunctional tissue and encourage a restoration of functional normality (Chaitow and DeLany, 2002; 2008). Alvarez and Rockwell (2002) suggested that myofascial pain syndrome is one of the most common causes of pain resulting from soft tissue dysfunction, and in particular, MTrPs. Explanations for the apparent existence of MTrPs incorporate a multitude of reasons, including: myofascial, postural and biomechanical imbalances; joint dysfunctions; trauma; overtraining; psychological and emotional issues (as may be associated with central sensitization); metabolic disorders; nutritional deficiencies; and conditions such as fibromyalgia (Chaitow, 2006). Any of these commonly presenting factors can contribute to hyperirritability, which is the hallmark of MTrPs, and while the actual aetiology and pathophysiology of MTrPs remains uncertain, what is certain is the multifactorial development aspect. Traditionally, MTrPs have been associated with dysfunctional motor end-plates, an excessive release of acetylecholine (ACh), local tissue hypoxia and low pH (Dommerholt, 2013). Quintner *et al.* (2014), however, in their review, suggest that the traditional theory for MTrP development is flawed and argue that there are two more plausible explanations for the development of localized muscle tenderness *'in structurally and physiologically unimpaired'* muscles. They propose that deep peripheral neurogenic inflammation may result in ectopic, spontaneous axonal discharge which can lead to sensitization of the innervated muscle; the authors do not, however, explain the underlying reasoning for such deep neuronal inflammation. Their second hypothesis designates an MTrP as *'a site of secondary allodynia reflecting altered central nociceptive mechanisms'*. The pathogenesis of MTrPs remains uncertain.

MTrPs have been described as being *active* (those that cause spontaneous and characteristically referred pain); and *latent* (those which have similar clinical features but without being currently responsible for pain) (Travell and Simons, 1998). Trigger point therapy (NMT or ischaemic compression) is presented as a technique utilizing palpatory assessment throughout delivery, communication and feedback from the patient, and continued modification of pressure application (which is usually intermittent). Applied pressure into a sensitive MTrP, which may be simply described as an area of local neuromuscular facilitation and chemical imbalance within a taut band of muscle, will typically cause referred pain to a site away from the local point (Simons, 2004). On first pressure there may be a 'twitch' response of the affected muscle (localized involuntary contraction); this is because the muscle fibres are facilitated and therefore have a reduced threshold for firing with mechanical stimulation. Trigger point therapy is delivered to generate a change in neuromuscular behaviour. Fritz (2005) notes that MTrPs may be identified during palpation by the presence of skin changes (tension and resistance to gliding; moisture from perspiration due to autonomic sympathetic facilitation; temperature changes; oedema), alongside deeper palpation which may evoke tenderness, and identify muscular tension or fibrosis. Gautschi (2008) explains that ischaemic compression to MTrPs can cause a reactive hyperaemia, which leads to an increase in local metabolism and a reflective detensioning of the taut band housing the MTrP. During trigger point therapy, direct manipulation may involve pushing the muscle belly together (to affect muscle spindles), pushing tendons apart (to affect golgi tendon organs – GTOs) and direct intermittent pressure (or squeezing together) of the MTrP (to affect local mechanoreceptors, including muscle spindles, and additionally to cause a circulatory effect). Chaitow and DeLany (2002; 2008) suggest gradually increasing local pressure applications of around eight seconds duration (staying within a maximum 7/10 subjective pain range) for between 30 seconds and two minutes at a time. The technique is deemed successful when any referral pain fades and when local pain and relaxation occurs in the affected muscle fibres. The therapist will maintain palpatory assessment during delivery, and it is essential that they maintain good working posture and protect their digits during treatment. It is recommended to deliver some form of lengthening of the locally affected connective tissues as part of the trigger point therapy, and obviously, as with all interventions, causative factors must be addressed and functional re-education employed (Gautschi, 2013).

Muscle energy technique

Muscle energy techniques (METs) are osteopathic in origin, and incorporate a number of approaches. They may be applied to both acute and chronic conditions, and aim to increase joint range of motion and soft tissue flexibility, reduce pain and decrease muscle spasm (Burns and Wells, 2006; Chaitow and DeLany, 2002). The basic principle of MET takes advantage of the relationship which exists between the peripheral nervous system and the muscles that they innervate, and how this relationship can be manipulated for therapeutic effect. More specifically, practitioners of MET will appreciate the reciprocal innervation of antagonistic muscle groups, and the specialized mechanoreceptors (GTOs) located at musculotendinous junctions. While the neuromuscular theory of reflex relaxation is plausible, no studies as yet show a decrease in electromyographic (EMG) activity following MET (Fryer, 2011). As the MET process typically takes a few minutes to perform, the techniques are highly likely to alter the pliability and length of the targeted myofascia due to its viscoelastic properties. Clearly, there are limitations to the MET evidence-base, as Fryer (2011) explains:

> like many manual therapeutic approaches, the efficacy and effectiveness of MET technique are under-researched, and there is little evidence to guide practitioners in the choice of the most useful technique variations (such as number of repetitions, strength of contraction or duration of stretch phase), causing frustration for those endeavouring to integrate relevant evidence into practice.

Hence, while being anecdotally useful, and objectively effective, further research is required to confirm effects and best applications. Post-isometric relaxation (PIR) and reciprocal inhibition (RI) are the most well-recognized examples of MET and may be used in combination with other soft tissue techniques (Chaitow, 2006).

Post-isometric relaxation

PIR MET follows the simple protocol that a gentle tensile stress (a stretch) is applied to muscle following a gentle isometric contraction. An isometric contraction is relatively static; tension is generated in the muscle, but the muscle length and joint angle does not alter. An isometric contraction is performed at a position of bind (the 'restriction barrier'), which is the position where the therapist first senses slight tensioning in the target tissue. This, it has been hypothesized, stimulates the GTOs and may cause a short-term relaxation (inhibition) of the involved muscle(s) and may contribute to resetting of the resting length (Norris, 2011; Vujnovich and Dawson, 1994). A 'window of opportunity' has also been described, where, following a low-intensity isometric contraction of the target muscle, a gentle stretch can be applied as the patient relaxes (and is instructed to breathe) (Chaitow, 2006) to make a change in the muscle length.

Application of PIR

Although a range of protocols are evident, for a general PIR strategy the therapist moves the affected tissues to a point where 'bind' is felt. The therapist then maintains this position for approximately ten seconds while the patient actively contracts against the therapist's resistance anywhere in the range 15–75 per cent of maximal contraction (Ballantyne *et al.*, 2003; Chaitow and DeLany, 2002; Smith and Fryer, 2008), although a simple gentle contraction (around 20 per cent) should suffice. The muscle is then relaxed, the patient encouraged to relax and breathe in and then out, and as they breathe out the limb is moved passively to the new position of bind. The process is usually repeated 2–5 times until no further increases are found (Burns and Wells, 2006; Chaitow and DeLany, 2002). Gibbons (2011) recommends that the final position is held for around 30 seconds in order to facilitate improved neuromuscular functioning.

Reciprocal inhibition

RI MET involves contraction of the antagonist muscle group, and deals with the reciprocal effects (relative inhibition of the target group) of an isometric contraction in the muscle group opposite to the target muscle group. Just as in PIR, the delivery of RI must incorporate appreciation and continued assessment of the 'bind' point, but often in RI, the isometric contraction will need to be performed back from the 'bind' point, in a mid-range joint position, due to the potential for cramp occurring in a biomechanically disadvantaged position (which relates to the length–tension relationship and active insufficiency in the contracting muscles). RI may be most useful when in acute or sub-acute situations where a degree muscle spasm is present – to help inhibit the hypertonic situation; and also where the contraction of an affected target muscle group may be uncomfortable or aggravating. When spasm or pain on contraction is not a feature, PIR and RI may be used in conjunction.

Positional release technique

Patients should ideally be effectively assessed in functional, loaded positions, if possible, so as to ascertain specific restrictions and symptomatic responses – which may not present as clearly in non-functional positions. Positional release technique (PRT) strategy can include having the patient's affected tissues relaxed, on stretch, contracted, in weight-bearing and during progressively loaded movement patterns, which are performed with the aim of producing and reducing, and therefore identifying, the symptomatic response. Once the restrictions or symptoms have been identified, the treatment strategy may incorporate PRT which may actually employ similar patient positioning. This approach is obviously used in conjunction with whatever else the sports therapist feels is appropriate. There are a number of techniques that involve placing the patient's body into a position of 'ease'. In a patient that presents with a distorted position caused by hypertonicity or spasm, the therapist may place the patient into a position that exaggerates the distortion (Chaitow, 2007). The hypothesis of PRT is that compensatory positions allow the resetting of physiological processes, which in turn can reduce the spasm and pain rather than antagonize the situation by causing the body to react with an increase in pain and resistance (Chaitow and DeLany, 2008). PRT aims to rectify somatic or musculoskeletal disturbances and may be effective in complex regional pain syndrome (Collins, 2007). It is postulated that its efficacy is due to causing a decrease in the commonly developed proprioceptive hyperactivity (Chaitow, 2007), coupled with a controlling influence on the neurophysiological propagation brought about by the overstimulation of muscle spindles and the related increase in neural discharge caused by mechanical strain (Collins, 2007). It has also been proposed that a 'circulatory flush' of previously ischaemic tissue will occur. PRT is an appropriate treatment when presented with a patient with either acute or chronic neuromuscular dysfunction (Chaitow and DeLany, 2002; Collins, 2007).

Application of PRT

The technique relies on precise palpatory and effective communication skill, so as to deliver a sensitive approach and to work with the patient to achieve a sense of ease. Hypersensitive tissue points may be relieved by working, one step at a time, to position the affected body part into its position of maximum relief (with full patient relaxation) for between 20 and 90 seconds (Chaitow and DeLany, 2008; Collins, 2007), while maintaining contact with the palpating finger. This typically involves very slight slackening of tissue, utilizing a sequential combination of subtle physiological and accessory movements (for example, at the glenohumeral joint, passive application of small degrees of abduction, lateral rotation, horizontal extension and cephalad movements) each time reassessing for change in sensitivity. Once in a position of ease, it is recommended that an integrated approach is utilized, and digital ischaemic compressions (NMT) are delivered. If the therapist has found a comfortable resting position, and if the tender point decreases by at least 70 per cent, the treatment is deemed a success (Chaitow, 2007; Collins, 2007).

Integrated neuromuscular inhibition technique

Using a combination sequence of NMT, PRT and MET in the form of integrated neuromuscular inhibition technique (INIT) has been advocated by Chaitow (2007), Hall (2014) and Nagrale *et al.* (2010). Such an approach may begin with NMT (using ischaemic compressions) to the affected points, then delivery of PRT; in the INIT approach, the therapist may continue delivery of ischaemic compression during the PRT. Following PRT, MET (PIR and/or RI) and MFR may be used to lengthen the (potentially desensitized) affected tissue.

Progressive soft tissue therapy approaches

Strategies and systematic approaches for delivery of STT, in terms of positions of application, intensity, repetition, duration and frequency have been generally presented as being technique specific and essentially with a large degree of operator (therapist) autonomy. There have been developments in recommendations for strategy in delivery of STT presented in recent years, yet as ever, more clinically reliable research is required. Progressive approaches for targeting soft tissue restrictions has been advocated and popularized by numerous authors; these include:

'Anatomy Trains' and 'Structural Integration Therapy' (Earls and Myers, 2010; Myers, 2008); 'Functional and Kinetic Treatment with Rehabilitation, Provocation and Movement' (FAKTR–PM) (Hyde *et al.*, 2011); 'Specific Soft Tissue Mobilization' (SSTM) (Hunter, 1994; 1998); and 'Therapeutic Stretching' (Lederman, 2014). Additionally, the field of neuromuscular therapy (including NMT, MET and PRT), which is subtly different to the more direct, mechanical approaches, and based on inhibitory, indirect and reflexive responses, is well established, with such authors as Chaitow (2006; 2007), Chaitow and DeLany (2002; 2008), Fritz (2005), Fryer (2011), Sharkey (2007) and Travell and Simons (1998). The traditional hypothesis for MTrPs has, however, been challenged by several authors (Quintner *et al.*, 2014). The INIT approach, combining digital ischaemic compression, positional release, MET (PIR and/or RI) and MFR, shows good evidence for achieving a reduction in MTrP sensitivity and increasing length in restricted soft tissue (Hall, 2014; Nagrale *et al.*, 2010). The understanding of INIT must include the structural and physiological intricacies of connective tissue and fascia as much as that of the muscular and neurovascular systems. It must also appreciate the many and various causes of dysfunction and adaptation (local and central; postural; traumatic; psychological; and respiratory). In the light of such appreciation, the practitioner will understand why STT is so useful, how it can work to influence positive changes (physically, physiologically and psychologically) and how it may be best applied. The mindful practitioner will, however, recognize that for long-term patient benefit an active, rather than passive, hands-on, approach may be far more appropriate.

Patient treatment positions and active involvement have been identified as being influential to the overall therapeutic potential for optimal improvement in tissue structure and function. Sports therapists should aim to consider, in remedial soft tissue treatments, the placing of patients into positions of function or provocation (which may be with affected soft tissues on stretch or in loaded contraction, such as with the use of theraband or free-weights) so as to be specific in their remedial delivery (Hyde *et al.*, 2011). Furthermore, the concept of SSTM recognizes the fact that soft tissues are anisotrophic, in that their properties alter according to the different directions of movement that are applied to them, and they are not loaded equally during any particular mechanical stress. Additionally, there is an 'order effect' in which joints may be moved by the practitioner in order to affect any targeted multi-articular muscle group (Hunter, 2006). The message here is that there are numerous ways of moving or affecting soft tissues, and that it is not always appropriate to use conventional or simply linear stretches to obtain the desired results. Even when a target muscle has been placed on a multi-directional stretch, employing the 'order effect' of a combination of joint movements, the practitioner still has the opportunity to perform what may be called 'accessory movements' of the already stretched fibres. Hence, there are a host of approaches to employ, and the therapist has to reason their way through their delivery while being sensitive to the response and feel of the tissues, the ranges of movement being employed at the involved joints, and the response of the patient themselves. Practitioners should aim to combine their soft tissue techniques into a seamless and comfortable STT session; they must also consider the best approach to integrating their soft tissue skills into the complete sports therapy session, which may also incorporate elements of manual therapy (joint mobilizations), possibly electrotherapy, taping, cryotherapy and especially exercise rehabilitation. Arguably, this is one of the main challenges that the sports therapist faces – how to optimize their therapeutic strategy; and practitioners should aim to recognize the notion of 'therapeutic intent' – having a clear vision in their own mind of what they are setting out to achieve. Andrade and Clifford (2008; 2012) have presented an 'outcome-based massage' (OBM) methodology, which incorporates a four-stage systematic decision-making process regarding: the identification of patient impairments associated with their condition or wellness goals; the specification of desired and relevant (client-centred) outcomes; the selection of most appropriate therapeutic techniques; and the application of selected techniques (incorporating psychomotor skills). Certainly, by 'throwing everything at the patient', the therapist is unable to be confident about which interventions are helping or hindering progress. Essentially, it is the combined employment of clinical reasoning strategy alongside the utilization of EBP which must be the dominant influences upon management planning. Being able to progress the patient/athlete from a purely passive approach to a more active and functionally relevant programme must be a priority in the majority of cases.

Table 3.5 General and local contraindications and precautions to soft tissue therapy

---

Acute injuries
Suspicion of complex injury
Inability to ascertain the nature of the complaint
General malaise and feeling unwell
Severe pain
Highly irritable conditions
Dizziness
'Red flag' signs
Significant 'yellow flag' signs (concerning biopsychosocial factors)
Infection
Febrile state (fever)
Congestive heart disease
Circulatory disorders
Hypertension
Recent surgery
Post-surgical pain
Recent inoculations (<24 hours)
Hypothermia / hyperthermia
Myositis ossificans
Hernia
Skin disorders
Tumours or unrecognizable lumps
Suspicion of melanoma
Suspicion of aneurysm
Haemophilia
Severe diabetes
Unstable epilepsy
Dysfunctional nervous system
Severe osteoarthritis / rheumatoid arthritis / osteoporosis / gout / bursitis / ankylosing spondylitis / spondylosis / spondylolysis / spondylolisthesis
Metal pins and plates
Pacemaker
Pregnancy
First two or three days of menstruation
Heavy meal
Alcohol / recreational drugs
Conditions requiring specialized medical supervision

Note: This list is not exhaustive; if there is any doubt regarding the suitability of patients for soft tissue therapy, then medical opinion must be sought.

Manual therapy
Principles of manual therapy

According to Cook (2012), the purpose of orthopaedic manual therapy is to apply techniques which *'reduce, centralize, or abolish the patient's signs and symptoms'*. While the fields of manual therapy are diverse and multifaceted, and potentially indicated for a range of health conditions, for the sports therapist the utility of manual therapy will be focused to support the management of the common neuromusculoskeletal injuries and conditions which present clinically. Due to the potential risk factors associated with this area of practice, it is essential that any manual therapy provided by a sports therapist must be within their scope of practice. Hence, the sports therapist must be qualified and insured: to be able to undertake effective neuromusculoskeletal assessment of their patients; to be able to make autonomous decisions regarding their patients' suitability to receive manual therapy; to be able to recognize when referral for medical assessment or other intervention must be recommended; and to be able to safely and effectively provide manual therapy when indicated.

In a pure sense, manual therapy may be described as being the application of an accurately directed and selected set of 'hands-on', non-invasive physical therapy techniques, with minimal equipment, and which are generally considered as being passively delivered treatments, but which may also be possibly offered in conjunction with certain active movements when appropriate. The techniques of manual therapy may include graded physiological and accessory joint mobilizations and manipulations, and neural mobilizations, as well as a vast range of soft tissue friction, stretching and muscle energy techniques. Hengeveld and Banks (2005) explain that, within the Maitland concept of manual therapy, 'mobilization' techniques are passive movements which are *'performed in such a manner and speed that at all times they are within the control of the patient'* and that 'manipulation' techniques are categorized as passive, high–velocity, short- or low-amplitude thrust techniques (HVLT) which are *'within the joint's anatomical limit performed at such a speed that renders the patient powerless to prevent it'*. It is generally accepted that manipulative techniques (Maitland grade V; Cyriax grade C) are not within the realm of a sports therapist unless appropriate post-graduate training has been undertaken. Manual therapy is not the sole domain of any one physical therapy profession, but is a primary component of the health care that orthopaedists, physiotherapists, osteopaths, chiropractors, manipulative therapists and sports therapists provide. Beyond this, Cook (2012) and others have explored the differences in underpinning manual therapy philosophy which are clearly apparent in the different professions. As Cook (2012) surmised, *'there is no direct evidence to determine which assessment philosophy reigns superiorly over another'*. There are a considerable number of influential manual therapy pioneers – practitioners who have contributed over the past 50 years to the understanding and general acceptance of manual therapy in clinical practice; these include: Butler (1991); Cook (2012); Cyriax and Cyriax (1982); Greenman (1996); Grieve (1988); Hartman (1997); Hengeveld and Banks (2005); Kaltenborn (1970; 1999); Magee (2008); Maitland *et al.* (2005); Mennell (1960); Mulligan (1993; 2004); and Paris (2012). Sports therapists must be recommended to develop their appreciation of the work of these recognized practitioners, in conjunction with a developing knowledge of ever-evolving contemporary EIP in this field. Clearly it is beyond the scope of this text to provide more than a brief overview of manual therapy and a discussion of the principles which underpin it, and as such sports therapists are directed towards the key reference material as presented in text.

Table 3.6 Terminology in manual therapy

Terminology	Definition
Physiological movement	A gross active or passive functional movement of a joint, such as flexion and extension (Hengeveld and Banks, 2005)
Accessory movement	A small movement of a joint which cannot be performed actively, but can be performed passively by the therapist. Accessory movements include the roll, spin and slide which accompany each joint's physiological movements (Magee, 2008). Also known as 'joint play' (Mennell, 1960)
Close-packed (synarthrodial) position	Where the associated articular joint surfaces are in maximal contact with each other; where primary static stabilizers may be on tension; and where a position of maximal congruency occurs (Magee, 2008). An unfavourable position for joint mobilization techniques
Loose-packed (resting) position	Where the associated articular joint surfaces are not in maximal contact with each other; where primary static stabilizers are not on full tension; and where the joint is less than maximally congruent (Magee, 2008). A favourable position for performing joint mobilization techniques
Mobilization techniques	Passive physiological, accessory or combination movements performed in such a manner and speed that at all times they are within the control of the patient. These are most commonly graded I–IV (Maitland *et al.*, 2005)
Manipulation techniques	Passive movements consisting of accurately localized high-velocity, small-amplitude thrust manoeuvres within the joint's anatomical limit. It may employ use of short or long leverages, and is performed at such a speed that it is beyond the control of the patient (Cook, 2012). In the Maitland system, these are grade 5 techniques (Maitland *et al.*, 2005)
Grades of joint mobilization	Systematically assessed and delivered, graded physiological or accessory, vertebral or peripheral, joint mobilizations. Several acknowledged grading systems exist, the most common being: Maitland grades of mobilization on a five-point scale (I–V) (Maitland *et al.*, 2005); Cyriax grades on a three-point scale (A–C) (Atkins *et al.*, 2010); and Kaltenborn grades, also on a three-point scale (I – loosening; II – tightening; III – stretching) (Kaltenborn, 1970; 1999)
MWM	'Mobilizations with movement', as first presented by Mulligan (1993; 2004); these may be applied to both vertebral and peripheral joints
NAGS	'Natural apophyseal glides'. Oscillatory spinal mobilizations performed with the patient in a seated, weight-bearing position (Mulligan, 2004). They are applied to facet joints antero-cranially in a pre-assessed mid- to end-range position
SNAGS	'Sustained natural apophyseal glides'. Spinal mobilizations performed with the patient in a seated, weight-bearing position (Mulligan, 2004). The combination of a sustained facet joint glide with active movement
Osteokinematics	A term used to describe the gross movements of body parts (bones at joints), described in terms of anatomical planes (i.e. frontal, sagittal and transverse), and what is occurring at the joint during the movement (for example, flexion or rotation)
Arthrokinematics	A term used to describe the movements occurring within the joint and between articular surfaces, and can be described as accessory movements

Table 3.6 continued

Terminology	Definition
Convex–concave rule	A functional anatomical concept indicating that joint movements are guided by the presence of a convex–concave congruency in the associated articulating surfaces. The movement of initiation dictates the direction of movement (Cook, 2012). If the moving surface is concave, the associated glide will occur in the same direction as the moving bone. If the moving surface is convex, the glide will occur in the opposite direction. The universal application of this theory, however, has been challenged
Glide (slide)	An accessory movement where the same area of one articular surface meets new areas on the opposing articular surface (for example, a PA glide)
Spin	An accessory rotational movement around a stationary axis
Roll	An accessory movement where one articular surface rolls on another. New areas on one articular surface will meet new areas on the opposing articular surface
Capsular pattern	A pattern of proportional joint movement limitation as described by Cyriax and Cyriax (1982), where the capsule of the joint is affected (Magee, 2008; Petty, 2011). The pattern, it is suggested, is a result of a total joint reaction to arthrosis, with muscle spasm, capsular contraction (the most common cause) and osteophyte formation being typical causative mechanisms. Although Cyriax and Cyriax (1982) suggest that all major joints have a particular common capsular pattern, the universality of the theory has been questioned
End-feel classifications	The quality of a joint's end-feel, which is sensed by the therapist as the joint is passively taken to the end of its available range of movement. Generic and normal end-feels include: bone to bone; soft tissue approximation; tissue stretch. Generic abnormal end-feels include: hard capsular; empty; early muscle spasm; springy block (Magee, 2008). Therapists must appreciate that each set of joint movements will have their own set of normal and abnormal end-feels
Hypomobility	A reduction in normal and expected mobility. May be congenital, developmental, acquired, age-related, local or general. It must be assessed and compared against contralateral regions and against published norms. May relate to joint restriction or soft tissue restriction.
Hypermobility	An increase in normal and expected mobility
Cavitation	The audible or palpable 'popping ' or 'cracking' that is a high-frequency vibration that may occur at a specific joint during a mobilization or manipulation technique (or spontaneously during functional movement). Cavitation is due to a sudden distention of the synovial joint capsule, and its effect on the associated negative intra-articular, vacuum-like pressure. Physiological changes may take place during a mobilization or manipulation in the absence of cavitation
PPIVM	Passive physiological intervertebral movements
PA	Posteroanterior
AP	Anteroposterior
MG	Medial glide
LG	Lateral glide
TG	Transverse glide

Terminology	Definition
PAIVM	Passive accessory intervertebral movements
Traction	Manual or mechanical tensile force which therapeutically is designed to produce a combination of distraction and gliding to relieve pain, increase joint range of movement and improve function. '*The terms traction and distraction have the same meaning in describing a force applied to produce separation of joint surfaces and widening of the joint space. There is a convention that traction is applied to spinal joints and distraction to peripheral joints, but this is not a hard and fast rule*' (Atkins *et al.*, 2010). The opposite of compression
Compression	Mobilization techniques delivered so as to cause reduction in space between articular surfaces. The opposite of traction
Cephalad	Mobilization directed towards the head (i.e. cranially or proximally)
Caudad	Mobilization directed away from the body, towards a distal end
Oscillations	The rhythmic repetitive movements performed during mobilization techniques. Start position, grade, velocity and amplitude may be varied

Effects of manual therapy

Manual therapy techniques used in sports therapy are employed variously to assist the management of soft tissue, joint and nerve-related pain and inflammation, to promote tissue repair, to improve soft tissue and joint range of motion and to promote improved functional biomechanics and the patient's kinaesthetic sense. The effects of manual therapy are multitudinous and involve neurophysiological (local, spinal and supraspinal), nutritional and mechanical responses (Houglum, 2010; McCreesh and O'Connor, 2012). Pain reduction may result initially via gate-control mechanisms, as stimulated larger-diameter A-beta mechanoreceptors may inhibit nociceptive messaging at the levels of the spinal cord and brainstem; and muscle spasm may relax in response to reduced nociceptive inputs. Descending inhibitory pathways have been shown to be activated for the generation of pain relief during the process of manual therapy (Vicenzino *et al.*, 1998). Particularly in early joint-related injury management, manual therapy can be used to help create an 'ideal environment' for optimal recovery, especially where patients may be reluctant to actively mobilize (Hengeveld and Banks, 2005). As a result, local synovial and circulatory increases may facilitate increased nutrient exchange and metabolic activity, which can contribute to improved healing processes. Carefully targeted mechanical forces can improve joint hypomobility; as Houglum (2010) highlights, hypomobile joints may lead to the development of collagenous adhesions in their associated soft tissues (capsule; capsular ligaments; fascia; tendons; and muscles) which may be stretched and loosened by manual therapy. McCreesh and O'Connor (2012) review the mechanical forces and resulting microtrauma to periarticular soft tissues, which may cause the required permanent change in length so as to observe significant increases in range of movement. Mechanotransduction is the process of tissue cells' response to mechanical loading (Khan and Scott, 2009); and in appreciating this, therapists can recognize the potential to positively stimulate structural adaptation. In manual therapy, the mechanotransduction process first involves 'mechanocoupling', where applied forces cause deformation and perturbation of cells; these forces are then transformed into chemical signalling by the affected cells. The second part of the process involves 'cell to cell communication', where same-region tissue cells, not necessarily nor initially directly in receipt of the mechanical stimuli, also register the signal (Wall and Banes, 2005). The third component of the mechanotransduction process is termed the 'effector cell response'; this occurs at the boundary between the tissue cells and their extracellular matrix (ECM) as mechanically induced protein expression from tissue cells leads to remodelling of the ECM (Khan and Scott, 2009). Other effects also obviously occur; at synovial joints, the intra-articular pressure influences their available range of movement; and the pressure itself depends upon fluid volume and joint position (Levick *et al.*, 1999). As where there is joint effusion, range of movement is usually limited; McCreesh and O'Connor (2012) explain that in such conditions, sustained end of available range positioning, in conjunction with appropriately graded mobilizations, can encourage reabsorption of excess fluid.

Finally, with regard to the effects of manual therapy, the potential for placebo effects (where patient beliefs may influence outcomes) must also be recognized. Bialosky *et al.* (2011) define the placebo effect in context as '*a mechanism likely accounting for some of the treatment effects of all interventions for pain, including manual therapy*'. The placebo effect is synergistically related to the patient, the clinician, the clinical intervention and the clinical environment; it is also '*beyond the specific mechanical parameters of the intervention*'. Clearly, although the placebo effect is challenging to quantify, it is a factor to consider both psychologically and physiologically with regard to optimizing patient outcomes.

Physiological and accessory joint movements

Physiological (osteokinematic) motion is defined as the gross body movements which the patient can perform actively, or which the therapist can perform passively. Active physiological movement is the result of concentric or eccentric muscle contractions, and where bones at joints move through their available ranges (Palastanga *et al.*, 2007). Depending on the joint concerned, physiological movements include: flexion, extension, lateral flexion, abduction, adduction, medial and lateral rotation, pronation, supination, plantarflexion, dorsiflexion, inversion, eversion and combinations of these. Physiological mobilizations may be performed in conjunction with accessory movements. Accessory (arthrokinematic) movements are the gliding, rolling and spinning movements which are necessary for normal physiological joint range of motion, but which cannot be isolated or actively performed independently of physiological movements, unless produced under external passive force (i.e. by the therapist). The reason that accessory movements cannot be performed actively is because humans do not have the intricate musculature or fine motor control to be able to glide, spin or roll independently of a physiological movement. If any of the accessory movements associated with a particular joint are deemed to be restricted (hypomobile), then it follows that normal full-range physiological movements are likely to be adversely affected; but obviously, other factors contribute to the quality of movement (pain, hypermobility, arthrosis and restricted soft tissue mobility for example). With such conditions, dyskinesia (gross abnormal movement pattern) will be observed.

Application of manual therapy

Any delivery of manual therapy must be preceded by the undertaking of a thorough patient history and subjective and objective assessment, and be based upon a clinically reasoned set of short-term therapeutic goals. Some patients, from the outset, will not be suitable candidates for manual therapy (due to identified contraindications) and must be managed accordingly. Importantly, the delivery of manual therapy must incorporate appreciation of patient (and symptom) response, hence practitioners must be recommended to work with care to observe and palpate all changes occurring in the target tissues. Indeed, Maitland *et al.* (2005) state that palpation is the most important and most difficult skill to learn. Sports therapists should also appreciate that there are issues of inter-rater reliability regarding palpation, particularly with regard to intervertebral segment movement (Schneider *et al.*, 2008). Maitland *et al.* (2005), cited in Banks and Hengeveld (2010), have presented a simple classification system for vertebral segment palpation: ideal (*'perfect in every way, asymptomatic and devoid of any palpable signs of movement impairment'*); average (*'disadvantaged, tolerable level of symptoms accepted by the person, accompanying signs of disadvantage or impairment are evident'*); abnormal (*'disordered, symptoms are unacceptable and there are clear palpable signs of tissue impairment'*). A sequence for palpation must also be considered to incorporate assessment of: local superficial skin temperature and conductance (sweating); local soft tissue changes; bony position and alignment; and symptom responses to passive movement. As the majority of manual therapy is passively performed, Cook (2012) describes this aspect of effective delivery as assessing for *'within-session changes'*, and refers to it as a *'patient response-based method'*. The therapist must aim to achieve a confident understanding of: what is normal or abnormal (with regard to the tissues and structures being treated); what is hypomobile or hypermobile (and the degree of such); what is symptomatic or relieving (i.e. pain producing, exacerbating or reducing, or the cause of other symptoms such as dysaesthesia); and what the continuing therapeutic objectives are. The use of 'clinical indicators' (objective markers) should be incorporated into this approach. Clinical indicators are movements that have been identified during assessment as being problematic or restricted; these movements should be re-tested 'within-session'. For the sports therapist, manual therapy is an essential intervention, but it must be underpinned by a comprehensive anatomical and pathological understanding, together with a strong appreciation of the principles of manual therapy (indications; contraindications; safety considerations; and practical applications). One other essential component of manual therapy, as highlighted by the International Federation of Orthopedic Manipulative Physical Therapists (IFOMPT, 2010), is its requirement to be 'patient-centred' – the patient must be at the centre of all clinical decision-making, and their understandings, beliefs and feelings must influence any resulting intervention.

Following patient assessment, the therapist is then challenged to select the most applicable therapeutic intervention. This requires considerable clinical reasoning, in the moment, and with regard to manual therapy, numerous considerations must present to the sports therapist: the current severity of symptoms; the state of tissue irritability; the main symptom–generating tissues (the 'genics'); the acuteness or chronicity of the condition; the pain mechanisms at play (i.e. nociceptive; peripheral neuropathic; centrally sensitized); the effect of pain and any inflammation on the muscles associated with the joint (i.e. inhibition; atrophy; spasm); the presence of hypomobilty (stiffness); the presence of hypermobility (laxity); the presence of articular surface degeneration; the presence of structural anomalies (i.e. cartilage; capsule; bone; cysts; fragmentation); the relationships between related regions and joints; beyond inhibition or spasm, the state of myofascial balance on the joint; clinical indicators (most problematic re-testable movements); and the presence of any psychosocial factors (yellow flags). Once all such considerations have been thought through, a treatment strategy must be formulated. This must include a plan for dosage of treatment, which will include identifying: joints to be treated (this must go beyond simply, for example, the elbow, or the thoracic spine) as the therapist must be anatomically specific); mobilizations to be employed (i.e. physiological or accessory, or combinations), and which specific types (or vectors) of mobilizations (for example, physiological flexion; accessory posteroanterior [PA] glide); grades of mobilizations (i.e. Maitland I–IV; Cyriax A–B, depending upon system employed); frequency of delivery (this includes consideration of the rhythm or speed of oscillations – which may be slow and gentle with one oscillation every one to two seconds (most appropriate for grade II and III, larger amplitude mobilizations), or sharp staccato – with two to three oscillations per second (most appropriate for grade I and IV, smaller amplitude mobilizations), or sustained without movement (Maitland *et al.*, 2005); duration of delivery of mobilizations – although evidence is lacking, 20–60 seconds of repetitions have been suggested for decreased range of motion, and 1–2 minutes for pain (however, this could be until a sense of symptom relief or reduction in stiffness or spasm is achieved, or simply a short set time frame, prior to any repeat application or re-testing); repetitions of a set of mobilizations (for example, the therapist may elect to perform one, two or three sets based on tissue and symptom response). Beyond this, further considerations to the successful delivery of manual therapy include: patient positioning; therapist position; handling and contact points; communication and feedback during application (visual, verbal and tactile); and assessment of efficacy (i.e. symptom relief; re-testing of clinical indicators). Cook (2012) presents a range of other subtle factors influencing delivery of mobilization therapy, including the fine-tuning of technique (such as altering the magnitude of forces, and the rate of any increase of force). When one considers the innumerable symptom-generating conditions that patients present with, in tandem with the variety of treatment strategies and techniques available to the sports therapist, it can be easily appreciated how exacting the practitioner must be from the outset.

Convex–concave rule

The shape of the articulating joint surfaces and direction of movement is defined to some degree by the convex–concave rule, which describes the directions of movement associated with a joint as being dependent upon the shape of the moving articular surfaces (Kaltenborn, 1999; Schomacher, 2009). Kessler and Hertling (1983) distinguished that as a concave surface

Table 3.7 Grades of mobilization (I–V Maitland; A–C Cyriax)

Grade	amplitude	Range of movement	Indication
I	Small	Start of range	Pain
II	Large	Across middle of range	Pain Stiffness
III	Large	Middle to end of range movement	Stiffness Pain
IV	Small	End of available range	Stiffness Momentary pain
V	Small, high velocity	A manipulation past end of presenting available range	Stiffness Pain
A	Small/large	Within pain-free elastic range. In peripheral joints. In mid-range at spinal joints	Pain
B	Small	At end of available range of peripheral and spinal joints. A sustained stretching technique to affect plastic deformation of connective tissues	Pain Stiffness
C	Small, high velocity	A manipulation past end of presenting available range	Stiffness Pain

Source: adapted from Atkins *et al.*, 2010; Maitland *et al.*, 2005.

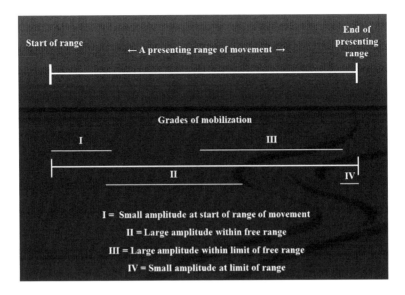

Photo 3.9 Grades of mobilization (source: adapted from Maitland *et al.*, 2005).

moves on a convex surface (where the convex surface is fixed), then accessory movement (roll and glide) will occur in the *same* direction to the angular physiological movement. In contrast, if the convex joint surface is moving on a fixed concave surface, then the accessory movement is in the *opposite* direction to the angular physiological movement. During flexion or extension of the knee in non-weight-bearing (seated or single-leg stance), the concave tibial condyles will glide in the same direction on the fixed convex femoral condyles. As explained, when a convex surface moves on a fixed concave surface, the accessory roll and glide occurs in the opposite direction to the physiological movement, such as with elevation of the glenohumeral joint through abduction; here, when the concave glenoid cavity is fixed, the convex surface of the humeral head translates inferiorly as the humerus physiologically travels superiorly. Some articulatory surfaces may be observed to be relatively flat, and have less obvious concavity and convexity, but where this is the case, the smaller, flatter joint surface will frequently present with intra-articular fibrocartilage contributing to form a degree of concavity. Recent literature has, however, questioned the universal clinical relevance of the convex–concave rule. Banks and Hengeveld (2010) place lesser credence on the model as an influence for planning manual therapy, particularly with regard to pain, and stipulate the use of the least painful accessory movement(s) as the starting point for joint mobilizations. Johnson *et al.* (2007) suggest that the direction of mobilization may be irrelevant in treatment where joint hypomobility is present.

Open- and close-packed positioning

Correct joint positioning will enhance the effectiveness of any mobilization technique. It is essential to be aware of the open- and close-packed positions of joints. In many cases, it is preferable to perform mobilizations with the target joint in an open (or loose)-packed position. The open-packed position indicates that the articulating surfaces are not maximally congruent, are separated, and the joint will exhibit a certain amount of joint play. This is the position in which the joint capsule and ligaments are less tense. In contrast, the close-packed position is where joint surfaces are most congruent and in maximal contact with each other, the main ligaments and joint capsule are in a taut state, and the joint is said to have maximum stability

Table 3.8 Considerations in manual therapy

Clinical indicators in manual therapy	A position, movement or test with an outcome measure which can provide criteria for evaluating progress in treatment. Essentially, a re-assessment method which can be used during a treatment session
Indications for manual therapy	In simple terms, indications for manual therapy include: hypomobile joints; capsular patterns; nerve root pain; peripheral neuropathic pain; joint and muscle-related somatic pain; muscle spasm or guarding. Each indication must be appraised further prior to any application, and furthermore it is essential that appropriate types and grades of mobilization are selected for the indicated condition
Contraindications to manual therapy	Clinically assessed reasons to either avoid manual therapy (absolute or general contraindications); or reasons to adapt or modify manual therapy and proceed with caution (local or precautionary contraindications). Examples include: red flag signs; yellow flag signs; patient unwell; underlying medical conditions (such as osteoporosis; cardiovascular disease; hypertension; acute inflammatory disease – such as rheumatoid arthritis; malignancy); fractures; VBI (see below); patient unstable on medications; infectious conditions; patient under the influence of alcohol or recreational drugs; undiagnosed lumps or lesions; varicose veins. Refer also to Table 3.5
Special questions in manual therapy	Due to the wide of range of causes of neuromusculoskeletal symptoms, the sports therapist must be able to ascertain all essential background information from the patient prior to the delivery of any objective assessment or manual therapy. Special questions are those which are required to help confirm the nature of the condition, the patient's suitability for manual therapy, and to guide what form the therapy will take in light of such. Special questions need to be asked regarding such presenting issues as: recent weight loss; recent illness (such as glandular fever, TB or meningitis); long-term illness (such as epilepsy, diabetes, multiple sclerosis, HIV, fibromyalgia, ankylosing spondylitis or rheumatoid arthritis); recent medical investigations (such as imaging scans or blood tests); recent or major operative interventions; and recent health care interventions (such as neurology; physiotherapy; osteopathy; or podiatry)
Precautions to manual therapy	Where it has been identified that a particular objective assessment or treatment technique may have the potential to produce an adverse effect, action should be taken in advance to protect against harm to the patient. This may simply involve: adapting procedures (such as reducing the intensity or duration of a technique or treatment session, or avoiding a body region); alternative patient positioning (such as performing techniques in seated positions); or considering alternative strategies to manual therapy
Vertebrobasilar insufficiency (VBI)	VBI is an essential consideration when dealing with patients who may have inadequate blood flow through the vertebral and basilar arteries which contribute to essential supply to the brain. Inadequate supply can initially cause such symptoms as dizziness, fainting, dysarthria, dysphagia, diplopia or nystagmus. VBI insufficiency can lead to TIA (transient ischaemic attack), CVA (cerebrovascular accident – a stroke) or even death. Practitioners must consider testing for VBI when considering applying manual therapy to the cervical spine, as insufficient vascularity is an absolute contraindication
Red flags in manual therapy	Warning signs of possible serious condition or pathology (such as cancer, significant and worsening unexplainable neural deficits or an unstable fracture). Sports therapists must be able to recognize such warning signs, which may present during the taking of a patient's history or during objective assessment. Example situations of where these must be considered include: unusual age of onset

	of a condition; history of violent trauma; constant non-mechanical pain (and which does not alter with position, movement or medication); night pain; thoracic pain; previous history of cancer; recent significant unexplained weight loss; systemically unwell; impaired bladder or bowel control, and dysaesthesia in the perianal region ('saddle anaesthesia') (both associated with cauda equina syndrome); blood in sputum; structural deformity; progressive neural deficits; bilateral radiculopathy; ulcer-type wounds which do not heal; abnormally presenting moles; clonus signs; long-term corticosteroid use; suspicion of DVT (deep vein thrombosis). This list is not exhaustive
Yellow flags in manual therapy	Warning signs to the biopsychosocial factors which may be predictors of chronicity. 'Bio' relates to the biological and pathological aspect of the presenting injury or condition; 'psycho' relates to the cognitive aspects, the patient's attitude, beliefs, emotions and behaviours regarding their condition; and 'social' relates to the patient's domestic, work, social and cultural environment and stressors thereof. By being vigilant and sensitive to any presenting yellow flag signs, the therapist is better able to support and advise the patient accordingly. Biopsychosocial factors can be the cause of stress, depression, work absenteeism, fear avoidance beliefs about activity and work and symptom exacerbation. Importantly, yellow flags may affect patient adherence to the therapeutic programme. There may also be additional considerations, such as compensation issues
Adverse effects of manual therapy	Undesirable effects of treatment, which may be short term and mild adverse effects (such as symptom exacerbation, muscle soreness or headache); or extremely rare major adverse effects (including vascular insults, neurological incapacity or death) (Carnes et al., 2010). Adverse effects can be the result of poor practice (in patient selection, assessment or treatment) or due to unforeseeable, unexpected patient responses to treatment
Patient-centred manual therapy	In manual therapy clinical decisions must be patient-centred. This means that patients' understandings, beliefs and feelings are considered and influence the resulting interventions. Patients must be encouraged to be active participants (IFOMPT, 2010)
Patient values	The recognition of the unique expectations, concerns and beliefs that each patient has in any clinical situation. The individualized aspect of any case must be considered and integrated into resulting clinical decisions (IFOMPT, 2010)
Placebo effect	The perceivable or expected after-effect of an intervention. It has been suggested that manual therapy may provide a powerful, short-term placebo effect (Cook, 2012)
Equipment in manual therapy	While the emphasis in manual therapy is the use of techniques delivered by hand, equipment to support such delivery may include: height-adjustable couch; bolsters; and mobilization belts
Manual therapy variables	The various ways in which the therapist may elect to deliver their treatment, which must be based on identified objectives and any precautionary contraindications. Variables may include: the positioning of the patient; the positioning of the target joint(s); the directions of mobilization techniques; the type of mobilization techniques employed (i.e. physiological; accessory; combination; oscillatory; sustained); the grades of mobilization (i.e. I–IV; A–C); the duration of application; the number of repeat applications
Proposed beneficial effects of manual therapy	Pain relief; improved specific mobility; increased local blood flow; break down of fibrous adhesions; elastic and/or plastic deformation of soft tissues; improved functional mobility; patient education

Table 3.9 Precautions and contraindications to manual therapy

Absolute contraindications
Contagious infection
Severe cardiovascular disease
Deep vein thrombosis
Phlebitis
Inflammatory arthritis
Malignancy
Bone disease
Fracture
Congenitally deformed bone
Vertebral artery insufficiency
Recent operative procedures
High severity or irritability
Unremitting night pain (preventing patient from falling asleep)
Conditions involving neurology (i.e. UMNL; spinal cord injury; cauda equina syndrome)
Significant neural symptoms (multi-level; worsening symptoms)
Patient under influence of alcohol or recreational drugs
Conditions requiring specialized medical supervision

Precautions
Significant joint laxity/instability
Pain exacerbated by lying down
Five Ds (dizziness; drop attacks; diplopia; dysarthria; dysphagia) – cervical manual therapy
contraindicated
History of cardiovascular disease
History of cancer
Medication that alters pain perception or circulatory response
Benign tumour
Acute injury/wound
Nerve root signs
Long-term steroid use
Systemically unwell
Recent manual or manipulative therapy from another health professional

Source: adapted from Cook, 2012; Maitland *et al.*, 2005; Prentice, 2011; Hengeveld and Banks, 2005; Greenhalgh and Selfe, 2007; Vizniak, 2012).

Note: This list is not exhaustive; if there is any doubt regarding the suitability of patients for manual therapy, then medical opinion must be sought.

(Mangus *et al.*, 2002). Initial mobilization is performed in an open–packed position; however, in some cases the position is determined by that which is least painful and most comfortable for the patient.

Safety, precautions, contraindications and adverse reactions in manual therapy

As with all manual therapies, the sports therapist must be fully conversant with red flag signs and precautions to treatment. Numerous authors (including Cook, 2012; Maitland *et al.*, 2005; Prentice, 2011; Hengeveld and Banks, 2005; Greenhalgh and Selfe, 2006; and Vizniak, 2012) have presented safety considerations and precautions and contraindications to manual therapy treatment.

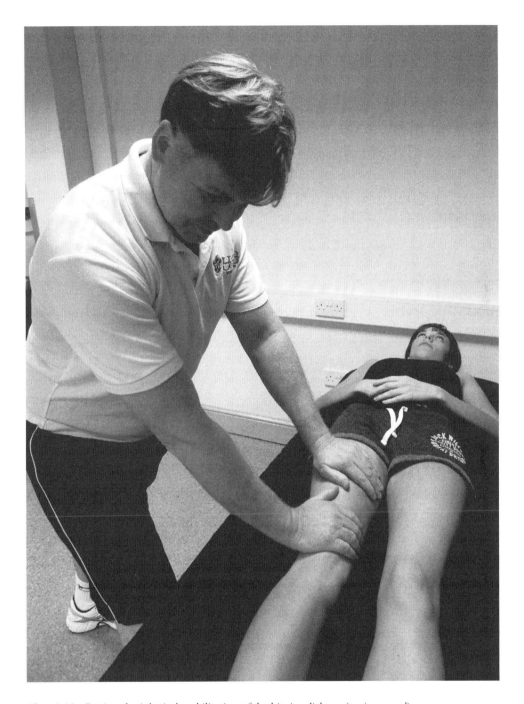

Photo 3.10 Passive physiological mobilization of the hip (medial rotation in neutral).

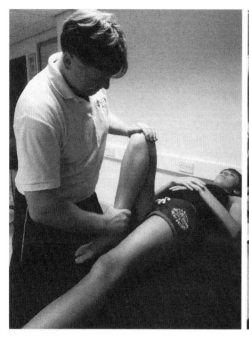

Photo 3.11 Passive physiological mobilization of the knee (flexion).

Photo 3.12 Accessory mobilization of the subtalar joint (AP glide).

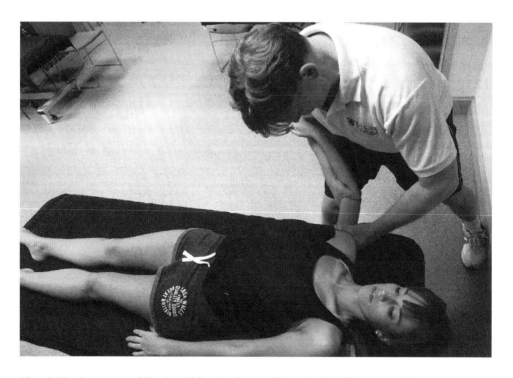

Photo 3.13 Accessory mobilization of the glenohumeral joint (caudad glide in 90° abduction).

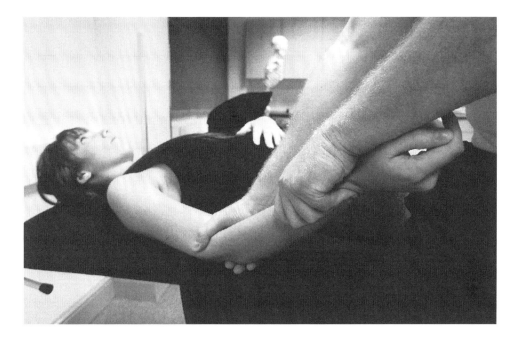

Photo 3.14 Accessory mobilization of the radiohumeral joint (caudad glide in 30° elbow flexion).

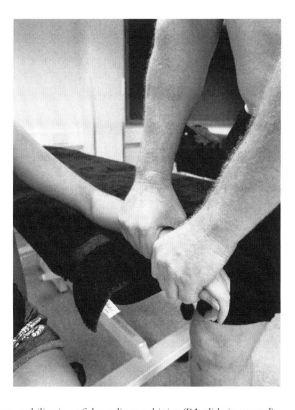

Photo 3.15 Accessory mobilization of the radiocarpal joint (PA glide in neutral).

Adverse effects may result from poor practice (in patient selection, assessment or treatment) or may be due to unforeseeable, unexpected patient responses to treatment. Carnes *et al.* (2010) identified that the risk of major adverse events within manual therapy is low, but that the prevalence of minor to moderate adverse events after treatment is more significant. Major adverse events (which may include vascular insults, neurological incapacity or even death) have been described as medium- to long-term duration, moderate to severe, and are considered unacceptable. They will also by nature normally require further medical care. Moderate adverse events differ from major simply in that they are less severe, but still require careful patient monitoring, such as with a worsening of symptoms. Mild events are described as being short-term and of low severity, and symptoms are transient and reversible; these may include mild inflammatory reactions, tissue tenderness, slight worsening of symptoms and post-treatment fatigue. In order to offset the potential for adverse events, sports therapists must recognize the significance of undertaking a detailed patient history, appreciating the history of the main complaint and, importantly for manual therapy, the severity, irritability and nature (SIN) of symptoms.

Neurodynamic mobilization

Butler (1991), Butler and Nee (2006), Coppieters and Nee (2012), Learman and Cook (2012), Ridehalgh and Barnard (2012) and Shacklock (1995; 2005) all discuss at length the specialized aspect of manual therapy which focuses on managing symptoms involving peripheral nervous tissue. The term 'neurodynamics' implies functional movement of the nervous system, and more explicitly, neurodynamics is the interaction between physiological and mechanical functions of the nervous system (Shacklock, 1995). In the clinical environment, neurodynamics must incorporate physical assessment of the functioning of the peripheral nervous system (sensory and motor). This includes (in addition to any other appropriate assessment methods) dermatomal, myotomal and reflex testing, and assessment of the mobility and irritability of peripheral nerves (via neurodynamic tests and nerve palpation). While neurodynamic therapy is indicated for peripheral neuropathic pain states (Coppieters and Nee, 2012), the nervous system must be viewed very much as a continuum, and any movements of the body will transmit forces along the system (Shacklock, 2005). Indeed, just as cervical flexion has been shown to alter the position and tension of the lumbar spinal cord and nerve roots, the straight leg raise (SLR) can exert tensioning and altered positioning via the sciatic nerve, spinal cord and thecal sac, up to the brain and its meninges (Breig, 1978). The tissues and structures found in close association with peripheral nerves as they pass through the body from nerve root to distal periphery may be described as mechanical interfaces; these include the fibro-osseous tunnels, muscles, tendons, joint capsules, ligaments, fibrous discs and fascia. The mechanical interfaces associated with each peripheral nerve may be considered as 'neighbouring' and 'container' tissues (NOI, 2010). It is important to recognize that local pathological states (such as with soft tissue inflammation, fibrosis or arthritic degeneration), as well as joint instability, can easily contribute to the irritation of peripheral nerves at mechanical interfaces during certain movements – and even simply at rest. The structure of the peripheral nerves themselves is complex and also varies throughout their length, and this in itself influences function (consider the perineurium, the distribution of the myelin sheath, the nodes of Ranvier and distribution of ion channels, the essential blood supply to the nerve and the 'nerve of the nerve' – the nervi nervorum). Shacklock (2005) explains that the perineurium *'is effectively the cabling in the peripheral nerve'* and *'the primary guardian against excessive tension'*. Formed from densely packed connective tissue, the perineurium contributes longitudinal strength and elasticity to the nerve, and has viscoelastic properties. Sunderland (1991) identified that peripheral nerves are able to withstand 18–22 per cent strain before failure. Simply, peripheral nerves, in addition to being directly affected by demyelinating disorders (such as Guillain-Barre syndrome), and indirectly by systemic conditions such as chronic diabetes, are also extremely vulnerable (sensitive) to the prolonged restrictive and compressive stresses associated with their mechanical interfaces. Such presenting conditions as carpal tunnel syndrome (CTS) or tarsal tunnel syndrome (TTS) often have a multifaceted aetiology, and practitioners should consider the local factors at the mechanical interfaces, as well as the 'double-crush' situation (where nerves are adversely affected at more than one site) (Schmid and Coppieters, 2010). Prolonged compression and restriction of a peripheral nerve can lead to local neural ischaemia, hypoxia, oedema, fibrosis, impaired axonal transport and ion channel alterations (and the development of abnormal impulse-generating sites – AIGS) (Coppieters and Nee, 2012). Symptomatically, these conditions can lead to local and diffuse, radiating pain, allodynia, hyperalgesia, dysaesthesias and, in resistant cases, muscle weakness and further limitations in functional ranges of movement.

Where positive signs and symptoms are present, specific neurodynamic therapy techniques may then be indicated and employed, obviously in conjunction with other treatment and advice. As Ridehalgh and Barnard (2012) emphasize *'there is no pure treatment for nerves, that is, treatment cannot be isolated to nerve alone: it will always, to a greater or lesser extent, affect joint and/or muscle tissues'*. Nerve mobilization is the passive (or active) delivery of movement to facilitate therapeutic effects in the nervous system. Techniques may involve gross movements which mobilize or tension the nervous system, or more localized movements employed to affect mechanical interfaces and neural connective tissue (Butler, 1991). Once a clinical impression of the patient has been ascertained, the sports therapist may elect to use neurodynamic techniques to reduce symptoms and improve function. It is obviously imperative that the therapist has a competent understanding of peripheral neural anatomy in order to both identify specific problems associated with it, and to also affect it safely, positively, locally and globally. Confident working knowledge of the peripheral nervous system is essential for this aspect of clinical therapy. Sports therapists must know the five peripheral nerve plexuses (cervical – C1–4; brachial – C5–T1; lumbar – L1–4; lumbosacral – L4–S3; and sacral – S3–5); the main peripheral nerves (and their segmental origins and peripheral distributions); and the more global interconnectedness of the nervous system, including the relationship of the peripheral nervous system to the central nervous system (spinal cord and brain) and to all other body tissues. The sports therapist must aim to know all of the main muscles supplied by each of the main peripheral nerves. In the upper limb, the main peripheral nerve routes to familiarize (from the brachial plexus) are the axillary, musculocutaneous, ulnar, median and radial nerves and their tributaries. In the lower limb, the obturator and femoral nerves originate from the lumbar plexus. The superior and inferior gluteal nerves, and the sciatic nerve and its branches (tibial, common, superficial and deep peroneal, medial and lateral plantar nerves), all originate from the lumbosacral plexus.

Following the clinical assessment, the therapist should have formulated a working hypothesis of the nature of the patient's problem, and the type and cause of their injury or pain. However, it is important to recognize that clinical assessment, including neurodynamic testing, cannot always irrefutably locate the precise source of symptoms; furthermore, asymptomatic patients may also experience positive limitations or discomfort during testing (Learman and Cook, 2012). Whether musculoskeletal and nociceptive, neuropathic, systemically pathological, acute or chronic, there may still be a good rationale for utilizing peripheral neural mobilization therapy. Just as with manual therapy applied to joint restrictions or pain, neural mobilization must be carefully planned, graded, delivered and evaluated. Particularly important to the assessment and ultimate mobilization of peripheral neural tissue are the recognized neurodynamic

Table 3.10 Terminology in neurodynamic mobilization

Neurodynamics	The interaction between physiological and mechanical functions of the nervous system (Shacklock, 1995)
Nerve mobilization	The active or passive delivery of movement to facilitate therapeutic effects in the nervous system. May involve gross movement techniques which mobilize or tension the nervous system, or more localized movements employed to affect mechanical interfaces and neural connective tissue (Butler, 1991)
Adverse neural tension	*'Any abnormal physiological or mechanical response from the nervous system that limits the nervous system's range or stretch or results in neurological symptoms through available range'* (Cook, 2012)
Sensitizing and desensitizing manoeuvres	Sensitizing manoeuvres involve delivery of systematic (sequenced) multipositional joint movements so as to evoke a carefully increased tensioning in neural tissue. May be used as a procedure in the assessment of patients with suspected adverse neural tension; or as part of a neural tensioning mobilization strategy. Desensitizing manoeuvres, which slacken neural tension to a degree, may be performed so as to reduce symptoms of neural tension during assessment; or as part of a neural gliding mobilization strategy
Neural glides	Slow, methodical, active or passive movements designed to mobilize neural tissue through its available range. These techniques have also been described as 'neurodynamic sliders' or 'nerve flossing'
Neural tensioners	Slow, methodical, active or passive movements designed to offer gentle tensile stress to neural tissue
Mechanical interfaces	The tissues and structures found in close association with peripheral nerve tissue (such as fibro-osseous tunnels, muscles, tendons, joint capsules, ligaments, fibrous discs and fascia). May be considered as 'neighbouring' 'container' tissues (NOI, 2010). It is important to recognize that pathological responses (inflammation; arthropathy) can contribute to irritation at mechanical interfaces

tests. While best approaches and methods used to assess the mobility and symptom response of neural tissue are under constant appraisal and development, the four main tests used to assess the main upper limb nerves are known simply as upper limb neurodynamic tests (ULNTs). These are sequential and individualized multipositional joint movements which are designed to carefully lengthen specific peripheral nerves to a point of gentle tension or very mild symptom response. ULNT1 predominantly affects the median nerve pathway; ULNT2a affects the median, musculocutaneous and axillary pathways; ULNT2b affects the radial pathway; and ULNT3 affects the ulnar pathway. In the lower limb, the most well-recognized tests are the: femoral nerve stretch (slump knee bend) test; slump test (which assesses for possible neural irritation at the level of the spinal cord or dura mater, or through the peripheral sciatic distribution); and the SLR test (for lumbar nerve root and sciatic irritation). All neurodynamic tests must be performed carefully (as by nature neural tissue is sensitive, responsive and irritable). Sensitizing manoeuvres individualize the assessment via systematic (sequenced) positioning of the patient so as to evoke an increased tensioning of neural tissue. Desensitizing manoeuvres are performed so as to reduce neural tension slightly and help to confirm assessment findings. Adverse neural tension may be considered as a symptomatic limitation in range of movement affected by the restrictions placed on neural pathways.

As well as being used to assess adverse neural tension, sensitizing manoeuvres may then be used as part of the neural mobilization strategy; such techniques have been described as 'neural tensioners' – which, although performed slowly and methodically and designed to offer gentle tensile stress to neural tissue, can be irritating to more acute or irritable conditions. In such cases, 'neural glides' (also known as 'neurodynamic sliders') are similarly slow and methodical movements, but are designed to mobilize neural tissue through a designated and non-provocative range. When performing tensioning neural mobilization, the approach utilizes sequential, individualized, multipositional, proximal and distal joint movements to move the targeted peripheral nerve to a point of gentle tension (essentially 'sensitizing' the tissue via nerve strain). Nee and Butler (2006) suggest that tensioning techniques are not nerve stretches, and that they *'are performed in an oscillatory fashion so as to gently engage resistance to movement that is usually associated with protective muscle activity'*. Coppieters and Nee (2012) have highlighted that many conditions are not amenable to such tensioning techniques. When glides are performed the target peripheral nerve pathway is mobilized (still using the sequential, multipositional, proximal and distal approach) through its available range, but importantly not to a point of potentially irritating tension – simply one end of the pathway (distal or proximal) is moved towards the other and vice versa in a series of repetitions. Coppieters and Nee (2012) explain that *'sliding techniques result not only in a larger longitudinal excursion of the nerve relative to surrounding structures, but are also not associated with significant increases in strain'*. The starting point for treatment is established via the assessment of where in the sequential range of joint positions the limitations, tensions or symptoms are apparent (via the neurodynamic tests). Neural mobilizations, therefore, move the target peripheral nerve, its nerve bed and all associated connective tissue, fascia, muscles, tendons, bones and joint surfaces through a range of movement, carefully, repetitively and non-provocatively, from a pre-assessed start position. It is important not to mentally separate neural mobilization from manual therapy as a whole; the method for mobilizing nerves may be enhanced locally via directed soft tissue techniques (such as myofascial release or frictions) to any restrictive connective tissues or muscles (using muscle energy, neuromuscular or STR techniques). Physiological and accessory spinal or peripheral joint mobilization techniques are also usually used in combination with neural mobilizations.

The most appropriate method and strategy to employ cannot be ascertained without an individualized clinical assessment. It may be that designated STT, followed by specified spinal and peripheral joint mobilizations, will pave the way for more effective neurodynamic mobilization, but this may not always be the case. Similarly, the sports therapist must also clinically reason their way through the actual delivery of the neural mobilizations – for a start position to mobilize the median nerve pathway, for example, the patient may be positioned in supine with shoulder depression, then shoulder abduction to 90° and lateral rotation to 85°, the elbow may be extended to perhaps 35° flexion, the forearm to 90° supination, the wrist to 70° extension and the cervical spine may remain in neutral. Some patients will not tolerate such positioning because of the symptom response (or because of comorbidities); for others this position will not provide sufficient tensioning to provide effective mobilization. However, as an example, from such a start position, to gently tension the tissues the sports therapist may then sensitize through cervical lateral flexion carefully to the contralateral side while at the same time increasing extension at the elbow or wrist (hence, tensioning at both ends of the chain). Potentially less provocatively, to glide through this range (without providing additional proximal and distal tension) from the previous starting position, the therapist may instead desensitize the neural pathway via cervical lateral flexion to the ipsilateral side, while at the same time further extending the elbow and/or wrist. This may sound complicated; but with practice these techniques can become easily employed. It is important to familiarize the ways in which each of the main peripheral nerve pathways may be mobilized.

Table 3.11 Delivering neurodynamic mobilizations

Modifier	Description
Grade of movement	Small-amplitude movement, short of resistance
	Larger-amplitude movement, short of resistance
	Large-amplitude movement into early resistance
	Small-amplitude movement into resistance
Direction of movement	May be longitudinal or transverse, but most likely will be a combination
Sequence of movement	The therapist may elect to emphasize the mobilizations via use of any of the proximal, middle or distal joint positions within the chain of involved joints, depending upon where the treatment is to be focused
Amplitude of oscillation	Movements may utilize short, sustained positions (tensioners) or slow, oscillatory techniques (gliders). These movements may be graded (as above)
Velocity and rhythm of movement	With gliding techniques, to avoid irritation, the velocity is generally slow or slightly faster through the graded range. Further, the rhythm may be smooth and steady, or staccato. With tensioning techniques, if indicated, the recommendation is to move towards neural strain slowly
Repetition of movement	The therapist should aim to provide neurodynamic mobilizations with a vigilant awareness of how the techniques are affecting the patient and their symptoms. If the patient is easily irritated, then techniques may need to be adjusted (by reducing the grade and position) or abandoned. If little or no provocation is apparent, then just as with joint mobilizations, the neurodynamic mobilizations may be continued, typically for between 20–60 seconds (although evidence is lacking)
Repeat applications	The therapist may elect to perform one, two or three sets of repetitions based on tissue and symptom response, and on ongoing clinical assessment
Progression methods	Progression is dependent on tissue, symptom and patient response. If there is no provocation, progressions in treatment can be maintained by altering joint positions (moving towards ends of ranges), increasing the direction and magnitude of force, reducing the amplitude of oscillation, increasing the duration of application, and also potentially (carefully) allowing more symptoms to be provoked
Regression methods	Regression is required when symptomatic irritation is apparent. The therapist may employ alterations to the ranges of joint movements involved, reduced direction and magnitude of force, increased amplitude of oscillation or reduced duration of application, all generally aimed at allowing fewer symptoms to be provoked

Source: adapted from Ridehalgh and Barnard, 2012.

Just as with all other interventions, the sports therapist must consider the full clinical impression of the patient and any potential contraindications or precautions prior to delivery. They must then consider grades of movement, repetitions of movement, duration of repetitions, re-testing movements for symptom changes, repeat applications and home care advice. Ridehalgh and Barnard (2012) suggest that the magnitude of force applied by the therapist should be related to their perception of resistance, and graded I–V. Such grades are related to those put forward by

Magarey (1986) and Maitland *et al.* (2005) for joint mobilizations. However, such a grading system for neural mobilizations has limitations; this is due in part to the fact that tensioning techniques are different to gliding techniques, and that there is also such a subtle flexibility in how neural mobilizations may be approached and performed. Probably the most important influence of the delivery of neurodynamic mobilizations is how irritable the patient's symptoms are, and how easily their symptoms are provoked. The evidence-base to support best practice in patients presenting with nerve-related symptoms is still evolving. A number of authors (Coppieters and Nee, 2012; Learman and Cook, 2012) have explored the limited evidence to support nerve gliding, nerve tensioning and the long-term clinical effectiveness, but conclude that further randomized trials with long-term follow-up are required.

Approaches to manual therapy delivery

In summary, manual therapy requires great care and process in delivery, and therapists must consider the following:

- patient history and prioritized objective assessment;
- the problem list and set of short-/long-term therapeutic goals prior to treatment;
- awareness of precautions and contraindications;
- main indications including local pain, hypomobility, dyskinesia and low-grade nerve irritation;
- main clinical indicators;
- type, range and grade of mobilizations required;
- patient positioning, patient handling, repetitions, duration and sets;
- patient, tissue and symptom response during treatment (visual, verbal and tactile);
- re-assessment of clinical indicators;
- selective use of additional interventions (such as STT or taping);
- patient home exercise and other advice;
- documentation of all assessment findings and specific management provided.

Cryotherapy

With Peter K. Thain

Within sports medicine environments, cryotherapy – literally meaning cold therapy – is a widely used therapeutic modality for the treatment of acute injuries, in addition to facilitating rehabilitation (Bleakley *et al.*, 2004; Knight, 1995; Knight *et al.*, 2000; MacAuley, 2001). In order to administer the most appropriate treatment for the athlete, it is imperative that the therapist understands the physiological effects of cryotherapy. This section therefore will outline the physiological effects of cryotherapy, before recommending specific modalities for use, dependent upon the aims of treatment.

Physiological effects of cold application

Analgesia

The immediate application of ice aims to provide a cold-induced analgesic effect, thereby reducing the appreciation of pain (Algafly and George, 2007; Bleakley and Hopkins, 2010; Saeki, 2002). Evidence suggests that cooling of peripheral nervous tissue prolongs the latency and duration of sensory action potentials, resulting in decreased nerve transmission (de Jong *et al.*, 1966). Additionally, a declining temperature suppresses nociceptive receptor sensitivity (Kunesch *et al.*, 1987), and may also act as a possible counterirritant (Saeki, 2002). Previous work examining the effect of ice application on analgesia has identified targeted skin temperatures to be 10–13.6 °C in order to provide an analgesic effect (Algafly and George, 2007; Bugaj, 1975). If these target temperatures are achieved, nerve conduction velocity can be reduced by 10–33 per cent (Algafly and George, 2007; McMeeken *et al.*, 1984). The rate at which the nerve conduction can be slowed, and thus how quickly analgesia will be experienced, is dependent entirely upon the modality's ability to reduce tissue temperature (Knight, 1995).

Metabolism

While there is unequivocal evidence to support the use of cryotherapy to provide an analgesic effect (Algafly and George, 2007; Bleakley *et al.*, 2004; Grant, 1964; Hayden, 1964; Knight *et al.*, 2000; Pincivero *et al.*, 1993), there is currently no research involving human subjects which supports the ability of ice application to reduce swelling. Until recently it was thought that ice application was fundamental in limiting the formation of oedema – typically referred to as swelling. When an injury occurs and there is structural damage, the swelling at the site of injury results from direct haemorrhaging and oedema (Knight, 1995). The swelling that occurs immediately with soft tissue injury is the result of haemorrhaging. Haemostasis can take place within minutes and by the time the extent of the injury has been determined, the haemorrhaging has probably stopped. Therefore, it is the delayed swelling, termed oedema, that therapists will be concerned with. The original premise of ice application by Knight (1995) was not to stop the initial haemorrhaging, but to reduce the effects of secondary hypoxic injury which causes disruption to healthy cells. The premise was that ice application would reduce metabolism, which in turn would limit the demands for oxygen in the tissue on the periphery of the injury, reducing secondary ischaemia and enzymatic injury and consequently oedema (Bleakley and Hopkins, 2010; Knight, 1995; Merrick, 2002).

A target temperature to reduce the oxygen demands of the injured tissue and reduce metabolic activity by 50 per cent is reported to be 10–11 °C (Sapega *et al.*, 1988). However, while these target temperatures are readily achievable at the level of the skin, such temperatures are yet to be reported at depths where the majority of musculoskeletal injuries occur – and where the reduction in temperature is typically required. Consequently, following the work of Bleakley and Hopkins (2010) and others, it is currently apparent that there is limited reliable evidence to support the notion that ice application plays an active role in reducing secondary hypoxic injury, and thus oedema. What does this mean for the future of ice and cryotherapy? First, ice is a fantastic, non-pharmacological modality for helping to reduce pain. Additionally, it may be argued that while it may not be possible to reduce deeper tissues to 10 °C, even if the temperature declines by 1 °C then perceivably this may still be of some benefit.

Skin temperature response to cold applications

When cryotherapeutic modalities are applied to the skin there is an immediate and rapid reduction in skin temperature (Dykstra *et al.*, 2009; Enwemeka *et al.*, 2002; Merrick *et al.*, 2003). Numerous studies have evaluated the effects of cooling skin temperature with a variety of application durations. Ice-based modalities consisting of crushed or cubed ice have been shown to reduce localized skin temperature to the required target temperature of 10–13.6 °C for analgesia within five minutes (Ebrall *et al.*, 1989; Ebrall *et al.*, 1992; Janwantanakul, 2006) and ten minutes (Jutte *et al.*, 2001; Kanlayanaphotporn and Janwantanakul, 2005; Merrick *et al.*, 2003). After the immediate sharp reduction in skin temperature, the rate of decline steadily

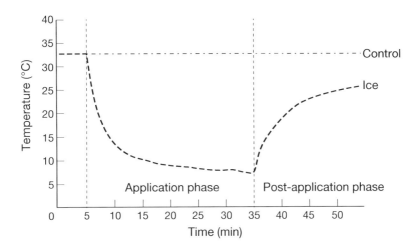

Figure 3.1 The effect of ice bag application on skin temperature (°C) throughout a 30-minute application to the anterior thigh (source: adapted from Merrick *et al.*, 1993).

slows after approximately five minutes (Jutte *et al.*, 2001; Merrick *et al.*, 2003) until eventually reaching a plateau just above the temperature of the modality (Knight, 1995). Following the cessation of ice application, skin temperature increases sharply – mirroring the initial decrease but to a lesser magnitude – before gradually returning to pre-application temperatures (Jutte *et al.*, 2001; Merrick *et al.*, 1993). Figure 3.1 illustrates the typical skin temperature response to cooling.

Subcutaneous and deep tissue response to cold applications

The rate of deep tissue cooling depends on the depth of the target tissue (Merrick *et al.*, 2003; Myrer *et al.*, 1998; 2001). The temperature decline in subcutaneous tissue (just beneath the surface) following ice application presents a similar temperature decline curve to that of the skin, although to a lesser magnitude (Knight 1995; Myrer *et al.*, 1998). At this level there is still an immediate rapid decline in temperature initially, followed by a more gradual decline throughout the remainder of the icing period (Enwemeka *et al.*, 2002; Myrer *et al.*, 1998). Likewise, the rewarming of superficial tissues replicates that of skin temperature (Myrer *et al.*, 1998), with a sharp increase in temperature followed by a more gradual increase to pre-application temperatures at ten minutes after the removal of application (Enwemeka *et al.*, 2002).

At increased depths, such as that of intramuscular tissue, a linear decline in temperature at a depth of 1 cm below the subcutaneous tissue is maintained throughout a 20- (Myrer *et al.*, 1998; 2000; 2001) and 30-minute application period (Merrick *et al.*, 1993; 2003). The decline is gradual and to a lesser magnitude than that of superficial tissues (see Figure 3.2), outlining that the deeper the target tissue, the slower the response and more limited the extent of cooling due to a diminishing thermal gradient (Enwemeka *et al.*, 2002; Jutte *et al.*, 2001; Merrick *et al.*, 2003). Merrick *et al.* (2003) illustrate this well as surface temperature declined by 25 °C following a 30-minute ice bag application to the anterior thigh, while at depths of 1 cm and 2 cm beneath the subcutaneous tissue, intramuscular temperature reduced just 8 °C and 4.5 °C, respectively. It is for this reason that the ability of cryotherapy modalities to reduce metabolism and thus limit secondary hypoxia injury has been questioned (Bleakley and Hopkins, 2010).

The target tissue temperature for a reduction in metabolism, which would most likely be at the equivalent depth of 2 cm beneath the subcutaneous tissue in the human model, has been reported to be approximately 10 °C (Sapega *et al.*, 1988). In the study by Merrick *et al.* (2003), the temperature at 2 cm sub-adipose tissue was 30.6 °C following 30 minutes of wet ice application. No study to date has achieved a muscle temperature below 20 °C in human tissue (Bleakley and Hopkins, 2010).

In contrast to superficial tissues, following the removal of ice bag application there is a continued decline in intramuscular temperature at subcutaneous depths of 1 cm (Merrick *et al.*, 1993; Myrer *et al.*, 1998; Zemke *et al.*, 1998), 2 cm (Dykstra *et al.*, 2009; Jutte *et al.*, 2001; Merrick *et al.*, 1993) and 3 cm (Myrer *et al.*, 2001). It has been reported that the temperature continually declined for five minutes after removal of the application (Merrick *et al.*, 1993), while Myrer *et al.* (1998) stated the decline was very minimal. Conversely, a decline in temperature for 15 minutes after the removal of ice application has been reported (Dykstra *et al.*, 2009). Such variances in results for ice bag application can be attributed to the depth of the thermistor (the temperature-sensitive resistor), with measurements obtained at 2 cm beneath the subcutaneous tissue by Dykstra *et al.* (2009), in comparison to 1 cm beneath the subcutaneous tissue by Merrick *et al.* (1993) and Myrer *et al.* (1998). These findings collectively underpin the thermodynamic principle regarding the conduction of thermal energy that the sports therapist needs to understand. The skin temperature will begin to rise by conduction of heat from the atmosphere, with superficial tissues subsequently warming via the absorption of thermal energy from the overlying warmed skin (Merrick *et al.*, 2003). This process continues, concluding that the deeper the tissue the greater the delay in heat absorption, thus resulting in prolonged temperature reductions.

Cryotherapy modalities

While cryotherapy is frequently used in sports environments, there is no consensus on the optimum modality (MacAuley, 2001; Merrick *et al.*, 2003). As previously discussed, there is a decline in skin temperature with continued application, until a temperature plateau is eventually reached just above the temperature of the modality (Knight, 1995). This would imply that the

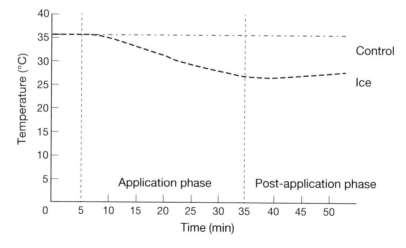

Figure 3.2   The effect of ice bag application on intramuscular (fat + 1 cm) temperature (°C) throughout a 30-minute application to the anterior thigh (source: adapted from Merrick *et al.*, 1993).

coldest modality would produce the greatest reduction in skin temperature and would therefore be the best modality at extracting heat from the body; however, this is not the case. When ice is applied to the skin, a thermal gradient exists between the modality and the temperature of the body (Knight, 1995). Basic thermodynamic principles suggest that the heat energy from the tissues is conducted into the modality. Over a period of time the modality will rise in temperature and become less effective as the thermal gradient decreases. Consequently, studies investigating the efficacy of different cryotherapy modalities at reducing skin temperature often compare ice bag application to that of commercially available gel packs (Belitsky *et al.*, 1987; Kanlayanaphotporn and Janwantanakul, 2005; Kennet *et al.*, 2007; Merrick *et al.*, 2003).

The temperature of an ice bag prior to application is often 0 °C, while a gel or cryogen pack may be as low as −14 °C, and therefore the packs tend to remain prevalent in sports clubs, with first aiders and therapists possibly believing that colder is better (Kennet *et al.*, 2007). Despite these commonly held beliefs, the evidence conclusively shows that after 15 (Belitsky *et al.*, 1987), 20 (Kanlayanaphotporn and Janwantanakul, 2005; Kennet *et al.*, 2007) and 30 minutes of application (Merrick *et al.*, 2003), there is a greater reduction in skin temperature when using an ice bag compared to a gel pack. This can be attributed to the greater heat capacity of ice (Knight, 1995), in addition to the need to overcome the latent heat of fusion (Merrick *et al.*, 2003). In other words, it takes a considerable amount of thermal energy to change one unit mass of a substance from solid to liquid without any change of temperature (Ellse and Honeywill, 2004). As a gel pack does not undergo a change in state, its ability to extract heat from tissue is significantly reduced in comparison to an ice pack. This is illustrated by Kennet *et al.* (2007) as the temperature of an ice bag throughout a 20-minute application period increased only 0.2 °C, in comparison to an increase of 12.3 °C seen in the gel pack. Furthermore, Merrick *et al.* (2003) observed a progressive decline in skin temperature throughout a 30-minute ice bag application, in contrast to a gel pack which reached its lowest skin temperature after just 11 minutes. Consequently, evidence suggests that ice-based modalities cause a greater reduction in skin temperature as a result of undergoing a change in state, therefore increasing the ability to absorb heat.

With regard to ice bag applications, ice is often delivered in non-porous bags in the form of cubed ice (Dykstra *et al.*, 2009; Hart *et al.*, 2005; Jutte *et al.*, 2001) or crushed ice (Dykstra *et al.*,

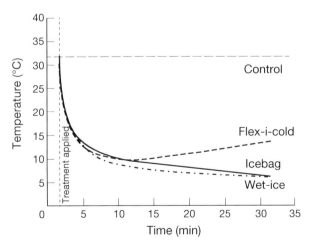

Figure 3.3 The effect of three different cryotherapy modalities on skin temperature (°C) throughout a 30-minute application to the anterior thigh (source: adapted from Merrick *et al.*, 2003).

2009; Hopkins *et al.*, 2006). Such methods are referred to as dry ice due to the non-porous nature of the bag and the dry interface (Belitsky *et al.*, 1987). Several studies have used wet ice, consisting of a fabric bag into which crushed ice is added (Belitsky *et al.*, 1987; Ebrall *et al.*, 1992; Kennet *et al.*, 2007; Merrick *et al.*, 2003). This porous material provides a wet interface to stop potential ice burn, while the water remains in contact with the skin. Based on the concept that cryotherapy modalities absorb heat through conduction and evaporation, wet ice exhibits a greater thermal conduction than that of its dry ice counterpart, and has therefore been shown to be superior at reducing skin temperatures (Belitsky *et al.*, 1987). After 15 minutes of application, the wet ice modality has been shown to reduce skin temperature by 12 °C in comparison to a reduction of 9.9 °C following dry ice bag application (Belitsky *et al.*, 1987). Additionally, in the literature reviewed, the lowest skin temperature reported after ten minutes of ice application was 3.6 °C, which utilized a wet ice method (Ebrall *et al.* 1992).

While recovery ice baths will be discussed later in this section, ice immersion techniques are also commonly used during early injury management (Kennet *et al.*, 2007; Myrer *et al.*, 1998) – mainly for peripheral extremities (ankle, foot, elbow, wrist and hand). The general consensus appears to be that the colder the water, the greater the reduction in tissue temperature (Knight *et al.*, 1981). However, there is a lack of high-quality research directly comparing wet ice application and ice immersion techniques. Recently, it has been identified that wet ice produces lower skin temperatures compared to immersion after 20 minutes of application to the ankle; however, the temperature of the immersion was 10 °C, with the effects of a colder ice bath such as 1–4 °C unknown (Kennet *et al.*, 2007). A comparison in temperature changes of the calf muscle following 20 minutes of either cold whirlpool immersion (10 °C), or crushed ice bag application identified that ice bag application reduced intramuscular (subcutaneous + 1 cm) temperature by a further 2 °C in comparison to the cold whirlpool immersion (Myrer *et al.*, 1998). Despite this, the rewarming rate of the crushed ice bag was significantly faster than that of the immersion technique, which showed a continued decline in intramuscular temperature 25 minutes after the removal of application. The subcutaneous temperature rewarmed in both modalities directly after the removal of the application (Myrer *et al.*, 1998). This ability of the intramuscular tissue to continue cooling long after the removal of cold whirlpool immersion, in contrast to the ice bag, can be accredited to the size of the contact area (Merrick *et al.*, 2003). With the conduction of thermal energy between the tissues, an enhanced thermal gradient may have been maintained when immersion was administered as the water absorbed heat from the full circumference of the ankle as opposed to just a focal area. Sports therapists can be recommended to utilize ice water immersion techniques during rehabilitation when extended periods of analgesia are required.

Cryokinetics

The ability of cryotherapy to provide an analgesic effect is the fundamental basis behind cryokinetics; aimed to better facilitate rehabilitation by reducing pain spasm and neural inhibition, enabling rehabilitation exercises to be performed earlier than would normally be possible (Bleakley *et al.*, 2004; Hopkins and Stencil, 2002; Knight *et al.*, 2000). First coined by Hayden (1964), cryokinetics (literally meaning 'cold' and 'motion') was shown to give marked improvements in soldiers' recovery time following injury (Grant, 1964; Hayden, 1964). Knight (1995) developed a sequence of exercises for the rehabilitation of a lateral ankle sprain using cryokinetics; Pincivero *et al.* (1993) identify that such protocols can enhance the return to activity.

Cryokinetic protocols generally involve an initial period of ten minutes of ice application to induce analgesia before exercise is performed (Hayden, 1964; Knight *et al.*, 2000; Pincivero *et al.*, 1993). Exercise is then undertaken until the analgesic effect diminishes (Barnes, 1979), typically for just two to three minutes (Knight, 1995). Subsequent ice applications of between three to five minutes are then re-administered before exercise is performed again (Barnes, 1979; Knight *et al.*, 2000). Cryotherapy does not remove all pain-sensing mechanisms, but may offset residual pain such as that caused by pressure from swelling on nerves and damaged tissue (Knight, 1995). Therapists may be concerned with cold water immersion (CWI) that the patient may not appreciate pain – a factor which could potentially contribute to further injury, yet this is not the case; such ice applications cause a degree of analgesia rather than complete anaesthesia. If an exercise becomes too advanced for the stage of rehabilitation, pain is still likely to be perceived, signalling the need to reduce the intensity (Knight 1995; Knight *et al.*, 2000).

During prescription of cryokinetic protocols, CWI is the modality of choice as it provides an optimal period of analgesia, thus increasing the window of opportunity to perform exercise (Knight, 1995). Although wet ice applications reduce skin temperature more quickly than immersion (Kennet *et al.*, 2007), it is the rate of re-warming which is paramount in cryokinetics, which is retarded following ice immersion (Myrer *et al.*, 1998). Cryokinetics is a powerful tool for the therapist. Initiation in the early phase of rehabilitation allows muscles to contract and therefore the ability to actively pump the swelling out of the area via the lymphatic drainage system (Knight, 1995). In the instance of an ankle sprain, by administering ice immersion, simple range-of-motion exercises can be performed earlier than normally would be possible, thus reducing swelling more quickly. Cryokinetics can be initiated in the sub-acute phase of rehabilitation right through until the athlete is ready to return to activity (Knight, 1995). Bleakley *et al.* (2012) have recommended a new early management acronym and methodology – POLICE (protection, optimal loading, ice, compression and elevation). The concept of optimal loading encourages incremental rehabilitation, whereby early activity promotes recovery. The implementation of cryokinetics allows for this optimal loading to take place more readily.

Ice massage

When implementing cryokinetic protocols, ice immersion is not always possible due to the anatomical location of the target tissue, for example at the knee, hip or shoulder. In such situations sports therapists may utilize wet ice bag applications or ice massage techniques. Ice massage consists of cubed ice applied directly to the skin in a typically gentle, stroking pattern parallel to the underlying muscle fibres (Knight, 1995). To protect the therapist's fingers, the 'tear-away cup method' can be utilized (characterized by water frozen in a polystyrene cup). Once frozen, the therapist tears away the lip of the cup to reveal the ice and then applies the massage directly to the target area. Alternatively, the 'lolly-stick method' may be preferred, characterized by a tongue-depressor placed into the polystyrene cup prior to freezing. This time, once frozen, the therapist removes the ice completely from the cup and applies the treatment by holding the tongue-depressor (acting as a handle). Duration of application should be between five and ten minutes to provide an analgesic effect (Grant, 1964; Halvorson, 1990; Hayden, 1964). The sports therapist should note that during the ice massage, the athlete will usually (obviously) experience a cold sensation, followed by a feeling of burning and aching (Grant, 1964). This period of discomfort should only present for a few minutes, yet is essential if analgesia is to ensue (Hayden, 1964). If ice massage is implemented for cryokinetic protocols, once the analgesia has been achieved the ice massage should be terminated and exercise should immediately follow. Subsequent two-minute applications are required every three minutes to maintain pain-free exercise (Bugaj, 1975). The ice massage modality is not only confined to use within cryokinetics, but is also recommended for pitch-side first aid when the athlete is to return to the field of play, and for quick analgesia where wet ice bags and ice machines may not be available. Ice massage is popular with sports therapists as it is inexpensive, immediately useful and can be administered by the athlete at home.

Cryotherapy: modality selection

The choice of cryotherapy modality should be made with reference to the physiological changes the sports therapist is trying to achieve. Following are three typical scenarios.

Scenario one: acute setting – return to play

When the athlete has received a trauma to the ankle/foot complex, but there is no obvious structural damage, the aim of the ice application is to provide quick pain relief before the athlete returns to activity. The best modality to use is an ice bag containing crushed ice, as it has been shown to reduce temperatures to critical levels required for analgesia within five minutes (Jutte *et al.*, 2001; Merrick *et al.*, 2003). Wet ice applications may be considered (where ice is applied through a fabric bag) as this method exhibits a greater thermal conduction than that of its dry ice counterpart. If wet ice is conceived as being messy or impractical in certain pitch-side situations, it is recommended that a mixture of cubed ice and water is put into a plastic bag and then applied (Dykstra *et al.*, 2009). However, during half-time, crushed ice can be placed into a thin wet cotton cloth and applied for fast pain relief for treating contusions following heavy tackles; such management may facilitate return to play.

Scenario two: acute setting – removal from play

When the athlete has received a significant trauma to the ankle – but where there is clear structural damage – the ice application will aim to provide pain relief, but more importantly, compression will need to be applied. In an effort to reduce oedema, compression will limit the available space for fluid to accumulate. As a result, wet ice application is of little use as the compression will not be consistent as the water escapes the porous bag. Instead, the dry ice method of crushed ice should be applied in a plastic bag and attached with a compression bandage. The ice is not the most important factor here, but rather the compression.

The ice may be applied intermittently – for ten minutes on, and then removed for ten minutes. In the rest period, the compression bandage should be reapplied. After the ten minutes of rest, the ice should be reapplied. Ideally, this cycle (ten minutes on, ten minutes off) will be continued for an appropriate period post-injury (over the following hours). Once icing is finished, before returning home, the injury should have the compression wrap reapplied.

The rationale for ten minutes on, ten minutes off, not only allows the skin a rest period from constant cold, but more importantly, the modality's ability to absorb heat is at its maximal for at least ten minutes before the modality temperature may begin to rise. Additionally, a thermal gradient is created between the skin and the intramuscular tissues, which allows cold to be reached at depth. When the ice is reapplied for a second ten-minute period, the tissue temperature at depth has not risen to pre-treatment levels and therefore can reach a lower temperature still. So, rather than the traditionally 20 minutes of continuous ice application – where the modality may start to warm after 15 minutes – here the athlete still receives a combined total of 20 minutes of ice application, but the tissue is maintained at a lower temperature for over 30 minutes.

Intermittent applications of ten minutes are superior at reducing skin temperature at the ankle (Ebrall *et al.*, 1992). Repeated ice applications of ten minutes on, ten minutes off, ten

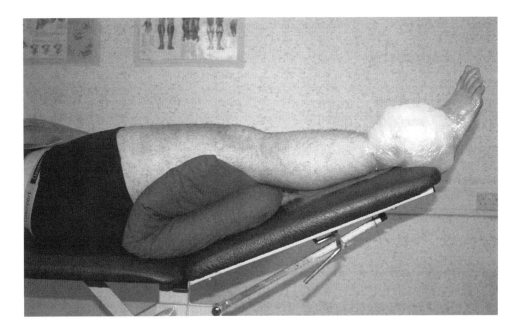

Photo 3.16   Clinical application of rest, ice, compression and elevation.

minutes on, not only have reduced skin temperature to below 3 °C following the second application, but have maintained temperatures below 15 °C for 33 minutes – 40 per cent longer than a 20-minute continuous application. Additionally, intermittent ice application significantly reduced pain on activity one week after a lateral ankle sprain injury (Bleakley *et al.*, 2006).

Scenario three: rehabilitation

During the rehabilitation setting, cryokinetic protocols should be implemented (Knight *et al.*, 2000; Pincivero *et al.*, 1993). Ice immersion should be the chosen modality here rather than wet ice bag application as it provides a longer period of analgesia. The consideration is less about how quickly the pain relief occurs, but more about how long it lasts. The longer the period of analgesia, the larger the window of opportunity to perform exercise.

Effect of cryotherapy on functional performance

With such a widespread use of cryotherapy in the sports medicine environment, sports therapists may have concerns regarding the possible detrimental effects ice applications may have on functional performance (Costello and Donnelly, 2010; Jameson *et al.*, 2001). Studies have examined the effects of cryotherapy on numerous functional tasks such as shuttle runs and vertical jump height (Cross *et al.*, 1996; Evans *et al.*, 1995; Richendollar *et al.*, 2006). Cross *et al.* (1996) reported that single-leg vertical jump height decreased, and that agility shuttle run times were slower following 20 minutes of ice immersion (13 °C) of the lower leg. Moreover, similar results were obtained when an ice bag application was applied for 20 minutes to the anterior thigh prior to maximal functional performance (Richendollar *et al.*, 2006). Furthermore, functional measures such as single-leg jumping have been shown to yield a decreased vertical impulse following full lower leg immersion (10 °C) for ten minutes (Kinzey *et al.*, 2000). In the only study to date to incorporate bilateral immersion, Patterson *et al.* (2008) identified jump height, peak power, agility T-test and a 40-yard dash were all impaired following immersion of the lower leg in a 10 °C cold whirlpool for 20 minutes. It was also reported that jump height and peak power remained significantly reduced for 32 minutes post application (Patterson *et al.*, 2008). In contrast, 20 minutes of immersion (1 °C) of the ankle complex (Evans *et al.*, 1995) and a ten-minute ice bag application to the lateral and medial aspects of the ankle (Atnip and McCrory, 2004) do not negatively affect functional performance. The contradictory results could be accredited to the surface area of tissue cooled. Whether unilateral (Cross *et al.*, 1996) or bilateral (Patterson *et al.*, 2008) immersion of the lower limb to the head of the fibula, the incorporation of muscle cooling was detrimental to functional performance. However, when ice application was focused specifically to a joint, no detriment in performance was apparent (Atnip and McCrory 2004; Evans *et al.*, 1995). In studies utilizing focal joint cooling rather than applications directly to muscle, no detriments in postural stability have been identified (Hart *et al.*, 2005; Jameson *et al.*, 2001). Jameson *et al.* (2001) examined ground reaction force (GRF) during landing from a vertical jump after subjects received crushed ice to either the ankle or knee, or a combination of both for 20 minutes. However, no significant difference in vertical GRF was identified between the experimental and control groups. Likewise, Hart *et al.* (2005) concluded that a 20-minute ice bag application to the knee did not alter peak vertical GRF or muscle activity of the gastrocnemius, hamstrings, quadriceps or gluteus medius during a single-leg landing. In fact, cooling of a joint, independent of a muscle, may be advantageous with a greater facilitation of the soleus motor neurone pool evident (Hopkins and Stencil 2002; Krause *et al.*, 2000). Whenever a detriment in functional performance has been identified, large muscle groups such as the quadriceps have been the target for cryotherapy. It is therefore prudent to suggest that cryotherapy to muscular tissue (Cross *et al.*, 1996; Patterson *et al.*, 2008; Richendollar *et al.*, 2006) provides greater detriment to functional performance than that of cryotherapy to a joint, such as the ankle (Atnip and McCrory, 2004; Evans *et al.*, 1995; Jameson *et al.*, 2001) or knee (Hart *et al.*, 2005; Jameson *et al.*, 2001). Despite this, where detriments in performance have been identified, ice application has been longer than that typically applied in the sporting environment. While longer application times may be present for cryokinetic protocols, the location of ice application is typically to a joint where detriments in performance have not been elicited. Consequently, the therapist should not be concerned with sending athletes immediately back to activity following cryotherapy treatment to provide analgesia.

Recovery ice baths

After the athlete competes, the musculoskeletal, nervous and metabolic systems can become fatigued, potentially leading to a detriment in subsequent performance (Ingram *et al.*, 2009). In an attempt to promote improved recovery, sports therapists may implement recovery cold water baths (also known as cold water immersion – CWI) up to the iliac crest or neck line (Bailey *et al.*, 2007; Wilcock *et al.*, 2006). Both water temperature and duration can vary from short bouts of 30 seconds (Mantoni *et al.*, 2007) to longer periods of ten minutes (Bailey *et al.*, 2007) in temperatures often below 15 °C (Bleakley and Davison, 2010). However, much of this modality's popularity comes from anecdotal evidence (Wilcock *et al.*, 2006), as the results from controlled laboratory experiments remain equivocal, with no consensus on an optimum treatment protocol (Bleakley and Davison, 2010; Cochrane, 2004). The sports therapist must understand that it is often challenging to get athletes to adhere to full immersion in cold water baths due to the intensity of the cold. Moreover, trying to implement extended periods of CWI immediately post-exercise can often be impossible in a team environment due to logistic constraints. However, when CWI is utilized, it is essential that athletes are monitored

---

Practitioner Tip Box 3.2

Patient home-care advice

It is recommended, for all areas of specified home-care advice – whether exercise, cryotherapy, heat therapy or any other – that clearly presented written/printed instructions are provided for patients. Photographic or video instruction demonstrating or coaching exercise techniques may also be provided using the patient's mobile phone. This will help to offset the potential for any harm or lack of progress due to misunderstanding of specific advice, and will also promote patient adherence.

---

throughout. With athletes who are unaccustomed to sudden entry into cold water, there is often a cold shock response – this consists of an inspiratory gasp, tachycardia and hyperventilation – which can quickly lead to unconsciousness (Lloyd, 1994; Tipton, 1989). Therefore it is recommended to implement habituation sessions for new athletes, where water temperatures are gradually lowered and the duration of applications are gradually increased.

Precautions and contraindications for cryotherapy

Patients with a fear or clear intolerance to ice applications should not be administered cryotherapy (Swenson *et al.*, 1996). Such conditions include Raynaud's phenomenon (where exposure to cold results in unduly reactive vasoconstriction of extremities, and most commonly affects fingers and toes [RSA, 2013]); and cryoglobulinaemia (where immune complexes precipitating at low temperatures are deposited onto vascular endothelial walls, and may cause a form of vasculitis [Patient Plus, 2011]). The risk of frostbite following cryotherapy is extremely rare but can be reduced by keeping application periods to less than 40 minutes (Knight, 1995). A barrier between the skin and the ice modality is advisable, such as with crushed ice placed in a plastic or fabric bag. Cryogen gel packs should be avoided as there are superior modalities to achieve the desired effects. Bleakley and Hopkins (2010) identified no cases of skin burns or untoward effects as a result of ice application in their review of over 35 laboratory-based cryotherapy studies.

Cryotherapy can be reliably administered to provide an analgesic effect, and therapists should consider the use of wet ice bag application to provide rapid pain relief. Cryokinetic protocols can be implemented in the sub-acute phase in order to provide optimal loading and aid the removal of swelling. Rest and ice application alone will not reduce swelling.

Heat therapy

Thermotherapy or heat therapy is the use of heat for therapeutic purposes, and may relate to any application of substance or device whose temperature is greater than body temperature. This allows the heat to pass from the device to the body. Heat is energy which is produced by the movement of atoms and molecules (Knight and Draper, 2008). The perception of heat is based primarily on subjective interpretation, and each individual will respond differently depending on the circumstances. The manner in which the body responds to the application of heat depends upon the type of heat therapy used, together with the duration and intensity of the application. It is also affected by the differing response of the tissues in different parts of the body. For a positive reaction to heat therapy, heat needs to be absorbed into the area and spread to adjacent tissues. For therapeutic use, it is important to apply the correct amount of heat; if too little is used, then no significant changes will occur, too much and tissues may be damaged (Prentice, 2009). Within sports therapy, heat may be used to boost blood flow to the area, where increasing local circulation improves the delivery of nutrients to the area and assists the removal of metabolites from the area. Such activity is likely to improve the healing rate of injured tissue, although evidence is limited (Knight and Draper, 2008).

Heat therapy may aid relaxation and general soreness, and anecdotally is often appreciated by patients. Heat therapy can be useful when used as a pre-treatment prior to STT. Laboratory studies have identified that warming of the musculotendinous unit will aid extensibility, and may decrease muscle strain (Knight *et al.*, 2001; Noonan *et al.*, 1993; Strickler *et al.*, 1990; Taylor *et al.*, 1995). The perception of pain may be decreased via the stimulation of A-beta thermoreceptors, as per the gate control theory of pain (Melzack and Wall, 1965; Prentice, 2009). The physiological effects of heat (vasodilation and hyperaemia) cause an increase in circulation (Knight and Draper, 2008), and this is thought to remove chemical irritants such as bradykinin away from the area. Metabolism of the site is increased; this benefits healing but must not be used during the initial phases as this will exacerbate bleeding and inflammatory responses (Knight and Draper, 2008). Heat may decrease pain by promoting a general sedative effect. This aids relaxation and is effective for general aches and pains (Knight and Draper, 2008). Muscle spasms, which may develop as a protective response to injury, can cause local ischaemia; these may be eased through the thermally induced increase in circulation and effect on the muscle spindles (Prentice, 2009). Joint stiffness may be decreased due to the 'gel to sol' effect on connective tissues induced by the increased local temperature (Burke *et al.*, 2001; Henricson *et al.*, 1984; Taylor *et al.*, 1995). Cross-linked fibres in collagen are also released to some degree. The combination of neural, vascular and mechanical effects allow connective tissues to become more elastic and enable more effective lengthening of soft tissues and mobilizing of joints to take place. Although heat is useful for relieving general aches and pains, it is not as effective as cold therapy when used with exercise in the early stages of sub-acute injury and may cause an exacerbation of pain (Knight and Draper, 2008). If pain becomes more dull and less sharp, heat may be better than cold in decreasing symptoms. Chronic injuries tend to respond well to heat therapy as it can be recommended for general pain relief, muscle soreness and tissue relaxation. Due to the gradual onset of chronic or overuse injuries, there is little effect on the circulation, therefore secondary metabolic injury is less of a concern. In such cases, pain may occur during activity and treatment may involve heat therapy prior to activity, and cold post-exercise (Knight and Draper, 2008).

Transference of heat

Conduction

Conduction is the transference of heat between two objects of uneven temperature, and requires direct contact between two objects. Hotter, faster-moving molecules interact with cooler atoms and molecules, transferring heat (energy) until the temperature becomes even (Knight and Draper, 2008). How quickly this occurs depends on the temperature of the modality and the exposure time. It is also affected by the quantity of blood flow in the area. Temperatures should not exceed 47 °C (116.6 °F), and great care should be taken with modalities above 45 °C (113 °F). These should not be used for longer than 30 minutes so that tissue damage can be prevented (Prentice, 2009). Conduction is the method of heat transfer most commonly used in sports and physical therapy, e.g. hot packs.

Convection

Convection is the transfer of heat indirectly through fluid or air as it passes its surface. This is a faster process than conduction. Convection is affected by the temperature of the modality and how fast the air (or fluid) is moved away from the body once it has become warm. If the air is moving slowly, then it will act as an insulator and continue to keep the body warm. It is also affected by how quickly the body part conducts heat. Hydrotherapeutic whirlpools use both convection and conduction to transfer heat (Knight and Draper, 2008).

Radiation

This may also be called radiant energy and uses the form of electromagnetic waves or rays to transfer heat. It transfers heat from one object to another through space without physical contact. Diathermy, laser, infrared and ultraviolet lamps use radiation to transmit heat (Knight and Draper, 2008).

Conversion

Deeper tissues may be selectively heated by conversion, a form of energy used by ultrasound and diathermy to increase tissue temperature, and therefore stimulate metabolic processes. Conversion relates to the generation of heat through other forms of energy (Prentice, 2009).

Heat therapy modalities

Hot packs

These are commonly used in sports therapy and superficially heat the tissues to help prepare the area for treatment (Starkey, 2004). They come in a variety of forms: they may be a dry, electrically heated pack; a simple hot water bottle; a gel–pack, warmed in hot water; a moist-heat pack – such as a 'wheat-bag', warmed in a microwave oven; or a hydrocollator pack. Medical standard electrically heated packs are heated to a temperature of 40–42 °C and can be controlled via a thermostat to maintain a constant temperature (Kitchen and Bazin, 2004). Hydrocollator packs are a form of moist heat, and are most commonly used in hospital settings or larger clinical environments. The packs are immersed in hot water in specialized cabinets at a temperature of approximately 75 °C. Hydrocollator packs contain silicate gel inside a cotton wrapping. Once heated, the packs are wrapped inside a towelling cover and applied to the affected area (most commonly osteoarthritic joints) for 20–30 minutes at a working temperature of 40–42 °C (Kitchen and Bazin, 2004; Prentice, 2010). It is essential that patients are carefully selected and monitored during the delivery of any direct heat application; patients must be instructed to report if the heat is too hot.

Infra-red lamps

Infra-red (IR) waves sit between visible light and microwaves on the electromagnetic spectrum. Most contemporary IR heat lamps use luminous 350–450 nm wavelengths (i.e. in addition to IR, they incorporate additional visible red light) with a light source of tungsten or carbon filament (Vizniak, 2012). Practitioners must observe the manufacturer's instructions regarding intensity output and recommended applications. Basic rules for delivery include appreciation of the inverse square law, which dictates the distance that the lamp should be positioned from the patient's body (the intensity of IR radiation increases as the distance from the patient decreases, and vice versa), but the actual intensity relates to the output of the lamp (Ward, 2004). The minimum recommended distance from the body is typically 50 cm. For even distribution of heat, the lamp and patient should be positioned so as to allow the rays to strike the body near to an angle of 90° (Vizniak, 2012). Radiant (luminous) IR can penetrate superficial skin layers to reach myofascial tissue. Treatment times are typically 10–20 minutes, and the patient should be free of any massage lotion or oil, have removed any jewellery and should avoid any eye exposure. Practitioners should always check equipment prior to use (i.e. the lamp, its stand, bulb, leads, plug and controls), and monitor patients' response during treatment.

Paraffin wax

Paraffin wax is a traditional physical therapy modality. The wax is heated in a thermostatically controlled container, and is maintained at a temperature of 42–54 °C (Kitchen and Bazin, 2004). While it has been used to treat smaller areas of the body such as the hands and feet, typically again for easing pain and stiffness associated with osteoarthritis, its popularity has waned in recent years. Treatment lasts 20–30 minutes. Application may be in the form of direct and repeated immersion (hands and feet), or molten wax may be brush-layered onto the affected area of the body. Usually, a thick layer of wax is built onto the body area, and then covered with plastic sheeting and towels to retain the heat. Due to the insulation quality of the wax, heat is maintained in the area, and superficial warming occurs. The procedure is less time-efficient than other modalities. Paraffin wax should not be used on broken skin, and caution should be used if there are any sensory or circulation impairments.

Hot water immersion

Hot water immersion (HWI) can include spas, hot tubs, whirlpools, hot water baths and showers. They are effective methods of providing general whole-body warming, which can generate a range of physiological and psychological responses, including, general relaxation, muscular relaxation, improved joint mobility and pain relief. Water temperature is recommended to be 36–41 °C.

Precautions with heat therapy

With acute injuries heat therapy will not normally be applied within the first two or three days. The increased metabolism created by the application of heat can increase secondary metabolic injury and delay healing. General and peripheral vascular disorders affect the body's ability to respond to increases in temperature and exacerbation of symptoms can occur. Sports therapists must take care also where the patient has impaired sensations. Overexposure or inability to sense changes in temperature can prevent the body's natural response to heat (thermoregulation), and may cause overheating; the body can be easily overheated, causing symptomatic hypotension and faintness. Skin mottling, burns and scalds can occur if practitioners are not careful. Furthermore, excessive heat therapy can cause transient hypotension, fainting and headache. Sports therapists must be responsibly vigilant to how any heat therapy affects the patient, taking care to gain verbal, visual and tactile feedback during treatment.

Electrotherapy
With Nick Gardiner
Principles of electrotherapy

Conclusive scientific evidence for electrotherapeutic modalities (electro-physical agents – EPAs) is lacking. However, there is a body of evidence which demonstrates significant physiological effects that may be of use therapeutically (Alexander *et al.*, 2010; Milne *et al.*, 2001; Watson, 1996; 2000).

Therapeutic ultrasound

Watson (2013a) provides an expansive review of the history, equipment, applications and evidence underpinning ultrasound (US) therapy:

> Ultrasound has been a part of clinical practice since the 1950s, and remains a popular and evidenced intervention for a range of clinical problems. Shah and Farrow (2012) provide an insight into its current clinical popularity as does the widely cited paper by Pope *et al.* (1995). General (textbook) reviews and explanations can be found in Watson and Young (2008) and Robertson *et al.* (2006), amongst others.

US machines use a piezoelectric transducer to produce mechanical vibrations, like sound waves but of a higher frequency; these are passed into the tissues via a coupling medium (gel or water) to avoid reflection of the waves. US absorption is greater for tissues with high protein content, so tendons, ligaments, fascia, joint capsules and scar tissue are the structures most commonly associated with US therapy (Vizniak, 2012), though a case for its use on muscle may still be made (Speed, 2001). US can be beneficial throughout the acute inflammatory, proliferative and maturation stages of healing, and the effects can be divided into non-thermal and thermal. US is proposed to accelerate the vascular and cellular events during the acute phase of healing (being pro-inflammatory); enhance fibroplasia and collagen synthesis during proliferation (being pro-proliferative); and improve the strength, elasticity and optimization of fibrous scar tissue during remodelling (Harr, 1999; Watson, 2013a).

The non-thermal benefits of US are utilized during the earlier stages of healing. Applications of US during the acute stage are proposed to enhance the inflammatory cascade (Watson, 2000). These effects occur by the ultrasonic mechanical vibrations interacting with specifically activated cells at the injury site (including platelets, mast cells, neutrophils and macrophages). It should be noted that there is conflicting evidence concerning this theory (Matsuzawa *et al.*, 2004). Acoustic streaming, which is the unidirectional movement of a fluid affected by the US field, can stimulate cell activity if it occurs at the boundary of the cell membrane and the surrounding interstitial fluid. This can affect membrane permeability, diffusion rates and the membrane potential. US causes 'cavitation' – the formation and implosion of gas-filled voids within the tissues and interstitial fluids. When the cavitation is 'stable', acoustic streaming is likely to be enhanced, and has potential to be therapeutic. 'Unstable cavitation' may occur where inappropriate US frequencies or intensities are employed, or when the treatment (transducer) head remains stationary during application, and this can cause tissue irritation. During the proliferative stage of healing it is proposed that US may promote both fibroblastic and endothelial cell activity, maximizing early scar tissue production and its quality (Watson, 2000). During proliferation US has been shown to increase the process of angiogenesis (Hogan *et al.*, 1982), along with an increase in protein synthesis. US has been shown to potentially stimulate cell division, fibroblast production and collagen synthesis during the active proliferative stage of ruptured rat tendons. This was hypothesized after the ultimate tensile strength was found to be greater compared to a control group (Ng *et al.*, 2003). Benefits that are seen during the remodelling phase occur primarily as a result of the thermal effects of US, and the indications for this are general musculoskeletal disorders such as muscle spasm and soft tissue fibrosis. General thermal effects of US may include increased extensibility of collagen-rich tissues (i.e. fascia; scar tissue), increased blood flow, increased nerve conduction velocity, increased muscle relaxation and reduced muscle spasm, pain and myofascial trigger points.

US dosage for non-thermal treatments uses a pulsed delivery of the waves which reduces the heat in the tissue; this is known as the 'duty cycle'. US machines will display this either as a ratio, such as 1:4 (one part US to four parts rest in each cycle), or as a percentage, i.e. 20 per cent. The ratio 1:4 is a relatively low dose of US, most commonly used in acute presentations. The other commonly pulsed ratios are 1:9 (extremely low dose), 1:2 (used more in the post-acute phase) and 1:1 (50 per cent). Thermal US treatments (for more chronic presentations) will use a continuous delivery, which may be displayed as CW (continuous wave) or as a percentage (100 per cent). A additional factor when prescribing US dosage is the target tissue depth. Most US machines will feature dual frequency options (1 MHz and 3 MHz). US energy decreases exponentially with depth. A frequency of 1 MHz is used for deeper tissues, and a half-value depth for this setting is approximately 4 cm. This means that half of the US energy will have been absorbed at 4 cm. Therefore, this is an essential factor when determining the intensity settings as this must allow for this absorption rate. As a general rule, a frequency of 3 MHz is used for more superficial structures, and its half-value depth is approximately 2.5 cm (Watson, 2000). The intensity of US application is measured in W cm^{-2} (watts per centimetre squared) and relates to the power output to the surface area via the transducer head. Again, as a general rule, the more acute the injury, the less power will be needed to excite the tissue (and vice versa for more chronic injuries).

To calculate the timing of a US treatment a simple calculation can be used; the number of treatment heads that cover the affected area can be multiplied by the sum of the duty cycle as a ratio. For example, if the area to be treated was the equivalent to two treatment heads and the duty cycle was to be 1:4, then the sum required would be $2 \times (1 + 4) = 10$ minutes. Another example may be that one treatment head was required for a duty cycle of 1:1; this sum would then be $1 \times (1 + 1) = 2$ minutes (Watson, 2013b).

Bone has a high content of protein but as an injured structure has not historically been considered an indication for US. Specialized units that deliver very low intensities (0.01 W cm^{-2}) have been shown to be most beneficial for fracture healing (LIPUS – low intensity pulsed ultrasound), but are expensive in comparison to conventional units (Warden et al., 2006). The shear forces applied to cellular membranes are thought to induce a cellular response and a 30–38 per cent acceleration rate for healing has been seen (Warden, 2003). There is research which suggests that lower intensity US may also be of benefit to soft tissue pathologies. It should also be noted that despite some comparisons between the results seen for the specialized units and standard LIPUS, it is thought that the accuracy of standard machines is not reliable enough to qualify their use for fracture healing. Another application of US is the use of phonophoresis, which is the driven migration of medication molecules from under the treatment head (as part of a coupling medium), offering superficial, non-invasive medication, and a potential synergistic relationship between US and medication (Wells, 1977). Phonophoresis has been most commonly used in clinical settings for the application of non-steroidal anti-inflammatory drugs (Hsieh, 2006; Sevier and Wilson, 1999).

Table 3.12 Different parameters for therapeutic ultrasound intensity

Stage of healing	Ultrasound intensity
Acute	0.1–0.3 W cm^{-2}
Sub-acute	0.2–0.5 W cm^{-2}
Chronic	0.3–0.8 W cm^{-2}

Source: adapted from Watson, 2013b.

Table 3.13 Contraindications for ultrasound, interferential and TENS

Contraindication	US (thermal)	US (Non-thermal)	IF and TENS
Pregnancy	LC	LC	LC
Malignancy	C	C	LC
Electronic implants (pacemaker)	LC	LC	C
Active epiphysis (aged <19)	LC	LC	LP
Metal implant	LC	LC	LP
Local circulatory insufficiency	LC	LC	LP
Devitalized tissue	LC	LC	LC
Epilepsy	–	–	LC
Bacterial infections	LC	LC	LC
Tissue bleeding	LC	LC	LC
Specialized (organ) tissue	LC	LC	LC

Source: adapted from Robertson *et al.*, 2006; Watson, 2011.

Note: LC, local contraindication; LP, local precaution; C, contraindication.

Contraindications to therapeutic ultrasound

Most US contraindications are related to its application for its thermal heat effect. In relation to soft tissue injuries, the main concerns include treatment over cancerous or infectious lesions, epiphyseal growth plates in children and adolescents, haemorrhagic regions, ischaemic peripheral regions, sensory disability, electronic (pacemaker) or metal implants and areas previously exposed to radiology (Belanger, 2002). As US has an effect on cellular activity and blood flow it means that local circulatory issues and pregnancy and are also contraindications, along with bacterial infections.

Safety issues with therapeutic ultrasound

Transient, or unstable, cavitation is a potential risk of US treatment. This occurs due to inappropriate application and results in rapid changes in the volume of bubbles, leading to their implosion which can cause temperature changes and cell damage (Wells, 1977). It is important to keep the treatment head moving at all times to minimize the risk of transient unstable cavitation. Another common danger is the creation of standing waves which can occur when two interfacing tissues of differing acoustic properties reflect the ultrasonic waves, creating 'hot spots'. This occurs when an incident wave meets a returning wave with the same amplitude, which results in a much stronger input than would be expected. This can cause endothelial damage through the release of free radicals. Endothelial cell metabolism and function is important for maintaining vascular integrity, thus rendering the micro-circulation a vulnerable component of soft tissue (Maxwell, 1992). For example, standing waves may be more likely to occur when US is applied to a tendon close to its attachment to a bony prominence. It is also important to perform a skin sensation test prior to the treatment in the form of a hot/cold test (typically using test tubes filled with water of different temperatures). Even though most potential benefits of US occur sometime after the treatment, it is still important to record an objective marker prior to treatment as this can be useful for recognizing if there has been any immediate negative impact from the treatment which may give reason to cease further treatments, or a justification to modify the treatment parameters.

Practitioner Tip Box 3.3

Therapeutic ultrasound application

1 Assess patient (suitability for ultrasound; therapeutic objectives; locality and size of treatment area)
2 Set machine up
3 Test machine (controls; leads; transducer head; function)
4 Work out application settings
5 Safety checks on patient (including all contraindications; hot/cold sensation)
6 Explain effects of treatment to patient
7 Position patient appropriately (for comfort; protect clothing)
8 Advise patient to mention any discomfort during treatment
9 Begin application (apply coupling gel, and apply transducer head to tissues prior to starting)
10 Keep transducer head slowly moving during application
11 Observe, monitor and communicate with patient

Interferential therapy

Interferential (IF) treatment is the application of alternating medium-frequency electrical currents which are then amplitude modulated to allow a mimicking of low-frequency currents to give therapeutic benefits. The amplitude modulated frequencies (AMFs) act as 'carrier' currents which deliver the low-frequency AMF to the affected area. The body then demodulates the AMF; the mechanisms for this are still to be fully established (De Domenico, 1982; Johnson and Tabasam, 2003). The reason this approach is used is because low-frequency stimulation of nerve and muscle fibres has been shown to have beneficial therapeutic effect on deep nerve tissue. Skin, however, has a naturally high resistance to the passage of low-frequency current so the delivery of two medium (IF) frequencies that summate means that a lower-frequency treatment can be delivered to provide potential pain relief (Kloth, 1991; Martin, 1994; Nelson, 1981). Most IF machines have a carrier frequency in the region of 4,000 Hz, and an adjustable frequency known as the interference frequency that ranges between 4,001 and 4,150 Hz. The resulting frequency is known as the AMF or the beat frequency, and is the low frequency that will be delivered to the tissues (Johnson and Tabasam, 2003). The main physiological (and psychological) benefit of applying IF is to address pain, reduce oedema, promote healing and improve neuromuscular activation (Johnson and Tabasam, 2003). Pain relief, in simple terms, may be explained and achieved through two main pathways; the pain gate mechanism (stimulating A-beta fibres), which is appropriate for acute symptoms, overriding A–delta and C fibres; and the stimulation of endogenous opioid mechanisms for more persistent presentation, which may influence C-fibre-generated nociception (De Domenico, 1982; Melzack and Wall, 1965). IF can also be used for muscle stimulation, which can be useful for inducing a pumping and flushing effect to increase blood flow to the area and reduce oedema, as well as neuromuscular re-education. This can be useful for reducing swelling and optimizing the healing process (Lamb and Mani, 1994; Noble *et al.*, 2000).

Due to the summation of the two medium frequencies, IF can deliver low-frequency treatments with less discomfort than traditional methods. IF can also treat deeper and larger areas of tissues than other common electrotherapy modalities. Two-pole and four-pole IF can

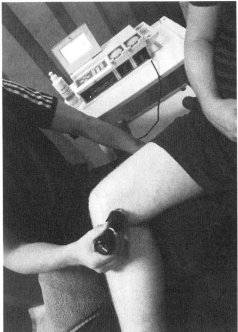

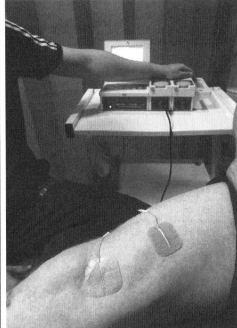

Photo 3.17   Therapeutic ultrasound.

Photo 3.18   Interferential therapy.

Table 3.14 Recommended interferential therapy parameters

Physiological effect	*Frequency*
Pain relief	90–150 Hz
Endogenous opioid mechanisms	1–5 Hz
Muscle stimulation	10–25 Hz

Source: adapted from De Domenico, 1982; Wadsworth and Chanmugam, 1980.

be used. Two-pole IF is 100 per cent amplitude modulated, which means it is efficient and produces perfectly formed beat frequencies. Four-pole, on the other hand, employs two circuits that are at right angles to each other, which produce a 'clover leaf' pattern where the interfering frequencies cross over (Kitchen and Bazin, 2004; Robertson *et al.*, 2006). Four-pole is well indicated for intra-articular joint pain due to its ability to target deep tissues. The actual delivery of electrical stimulation is via either re-useable or disposable single-patient electrodes (pads). These are rubber-coated, and the re-usable pads require water-dampened sponge covers to allow conduction to the patent's tissues. Re-useable electrodes need to be fixed in place using elasticated strapping. Disposable electrodes are slightly more costly, but much easier to apply, and arguably more hygienic. Suction pads are also available, which may also be easier to apply over irregular surfaces, and may aid the muscle pump action. Timings for treatments range from 10 to 20 minutes and the intensity of the machine should be set at the maximum within the patient's comfort level (Savage, 1984; Goats, 1990; Wadsworth and Chanmugam, 1980). It is important to check with the patient that the level of intensity feels the same throughout the treatment as this may need to be turned up to account for accommodation to the level of

Practitioner Tip Box 3.4

Interferential application

1　Assess patient (suitability for IF; therapeutic objectives; locality and size of treatment area)
2　Set machine up
3　Test machine (controls; leads; electrodes; function)
4　Work out application settings
5　Safety checks on patient (including all contraindications; sharp/blunt sensation)
6　Explain effects of treatment to patient
7　Position patient appropriately (for comfort)
8　Advise patient to mention any discomfort during treatment
9　Begin application (start on minimum intensity and turn up to maximal comfortable intensity)
10　Observe, monitor and communicate with patient

stimulation. Most IF machines have a sweep setting available, and some are automatic. Sweep means that the AMFs that have been set will rise and fall between the two parameters over a number of seconds, for example, 90–150 Hz over a period of six seconds (Kitchen and Bazin, 2004). There is some research to suggest that applying a sweep may allow a greater stimulation of excitable tissues (Low and Reed, 2004; Savage, 1984).

Contraindications to interferential therapy

Most contra-indications for IF are nerve-related due to the type of stimulation IF delivers, so this includes conditions such as epilepsy, pacemakers and devitalized tissue. However, as IF also has the potential to stimulate blood flow, circulatory conditions must also be included.

Safety issues with interferential therapy

IF dangers include overstimulation of nerve fibres if intensity is set too high, and irritation to tissues if the athlete's sensitivity is impaired. This is why it is important to carry out a skin sensation test in the form of a sharp/blunt test. Placement and positioning of the pads is important as poor electrode contact with the skin will lead to an ineffective treatment. It is also important to ensure that there are no short wave diathermy (SWD) machines in use within five metres at the same time (Goats, 1990). An appropriate objective marker should be recorded prior to the treatment for comparison afterwards.

Transcutaneous electrical nerve stimulation

Transcutaneous electrical nerve stimulation (TENS) is designed to provide pain relief by specifically exciting sensory nerves (Denegar, 2000). While there are some claims that TENS will aid management of inflammation and neuromuscular dysfunction, the most widely recognized indication is for the management of acute and chronic pain. This includes all manner of sports-related injuries such as low back pain, musculoskeletal pain, post-surgical pain and arthritic pain (Pengel *et al.*, 2002; Topuz *et al.*, 2004). The two main ways that TENS affects pain is via the pain gate mechanism, and through activation of the endogenous opioid system (i.e. stimulation of endorphin release) (Melzack and Wall, 1965; Ignelzi and Nyquist, 1979; Sjölund *et al.*, 1977; Andersson *et al.*, 1977; Topuz *et al.*, 2004). Conventional TENS activates the pain gate mechanism, and it does this using high-frequency (50–100 Hz), low-intensity (just above the patient's sensation threshold) and short pulse width (50 us) parameters (Kitchen and Bazin, 2004; Walsh *et al.*, 2000; Watson, 2011). Treatment times for conventional TENS range from 15–20 minutes to hours (Kitchen and Bazin, 2004; Robertson *et al.*, 2006; Walsh *et al.*, 2000). To activate the endogenous opioid system, an acupuncture-like setting is used (AL-TENS), which is effectively the opposite setting to that of conventional TENS. This uses a low-frequency (2–4 Hz), high-intensity (maximum for patient comfort) and long pulse width (200 us) (Walsh *et al.*, 2000; Watson, 2011). AL-TENS produces a much more stimulatory treatment and feels like a rhythmical 'thudding'. Consequently, the treatment times should be lower to reduce the risk of fatiguing muscle fibres, using an upper limit of 45 minutes to an hour (Robertson *et al.*, 2006). AL-TENS stimulates the release of endorphins and encephalins (Zadina *et al.*, 1997). There are also modulated and burst settings (Kitchen and Bazin, 2004) that can be used if accommodation to the currents becomes an issue. Modulated TENS may be a viable option if the efficacy of conventional TENS is wearing off. It uses parameters of 40–150 Hz. Burst TENS is more of a 'jack of all trades', addressing pain through both pathways using a frequency of 50–100 Hz (Watson, 2011). It is the type of pain that is key when deciding what mode of TENS to apply. As a first treatment for sharp, localized pain, conventional TENS would be the most appropriate choice, and for deeper, more poorly localized aches AL-TENS would be the best choice. Dual-channel TENS can be applied if required, which means that two channels of current are delivered simultaneously through four electrodes. This is of use when treating a large area of tissue, or for addressing referred pain, for example, placing two electrodes paraspinally in the L4–S3 region, and two electrodes at the site of referred pain in the leg. TENS electrodes are normally self-adhesive and easy to apply. The most common approach to electrode placement is to apply them directly over the injured area, but it is possible to use peripheral nerves, spinal nerve roots, trigger points and acupuncture points (Robertson *et al.*, 2006).

Contraindications to TENS

Due to the electrical stimulation that TENS delivers, patients with pacemakers and/or a history of epilepsy should not be treated. Inconclusive research means that the safest approach to treating pregnant patients is to consider pregnancy at least a local contraindication. Skin-related conditions such as bacterial infections should be avoided to reduce the chance of cross-infection.

Safety issues with TENS

The athlete must have normal skin sensation for the use of TENS to be safe, so a sharp/blunt test is required prior to all treatments. The small size, low cost and portable nature of the TENS units means they are especially good for home use. However, giving clear instructions for using the unit outside the clinic is essential. This includes dispensing advice such as not to use TENS while driving, operating machinery, sleeping or showering. It is also important to point out that prolonged use may result in irritation and a reddening of the skin beneath the electrodes. This will normally settle without complication. The athlete should be advised to adjust the exact positioning of the pads on a regular basis to avoid this. It is important to remember that TENS addresses more the symptoms of an injury rather than the cause. The patient should be made aware of this and understand that during TENS treatments, symptoms of pain may be masked which can increase the chance of worsening the injury through the performance of aggravating activities. Taking some form of objective marker and recording the patient's pain VAS score will allow for a comparison of symptoms before and after the treatment.

Athletic taping and strapping
Principles of taping

Taping is a commonly utilized, temporary, adjunctive intervention (Birrer and Poole, 2004). It is used within all stages of the rehabilitation process for a host of therapeutic objectives, including: prophylactic or protective taping (to prevent injury); proprioceptive and joint positional sense taping (typically in repair stage recovery activities); compression taping to minimize swelling (such as in the presence of acute soft tissue injury); athletic taping to restrict specific movements during activity (such as restricting inversion in the presence of ankle instability); taping to improve motion control; taping to 'offload' irritable structures (such as with some reactive tendinopathies); taping to reduce biomechanical malalignment (such as with maltracking patella); taping to influence lymphatic drainage (such as with acute soft tissue injury); taping to stimulate muscle recruitment (facilitation) (such as with joint positional sense and postural re-education); taping to inhibit muscle recruitment; taping to relieve pain; taping to improve athletes' confidence on returning to functional activities following injury; taping to hold splints, pads or packs in place (Abell, 2010; Anderson *et al.*, 2009; Bahr and Engebretsen, 2009; Macdonald, 2004; Norris, 2011; Prentice, 2009; Vizniak, 2012).

Although taping in athletic and rehabilitation settings is widespread, evidence to support its use is somewhat limited, and particularly during sports, the desired effect of taping procedures can soon decrease as physically stressful activity takes place. Of the numerous published applications, the most common indications for athletic taping include: anterior glenohumeral instability; acromioclavicular sprain; elbow joint sprain; medial and lateral elbow epicondylalgia; wrist sprain; thumb medial ligament sprain; interphalangeal ligament sprain; adductor tears; quadriceps tears; hamstring tears; medial and lateral collateral ligament sprain; patellofemoral pain syndrome; patellar tendinopathy; medial tibial stress syndrome; calf tears; Achilles tendinopathy; medial and lateral ankle sprain; plantar fasciitis; turf toe (compressed and hyperextended first metatarsophalangeal joint); and a range of postural conditions (such as exaggerated thoracic kyphosis or lumbar lordosis, or 'winging' scapula). From an efficacy point of view, the sports therapist will be expected to consider the most appropriate taping application for the tissues involved, the severity and stage of healing, and the level of functional activity expected of the patient or athlete following the taping application. Beyond this, therapists must also consider when alternative methods of providing stability may be preferable. Purpose-designed products such as ankle and knee braces, lumbar and pelvic support belts, and epicondylalgia clasps are readily available and do have their place in early rehabilitation, and hence, the sports therapist will be expected to make informed decisions regarding their use. Braces, particularly when designed for the ankle, tend to fall into one of three categories: sleeves (provide compression and proprioception, but no stability); non-rigid (constructed from either elastic, nylon, canvas or neoprene with laces and/or elastic straps; these provide proprioception and minimal stability); and semi-rigid (similar to non-rigid, but with additional moulded medial and lateral support struts or air cushions; these may be used when greater stability is required) (Bahr and Engebretsen, 2009). By way of simple comparison, taping can be a cheaper short-term strategy, and can be more individualized. Bracing may be preferable when numerous repeat applications are required, and can also be re-tightened during activity (Abell, 2010). Bracing can be easily performed by the athlete, whereas taping is therapist-dependent. Certainly, athletes with a history of ankle sprains who regularly use either taping or bracing have been shown to have a lower incidence of re-injury (Quinn *et al.*, 2000). The specific efficacy and indications for both, however, still require far more investigation.

Bandyopadhyay and Mahapatra (2012) provided an update and review of the use of tape in sports. They note that, as part of an injury-prevention strategy, athletic taping must be viewed as a major procedure. In contact and collision sports, tape may contribute to a reduction in extrinsic aetiology. Overuse injuries may be protected against and reduced. Taping is also commonly used to help return athletes earlier to their sports after injury, as taping provides the stability and support to injured structures. Butterwick *et al.* (2004) indicated that taping can reduce both incidence and intensity of injury in many sporting environments. Certainly, in clinical sports therapy practice, there is scope to explore the use of taping in the post-acute and early stages of rehabilitation, and also importantly as an intervention to reduce pain. McConnell (2000; 2002) has undertaken significant work in this area, particularly with regard to patellofemoral pain syndrome (PFPS). Of the possible disadvantages associated with taping, and not least the delivery of inappropriate, ineffective or, worse, harmful taping procedures, Birrer and Poole (2004) highlight the potential for the athlete developing a psychological dependency on the external support. Both Cordova *et al.* (2000) and Quirke and Harrison (2000) have identified the limited duration of effect from ankle taping applications in sports, suggesting that the effectiveness of tape may actually only last for 10–20 minutes. In a PEDro systematic review of ankle taping and bracing for proprioception Janssen and Kamper (2013) concluded, in light of the established evidence-base, that it should not be discouraged. This is clearly an area for further investigation, where both taping techniques and technologies must be evaluated.

Just as there are innumerable taping indications and applications, there are also a wide range of taping products and materials. While taping is generally seen as a useful adjunct to other therapeutic modalities, a strong understanding of anatomy, biomechanics, mechanisms of injury, pathology, progressive treatment and rehabilitation techniques, and individual sports, as well as the athlete or patient themselves, is required to guide the sports therapist in the choice of technique. Thorough clinical assessment should provide the therapist with necessary information to decide, for example, which structures need to be supported, which movements needs to be restricted and what are the most suitable taping materials needed for the athlete and the sporting environment. Sports therapists will recognize that practise is the key to the delivery of proficient taping techniques. Although there are specific guidelines on correct taping techniques, practitioners must be open and flexible to experiment to adapt individual techniques to suit each situation and athlete. It is also important to bear in mind that taping applied incorrectly may aggravate an existing injury, or even cause a new one.

Taping equipment

There is a wide variety of taping equipment available, with products being developed for a range of uses. Birrer and Poole (2004) explain that athletic tape is graded on a number of technical characteristics, including: the number of vertical and horizontal threads per square inch; the tensile strength; whether the tape is cotton, synthetic or a combination; and its adhesive properties. Taping products can be expensive, and most are single-use and disposable, hence it is important to ensure that whichever products are selected, they must be the most appropriate for the therapeutic objectives and the environment. Taping materials should be stored hygienically in a dry, cool place. Some of the most common taping and strapping products are discussed below.

Table 3.15 Athletic taping application terminology

Anchor	A strip of adhesive rigid tape applied to provide a firm base to attach other tapes to
Basketweave	A series of alternate interweaving stirrup and spur strips applied in a half overlapping pattern. Used at the ankle to restrict movement following sprain
Buddy tape	Circumferential adhesive non-elastic taping strips applied around two fingers proximal and distal to a sprained interphalangeal joint. May have a splint inserted between the two fingers
Butterfly	Strips of tape which fan out from a single anchor strip
Check-rein	One or more strips of tape which run between two anchor strips
Fan strip	Three or more strips of tape produced as an 'X' pattern. Applied between two anchor strips. The strips are then reinforced with additional locking anchor strips. Used to restrict joint movement
Figure of eight	Continuous loop of crepe, cohesive or elastic adhesive tape in a figure-of-eight pattern. Used to provide compression to control swelling, or to reinforce stability at a joint
Lock	A strip of rigid tape applied to provide final reinforcement and complete a tape application
McConnell technique	A specific application using strong, rigid tape (over hypoallergenic adhesive fleece tape) which aims to relieve pain and improve patellofemoral alignment and neuromuscular recruitment
Reinforcing strips	A series of overlapping strips which reinforce the underlying strips
Spica	A repeated figure of eight. Most commonly utilizes wide elastic tape, which may be applied over clothing. It is used mainly for restricting thumb, ankle, knee and hip movements. It may be reinforced by strips of adhesive rigid tape
Spiral	A winding, continuous elastic or cohesive strapping applied circumferentially around a limb to provide compression or restrict muscular movement. Each continued application overlaps the previous one by a half-width. May be reinforced by strips of rigid tape
Spur	Horizontal strips of tape which hold stirrups in place. May form part of a 'basketweave' pattern
Stirrup	A vertical U-shaped piece of tape supporting the lateral aspects of a joint. Stirrups run from one side of the joint and up the other

Zinc oxide

Zinc oxide (ZO) is adhesive, inelastic and hand-tearable, and is intended to provide certain rigid support to inert injured structures such as ligaments and joint capsules, and to also subtly reinforce other taping applications. ZO can be used as anchors at musculotendinous junctions, and is commonly indicated for prophylactic purposes. As it is inelastic, it should never be applied circumferentially. Depending on the anatomical area, ZO comes in a variety of sizes. To tear ZO, the sports therapist should pull the tape apart and perform a short, firm and quick twisting movement. ZO comes in a variety of widths (typically in rolls from 1.25 cm to 7.5 cm wide, and 5 m to 10 m long); and also a selection of densities and adhesive properties are available.

Micropore

A rigid, conformable, inelastic, non-woven viscose fabric which is coated with an acrylic adhesive (rather than, for example, a ZO adhesive). As it is microporous, it will withstand limited exposure to water without losing all of its adhesive properties, and also offers some protection against maceration.

Elastic adhesive bandage

Elastic adhesive bandaging (EAB) conforms to the contours of the body, and allows for normal tissue expansion, particularly involving musculature. It is adhesive and offers elasticity. EAB is usually non-tearable (requires cutting); however, there now are lighter-weight stretch tapes which can be torn by hand. EAB provides compression, and can also be used as an anchor around a muscle belly. If some give in the tape application is required, then EAB is indicated. It will not provide effective mechanical support to ligaments, but can be used in conjunction with ZO or other rigid tape. EAB is commonly available in a range of widths from 1.25 cm to 10 cm.

Cohesive bandage

Cohesive bandage has elastic properties and may be tearable or non-tearable. Cohesive is non-adhesive but sticks to itself. It is used to provide compression and support to tissues (particularly in acute situations), and can be easily removed and reapplied. Cohesive tapes tend to come in widths of between 5 cm and 10 cm.

Hypoallergenic adhesive fleece mesh

Hypoallergenic adhesive mesh (such as 'hypafix' or 'mefix') is a flexible, adhesive and breathable underwrap, which can provide skin protection when applied under other taping products, such as ZO. Because of the tape's permeability, the skin is less vulnerable to maceration.

Underwrap

Underwrap is a light, non-adhesive, non-restricting polyurethane foam material which may be applied under EAB, ZO or micropore. It is also commonly used in conjunction with heel and lace pads, and essentially can help to reduce areas of skin contact with tape, which may otherwise cause skin irritation. When underwrap is applied, however, the actual tape application may loosen off more quickly with activity.

Heel and lace pads

Heel and lace pads are thin foam squares which are designed to help reduce friction around the ankle and foot. They are commonly used together with tape adhesive and lubrication (petroleum jelly).

Padding and felt

A foam, or rubberized, material must be cut to shape and used to pad out uneven regional contours or to apply specific compression to tissue. Examples include the use of a 'horseshoe' pad applied inferiorly to the medial or lateral malleoli for post-acute ankle support.

Tape adhesive spray

Adhesive spray (such as 'Tuff skin') may be applied directly to the skin prior to any tape application to reinforce the adhesion of tape. This can be useful when repetitive body movements or excessive sweating may cause loosening of the tape; also when the conditions are wet, or when the athlete has oily skin.

Tape remover

Tape remover (dehesive) works to dissolve the adhesive on EAB, ZO, micropore or fleece mesh. This is generally available in both lotion and spray form.

Tape scissors

Taping scissors are unique in that they are specifically designed with stubbed ends, for safety when attempting to remove tape. 'Sharks' are frequently used to take tape off, these specifically designed scissors minimize the chance of skin cuts, and are also easier to use for this purpose.

Practitioner Tip Box 3.5

Taping applications

- Assess patient/athlete (suitability for taping; therapeutic objectives; therapeutic technique)
- Consider all possible contraindications (including undetermined injury; compromised skin sensation or blood flow; allergy to taping materials)
- Do not tape acute injury (compression may be considered as a first aid measure)
- Do not apply tape to any area which has just received cryotherapy or heat therapy
- Tape will not stick to skin which has had massage lubricant applied
- Ensure all required material is at hand
- Clean (using antiseptic soap) and dry area to be taped
- Shave hair (in a downward direction) from any areas where tape will be applied directly to the skin (unless using underwrap or non-adhesive tape)
- Position the athlete appropriately and maintain this position throughout application
- Protect areas likely to experience friction
- Attend to and protect any skin lesions (blisters; grazes; cuts)
- Apply adhesive spray where increased adherence of tape is required
- Apply underwrap for sensitive skin
- Apply adhesive fleece tape under zinc oxide to protect skin in absence of underwrap
- Apply tape smoothly and firmly, avoiding wrinkles and gaps which could cause friction, blisters or skin breakdown
- Avoid using continuous taping tightly around a limb as this may cause a tourniquet effect
- Use strips of tape which are slightly angled to conform to the limb contours
- Always check that the taping is comfortable, avoiding undue pressure or tension. Remove if any discomfort arises
- Once tape has been applied, check that the technique has achieved its objective without limiting desired function
- Assess circulation, sensation and comfort local and distal to the area of application
- Alterations in skin colour, temperature or other sensory changes indicate that the tape is too tight and should be removed immediately
- Remember that gaps in tape applications can trap skin; creases can cause friction irritation
- Advise patient/athlete regarding how long to keep the taping application on, how to remove it and any follow-up treatment

---

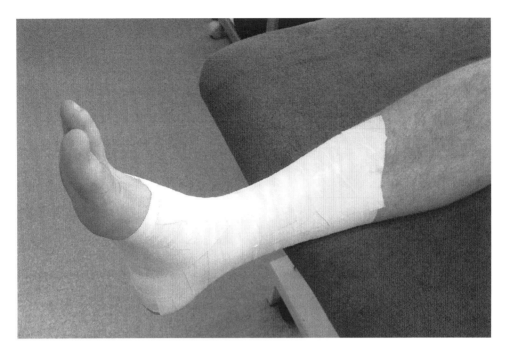

Photo 3.19 Closed basketweave for the ankle (courtesy of Greg Littler and Lee Young).

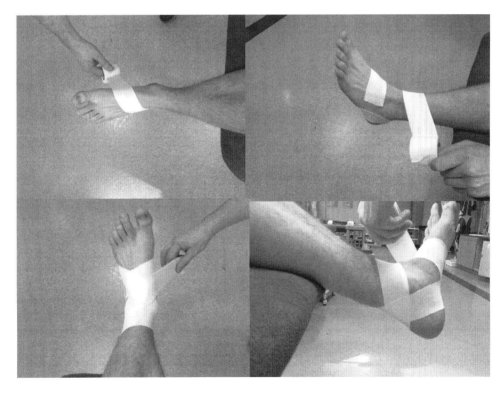

Photo 3.20 Heel lock for the ankle (courtesy of Greg Littler and Lee Young).

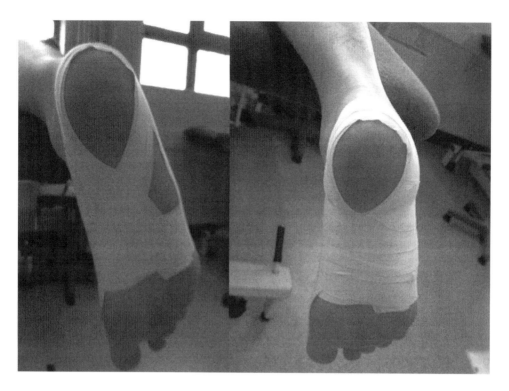

Photo 3.21   Plantar fascia taping support (courtesy of Greg Littler and Lee Young).

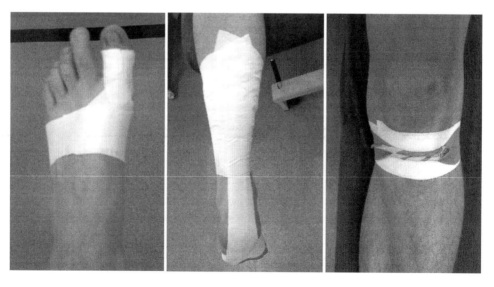

Photo 3.22   Turf toe taping (courtesy of Greg Littler and Lee Young).

Photo 3.23   Achilles tendinopathy support (courtesy of Greg Littler and Lee Young).

Photo 3.24   Patella tendon off-load taping (courtesy of Greg Littler and Lee Young).

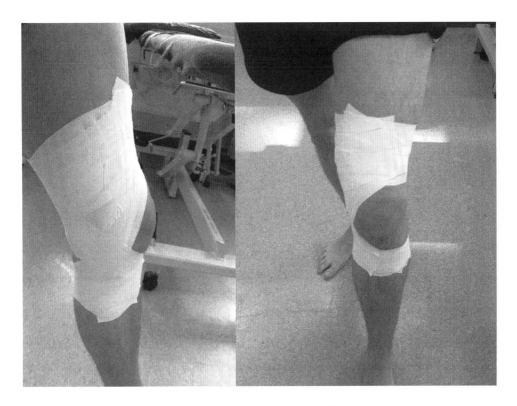

Photo 3.25   Medial collateral ligament taping (courtesy of Greg Littler and Lee Young).

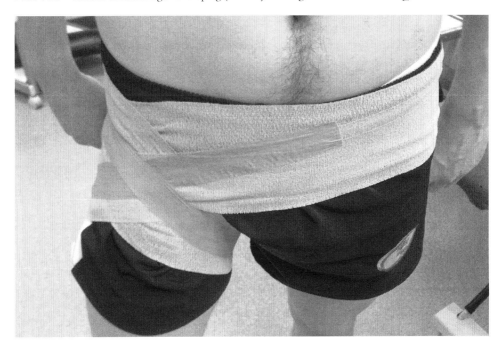

Photo 3.26   Hip spica taping (courtesy of Greg Littler and Lee Young).

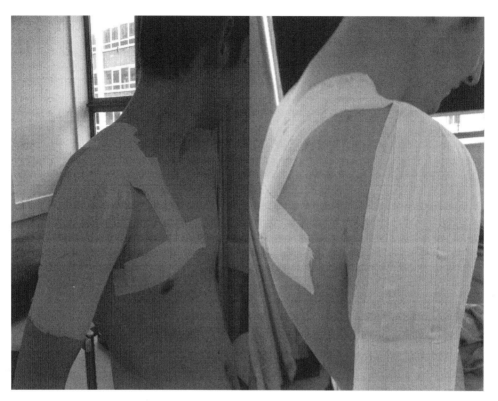

Photo 3.27 Acromioclavicular joint support (courtesy of Greg Littler and Lee Young).

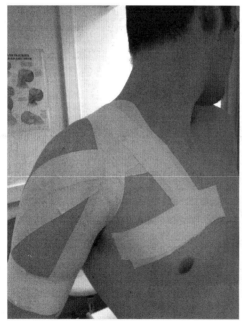

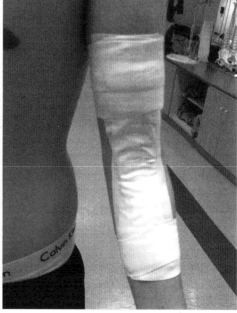

Photo 3.28 Anterior glenohumeral instability support (courtesy of Greg Littler and Lee Young).

Photo 3.29 Elbow hyperextension restriction taping (courtesy of Greg Littler and Lee Young).

Precautions for taping and strapping

There are certain instances when the application of taping and strapping are not applicable. The main contraindications to taping and strapping include where: a complete assessment has not been performed; the therapist is unsure of the nature of the problem; serious injury is suspected; and urgent referral for medical assessment is required (first aid applications must still apply). Taping should never be used as a substitute for treatment. When the patient or athlete complains of discomfort, the therapist must use their professional judgement to determine the suitability of taping. It is considered a contraindication to tape (beyond first aid compression strapping) during acute stages of injury, where there are open wounds or where the joint is clearly unstable. Similarly, if the area is extremely swollen and irritable, shows signs of infection or there is a suspected fracture, poor circulation or known allergy to taping materials, or poor skin integrity, such as that which may follow local steroid therapy. Itching, blisters and other signs of allergy may present immediately following taping, or might be latent. Considerations must also be given regarding taping on or over areas where friction can occur during movement (particularly during exercise). Excessively tight taping applications or incorrectly taped areas may be identified by any circulatory changes such as oedema, changes in skin colour or failure of capillary refill (a pinch of the nail beds of fingers and toes can assess for this).

Tape should always be removed carefully using tape cutters or bandage scissors wherever necessary or possible. A lubricant may be applied to the tip of tape cutters to assist its gliding under the tape. The sports therapist must be careful to not nip the skin or any bony prominences. Tape may be more easily removed following a soak in the bath. Adhesive tape should be peeled back (preferably in line with hair growth) while supporting the adjacent skin; this will help reduce skin traction; a dehesive spray or lotion may be used and tape should never be ripped off. The sports therapist should always check the area after tape removal for any signs of allergy or irritation. All soiled taping materials must be disposed of hygienically, ideally into a clinical waste container. Tape should never be left on for too long, as this can lead to skin soreness and possible skin breakdown (maceration). Different taping products, applications and situations will determine how long a taping application should remain on the athlete or patient. As mentioned, athletic taping, where the athlete is taped prior to the game (whether for standard prophylactic purposes or for specific support to an existing injury) may only remain effective for a relatively short functional time frame, and re-application may be required at half-time. Athletic taping applications are usually removed immediately following the activity. Taping for other objectives may require tape to remain in-situ for 20 hours or so – any longer than this and there is potential for maceration and possible infection (particularly bacterial or fungal). Kinesiology applications, however, may in some circumstances be indicated to remain in place for two to three days.

Kinesiology taping

Kinesiology tape and its associated taping techniques were first developed in Japan in the 1970s, and have steadily gained popularity with athletes and practitioners over the past 20 years. While Dr Kenzo Kase first patented 'Kinesio taping' and 'Kinesio Tex tape' (Kinesio UK, 2013), there are now a number of established kinesiology-style taping methodologies in general usage. One of the original theories for the use of kinesiology tape was that the tape should mimic some of the movement, flexibility and function of human skin, hence the functional properties of kinesiology tape include an elasticity and thickness which resembles that of the epidermis (Kase *et al.*, 2003). Kumbrink (2012) explains that kinesiology tapes are applied to follow the course of tissues and may be applied to almost any region of the body. In addition, there are lymphatic applications designed to help improve local circulation; hence, kinesiology taping is proposed as a treatment method.

Although there are variant specifications, kinesiology tape is made predominantly from cotton, which surrounds its polymer elastic strands, and its porosity allows for evaporation of body moisture and quick drying. Most tapes are latex-free, hypoallergenic and water-resistant. They are backed by an acrylic adhesive, which is heat activated (by the gentle manual rubbing of the tape once in position). The adhesive is applied to the back of the tape in a wave-like pattern, similar to that of the fingerprint, and this, in combination with its elastic properties, is purported to facilitate the escape of moisture and to assist the tape's ability to lift the skin. The tape is applied to a backing paper and supplied in rolls. Kinesiology tape's elasticity allows for it to be stretched longitudinally by 100 per cent (or more) of its resting length, and most are applied to their backing paper in a state of slight tension (typically 10 per cent of available tension) (Kase *et al.*, 2003; Kumbrink, 2012). This means that the tape 'comes off the roll' in slight tension. Traditional forms of kinesiology tape are only able to be stretched longitudinally, although there are now tapes which also provide for horizontal elasticity. Kinesiology tape is by definition ultra-flexible and mouldable to body contours (Gibbons, 2014). The tape is non-tearable and requires cutting prior to application; there are 'pre-cut' tapes available which are designed for specific applications, and these may save time, particularly in team settings or large departments. Original kinesiology tape came in four colours (cyan, magenta, beige and black), but there are now a host of different colours (and patterns) available. While there is no difference in the structure or properties of the traditional tapes, the four original colours were chosen to utilize potential additional benefits of 'colour therapy' (Gibbons, 2014; Kumbrink, 2012).

Just as with athletic taping, prior to any application the therapist must consider what the therapeutic objectives are, where the tape(s) will be applied and what degree of tension will be applicable. It is generally proposed that kinesiology tape may:

- aid the body's natural healing processes;
- stimulate neurological and circulatory activity (thereby reducing pain and improving lymphatic drainage);
- facilitate either muscle activation or inhibition;
- provide support to injured muscles, tendons or ligaments;
- provide fascial, anatomical space or joint alignment correction ('lift' tapes).

The correction application techniques as described by Kase *et al.* (2003) have yet to be effectively evidenced. Kinesiology taping is not designed to provide rigid support for severe injury or to stabilize an unstable joint; the elastic properties will not efficiently facilitate this. However, it may be used to help prevent potentially harmful ranges of motion (Athletic Tape Info, 2013). Kinesiology tape is designed to provide support and stimulation to tissue while allowing the available range of motion; and the actual effect may be considered as offering a continuous and uninterrupted stimulation, which may then lead to favourable structural adaptation (Hyde *et al.*, 2011). The four main applications for kinesiology taping are as follows (adapted from Kumbrink, 2012):

1. Muscle applications: stimulation and inhibition techniques – these typically use 'I' and 'Y' strips applied with the target muscle in an elongated position, and with the tape on around 10–20 per cent stretch.

2. Support applications: applied to ligaments, tendons, muscle tears and spinal segments – these typically use an 'I' strip applied with between 70–90 per cent tape tension over the target tissue.
3. Correction ('lift') applications: applied to address myofascial tensions, localized pain points, myofascial trigger points, or bony misalignments. These typically use 'I' or 'Y' strips applied with tape tensions of 50–70 per cent.
4. Lymphatic applications: used to gently lift skin and thereby support lymphatic drainage – these may utilize 'fan' strips or 'web' patterns applied with the patient's target region on stretch, and with typically around 25 per cent tape tension.

The general recommendation for muscle inhibition has been for the tape to be applied from insertion to origin; for muscle facilitation the tape may be applied from origin to insertion (both applications should have the target muscle on stretch) and with around 10–20 per cent tape tension. While athletes may perceive benefit, and clinicians anecdotally report positive outcomes, Gómez-Soriano and colleagues (2014) looked at applications of kinesiology tape applied to influence the gastrocnemius muscle in a double-blind, placebo-controlled crossover trial involving 19 healthy participants using a range of outcome measures (muscle tone, extensibility, electromyography and strength) and found *'no effect on healthy muscle tone, extensibility nor strength'*. They did identify a short-term increase of gastrocnemius EMG activity after taping, which *'suggests the activation of central nervous system mechanisms, although without a therapeutic implication'*. As ever, further research is require to substantiate the positive influence of kinesiology taping applications for muscle tone. Another of the aims (or claims) of kinesiology taping for injured ligaments and tendons is to increase stimulation of local mechanoreceptors to facilitate improved responsive proprioception (Kase *et al.*, 2003). Typically, these tapes are applied with a high degree of tension (50–100 per cent). For localized areas of pain associated with muscular injury or MTrPs, a 'lift' or 'star' technique may be applied; this simply involves two or more short strips applied with high tension in a cross-type (X) pattern. In acute injury, kinesiology tape is purported to assist lymphatic circulation. As lymphatic applications are applied in a state of minimal tension (10–15 per cent), the tape's elastic properties are designed to cause a lifting effect on the epidermis which may decrease pressure on superficial lymphatics and blood vessels. Applications to support this include the use of 'fan' strips or 'web' patterns. The base of the fan or web should be located in a direction towards the nearest proximal lymph nodes to which the therapist would like to encourage drainage. Bleakley (2013) interestingly identifies a challenge to the sports therapist's clinical reasoning process in terms of how the oedema associated with many acute soft tissue injuries may be managed: *'The revolutionary science of using kinesiotape to microscopically "lift" the skin to potentially enhance vascular and lymphatic function post-injury is tantamount to "anti-compression" and indicates the current ambiguity in this field of study.'*

When kinesiology tape is applied with the skin and tissues in a position of stretch, and with the tape in a 'resting tension', 'convolutions' of the tape will appear as the patient returns to a neutral position following the tape application. It is the convolutions (resulting from the gentle elastic-recoil effect of the tape) which lift the skin. As the skin is 'lifted', and subcutaneous tissue pressure reduced, then any excessive interstitial fluid and channelling lymphatic fluid may be more effectively dispersed. Osmolarity gradients are altered and the direction of fluid flow runs from areas of high pressure to lower pressure (Hyde *et al.*, 2011). This effect, it is proposed, can reduce fluid stasis, and therefore swelling and oedema, which in turn can assist the removal of chemical (locally noxious) irritants from the injured area and accelerate tissue healing. For its potential effect regarding pain relief, the consideration is that the tape can provide enhanced sensory (mechanical and innocuous) inputs, and as such will stimulate A-beta fibres, which may then offset the previously stimulated nociceptive A-delta and C-fibre inputs. With taping applications that are aiming to affect neurosensory systems, the therapist will usually place the affected muscle onto a position of stretch, rather than the tape during the tape's application.

Tapes are generally individually cut from standard 5 cm × 5 m tape rolls by the practitioner (although wider and longer tapes are available, as well as 'pre-cut' tapes). The patterns that may be employed include 'I', 'X', 'Y' and 'fan' strips. When applying the tape, the skin should be dry and free of oil, and excessively hairy areas may need to be trimmed or shaved; tape adhesive spray can also be used where effective adhesion may be compromised.

Prior to the application of kinesiology tape, the sports therapist must determine the appropriate tape size and shape, joint positioning and tape tension required. It is advisable to 'round the edges' of the tape (using scissors) so as to reduce the potential for the tape edges to start to peel off. Both the proximal base and distal ends should be applied without tension. Once tape has been applied, the patient/athlete should be observed performing functional activity.

When exploring the effects of kinesiology taping on scapular kinematics, muscle performance and shoulder impingement, Hsu *et al.* (2008) found positive changes in both scapular motion

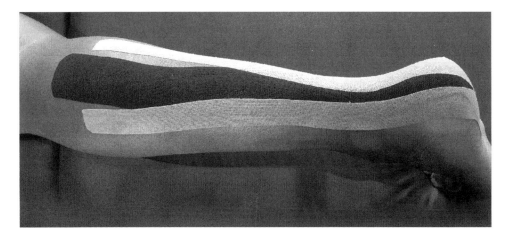

Photo 3.30 Kinesiology 'muscle' technique.

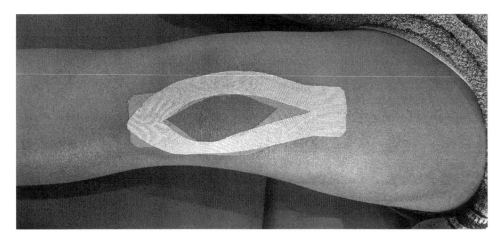

Photo 3.31 Kinesiology 'support' technique.

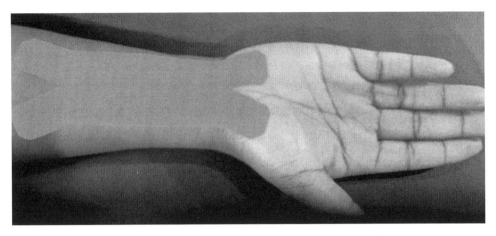

Photo 3.32 Kinesiology 'lift' technique.

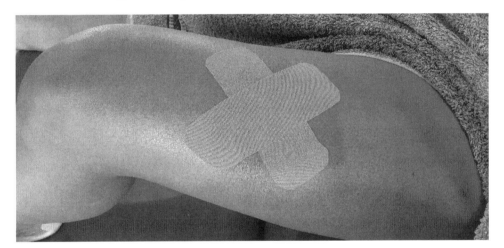

Photo 3.33 Kinesiology 'star' technique.

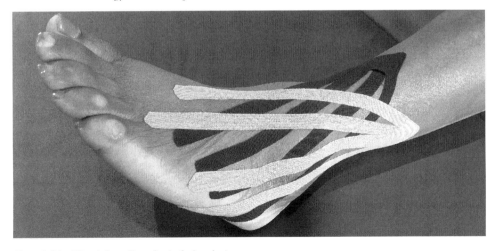

Photo 3.34 Kinesiology 'lymphatic fan' technique.

and muscle performance which supports its use as a treatment aid in managing shoulder impingement. In a randomized controlled study by Thelen and colleagues (2008), shoulder patients with rotator cuff conditions who were treated with kinesiology tape also demonstrated improved pain-free range of movement. Irrefutable evidence to support the use of all kinesiology taping applications is clearly lacking. Williams *et al.* (2012) concluded that, while there is significant case study and anecdotal support for the method, it is essential that more high-quality research is required, particularly regarding sports injuries.

The demand for and use of taping in sports therapy continues to grow; and while there are a wide range of taping techniques, applications, methodologies and technologies, it is essential now that the evidence-base for each of these interventions is expanded further so as to better guide practice and optimize therapeutic outcomes.

This chapter has attempted to present an introductory and informed discussion of the main contemporary clinical sports therapy interventions. In so doing, the authors have highlighted key principles and applications and essential safety issues, and provided evidence to support clinical decision making. It has been beyond the scope of this chapter to present a multitude of example treatment applications, but the sports therapist, as ever, is recommended to reflect on the information presented, and to review the main reference sources for each intervention. Finally, clinicians must be advised to think carefully and be very considerate in their use of modalities; as such, an educated internal dialogue (metacognitive reasoning) should always be employed (see Practitioner Tip Box 3.6).

Practitioner Tip Box 3.6

Important questions to ask prior to delivery of any therapeutic modality

- What specific goals am I attempting to achieve with this modality today?
- Am I using the best available modality (and correct application technique) to achieve these goals?
- What specific criteria must I consider to indicate that I should stop using this modality?
- What specific criteria must I consider to indicate that I have finished using this modality as part of this patient's management plan?

Source: adapted from Merrick, 2012.

References

Abell, B.A. (2010) *Taping and wrapping made simple*. Lippincott, Williams and Wilkins. Philadelphia, PA

Alexander, L.D, David, R.D, Gilman, D.R, Brown, J.L and Houghton, P.E. (2010) Exposure to low amounts of ultrasound energy does not improve soft tissue shoulder pathology: A systematic review. *Physical Therapy*. 90 (1): 14–25

Algafly, A.A. and George, K.P. (2007) The effect of cryotherapy on nerve conduction velocity, pain threshold and pain tolerance. *British Journal of Sports Medicine*. 41 (6): 365–369

Alter, M. (2004) *Science of flexibility*. Human Kinetics. St Louis, MO

Alvarez, D. and Rockwell, P. (2002) Trigger points: Diagnosis and management. *American Family Physician*. 65 (4): 653–657

Anderson, M., Parr, G. and Hall, S. (2009) *Foundations of athletic training: Prevention, assessment and management*, 4th edition. Lippincott, Williams and Wilkins. Philadelphia, PA

Andersson, S.A., Holmgren, E. and Roos, A. (1977) Analgesic effects of peripheral conditioning stimulation: Importance of certain stimulation parameters. *Acupuncture and Electrotherapy Research.* 2: 237–247

Andrade, C.K. and Clifford, P. (2008) *Outcome-based massage: From evidence to practice*, 2nd edition. Lippincott, Williams and Wilkins. Philadelphia, PA

Andrade, C.K. and Clifford, P. (2012) Qualitative research methods. In Dryden, T. and Moyer, C.A. (eds) *Massage therapy: Integrating research and practice.* Human Kinetics. Champaign, IL

Athletic Tape Info (2013) *Archive for the 'Health Professionals' Category* www.athletictapeinfo.com/category/health-professionals, accessed May 2013

Atkins, E., Kerr, J. and Goodlad, E. (2010) *A practical approach to orthopaedic medicine: Assessment, diagnosis and treatment*, 3rd edition. Churchill Livingstone, Elsevier. London, UK

Atnip, B.L. and McCrory, J.L. (2004) The effect of cryotherapy on three dimensional ankle kinematics during a sidestep cutting manoeuvre. *Journal of Sports Science and Medicine.* 3: 83–90

Bahr, R. and Engebretsen, L. (2009) *Sports injury prevention (Olympic handbook of sports medicine).* Wiley-Blackwell. Oxford, UK

Bailey, D.M., Erith, S.J., Griffin, P.J., *et al.* (2007) Influence of cold-water immersion on indices of muscle damage following prolonged intermittent shuttle running. *Journal of Sports Sciences.* 25 (11): 1163–1170

Ballantyne, F. Fryer, G. and McLaughlin, P. (2003) The effect of muscle energy technique on hamstring extensibility: The mechanism of altered flexibility. *Journal of Osteopathic Medicine.* 6 (2): 59–63

Bandyopadhyay, A. and Mahapatra, D. (2012) Taping in sports. *Journal of Human Sport and Exercise.* 547 (2): 544–552

Banks, K. and Hengeveld, E. (2010) *Maitland's clinical companion: An essential guide for students.* Churchill Livingstone, Elsevier. London, UK

Barnes, J.F. (1990) *Myofascial release: The search for excellence.* Rehabilitation Services Inc. MFR Treatment Centers and Seminars. Pennsylvania, USA

Barnes, L. (1979). Cryotherapy: Putting injury on ice. *Physician and Sportsmedicine.* 7(6): 130–136

Belanger, A.Y. (2002) *Evidence-based guide to therapeutic physical agents.* Lippincott, Williams and Wilkins. Philadelphia, PA

Belitsky, R.B., Odam, S.J. and Hubley-Kozey, C. (1987) Evaluation of the effectiveness of wet ice, dry ice, and cryogen packs in reducing skin temperature. *Physical Therapy.* 67 (7): 1080–1084

Belsey, J. and Snell, T. (2009) *What is evidence-based medicine?*, 2nd edition. Hayward Medical Communications. Oxford, UK

Benjamin, P.J. and Lamp, S.P. (2005) *Understanding sports massage*, 2nd edition. Human Kinetics. Champaign, IL

Bialosky, J.E., Bishop, M.D., George, S.Z. and Robinson, M.E. (2011) Placebo response to manual therapy: Something out of nothing? *Journal of Manual and Manipulative Therapy.* 19 (1): 11–19

Birrer, R.B. and Poole, B. (2004) General principles and specifics for the ankle-taping of sports injuries: Review of a basic skill. *Journal of Musculoskeletal Medicine.* 21: 197–211

Bleakley, C.M. (2013) Acute soft tissue injury management: Past, present and future. *Physical Therapy in Sport.* 14: 73–74

Bleakley, C.M. and Davison, G.W. (2010) What is the biochemical and physiological rationale for using cold-water immersion in sports recovery? A systematic review. *British Journal of Sports Medicine.* 44: 179–187

Bleakley, C.M. and Hopkins, J.T. (2010). Is it possible to achieve optimal levels of tissue cooling in cryotherapy? *Physical Therapy Reviews.* 15 (4): 344–350

Bleakley, C.M., McDonough, S.M. and MacAuley, D.C. (2004) The use of ice in the treatment of acute soft-tissue injury. *American Journal of Sports Medicine.* 32 (1): 251–261

Bleakley, C.M., McDonough, S.M. and MacAuley, D.C. (2006) Cryotherapy for acute ankle sprains: A randomised controlled study of two different icing protocols. *British Journal of Sports Medicine.* 40 (8): 700–705

Bleakley, C.M., Glasgow, P. and MacAuley, D.C. (2012) PRICE needs updating: Should we call the POLICE? *British Journal of Sports Medicine.* 46 (4): 220–221

Bogduk, N. and Twomey, L.T. (1987) *Clinical anatomy of the lumbar spine.* Churchill Livingstone. New York

Breig, A. (1978) *Adverse mechanical tension in the central nervous system.* Almqvist and Wiksell. Stockholm, Sweden

Briggs, J. (2001) *Sports Therapy: Theoretical and practical thoughts and considerations*. Corpus Publishing. Chichester, UK

Brummitt, J. (2008) The role of massage in sports performance and rehabilitation: Current evidence and future direction. *North American Journal of Sports Physical Therapy*. 3 (1): 7–21

Bugaj, R. (1975). The cooling, analgesic, and rewarming effects of ice massage on localized skin. *Physical Therapy*. 55 (1): 11–19

Burke, D., Holt, L., Rasmussen, R., MacKinnon, N., Vossen, J. and Pelham, T. (2001) Effects of hot or cold water immersion and modified proprioceptive neuromuscular facilitation flexibility exercise on hamstring length. *Journal of Athletic Training*. 36 (1): 16–19

Burns, D.K. and Wells, M.R. (2006) Gross range of motion in the cervical spine: The effects of osteopathic muscle energy technique in asymptomatic subjects. *Journal of American Osteopathic Association*. 106 (3): 137–142

Butler, D. (1991) *Mobilisation of the nervous system*. Churchill Livingstone. Melbourne, Australia

Butler, D and Nee, R.J. (2006) Management of peripheral neuropathic pain: Integrating neurobiology, neurodynamics, and clinical evidence. *Physical Therapy in Sport*. 7: 36–49

Butterwick, D.J., Nelson, D.S., Lafave, M.R. and Meeuwisse, W.H. (2004) Epidemiological analysis of injury in one year of Canadian professional rodeo. *Clinical Journal of Sports Medicine*. 6: 171–177

Callaghan, M.J. (1993) The role of massage in the management of the athlete: A review. *British Journal of Sports Medicine*. 27 (1): 28–33

Carnes, D., Mars, T., Mullinger, B., Froud, R. and Underwood, M. (2010) Adverse events in manual therapy: A systematic review. *Manual Therapy*. 15 (4): 355–363

Cash, M. (2012) *Advanced remedial massage and soft tissue therapy*. Ebury Press. London, UK

CASP (Critical Appraisal Skills Programme) (2014) *CASP Checklists*. www.casp-uk.net/#!casp-tools-checklists/c18f8, accessed August 2014

Chaitow, L. (2006) *Muscle energy techniques*, 3rd edition. Churchill Livingstone, Elsevier. London, UK

Chaitow, L. (2007) *Positional release techniques*, 3rd edition. Churchill Livingstone, Elsevier. London, UK.

Chaitow, L. and DeLany J.W. (2002) *Clinical application of neuromuscular techniques. Volume 2: The lower body*. Churchill Livingstone, Elsevier. London, UK.

Chaitow, L. and DeLany, J. (2008) *Clinical application of neuromuscular techniques. Volume 1: The upper body*, 2nd edition. Churchill Livingstone, Elsevier. Edinburgh, UK

Cochrane, D.J. (2004) Alternating hot and cold water immersion for athlete recovery: A review. *Physical Therapy in Sport*. 5: 26–32

Collins, C.K. (2007) Physical therapy management of complex regional pain syndrome in a 14-year old patient using strain counter strain: A case report. *Journal of Manual and Manipulative Therapy*. 15 (1): 25–41

Cook, C.E. (2012) *Orthopedic manual therapy: An evidence-based approach*, 2nd edition. Pearson Health Science. Upper Saddle River, NJ

Coppieters, M.W. and Nee, R.J. (2012) Neurodynamics: Movement for neuropathic pain states. In Schleip, R., Findlay, T.W., Chaitow, L. and Huijing, P.A. (eds) *Fascia: The tensional network of the human body*. Churchill Livingstone, Elsevier. Edinburgh, UK

Cordova, M.L., Ingersoll, C.D. and Le Blanc, M.J. (2000) Influence of ankle support on joint range of motion before and after exercise: A meta-analysis. *Journal of Orthopedic Sports Physical Therapy*. 30 (4): 170–182

Costello, J.T. and Donnelly, A.E. (2010) Cryotherapy and joint position sense in healthy participants: A systematic review. *Journal of Athletic Training*. 45 (3): 306–316

Cross, K.M., Wilson, R.W. and Perrin, D.H. (1996) Functional performance following an ice immersion to the lower extremity. *Journal of Athletic Training*. 31 (2): 113–116

Cyriax, J. and Coldham, M. (1984) *Textbook of orthopaedic medicine: Volume 2 – Treatment by manipulation, massage and injection*, 11th edition. Baillière Tindall. London, UK

Cyriax, J. and Cyriax, P. (1982) *Cyriax's illustrated manual of orthopaedic medicine*. Butterworth-Heinemann. Oxford, UK

De Domenico, G. (1982) Pain relief with interferential therapy. *Australian Journal of Physiotherapy*. 29 (3): 14–18

de Jong, R.H., Hershey, W.N. and Wagman, H.I. (1966). Nerve conduction velocity during hypothermia in man. *American Society of Anesthesiologists*. 27 (6): 805–810

Dejung, B., Lewit, K., Irnich, D. and Schleip, R. (2013) Manual therapy and physiotherapy. In Irnich, D. (ed.) *Myofascial trigger points: Comprehensive diagnosis and treatment*. Churchill Livingstone, Elsevier. Edinburgh, UK

Denegar, C.R. (2000) *Therapeutic modalities for athletic injuries*. Human Kinetics. Champaign, IL

Dinsdale, N. (2008) Research skills: EBP. *SportEX Dynamics*. 18: 10–13

Dinsdale, N. (2012) *Evidence-based practice*. www.njdsportsinjuries.co.uk/Evidence-Based-Practice.htm, accessed January 2014

Dommerholt, J. (2013) Trigger point therapy. In Schleip, R., Findlay, T.W., Chaitow, L. and Huijing, P.A. (eds) *Fascia: The tensional network of the human body*. Churchill Livingstone, Elsevier. Edinburgh, UK

Donaldson, M. (2012) Soft-tissue mobilization. In Cook, C.E. (ed.) *Orthopedic manual therapy: An evidence-based approach*, 2nd edition. Pearson Health Science. Upper Saddle River, NJ

Dykstra, J.H., Hill, H.M., Miller, M.G., Cheatham, C.C., Michael, T.J. and Baker, R.J. (2009) Comparison of cubed ice, crushed ice, and wetted ice on intramuscular and surface temperature changes. *Journal of Athletic Training*. 44 (2): 136–141

Earls, J. and Myers, T. (2010) *Fascial release for structural balance*. Lotus Publishing. Chichester, UK

Ebell, M.H., Siwek, J., Weiss, B.D., Woolf, S.H., Susman, J., Ewigman, B. and Bowman, M. (2004) Strength of Recommendation Taxonomy (SORT): A patient-centered approach to grading evidence in the medical literature. *American Academy of Family Physicians*. 69: 548–556

Ebrall, P., Moore, N. and Poole, R. (1989) An investigation of the suitability of infrared telethermography to determine skin temperature changes in the human ankle during cryotherapy. *Chiropractic Sports Medicine*. 3 (4): 111–119

Ebrall, P.S., Bales, G.L. and Frost, B.R. (1992) An improved clinical protocol for ankle cryotherapy. *Journal of Manual Medicine*. 6 (5): 161–165

Ellse, M. and Honeywill, C. (2004) *Electricity and thermal physics*. Nelson Thornes. Cheltenham, UK

Enwemeka, C.S., Allen, C., Avila, P., Bina, J., Konrade, J. and Munns, S. (2002) Soft tissue thermodynamics before, during and after cold pack therapy. *Medicine and Science in Sports and Exercise*. 34 (1): 45–50

Evans, T., Ingersoll, C., Knight, K. and Worrell, T. (1995) Agility following the application of cold therapy. *Journal of Athletic Therapy*. 30 (3): 231–234

Field, T.M., Hernandez-Reif, M., Diego, M., Schanberg, S. and Kuhn, C. (2005) Cortisol decreases and serotonin increase following massage therapy. *International Journal of Neuroscience*. 1515: 1397–1413

French, R.M. (2011) *Milady's guide to lymph drainage massage*, 2nd edition. Delmar Cengage Learning. New York

Fritz, S. (2005) *Sports and exercise massage: Comprehensive care in athletics, fitness and rehabilitation*. Elsevier, Mosby. Philadelphia, PA

Fryer, G. (2011) Muscle energy technique: An evidence-informed approach. *International Journal of Osteopathic Medicine*. 14 (1): 3–9

Galloway, S., Hunter, A. and Watt, J.M. (2012) Athletes. In Dryden, T. and Moyer, C.A. (eds) *Massage therapy: Integrating research and practice*. Human Kinetics. Champaign, IL

Gautschi, R. (2013) Treatment plan for myofascial trigger point therapy. In Irnich, D. (ed.) *Myofascial trigger points: Comprehensive diagnosis and treatment*. Churchill Livingstone, Elsevier. Edinburgh, UK

Gibbons, J. (2011) *Muscle energy techniques: A practical guide for physical therapists*. Lotus Publishing. Chichester, UK

Gibbons, J. (2014) *A practical guide to kinesiology taping*. Lotus Publishing. Chichester, UK

Goats, G.C. (1990) Interferential current therapy. *British Journal of Sports Medicine*. 24 (2): 87–92

Goats, G.C. (1994a) Massage: The scientific basis of an ancient art: Part 1 – the techniques. *British Journal of Sports Medicine*. 28 (3): 149–152

Goats, G.C. (1994b) Massage: The scientific basis of an ancient art: Part 2 – physiological and therapeutic effects. *British Journal of Sports Medicine*. 28 (3): 153–156

Goldberg, J., Sullivan, S.J. and Seaborne, D.E. (1992) The effect of two intensities of massage on H-reflex amplitude. *Physical Therapy*. 72 (6): 449–457

Gómez-Soriano, J., Abián-Vicén, J., Aparicio-García, C., Ruiz-Lázaro, P., Simón-Martínez, C., Bravo-Esteban, E. and Fernández-Rodríguez, J.M. (2014) The effects of Kinesio taping on muscle tone in healthy subjects: A double-blind, placebo-controlled crossover trial. *Manual Therapy*. 19 (2): 131–136

Grant, A.E. (1964) Massage with ice (cryokinetics) in the treatment of painful conditions of the musculoskeletal system. *Archives of Physical Medicine and Rehabilitation*. 45: 233–238

Gratton, C. and Jones, I. (2010) *Research methods for sports studies*, 2nd edition. Routledge. Oxon, UK

Greenhalgh, S. and Selfe, J. (2006) *Red flags: A guide to identifying serious pathology of the spine*. Churchill Livingstone, Elsevier. Edinburgh, UK

Greenhalgh, T. (1997) How to read a paper: Getting your bearing. Deciding what the paper is about. *British Medical Journal*. 3 (15): 243–246

Greenhalgh, T. (2012) Why do we always end up here? Evidence-based medicine's conceptual cul-de-sacs and some off-road alternative routes. *Journal of Primary Health Care*. 4: 92–97

Greenhalgh, T., Howick, J. and Maskrey, N. (2014) Evidence based medicine: A movement in crisis? *British Medical Journal*. 348: g3725

Greenman, P.E. (1996) *Principles of manual medicine*, 2nd edition. Williams and Wilkins. Baltimore, MD

Grieve, G. (1988) *Common vertebral joint problems*, 2nd edition. Churchill Livingstone. Edinburgh, UK

Hall, K. (2014) *Evidence-based soft tissue skills*. Kevin Hall Physiotherapy Course Manual. UK

Hall, S. and Getchell, N. (2014) *Research methods in kinesiology and the health sciences*. Wolters Kluwer. Philadelphia, PA

Halvorson, G.A. (1990) Therapeutic heat and cold for athletic injuries. *The Physician and Sports Medicine*. 18 (5): 87–94

Hammer, W. (2008) The effect of mechanical load on degenerative soft tissue. *Journal of Bodywork and Movement Therapies*. 12: 246–256

Hammer, W. (2012) Graston technique: A contemporary instrument assisted mobilization method for the evaluation and treatment of soft tissue lesions. In Schleip, R., Findlay, T.W., Chaitow, L. and Huijing, P.A. (eds) *Fascia: The tensional network of the human body*. Churchill Livingstone, Elsevier. Edinburgh, UK

Harr, G. (1999) Therapeutic ultrasound. *European Journal of Ultrasound*. 9 (1): 3–9

Hart, J.M., Leonard, J.L. and Ingersoll, C.D. (2005) Single-leg landing strategy after knee-joint cryotherapy. *Journal of Sports Rehabilitation*. 14: 313–320

Hartman, L. (1997) *Handbook of osteopathic technique*, 3rd edition. Singular Publishing Group. San Diego, CA

Hayden, C.A. (1964) Cryokinetics in an early treatment program. *Journal of American Physical Therapy Association*. 44 (11): 990–993

Haynes, R.B., Devereaux, P.J. and Guyatt, G.H. (2002) Clinical expertise in the era of evidence-based medicine and patient choice. *Evidence Based Medicine* 7: 36–38

Hemmings, B. (2001) Physiological, psychological and performance effects of massage therapy in sport: A review of the literature. *Physical Therapy in Sport*. 2: 165–170

Hengeveld, E. and Banks, K. (2005) *Maitland's peripheral manipulation*, 4th edition. Elsevier, Butterworth Heinemann. London, UK

Henricson, A.S., Fredriksson, K., Persson, I., Pereira, R., Rostedt, Y. and Westlin, N.E. (1984) The effect of heat and stretching on the range of hip motion. *Journal of Orthopedic Sports Physical Therapy*. 6 (2): 110–115

Hilbert, J.E., Sforzo, G.A. and Swensen, T. (2003) The effects of massage on delayed-onset muscle soreness. *British Journal of Sports Medicine*. 37: 72–75

Hogan, R.D., Burke, K.M. and Franklin, T.D. (1982) The effect of ultrasound on microvascular hemodynamics in skeletal muscle: Effects during ischemia. *Micro Research*. 23: 370–379

Hopkins, J.T. and Stencil, R. (2002) Ankle cryotherapy facilitates soleus function. *Journal of Orthopaedic and Sports Physical Therapy*. 32 (12): 622–627

Hopkins, J.T., Hunter, I. and McLoda, T. (2006) Effects of ankle joint cooling on peroneal short latency response. *Journal of Sports Science and Medicine*. 5 (2): 333–339

Houglum, P.A. (2010) *Therapeutic exercise for musculoskeletal injuries*, 3rd edition. Human Kinetics. Champaign, IL

Hsieh, Y.L. (2006) Effects of ultrasound on Diclofenac phonophorosis on inflammatory pain relief: Suppression of inducible nitric oxide synthase in arthritic rats. *Physical Therapy*. 86 (1): 39–49

Hsu, Y.H., Chen, W.Y., Lin, H.C., Wanga, W.T.J. and Shih, Y.F. (2008) The effects of taping on scapular kinematics and muscle performance in baseball players with shoulder impingement syndrome. *Journal of Electromyography and Kinesiology*. 19: 1092–1099

Hunter, G. (1994) Specific soft tissue mobilisation. *Physiotherapy*. 80 (1): 15–21

Hunter, G. (1998) The use of specific soft tissue mobilisation in the management of soft tissue dysfunction. *Manual Therapy*. 3 (1): 2–11

Hunter, G. (2006) *Specific soft tissue mobilisation (SSTM): Lower limb*. Course manual. Wellbeing CPD Limited. UK

Hyde, T., Doerr, G., Hammer, W., de Bono, V., Strachan, D. and Pearce, K. (2011) *FAKTR-PM: Functional and kinetic treatment with rehab, provocation and movement.* Course manual. UK

ICAHE (International Centre for Allied Health Evidence) (2014) *Evidence-based practice glossary.* www.unisa.edu.au/Research/Sansom-Institute-for-Health-Research/Research-at-the-Sansom/Research-Concentrations/Allied-Health-Evidence/Resources/Glossary, accessed February 2014

IFOMPT (International Federation of Orthopedic Manipulative Physical Therapists) (2010) *Standards committee glossary of terminology.* www.ifompt.com/Standards/SC+Glossary.html, accessed May 2013

Ignelzi, R.J. and Nyquist, J.K. (1979) Excitability changes in peripheral nerve fibers after repetitive electrical stimulation: Implications in pain modulation. *Journal of Neurosurgery.* 51: 824–833

Ingraham, P. (2013) *Does fascia matter? A detailed critical analysis of the clinical relevance of fascia science and fascia properties.* http://saveyourself.ca/articles/does-fascia-matter.php#sec_tough, accessed April 2014

Ingram, J., Dawson, B., Goodman, C., Wallman, K. and Beilby, J. (2009) Effect of water immersion methods on post-exercise recovery from simulated team sport exercise. *Journal of Science and Medicine in Sport.* 12 (3): 417–421

Ioannidis, J.P.A. (2005) Why most published research findings are false. *PLoS Medicine.* 2 (8): e124

Jameson, A.G., Kinzey, S.J. and Hallam, J.S. (2001) Lower-extremity-joint cryotherapy does not affect vertical ground-reaction forces during landing. *Journal of Sports Rehabilitation.* 10: 132–142

Janssen, K.W. and Kamper, S.J. (2013) Ankle taping and bracing for proprioception. *British Journal of Sports Medicine.* 47: 527–528

Janwantanakul, P. (2006) Cold pack/skin interface temperature during ice treatment with various levels of compression. *Physiotherapy.* 92 (4): 254–259

Jelveus, A. (2011) *Integrated sports massage therapy.* Churchill Livingstone, Elsevier. Edinburgh, UK

Johnson, A.J., Godges, J.J., Zimmerman, G.J. and Ounanian, L.L. (2007) The effect of anterior versus posterior glide joint mobilization on external rotation range of motion in patients with shoulder adhesive capsulitis. *Journal of Orthopaedic and Sports Physical Therapy.* 37 (3): 88–99

Johnson, M.I. and Tabasam, G. (2003) An investigation into the analgesic effects of interferential currents and transcutaneous electrical nerve stimulation on experimentally induced ischemic pain in otherwise pain-free volunteers. *Physical Therapy.* 83 (3): 208–223

Jutte, L.S., Merrick, M.A., Ingersoll, C.D. and Edwards, J.E. (2001) The relationship between intramuscular temperature, skin temperature, and adipose thickness during cryotherapy and re-warming. *Archives of Physical Medicine and Rehabilitation.* 82 (6): 845–850

Kaltenborn, F.M. (1970) *Mobilization of the spinal column.* New Zealand University Press. Wellington, New Zealand

Kaltenborn, F.M. (1999) *Manual mobilisation of the joints: The Kaltenborn method of joint mobilisation and treatment,* 5th edition. Olaf Norlis Bokhandel. Oslo, Norway

Kanlayanaphotporn, R. and Janwantanakul, P. (2005) Comparison of skin surface temperature during the application of various cryotherapy modalities. *Archives of Physical Medicine and Rehabilitation.* 86 (7): 1411–1415

Kase, K., Wallis, J. and Kase, T. (2003) *Clinical therapeutic applications of the Kinesio taping method,* 2nd edition. Kinesio Taping Association. Tokyo, Japan

Kennet, J., Hardaker, N., Hobbs, S. and Selfe, J. (2007). Cooling efficiency of 4 common cryotherapeutic agents. *Journal of Athletic Training.* 42 (3): 343–348

Kessler, R.M. and Hertling, D. (1983) *Management of common musculoskeletal disorders: Physical therapy, principles and methods.* Harper and Row, Publishers Inc. Philadelphia, PA

Khan, K.M. and Scott, A. (2009) Mechanotherapy: How physical therapists' prescription of exercise promotes tissue repair. *British Journal of Sports Medicine.* 43: 247–251

Kidd, R.F. (2009) Why myofascial release will never be evidence-based. *International Musculoskeletal Medicine.* 31 (2): 55–56

Kinesio UK (2013) *A brief history of Kinesio Tex taping.* www.kinesiotaping.co.uk/history.jsp, accessed May 2013

Kinzey, S.J., Cordova, M.L., Gallen, K.J., Smith, J.C. and Moore, J.B. (2000) The effects of cryotherapy on ground-reaction forces produced during a functional task. *Journal of Sports Rehabilitation.* 9: 3–14

Kitchen, S. and Bazin, S. (2004) *Electrotherapy: Evidence-based practice,* 11th edition. Elsevier. Edinburgh, UK

Kloth, L.C. (1991) Interference current. In Nelson, R.M. and Currier, D.P. (eds) *Clinical electrotherapy,* 2nd edition. Appleton and Lange. Norwalk, CT

Knight, C.A., Rutledge, C.R., Cox, M.E., Acosta, M. and Hall, S.J. (2001) Effect of superficial heat, deep heat, and active exercise warm-up on the extensibility of the plantar flexors. *Physical Therapy*. 81 (6): 1206–1214

Knight, K.L. (1995) *Cryotherapy in sports injury management*. Human Kinetics. Champaign, IL

Knight, K.L. and Draper, D.O. (2008) *Therapeutic modalities: The art and science*. Lippincott, Williams and Wilkins. Philadelphia, PA

Knight, K.L., Bryan, K.S. and Halvorsen, J.M. (1981) Circulatory changes in the forearm in 1, 5, 10, and 15°C water. *International Journal of Sports Medicine*. 4 (281): abstract

Knight, K.L., Brucker, J.B., Stoneman, P.D. and Rubley, M.D. (2000) Muscle injury management with cryotherapy. *Athletic Therapy Today*. 5 (4): 26–30

Krause, B.A., Hopkins, J.T., Ingersoll, C.D., Cordova, M.L. and Edwards J.E. (2000). The relationship of ankle temperature during cooling and rewarming to the human soleus H reflex. *Journal of Sports Rehabilitation*. 9: 253–262

Kumbrink, B. (2012) *K-taping: An illustrated guide*. Springer-Verlag. Berlin, Germany.

Kunesch, E., Schmidt, R., Nordin, M., Wallin, U. and Hagbarth, K.E. (1987) Peripheral neural correlates of cutaneous anaesthesia induced by cooling in man. *Acta Physiologica Scandinavica*, 129 (2): 247–257

Lamb, S. and Mani, R. (1994) Does interferential therapy affect blood flow? *Clinical Rehabilitation*. 8: 213–218

Law, M. and MacDermid, J. (2008) *Evidence-based rehabilitation: A guide to practice*, 2nd edition. SLACK Incorporated. Thorofare, NJ

Learman, K. and Cook, C.E. (2012) Neurodynamics. In Cook, C.E. (ed.) *Orthopedic manual therapy: An evidence-based approach*, 2nd edition. Pearson Health Science. Upper Saddle River, NJ

Lederman, E. (2014) *Therapeutic stretching: Towards a functional approach*. Churchill Livingstone, Elsevier. London, UK

Levick, J.R., Mason, R.M., Coleman, P.J., *et al*. (1999) Physiology of synovial fluid and trans-synovial flow. In Archer, C.W., Caterson, B., Benjamin, M., *et al*. (eds), *Biology of the synovial joint*. Harwood Academic Publishers. Australia

Lewis, M. and Johnson, M.I. (2006) The clinical effectiveness of therapeutic massage for musculoskeletal pain: A systematic review. *Physiotherapy*. 92: 146–158

Lloyd, E.L. (1994) ABC of sports medicine: Temperature and performance – cold. *British Medical Journal*. 309: 531–534

Loghmani, M.T. and Warden, S.J. (2009) Instrument-assisted cross-fibre massage accelerates knee ligament healing. *Journal of Orthopaedic and Sports Physical Therapy*. 39 (7): 506–514

Looney, B., Srokose, T., Fernandez-de-las-Penas, C. and Cleland, J.A. (2011) Graston instrument soft tissue mobilization and home stretching for the management of plantar heel pain: A case series. *Journal of Manipulative and Physiological Therapeutics*. 34 (2): 138–142

Low, J. and Reed, A. (2004) *Electrotherapy explained: Principles and practice*, 3rd edition. Butterworth Heinemann. Oxford, UK

MacAuley, D.C. (2001) Ice therapy: How good is the evidence? *International Journal of Sports Medicine*. 22 (5): 379–384

Macdonald, R. (2004) *Taping techniques: Principles and practice*. Butterworth Heinemann. London, UK

Magarey, M.E. (1986) Examination and assessment in spinal joint dysfunction. In Grieve, G.P. (ed.) *Modern manual therapy of the vertebral column*. Churchill Livingstone. Edinburgh, UK

Magee, D. (2008) *Orthopedic physical assessment*, 5th edition. Saunders. Philadelphia, PA

Maitland, G.D., Hengeveld, E., Banks, K. and English, K. (2005) *Maitland's vertebral manipulation*, 7th edition. Elsevier, Butterworth Heinemann. London, UK

Mangus, B.C., Hoffman, L.A., Hoffman, M.A. and Altenburger, P. (2002) Basic principles of extremity joint mobilization using a Kaltenborn approach. *Journal of Sports Rehabilitation*.11: 235–250

Manheim, C.J. (2008) *The myofascial release manual*, 4th edition. Slack Incorporated. Thorofare, NJ

Manske, R.C. and Lehecka, B.J. (2012) Evidence-based medicine/practice in sports physical therapy. *International Journal of Sports Physical Therapy*. 7 (5): 461–473

Mantoni, T., Belhage, B., Pedersen, L.M. and Pott, F.C. (2007) Reduced cerebral perfusion on sudden immersion in ice water: A possible cause of drowning. *Aviation, Space, and Environmental Medicine*. 78 (4): 374–376

Martin, D. (1994) Interferential for pain control. In Kitchen, S. and Bazin, S. (eds) *Clayton's electrotherapy*, 10th edition. W.B. Saunders. London, UK

Matsuzawa, T., Meguro, T., Eguchi, K., Yoshida, T., Maejima, T., Suda, M., Ohsawa, H., Noguchi, E. and Kobayashi, S. (2004) The effects of ultrasound stimulation on muscle blood flow in the hind limb and related neural mechanism in anesthetized rats. *Journal of Physical Therapy Science*. 16 (1): 33–37

Maxwell, L. (1992) Therapeutic ultrasound: Its effects on the cellular and molecular mechanisms of inflammation and repair. *Physiotherapy*. 78 (6): 421–425

McAtee, B. (2013) An overview of facilitated stretching. *SportEx Dynamics*. 36: 30–34

McConnell, J. (2000) A novel approach to pain relief: Pre-therapeutic exercise. *Journal of Science and Medicine in Sport*. 3: 325

McConnell, J. (2002) Racalcitrant chronic low back and leg pain: A new theory and different approach to management. *Manual Therapy*. 7: 183–192

McCreesh, K. and O'Connor, A. (2012) Principles of joint treatment. In Petty, N.J. (ed.) *Principles of neuromuscoloskeletal treatment and management: A handbook for therapists*, 2nd edition. Churchill Livingstone, Elsevier. Edinburgh, UK

McKenney, K., Sinclair-Elder, A., Elder, C. and Hutchins, A. (2013) Myofascial release as a treatment for orthopaedic conditions: A systematic review. *Journal of Athletic Training*. 48 (4): 522–527

McMeeken, J., Lewis, M. and Cocks, S. (1984). Effects of cooling with simulated ice on skin temperature and nerve conduction velocity. *Australian Journal of Physiotherapy*. 30 (4): 111–114

Melzack, R. and Wall, P.D. (1965) Pain mechanisms: A new theory. *Science*. 150: 971–979

Mennell, J. (1960) *Back pain: Diagnosis and treatment using manipulative techniques*. Little, Brown. Boston, MA

Merrick, M.A. (2002) Secondary injury after musculoskeletal trauma: A review and update. *Journal of Athletic Training*. 37 (2): 209–217

Merrick, M.A. (2012) Therapeutic modalities as an adjunct to rehabilitation. In Andrews, J.R., Harrelson, G.L. and Wilk, K.E. (eds) *Physical rehabilitation of the injured athlete*, 4th edition. Elsevier, Saunders. Philadelphia, PA

Merrick, M.A., Knight, K.L., Ingersoll, C.D. and Potteiger, J.A. (1993) The effects of ice and compression wraps on intramuscular temperatures at various depths. *Journal of Athletic Training*. 28 (3): 241–245

Merrick, M.A., Jutte, L.S. and Smith, M.E. (2003) Cold modalities with different thermodynamic properties produce different surface and intramuscular temperatures. *Journal of Athletic Training*. 38 (1): 28–33

Milne, S., Welch, V., Brosseau, L., *et al.* (2001) Transcutaneous electrical nerve stimulation (TENS) for chronic low back pain. *Cochrane Database Systematic Review*. 2: CD003008

Moraska, A. (2005) Sports massage: A comprehensive review. *Journal of Sports Medicine and Physical Fitness*. 45: 370–380

Moyer, C.A., Seefeldt, L., Mann, L.S. and Jackley, L.M. (2011) Does massage therapy reduce cortisol? A comprehensive quantitative review. *Journal of Bodywork and Movement Therapies*. 15: 3–14

Mulligan, B. (1993) Mobilisations with movement (MVMs). *Journal of Manual and Manipulative Therapy*. 1: 154–156

Mulligan, B. (2004) *Manual therapy: NAGS, SNAGS, MWMs etc.*, 5th edition. Plane View Services Limited. Wellington, New Zealand

Myers, T. (2008) *Anatomy trains: Myofascial meridians for manual and movement therapists*, 2nd edition. Churchill Livingstone. Edinburgh, UK

Myers, T. and Frederick, C. (2012) Stretching and fascia. In Schleip, R., Findlay, T.W., Chaitow, L. and Huijing, P.A. (eds) *Fascia: The tensional network of the human body*. Churchill Livingstone, Elsevier. Edinburgh, UK

Myer, J.W., Measom, G.J. and Fellingham, G.W. (1998) Temperature changes in the human leg during and after two methods of cryotherapy. *Journal of Athletic Training*. 33: 25–29

Myer, J.W., Measom, G.J. and Fellingham, G.W. (2000) Exercise after cryotherapy greatly enhances intramuscular rewarming. *Journal of Athletic Training*. 35 (4): 412–416

Myer, J.W., Myer, K.A., Measom, G.J., Fellingham, G.W. and Evers, S.L. (2001) Muscle temperature is affected by overlying adipose when cryotherapy is administered. *Journal of Athletic Training*. 36 (1): 32–36

Nagrale, A.V., Glynn, P., Joshi, A. and Ramteke, G. (2010) The efficacy of an integrated neuromuscular inhibition technique on upper trapezius trigger points in subjects with non-specific neck pain: A randomized controlled trial. *Journal of Manual and Manipulative Therapy*. 18 (1): 37–43

Nee, R.J. and Butler, D. (2006) Management of peripheral neuropathic pain: Integrating neurobiology, neurodynamics, and clinical evidence. *Physical Therapy in Sport*. 7: 36–49

Nelson, B. (1981) Interferential therapy. *Australian Journal of Physiotherapy*. 27: 53–56

Ng, C.O.Y, Ng, G.Y.F., See, E.K.N and Leung, M.C.P (2003) Therapeutic ultrasound improves strength of Achilles tendon repair in rats. *Ultrasound in Medicine and Biology*. 29 (10): 1501–1506

Nielsen, A. (1995) *Gua Sha: Traditional technique for modern practice*. Churchill Livingstone. Edinburgh, UK

Noble, J.G., Henderson, G., Cramp, A.F., *et al.* (2000) The effect of interferential therapy upon cutaneous blood flow in humans. *Clinical Physiology*. 20 (1): 2–7

NOI (Neuro Orthopaedic Institute) (2010) *Mobilisation of the nervous system*, 22nd edition *(course manual)*. NOI Group. Dublin, Republic of Ireland

Noonan, T.I., Best, T.M., Seaber, A.V. and Garrett, W.E. (1993) Thermal effects on skeletal muscle tensile behavior. *American Journal of Sports Medicine*. 21 (4): 517–522

Norris, C.M. (2011) *Managing sports injuries: A guide for students and clinicians*, 4th edition. Churchill Livingstone, Elsevier. London, UK

Orton, D. (2013) Using the spoon: An introduction to instrument-assisted soft tissue manipulation. *SportEx Dynamics*. 36: 7–8

Palastanga, N., Field, D. and Soames, R. (2007) *Anatomy and human movement structure and function*, 5th edition. Butterworth Heinemann. Edinburgh, UK

Paris, S.V. (2012) *Past, present and future of joint manipulation*. American Academy of Orthopaedic Manipulative Therapy (AAOMPT) Presentation. www.aaompt.org/education/conference11/handouts/distinguished_lecture_paris.pdf, accessed May 2013

Patient Plus (2011) *Cryoglobulinaemia*. www.patient.co.uk/doctor/Cryoglobulinaemia.htm, accessed November 2013

Patterson, S.M., Udermann, B.E., Donerstein, S.T. and Reineke, D.M. (2008) The effects of cold whirlpool on power, speed, agility and range of motion. *Journal of Sports Science and Medicine*. 7: 387–394

Pengel, H.M., Maher, C.G. and Refshauge, K.M. (2002) Systematic review of conservative interventions for subacute low back pain. *Clinical Rehabilitation*. 16: 811–820

Petty, N.J. (2011) *Neuromusculoskeletal examination and assessment*, 4th edition. Churchill Livingstone, Elsevier. Edinburgh, UK

Pincivero, D., Gieck, J.H. and Saliba, E.N. (1993) Rehabilitation of the lateral ankle sprain with cryokinetics and functional progressive exercise. *Journal of Sports Rehabilitation*. 2: 200–207

Pope, G.D., Mockett, S.P. and Wright, J.P. (1995) A survey of electrotherapeutic modalities: Ownership and use in the NHS in England. *Physiotherapy*. 81 (2): 82–91

Prentice, W.E. (2009) *Arnheim's principles of athletic training: A competence-based approach*, 13th edition. McGraw-Hill. New York

Prentice, W.E. (2010) *Essentials of athletic injury management*, 8th edition. McGraw-Hill. New York

Prentice, W.E. (2011) Joint mobilisation and traction techniques in rehabilitation. In Prentice, W.E. (ed.) *Rehabilitation techniques for sports medicine and athletic training*, 5th edition. McGraw-Hill. New York

Quinn, K., Parker, P., de Bie, R., Rowe, R. and Handoll, H. (2000) Interventions for preventing ankle ligament injuries. *Cochrane Database of Systematic Reviews (Online)*. 2: CD000018

Quintner, J.L., Bove, G.M. and Cohen, M.L. (2014) A critical evaluation of the trigger point phenomenon. *Rheumatology*. 53 (12): 270–278

Quirke, M. and Harrison, A.J. (2002) A kinematic analysis of the effects of ankle taping on joint function. In *Proceedings of the Royal Academy of Medicine in Ireland, Biomedical Meeting*, Trinity College Dublin, Republic of Ireland

Richendollar, M.L., Darby, L.A. and Brown, T.M. (2006) Ice bag application, active warm-up, and 3 measures of maximal functional performance. *Journal of Athletic Training*. 41 (4): 364–370

Ridehalgh, C. and Barnard, K. (2012) Principles of nerve treatment. In Petty, N.J. (ed.) *Principles of neuromusculoskeletal treatment and management: A handbook for therapists*, 2nd edition. Churchill Livingstone, Elsevier. Edinburgh, UK

Rinder, A.N. and Sutherland, C.J. (1995) An investigation of the effects of massage on quadriceps performance after exercise fatigue. *Complementary Therapies in Nursing and Midwifery*. 1 (4): 99–102

Robertson, A., Watt, J.M. and Galloway, S.D.R. (2004) Effects of leg massage on recovery from high intensity cycling exercise. *British Journal of Sports Medicine*. 38: 173–176

Robertson, V.J., Ward, A., Low, J. and Reed, A. (2006) *Electrotherapy explained: Principles and practice*. Elsevier. Oxford, UK

Rolf, I.P. (1977) *Rolfing: The integration of human structures*. Dennis Landman. Santa Monica, CA

RSA (Raynaud's and Scleroderma Association) (2013) *Raynaud's phenomenon.* www.raynauds.org.uk/images/stories/PDF/raynauds08.pdf, accessed November 2013

Sackett, D.L., Rosenberg, W.M.C., Gray, J.A.M. and Haynes, R.B. (1996) Evidence-based medicine: What it is and what it isn't. *British Medical Journal.* 312: 71–72

Sackett, D.L. Straus, S.E., Richardson, W.S., Rosenberg, W.M.C. and Haynes, R.B. (2000) *Evidence-based medicine: How to practice and teach EBM,* 2nd edition. Churchill Livingstone. Edinburgh, UK

Saeki, Y. (2002). Effect of local application of cold or heat for relief of pricking pain. *Nursing and Health Sciences.* 4 (3): 97–105

Sanderson, M. (2012) *Soft tissue release: A practical handbook for physical therapists,* 3rd revised edition. Lotus Publishing. Chichester, UK

Sapega, A.A., Quendenfeld, T.C. and Moyer, R.A., *et al.* (1981) Biophysical factors in range of motion exercise. *The Physician and Sports Medicine.* 9 (12): 57–65

Sapega, A.A., Heppenstall, R.B., Sokolow, D.P., *et al.* (1988) The bioenergetics of preservation of limbs before replantation. *Journal of Bone and Joint Surgery.* 70 (10): 1500–1513

Savage, B (1984) *Interferential therapy.* Faber and Faber. London, UK

Schleip, R. (2003) Fascial plasticity: A new neurobiological explanation: Part 1. *Journal of Bodywork and Movement Therapies.* 7 (1): 11–19

Schmid, A. and Coppieters, M. (2010) The double crush syndrome revisited: A Delphi study to reveal current expert views on mechanisms underlying dual nerve disorders. *World Conference of the International Association for the Study of Pain (IASP).* Montreal, Canada

Schneider, M., Erhard, R., Brach, J., Tellin, W., Imbarlina, F. and Delitto, A. (2008) Spinal palpation for lumbar segmental mobility and pain provocation: An inter-examiner reliability study. *Journal of Manipulative and Physiological Therapeutics.* 31 (6): 465–473

Schomacher, J (2009) The convex–concave rule and the lever law. *Manual Therapy.* 14 (5): 579–582

Scott, A., Docking, S., Vicenzino, B., *et al.,* (2013) Sports and exercise-related tendinopathies: A review of selected topical issues by participants of the second International Scientific Tendinopathy Symposium (ISTS), Vancouver, 2012. *British Journal of Sports Medicine.* 47: 536–544

Sevier, T.L and Wilson, J.K (1999) Treating lateral epicondylitis. *Sports Medicine.* 28 (5): 375–380

Shacklock, M. (1995) Neurodynamics. *Physiotherapy.* 81: 9–16

Shacklock, M. (2005) *Clinical neurodynamics: A new system of musculoskeletal treatment.* Butterworth Heinemann, Elsevier. Edinburgh, UK

Shah, S.G.S. and Farrow, A. (2012) Trends in the availability and usage of electrophysical agents in physiotherapy practices from 1990 to 2010: A review. *Physical Therapy Reviews.* 17 (4): 207–226

Sharkey, J. (2007) *The concise book of neuromuscular therapy: A trigger point manual.* Lotus Publishing, Chichester, UK

Simons, D.G. (2004) Review of enigmatic MTrPs as a common cause of enigmatic musculoskeletal pain and dysfunction. *Journal of Electromyography and Kinesiology.* 14 (1): 95–107

Sjölund, B., Terenius, L. and Eriksson, M. (1977) Increased cerebrospinal fluid levels of endorphins after electro-acupuncture. *Acta Physiologica Scandinavica.* 100: 382–384

Smith, M. and Fryer, G. (2008) A comparison of two muscle energy techniques for increasing flexibility of the hamstring muscle group. *Journal of Bodywork and Movement Therapies.* 12: 312–317

Smith, R. (2005) A POEM a week for the BMJ. *British Medical Journal.* 2 (325): 983

Speed, C.A. (2001) Therapeutic ultrasound in soft tissue lesions. *Rheumatology.* 40: 1331–1336

Starkey, C. (2004) *Therapeutic modalities,* 3rd edition. F.A. Davis Company. Philadelphia, PA

Straus, S.E., Richardson, W.S., Glasziou, P. and Haynes, R.B. (2005) *Evidence-based medicine: How to practice and teach it,* 3rd edition. Churchill Livingstone. Edinburgh, UK

Strickler, T., Malone, T., Garrett, W.E. (1990) The effects of passive warming on muscle injury. *American Journal of Sports Medicine.* 18: 141–145

Sullivan, S.J., Williams, L.R., Seaborne, D.E. and Morelli, M. (1991) Effects of massage on alpha motor neuron excitability. *Physical Therapy.* 71: 555–560

Sunderland, S. (1991) *Nerve injuries and their repair: A critical appraisal.* Churchill Livingstone. Edinburgh, UK

Swenson, C., Swård, L. and Karlsson, J. (1996) Cryotherapy in sports medicine. *Scandinavian Journal of Medicine and Science in Sports.* 6 (4): 193–200

Taylor, B., Waring, C. and Brashear, T. (1995) The effects of therapeutic application of heat or cold followed by static stretch on hamstring muscle length. *Journal of Orthopedic Sports Physical Therapy.* 21 (5): 283–286

Thelen, M.D., Dauber, J.A. and Stoneman, P.D. (2008) The clinical efficacy of kinesio tape for shoulder pain: A randomized double-blinded, clinical trial. *The Journal of Orthopaedic and Sports Physical Therapy* 38 (7): 389–395

Thomas, J.R., Nelson, J.K. and Silverman, S.J. (2005) *Research methods in physical activity*. Human Kinetics. Champaign, IL

Tiidus, P.M. (2000) A review of human massage therapy: Assessing effectiveness primarily from empirical data in the human species. *Proceedings of the Annual Convention of the AAEP 2000.* www.ivis.org/proceedings/aaep/2000/302.pdf, accessed June 2013

Tipton, M.J. (1989) The initial responses to cold-water immersion in man. *Clinical Science.* 77 (6): 581–588

Topuz, O., Ozfidan, E., Ozgen, M. and Ardic, F. (2004) Efficacy of transcutaneous electrical nerve stimulation and percutaneous neuromodulation therapy in chronic low back pain. *Journal of Back and Musculoskeletal Rehabilitation.* 17: 127–133

Travell, J.G., and Simons, D.G. (1998) *Travell and Simons' myofascial pain and dysfunction: v. 1 and v. 2: The trigger point*, 2nd revised edition. Lippincott Williams and Wilkins. Philadelphia, PA

Vicenzino, B., Collins, D., Benson, H. and Wright, A. (1998) An investigation of the interrelationship between manipulative therapy-induced hypoalgesia and sympathoexcitation. *Journal of Manipulative Physiological Therapeutics.* 21 (7): 448–453

Vizniak, N.A. (2012) *Quick reference evidence-based physical medicine*. Professional Health Systems. Canada

Vujnovich, A.L. and Dawson, N.J. (1994) The effects of therapeutic muscle stretch on neural processing. *Journal of Orthopedic Sports Physical Therapy.* 20: 145–153

Wadsworth, H. and Chanmugam, A.P.P (1980) *Electrophysical agents in physiotherapy*. Science Press. New South Wales, Australia

Wall, M.E. and Banes, A.J. (2005) Early responses to mechanical load in tendon: Role for calcium signalling, gap junctions and intercellular communication. *Journal of Musculoskeletal and Neuronal Interactions.* 5: 70–84

Walsh, D.M., Noble, G., Baxter, G.D. and Allen, J.M. (2000) Study of the effects of various transcutaneous electrical stimulation (TENS) parameters upon the RIII nociceptive and H-Reflexes in humans. *Clinical Physiology.* 20 (3): 191–199

Ward, K. (2004) *Hands-on sports therapy*. Cengage Learning, London, UK

Warden, S.J. (2003) A new direction for ultrasound therapy in sports medicine. *Sports Medicine.* 33 (2): 95–107

Warden, S.J. Fuchs, R. K. Kesler, C. K. Avin, K. G. Cardinal, R.E and Stewart, R.L (2006) Ultrasound produced by a conventional therapeutic ultrasound unit accelerates fracture repair. *Physical Therapy.* 86 (8): 1118–1127

Watson, T. (1996) Electrotherapy research developments and their relevance to women's health. *Journal of the Association of Chartered Physiotherapists in Women's Health.* 78: 7–12

Watson, T. (2000). The role of electrotherapy in contemporary physiotherapy practice. *Manual Therapy.* 5 (3): 132–141

Watson, T. (2011) Electrotherapy on the web: *Contraindications.* www.electrotherapy.org/modalities/contragrid.htm#interferential, accessed January 2011

Watson, T. (2013a) *Therapeutic ultrasound.* www.electrotherapy.org/downloads/Modalities/Therapeutic%20Ultrasound%20april%202013.pdf, accessed April 2013

Watson, T. (2013b) *Ultrasound dose calculations.* www.electrotherapy.org/assets/Downloads/Ultrasound%20Dose%20Calculations%20handout%20april%202013.pdf, accessed June 2013

Watson, T. and Young, S. (2008) Therapeutic ultrasound. In Watson, T. (ed.) *Electrotherapy: Evidence-based practice.* Churchill Livingstone, Elsevier. Edinburgh, UK

Watt, J.M. (2008) Massage. In Porter, S. (ed.) *Tidy's physiotherapy*, 14th edition. Churchill Livingstone, Elsevier. Edinburgh, UK

Weerapong, P., Hume, P.A. and Kolt, G.S. (2005) The mechanisms of massage and effects on performance, muscle recovery and injury prevention. *Sports Medicine.* 35 (3): 235–256

Wells, P.N.T. (1977) Ultrasonics in medicine and biology. *Physics in Medicine and Biology.* 22: 629–669

Wilcock, I.M., Cronin, J.B. and Hing, W.A. (2006) Physiological response to water immersion: A method for sport recovery? *Sports Medicine.* 36 (9): 747–765

Williams, S., Whatman, C., Hume, P.A. and Sheerin, K. (2012) Kinesio taping in treatment and prevention of sports injuries: A meta-analysis of the evidence for its effectiveness. *Sports Medicine.* 42 (2): 153–164

Ylinen, J. (2008) *Stretching therapy for sport and manual therapies*. Churchill Livingstone, Elsevier. London, UK

Zadina, J.E., Hackler, L., Ge, L.J. and Kastin, A.J. (1997) A potent and selective endogenous agonist for the μ-opiate receptor. *Nature*. 386: 499–502

Zainuddin, Z., Newton, M., Sacco, P. and Nosaka, K. (2005) Effects of massage on delayed-onset muscle soreness, swelling and recovery of muscle function. *Journal of Athletic Training*. 40: 174–180

Zemke, J.E., Andersen, J.C., Guion, W.K., McMillan, J. and Joyner, A.B. (1998) Intramuscular temperature responses in the human leg to two forms of cryotherapy: Ice massage and ice bag. *Journal of Orthopaedic and Sports Physical Therapy*. 27 (4): 301–307

4

PITCH-SIDE TRAUMA CARE

Lee Young and Tim Trevail

It is well recognized and documented that, independent of the level and type of sport, emergency situations occur in the sporting environment. Sports therapists are often required to work 'pitch-side', and can be at the centre of any emergency care provided. Although the sports therapist's role requires extensive knowledge of anatomy, physiology and sports injury pathology (including immediate assessment and management), the successful practical delivery of emergency care in sporting situations is often challenging. While it is an essential professional competency requirement to obtain and update first aid and cardiopulmonary resuscitation (CPR) qualifications, these do not necessarily guarantee proficiency in dealing with the multitude of situations and potential complications that so commonly present as a sporting emergency. Standard first aid qualifications teach basic life support skills and minor injury intervention, but for the successful management (and optimal outcome) of many sporting emergencies, an advanced level of knowledge, skill, qualification and practice is required. As this area of professional practice in sport has steadily evolved, graduate practitioners are now expected to achieve advanced competency. There are a number of recognized advanced trauma management and sports-specific first aid courses in existence, and practitioners should investigate which is most applicable to their area of practice. Once qualified, the sports therapist, rehabilitator or sports physiotherapist must continue to develop and update their skills and proficiency through validated training and assessment. It is essential for the sports therapist working in pitch-side environments to have understanding of the potentially unique emergency situations that can arise, and possess the knowledge and skills, and gain the experience and develop the expertise in emergency care, so as to be able to triage (prioritize injury management) and deliver optimal interventions. Just one mistake in the decision-making process or physical management of the injury could prolong the length of time required for rehabilitation and return to sport, or worse, potentially create a life-threatening situation for the athlete. This chapter aims to support and develop the knowledge of the graduate sports therapist working in pitch-side environments by outlining key areas, principles, methods and specialized techniques. For clarity, in this chapter 'continuation of play' decisions refer to whether the athlete can continue in the same game or event; 'return to play' (RtP) decisions involve decisions on returning to full activity following an injury-induced time away from sport. The term 'pitch-side' is used, which is a reference to working directly in the sporting environment, where the sports therapist is expected to deliver emergency care, whether on or off the football pitch, at court-side for a basketball game or pool-side for a water polo team.

Preparation for working in a pitch-side environment
Preparation

The sports therapist has a number of roles and responsibilities when working in a pitch-side environment providing emergency care. The role of a sports therapist in this setting is inevitably diverse, depending on the individual circumstances, which does make the role difficult to specify. For example, the therapist's role may consist of a wider remit if they are working autonomously and independently in the sports setting, compared to their duties if employed as part of a multidisciplinary team. It must be stressed that the sports therapist's role in either setting is ultimately defined by the parameters and scope of practice as defined by the competencies of their professional governing body. The role of a sports therapist not only entails preparation for injury management, but also the prevention of injury (SST, 2012). Preparation for pitch-side care begins by ensuring the suitability of the venue for safe participation, and assisting with or advising on appropriate warm-up and cool-down. The therapist may oversee appropriate fluid intake pre-, during and post-event to aid recovery and hydration. To aid these goals, the sports therapist will require an understanding of the rules of the game, especially with regard to any regulations affecting injury prevention methods (for example, the use of appropriate sports equipment, taping and bracing) and procedural rules regarding access to injured players during the game. Preparation is of paramount importance to achieve successful acute injury care and trauma management. The graduate sports therapist must currently, at a minimum, hold, in addition to their primary degree qualification, an appropriate first aid qualification which must be kept up-to-date in line with current Health and Safety Executive guidelines (HSE, 2009). In addition to this, certain sports governing associations have further recommendations or stipulations regarding practitioners' training and competency for practice in that particular sport. All graduate health care practitioners working in sporting situations (including sports therapists, rehabilitators and physiotherapists) additionally have clearly identified professional competencies and proficiencies, and codes of conduct and ethics. These are mandatory and are constantly being re-evaluated, agreed and presented by the appropriate professional governing body to their members. It is a professional requirement of all said professionals to adhere to such rules, regulations and formal guidelines. The setting of professional competencies for practitioners involved in first aid and sports trauma care is particularly important – such competencies differentiate said professionals from those who do not work in sporting situations. The therapist must have the essential and updated skills to deliver an emergency action plan, and be able to provide effective crisis management with correct techniques applied for the care of life threatening injuries. This is fundamental, as the pitch-side sports therapist is likely to be the first health care professional on scene. The sports therapist must always be aware of their professional limitations and scope of practice, and work within their remit.

Equipment

The majority of injuries that the sports therapist will manage pitch-side will be relatively minor; however, serious and catastrophic injuries are unpredictable and can occur without warning. The management of such serious injuries may require specific equipment to provide the best possible pre-hospital care for the athlete – within the financial constraints of the organization involved. Following any incident, medico-legal parties may be required to ascertain the suitability of the sports therapist's qualifications, and also the appropriate use of equipment and techniques. The sports therapist therefore should recognize their duty in ensuring that they have the training and knowledge to use the appropriate equipment in case of such emergencies. There are currently no set requirements for the contents of a first aid kit (HSE, 2009); however, the demands of the environment and the sport must be considered when equipping the medical room and first aid kit and bag. The contents of a medical room and first aid kit will vary depending on numerous factors, including the sport, the equipment that the therapist is competent and able to use and the financial constraints of the club or organization. Table 4.1 provides a suggested list of equipment that should be available for use; the techniques for use of such should fall under the remit of the graduate sports therapist. All medical equipment should be stored within the medical room in an organized manner so as to be readily available in any emergency. Some kit should be carried with the therapist at all times so as to be available for use in an emergency situation (in Table 4.1, this is listed as 'kit bag equipment'). Other items should be readily available pitch-side during periods of competition (in Table 4.1, these are listed as 'pitch-side') and other items should be stored in the medical room (in Table 4.1, these are listed as 'medical room'). The following sections highlight the specialized equipment required for the management of emergency situations. Specific use of such equipment is discussed later in the chapter.

Spinal boards

Spinal boards are currently used in Advanced Trauma Life Support (ATLS) systems to immobilize the spine allowing for extrication of the athlete from the playing field to a suitable environment for further assessment and treatment of their injuries. Butman *et al.* (1986, cited in Vickery, 2001) state that the spinal board is the gold standard for spinal immobilization during the pre-hospital phase of trauma management. Main and Lovell (1996) assessed other methods of protection for the spinally injured and demonstrated that a vacuum type of support surface should be the preferred method. In a study conducted by Luscumbe and Williams (2003), a comparison of spinal board and vacuum mattress immobilization was undertaken. It was concluded that scrutiny of the advantages and disadvantages of both methods of immobilization should be undertaken prior to disregarding one over the other.

Cervical collars

Rigid cervical collars are used alongside spinal boards and side supports with strapping for the stabilization of the cervical spine (British Trauma Society, 2003; Driscoll and Houghton, 1999). Restriction of cervical range of motion helps to minimize the potential of causing further injury to an athlete with suspected cervical spine pathology (British Trauma Society, 2003; Driscoll and Houghton, 1999). Colleen *et al.* (2004) compared four different types of commercially available cervical collar and their ability to immobilize cervical spine motion. They determined that 'stiff neck' and 'stiff neck select' types of collar were the most effective at reducing range of motion.

Splints

Splint applications are an essential aspect for the management of fractures and dislocations. There are many types of commercially available splints, including: 'SAM® splints'; inflatable air splints; vacuum splints; box splints; and traction splints. They each come in a range of sizes and are used to immobilize an injured joint or limb with the main aim of reducing risk of further injury. Other benefits of splintage include reducing: pain; blood loss; pressure on skin; pressure on surrounding neurovascular structures; and the risk of fat embolism (Lee and Porter, 2005). A 'SAM splint' is an aluminium and foam mouldable splint used for a variety of extremity and skeletal injuries. A box splint consists of three long padded boards which, once placed around

Table 4.1 Suggested contents of a pitch-side bag and medical room

Equipment	No.	Use	Kit bag (K)	Pitch-side (P)	Medical room (M)
Wound and soft tissue injury management					
Disposable latex gloves	5 pairs	For maintaining a barrier against cross infection	•		•
Sterile gauze	10–15	For stemming bleeds and bathing wounds	•		•
Non-adherent dressing (various sizes)	5	For wound dressing	•		•
Steri-strips	1	Used as wound closure strips	•		•
Plasters (assorted)	Box	To cover small wounds	•		•
Antiseptic wipes/spray	1	For cleaning wounds	•		•
Sterile eyewash	2	For removing foreign bodies and irritants from eye	•		•
Eye pad	1	For eye protection following trauma	•		•
Nasal tampons	10	To stem epistaxis bleeds	•		•
Blister pads	10	To reduce friction over blisters	•		•
Sterile irrigation solution	2	For wound irrigation	•		•
Tweezers	1	To remove splinters (sterile or disposable)	•		•
Medical waste bag	10	To dispose of bodily fluids safely	•		
Shearing scissors	1	For cutting tough materials	•		
Rubber ice bag	1	To apply ice during match play	•		
Crushed ice		For making ice packs		•	•
Plastic bags	5–10	To make ice packs			•
Chemical ice pack	20	To apply to acute injury		•	•
Cling film roller wrap	1	To apply compression to ice packs and prevent infection after burns		•	
Cool bag	1	To maintain ice temperature pitch-side		•	
Taping and strapping supplies					
Disposable razors and gel	5–10	For hair removal prior to taping			•
Tape adhesive spray	1	To prepare skin for tape			•
Underwrap	5–10	For sensitive skin or can be used for light padding			•

Table 4.1 continued

Equipment	No.	Use	Kit bag (K)	Pitch-side (P)	Medical room (M)
Adhesive padding	1 roll	To pad bony areas or apply specific pressure (such as AC joint) or take pressure off an area	•		•
Tape scissors	1	For tape cutting and removal	•	•	
Rigid zinc oxide (ZO) strapping tape	5–10 25 mm	For mechanical support taping	•	•	
	5–10 38 mm			•	
Elastic adhesive bandage (EAB)	5–10 25 mm	To provide mechanical and compressive support	•	•	•
	5–10 38 mm			•	
Cohesive bandage	5–10 38 mm	To provide compressive support	•	•	•
	5–10 50 mm			•	
Electrical tape	2 rolls	To secure tape around head, ears, wrists, etc.	•	•	
Splints and braces					
Triangular bandage	2	To use as an arm sling or as a compression bandage	•	•	•
Safety pins	10	To secure slings and bandages	•	•	
Leg splint	2	To stabilize suspected fractures and dislocations	•	•	
Neck collar	1	To stabilize suspected spinal injuries		•	
Finger splints	1 pack	Stabilize dislocations and PIP/DIP sprains	•	•	
Soft neck collar	1	To protect soft tissue neck injuries	•	•	
Mouldable splint	1	To stabilize suspected fractures and dislocations	•	•	•
Miscellaneous					
Freezer/ice machine	1	To produce and store ice	•	•	
Couch	1	To support athletes during assessment and treatment	•	•	
Stretcher	1	For removal of NWB athlete			•
Spinal board	1	To stabilize suspected spinal injuries			•
Sink area	1	For hand washing and water access			
Athlete records	1	Including PMH and allergies stored in lockable cabinet (taken from pre-season screening)	•	•	

Equipment	No.	Use	Kit bag (K)	Pitch-side (P)	Medical room (M)
Foil blanket	1	To prevent hypothermia and shock	•		•
Water bottle	1	For hydration and fluid replacement (not to be shared by athletes)	•	•	•
Airway adjunct	Assorted	Naso/oropharyngeal airways for CPR	•		•
CPR face mask	1	For CPR	•	•	•
Vaseline	1	To prevent chafing and rubbing	•		•
Water spray	1	To cleanse wounds	•		•
Sunscreen (20+)	1	To protect from UV rays	•	•	•
Pen	1	For record keeping including 'SAMPLE' hx for patient handover	•		•
Cold box	1	To maintain ice temperature pitch-side	•	•	
Banned substances list	1	To advise athletes on legal and illegal substances	•		•
Mobile phone	1	For emergency calls	•		•
Massage cream or oil	1	For pre-event preparation or treatment	•		•
Heat lotion	1	For pre-event soft tissue treatment	•		
Pen light	1	For assessing pupil reactions	•		•
Insect repellent	1	For mosquitos, etc.	•		
Contact lens container	1	To carry spare contact lenses	•		•
Thermal blanket	1	For hypothermia, shock	•		
Sugar sweets	1 pack	For diabetics	•		•
Carry bags	Assorted	To store and carry first aid supplies on field and side of field	•		
Packet tongue depressors	1 pack	For oral examination	•	•	•
Gases	1	O_2 and Entonox	•		
Automatic external defibrillator (AED)	1	For use in CPR	•		
Disposable suture kit	2	To be used by on-site doctor if present	•		•
First-Aid Handbook (must be current and appropriate level)	1	For guidance and clarification	•		•

the injured limb, are secured with Velcro straps. Vacuum splints are made of strong plastic material containing polystyrene beads. Removal of air from the bag makes the splint rigid and allows it to conform to a deformed limb, providing support. Traction splints may be used on open or closed fractures. Application of the splint provides support in a near-reduced position. Dislocations are contraindications for use, and if used the sports therapist should always assess the neurovascular status of the distal limb. All splintage methods have advantages and disadvantages, and should be selected upon appropriateness to injury, experience and training of the sports therapist or the emergency medical team (Lee and Porter, 2005).

Airway adjuncts

Airway adjuncts are used for the maintenance of airways for the unconscious and non-breathing injured athlete. Standard equipment for this includes pharyngeal airway adjuncts (oropharyngeal and nasopharyngeal), endotracheal intubators and laryngeal mask airways (Lloyd, 2000). The applications of airway adjuncts are discussed in the airway management section of this chapter.

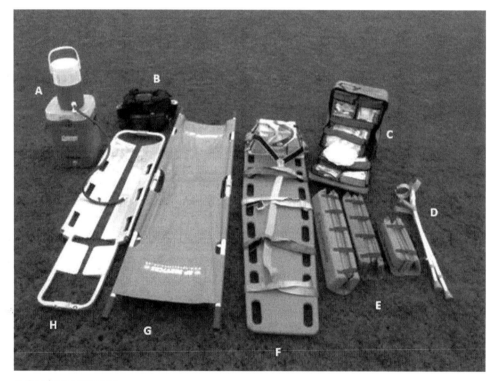

A: Cryotherapy equipment
B: Pitch-side running-on bag
C: Emergency medical equipment bag (advanced trauma life support/AED)
D: Crutches
E: Frac-pac immobilizer (various sizes)
F: Spinal board/ spider strap/head immobilizer/cervical collar
G: Soft stretcher
H: Scoop stretcher

Photo 4.1 Specialized emergency medical equipment.

Table 4.2 Equipment for airway maintenance

- CPR mask, tight-fitting transparent face mask
- High-flow oxygen
- Self-inflating bag and mask (selection of sizes)
- Selection of laryngoscopes
- Selection of oropharyngeal and/or nasopharyngeal airways or laryngeal mask airways

---

Source: adapted from Ollerton *et al.*, 2006; Rehberg, 2007.

Emergency action plan

The sports therapist must be prepared to deal with the management of sporting emergencies. Due to the unpredictable nature of accidents, an organized approach is needed to ensure that any incident can be managed quickly and effectively. Critical management of time could mean the difference between life and death, or permanent disability of an athlete (Courson and Henry, 2005). It is therefore crucial that, as the sports therapist is working in an environment where first aid is going to be administered, an Emergency Action Plan (EAP) is designed and utilized. The EAP is a written document which identifies key factors for implementation when managing a sporting emergency. Sports therapists should prepare, practice and review their EAP, and this should be done, as a minimum, at the start of every new season and also intermittently throughout the year. The EAP will be specific to the venue, taking into consideration any legal implications for the club, organization or institute (Courson *et al.*, 2005b; Fincher, 2001) (see Figure 4.1 and Table 4.3).

Emergency medical team

The sports therapist, as part of the sports medicine team, will often be the first responder in any emergency situation. As an individual, the sports therapist will be unable to manage every medical situation, so it is vital that an emergency medical team (EMT) is formed to support them (Anderson *et al.*, 2002). Careful consideration should be given to the members of the team to be included, as members may change between training and game situations due to availability. For example, a doctor may not be present for every training session; with injuries being just as likely to occur here as in a game situation (Fu *et al.*, 2007); it is important to consider this when forming an EMT. Often, the level of sport will dictate the level and range of medical qualifications of the EMT (see Table 4.4 for a list of possible members of an EMT), and this will also dictate the level of emergency care which can be offered.

Courson *et al.* (2005a) describe four basic roles of the EMT. The first is to ensure the immediate care of the athlete. This role will be fulfilled by the most qualified member of the EMT present, and will in many cases be the sports therapist. The second involves contacting the emergency medical services with a 999/112 call, relaying the necessary information. The third role described is a retrieval role, where the designated person brings any necessary equipment to the scene, for example the spinal board with cervical collar and stabilizing head blocks. The fourth role is to ensure that the emergency medical services are brought to the correct location of the injured athlete. There are additional situations in which an EMT is necessary, which need to be discussed. For example, when suspecting cervical spine injury, a neurological examination is required to rule out serious cervical spine pathology. This should be performed while the cervical spine is manually immobilized, and requires two people – one to stabilize and one to perform the examination; it is impossible for the solo sports therapist to perform this exercise on their own. In such instances, it may be decided to teach a member of

---

Emergency Action Plan for Medical Emergencies (example)

Emergency Medical Personnel: *sports therapist (ST)*
Emergency Medical Team:
sports therapist (ST); team manager (TM); coach (C); other team member (OTM)
Emergency Communication:
fixed telephone line (tel. no.) is located in the clubhouse in the entrance, pitch-side; mobile phones carried by ST (tel. no.) and TM (tel. no.)
Emergency Equipment:
spinal board, cervical collar, splints, oxygen, soft stretcher. Locations:
Match days - *home technical area*   Training sessions - *medical room*
Roles of Emergency Medical Team:
ST: *First responder & immediate care of the athlete. To provide medical care until arrival of a paramedic or other emergency care assistant.*
TM: *To dial 999*
> ➤ *To provide information to the emergency medical dispatcher*
>> • *Name address and telephone number of caller*
>> • *Number of victims involved*
>> • *Details of incident*
>> • *Age of victim(s)*
>> • *Condition of victim(s) with specific details*
>> • *First-aid treatment given by first responder*
>> • *Specific directions for location of the victim at the venue: instruct ambulance crew to meet _____ at _____*

> ➤ *To direct ambulance to scene*
>> i.   *To unlock/open gates*
>> ii.   *To meet ambulance at stated meeting point and direct to incident*
>> iii. *To 'crowd' control at scene*

C: *To retrieve emergency equipment; Cx stabilization; perform log roll*

Venue Directions:
The first team play on the main pitch next to the clubhouse.
The clubhouse is accessed via the gateway off Top Road. Once through the main gate, access to the main pitch is via the emergency road to the right at the rear of the clubhouse. Follow the drive to the car park, pass the clubhouse on your right, then onto the access road.

Emergency Communication
Additional Telephone Numbers
Hospital-   A&E department-   Clubhouse-

Notes
• if possible, member of sports medical team to accompany athlete
• obtain athlete's medical history
• notify parents or next of kin
• document incident including any interventions provided

Figure 4.1   Example EAP.

Table 4.3 Contents of an emergency action plan

• Involved personnel
• Emergency equipment
• Emergency medical team
• Lines of communication
• Chains of command
• Transportation or removal of the injured athlete

Table 4.4 Members of an emergency medical team

- Doctor
- Physiotherapist
- Sports therapist
- Coach
- Manager
- Sports massage practitioner
- Other staff
- Athletes

Table 4.5 Dialling 999 (or 112): required information for the emergency medical services

- Name, address and telephone number of caller
- Number of victims involved
- Details of incident
- Age of victim(s)
- Condition of victim(s) with specific details
- Firs aid treatment given by first responder
- Specific directions for location of the victim at the venue

the EMT a change-over technique prior to an incident. This would enable the sports therapist to administer the neurological exam and any other following interventions. Otherwise, the sports therapist may decide to stabilize and wait for the ambulance crew to arrive. Another situation in which an EMT is required is when the decision is made to stabilize and move an athlete using a spinal board. For this procedure it is necessary to perform a log roll manoeuvre, which requires a minimum of five people, demonstrating the need for assistance when working as the sole sports therapist.

Equipment for emergency care

The equipment necessary for emergency care will be listed in your EAP along with the precise location. It is essential that emergency equipment is easily accessible and, as necessary, pitch-side. When not in use the equipment should still be readily available and stored in a clean, secure environment. The equipment should be checked regularly, ensuring it is in good working order; this can be done prior to any athletic event and when practising the EAP. The sports therapist will need to assess what type of equipment is required to manage any possible emergency situation. In doing this, several factors must be considered: the sport, level and age of participants; types of prevalent injury; qualifications of the EMT; and rules pertaining to equipment and protective wear. For example, if the sport involves contact, such as rugby, there is a higher risk of spinal injury (McIntosh and McCrory, 2005), and therefore it is necessary to have a rigid cervical collar and spinal board as part of the pitch-side equipment. A simple risk analysis will ensure that the most appropriate equipment is available. Consideration should be given to ensure that the equipment is of an appropriate level to the most highly qualified member of the emergency team, and all personnel should be familiar with its function and use.

Communication

Courson and Henry (2005) state that communication is a critical element when preparing the EAP, and a full understanding of individual roles within the EMT will facilitate clear

233

communication channels. During an emergency situation, communication between members of the EMT must be calm and clear, hence allowing each to fulfil their role. A clear, structured chain of command should be established and followed, ensuring that the least qualified always secedes to the most qualified member of the EMT when providing first aid assistance. It may be necessary for the EMT to devise hand signals which will allow communication at a distance to pitch-side if radios are unavailable. When a change of environment occurs, such as with an away game, communication with the opposition team's medical staff is necessary. This allows the sports therapist to confirm their EAP and protocols. A warm and friendly introduction with a few simple questions is good practice. Building rapport with the opposition team's medical staff can strengthen the sports therapist's management of emergency situations, as their EMT can assist with this. Another communication consideration is how information is relayed to the emergency medical services. This information will be delivered at two differing stages. The first stage is upon dialling 999/112, and on request, the operator will connect the call maker to an ambulance control room. The information provided at this stage is required so as to facilitate smooth, prioritized and appropriate emergency medical dispatch. The accuracy of information conveyed is crucial at this stage (see Table 4.5 for required information). The second stage of information relay to the emergency medical services will be at handover to them at the scene of the incident; this should include any pertinent information, including the condition of the athlete and a 'SAMPLE' history (see secondary survey) for a conscious athlete, or for an unconscious athlete, a medical card which contains the athlete's relevant medical history.

Practice and review

Once an EAP has been established for the venue, it is vital that it is practised. The use of simulated emergencies is an ideal way to do this (Anderson *et al.*, 2002). The implementation of simulated emergencies is essential for the review and development of the EAP, but it also ensures that all members of the emergency medical team are prepared for real emergencies when they do occur. Even the most well-developed EAP will only be as good as the ability of the EMT to carry it out during an emergency. Potter and Martin (2009) expand on this idea, providing detailed information on designing a simulated emergency.

Emergency aid

Assessing the situation

Primary care is delivered by doctors and paramedics, but as already established, in a sporting environment the sports therapist will often be the first responder to a medical emergency. A systematic assessment protocol will enable the sports therapist to manage a medical emergency, delivering the appropriate medical care. The primary/secondary survey protocol is used by doctors and paramedics alike to accomplish a proficient assessment of the victim, thus enabling the appropriate medical care. This protocol can be applied and utilized by the sports therapist in the sporting environment. The primary survey will always take priority to the secondary survey as it allows for the assessment of immediate life-threatening conditions. On completion of this assessment, the sports therapist is able to provide the appropriate immediate basic life support (BLS) to the athlete as warranted. Once any necessary BLS has been administered and the athlete has been stabilized, the secondary survey can be undertaken. The secondary survey completes the immediate picture, providing the sports therapist with specific information regarding the injury and enabling detection of any other life- or health-threatening problems. The secondary survey is undertaken by assessing the athlete's vital signs (pulse, heart rate, blood pressure quality and rate of breathing), taking a subjective history ('SAMPLE') and completing a physical examination (Courson *et al.*, 2005a; Driscoll *et al.*, 2004).

It is pertinent to present a short discussion on considerations and decision modifiers prior to commencement of a primary/secondary survey protocol and first aid provision. First, the safety of the sports therapist is paramount, and it is essential that no danger is brought to the sports therapist while providing any intervention to the injured athlete. In many athletic emergency situations it is likely that there will be exposure to potentially infectious fluids, such as blood or other bodily fluids, and so appropriate barriers must be used. The use of disposable gloves is essential; the sports therapist should ensure that these are readily available and worn when dealing with any medical situation which may involve contact with any bodily fluid. In pitch-side situations two gloves can be worn; this can ensure that the therapist is able to deal with any life threatening situations rapidly. An example of this would be when dealing with a severe bleed; time could be lost if the injured athlete was waiting for the sports therapist to put on their gloves. It is easier to take the gloves off for a non-life threatening incident (for example, taping a joint), where time is not critical. Other protective equipment, such as face shields, should be kept readily available. In the medical room, further protective equipment may be stored, including face masks, goggles, sharps bins and clinical waste bags. The safety of the sports therapist on the field of play is essential. It is necessary for the sports therapist to understand the rules of the sport for which they are providing first aid cover, and to have an understanding of how the game is played (certainly in terms of plays and patterns). In a sport such as rugby, the sports therapist may enter the field of play while the game continues. Knowledge and understanding of the game will enable the therapist to do this without endangering themselves (or others). Consideration can be given as to when the assessment of an injured athlete truly begins. In reality, when working pitch-side the sports therapist is likely to witness the incident and observe the mechanism of injury. This observation should enable the sports therapist to gain an appreciation of the type and potential extent of the injury(s) sustained by the athlete, immediately providing them with an understanding of the possible assessment and aid the player may require, thus enhancing the speed of delivery of emergency care when time may be a crucial factor. With this in mind, the sports therapist should always try to place themselves in advantageous positions to be able to observe the game closely and to be able to have easy and safe access to the field of play. It is also important to note that 'ball watching' should be avoided; the sports therapist should ensure player safety even if play has moved on. For example, in rugby it may be necessary to observe any ruck, maul or tackle situation, ensuring all players return to play even after the ball and play has continued, or close observation given to the tackle situation. These situations have been highlighted in this example as they are the situations in which the injury is most likely to occur during a game of rugby union (Brooks *et al.*, 2005; Heady *et al.*, 2007).

Primary survey

Driscoll *et al.* (2004) identified that the aim of this survey is to assess whether the injured athlete can be categorized as 'primary survey positive', i.e. do they have an immediate life-threatening condition? This vital survey should take a maximum of 30 seconds to ensure quick delivery of immediate care. In approaching the injured athlete, a general impression of the victim's condition can be quickly gained as the therapist initiates their primary survey. Life-threatening problems take precedence over all other injuries. Driscoll *et al.* (2004) identify a criterion with which exclusion from this category can be made, and immediate resuscitation identified as unnecessary. The criteria presented are as follows:

- the athlete can talk;
- they are fully alert;
- their respiratory rate is between 10 and 29 breaths per minute;
- their pulse is between 50 and 120 beats per minute;
- the athlete is not cold, clammy or sweaty.

To assess these basic functions, therapists can use the 'ABCDE' approach; taking into account the points discussed earlier, 'DR' can be added: 'DR ABCDE' (see Practitioner Tip Box 4.1). When using the 'DR ABCDE' protocol, an intervention must be given at any stage that is found to be positive. For example, if at D a danger is found, this should be removed so that the sports therapist can work in a safe environment. At R, if no response is given, the therapist needs to get further help – i.e. shout for help, moving on to the assessment of the airway, and so on.

Danger

A quick scene survey is performed, assessing the situation of the incident and any potential additional dangers to the therapist or the athlete. The sports therapist should remember the use of protective barriers and safety when entering the field of play.

Response

The type of response given by an injured athlete can give information on their condition. The sports therapist should ensure a clear and loud tone when communicating verbally. If on reaching an injured athlete they are found to be alert and conversing normally, then it is known that the athlete will have an airway, will be breathing and will have a pulse. Here, a secondary survey can be undertaken using the 'TOTAPS' protocol (see the *Pitch-side assessment* section). However, if they are unresponsive to verbal communication, the sports therapist may try to elicit a response by using the following, in the order described: speaking clearly and loudly to the athlete in closer proximity; a gentle tap on the shoulders (this will be omitted if cervical spine injury is suspected); and then a light pinch (perhaps a pinch of the ear lobe). If a response is not gained, then a primary survey will be initiated immediately, beginning with the assessment of the airway.

Airway

The sports therapist assesses for any evidence of airway obstruction. The injured athlete may display any of the following signs and symptoms: noisy breathing; stridor (high-pitched

---

Practitioner Tip Box 4.1

'DR ABCDE'

Danger – scene survey
Response – verbal and tactile checks
Airway – open considering possible cervical spine injury
Breathing – with adequate ventilation
Circulation – with haemorrhage control
Disability – (e.g. neurological dysfunction)
Exposure and environment

wheezing); or other altered respiratory pattern. These may be present due to tongue displacement, foreign bodies (such as teeth, or protective equipment such as gum shields). If the athlete is unconscious there may be failure to protect the airway i.e. a loss of the ability to swallow which in turn may cause a pooling of secretions blocking the airway, therefore being another causative factor for the disruption of the airway. If during assessment the sports therapist decides the airway needs to be opened, then two techniques can be used: the head tilt chin lift method; and the jaw thrust. The latter is used if cervical spine injury is suspected. Both techniques lift the tongue from the back of the throat and attempt to unblock the airway. If any foreign bodies are found to be obstructing the airway they must be removed using a simple finger scoop of the mouth. The head tilt chin lift involves two steps:

1. the sports therapist places one hand on the player's forehead and gently tilts their head back;
2. with their fingertips under the player's chin, the sports therapist lifts the player's chin to open the airway.

Breathing

When assessing whether the injured athlete is breathing, the sports therapist observes for: evidence of increased work for breathing (tachypnoea; accessory muscle use; recession); evidence of hypoxia or fatigue (cyanosis; feeble respiratory effort); and evidence of pneumothorax; asthma; anaphylaxis; or heart failure. To determine each of these, while maintaining the open airway, the sports therapist should kneel to the side of the athlete and turn their head to face the athlete's feet; while placing their ear above the athlete's mouth, the therapist should look, listen and feel for normal breathing. This assessment should take no more than ten seconds.

   If there is any doubt as to whether normal breathing is occurring then the sports therapist must act as though it is not normal. This is essential, as in the event of a cardiac arrest, during the first few minutes it is possible for the victim to take infrequent noisy gasps ('agonal gasps') – these must not be mistaken for a normal breathing pattern, and are an indication for immediate CPR.

Circulation

When assessing the circulation of the injured athlete, the sports therapist should consider a number of factors. Does the injured athlete have any evidence of bleeding? Bleeding can be obvious, or it can include: haematemesis – vomiting of blood, generally from the upper digestive

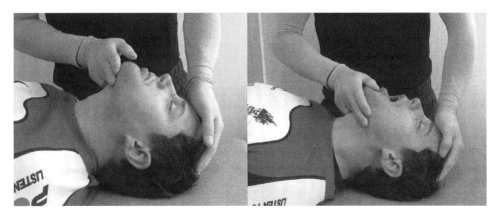

Photo 4.2   Opening the airway: head tilt chin lift method.

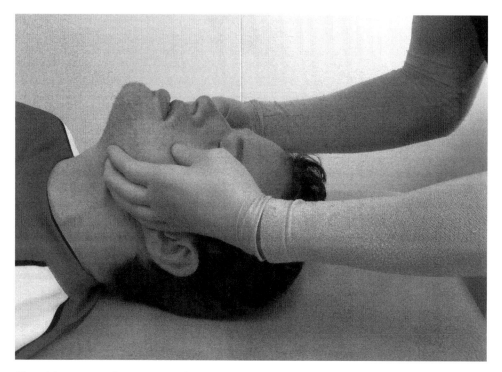

Photo 4.3　Opening the airway: jaw thrust method

Practitioner Tip Box 4.2

Assessing for breathing in the injured athlete

- Look for chest movement
- Listen at mouth for breathing sounds
- Feel for expired air on your cheek

---

tract; epistaxis – a nose bleed or nasal bleeding from the ear; and the possibility of concealed internal bleeding. Is there any evidence of shock? Signs of shock can include: tachycardia; prolonged capillary refill time; low blood pressure; or increased respiratory rate. The therapist should also check for evidence of acute coronary syndrome or heart failure. The pulse is a direct extension of a functioning heart, therefore an alteration from normal may indicate the presence of a pathological condition, and a disruption in circulatory function. In emergency situations this is usually determined by initially taking the carotid pulse; however, assessment of the radial pulse is also a useful diagnostic tool, and other pulses (femoral and dorsalis pedis) are used for severe injuries to the lower extremity. Normal pulse rates for adults range between 60 and 80 beats per minute (bpm), and children from 80 to 100 bpm. However, it should be noted that athletes generally have slower pulse rates than the average population. The rate is best assessed by counting the number of beats for 30 seconds and multiplying by two to determine the bpm. The strength of the pulse should also be noted as this may be indicative of types of pathological conditions. The pulse may be strong or weak (see Practitioner Tip Box 4.3).

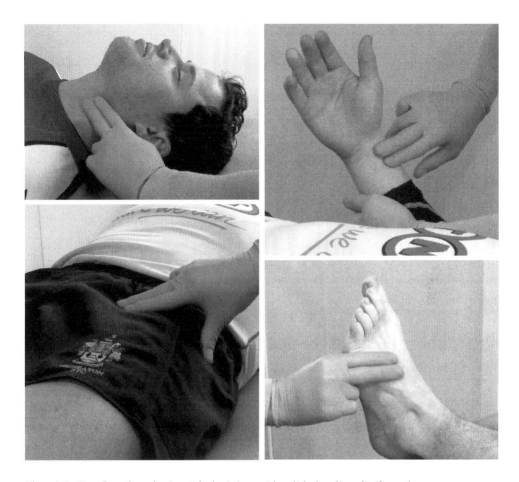

Photo 4.4   Sites for pulse palpation: (clockwise) carotid; radial; dorsalis pedis; femoral.

Practitioner Tip Box 4.3

Pathological conditions which may be indicated by an altered pulse rate

Rapid weak pulse – shock, bleeding, diabetic coma, heat exhaustion
Rapid strong pulse – heatstroke, severe fright
Strong but slow pulse – skull fracture, stroke
No pulse – cardiac arrest, death

The following are anatomical descriptions for the palpation of pulse sites. The carotid pulse can be palpated on either side of the thyroid cartilage deep to the sternocleidomastoid muscle. Moving the muscle laterally allows for the fingers to be slipped into the cleft between the cartilage and the muscle, allowing for ease of palpation of the pulse (Field, 1997). The radial artery and pulse can be palpated in the groove between flexor carpi radialis and the anterior border of the radius (Field, 1997). The pulsation of the femoral artery can be palpated in the groin below the mid-point (halfway between the anterior superior iliac spine and the pubic tubercle) of the inguinal ligament, directly anterior to the head of the femur at the hip joint (Field, 1997). The dorsalis pedis is at the distal section of the anterior tibial artery and can be palpated distal to the extensor retinaculum in a space between the first and second metatarsals (Field, 1997).

Disability

A basic neurological assessment process can be made using the mnemonic 'AVPU' (alert, verbal, pain, unresponsive). The level of consciousness is assessed with a response to differing stimuli. Is the injured athlete alert? Do they respond to verbal stimuli? Do they respond to a pain stimulus (for example, a squeeze or pinch of their upper trapezius)? Or are they unresponsive to all of the previous stimuli? A more detailed neurological assessment may be performed as part of the secondary survey once in a more suitable environment, such as the medical room, typically using the Glasgow Coma Scale (GCS). The GCS is a quick and recognized method of determining the level of consciousness and is predictive of patient outcome; it incorporates a totalled 15-point score which evaluates the individual's motor responsiveness, verbal performance and eye opening (Teasdale and Jennet, 1974). The sports therapist must also consider if the patient is 'fitting' (having a seizure) or if they are hypoglycaemic.

Exposure and environment

The sports therapist must ensure adequate exposure of and access to the injured athlete is sought to fully assess their condition. This may require the removal of items of kit, such as boots or head gear, to be able to do this. The sports therapist must also consider whether the athlete is in an appropriate environment to assess them or to provide further intervention. Consideration must be given to the physiological effects of the environmental conditions, especially cold temperatures (so as to avoid hypothermia), and decisions must be made regarding the possible removal of the athlete from the given environment. Blankets or silver foil survival covers may be used to cover the injured athlete and keep them warm. If removal is deemed necessary, then the necessary equipment and methods are utilized, ensuring no further injury is caused to the athlete, such as the use of splints and a stretcher if fracture is suspected.

Secondary survey

The secondary survey follows the primary survey, and also follows the delivery of any appropriate BLS. It must aim to ensure that the athlete is in a stable condition and seek to establish the findings of the complete (initial) assessment. It consists of: taking a history for the injured athlete; completing a physical examination; re-evaluating the complete assessment; and documenting all required findings.

History

The 'SAMPLE' acronym can help to systematically collect pertinent information with regard to the injured athlete in a medical emergency. The information collected can be communicated to the attending ambulance crew. This information will aid safe, prompt and effective management of the athlete by the ambulance crew and in the accident and emergency department. Table 4.6 presents the type of questions that can be asked when attempting to attain the history of the incident and explains the required information. The subjective information provided assumes that the athlete is conscious and able to provide information. In situations where the athlete is unable to provide such information, the organized sports therapist will hold key background personal information on players under their care, which can be easily conveyed to the medical services. Alternatively, a family member or friend may be able to provide the required information.

Table 4.6 'SAMPLE' history

SAMPLE history	Questions	Looking for
Signs and symptoms	What can you feel? Where is the discomfort?	Signs: rapid visual inspection. Symptoms: reported by injured athlete (e.g. type of pain; severity; movement; sickness)
Allergies	Have you any known allergies?	Specific allergies: medications (e.g. penicillin); food (e.g. nuts); seasonal (e.g. hay fever); bee stings; materials (e.g. elastoplast; latex)
Medication	Have you taken any medications and/ or supplements? If so, when? How much?	Specific medications (prescription and over-the-counter). Other (e.g. vitamins; herbal remedies; supplements)
Past medical history	Have you had any recent illnesses or injuries? If so, what and when?	Recent major illnesses; significant injuries; recent surgery; recent hospitalization
Last intake	When did you last eat or drink? What did you have? (Quantity)	To include: food; drink; medications
Events and environment	Can you remember what happened?	Prior to presenting injury or illness; mechanism of injury; bystanders

Physical examination

The physical examination will include a rapid head-to-toe check to decide if there are any other injuries sustained by the athlete. Once the injury site, or sites, have been confirmed then it is necessary to examine the areas for any musculoskeletal examination. The pitch-side 'TOTAPS' protocol can be used to do this, enabling the sports therapist to recognize and evaluate whether the athlete is able to return to play (the 'TOTAPS' protocol is discussed in the *Emergency trauma* section).

Re-evaluation

A second primary survey is undertaken and utilized to re-evaluate the injured athlete following any secondary assessment or intervention given to the injured athlete, or any of the other points outlined in Table 4.7 are present. This always ensures that the athlete is in a stable state and with no life-threatening conditions.

Documentation

Observations taken from the re-evaluation of the injured athlete should be documented by the sports therapist. This will include respiratory rate, heart rate and level of consciousness. The 'SAMPLE' history must also be noted with details of any intervention provided. It is likely to be recorded on several documents – certainly one copy should be passed on to the attending emergency services, and one copy placed in the athlete's medical records.

Basic life support

Figure 4.2 demonstrates the appropriate assessment pathways for the responsive and unresponsive injured athlete. BLS will be given to a primary survey positive athlete and will follow one of two pathways, depending on whether they are breathing or not. Figure 4.3 shows the pathway

Table 4.7 Re-evaluation of the injured athlete

MUST OCCUR IF:
- Any **INTERVENTION** has been undertaken
- The injured athlete shows any signs of **DETERIORATION**
- There is any other **CAUSE for CONCERN**
- There is any **UNCERTAINTY**

for an unresponsive, breathing injured athlete, while Figure 4.4 shows the pathway for an unresponsive non-breathing athlete. If it has been established that the injured athlete is primary survey positive and not breathing, the initial action by the sports therapist must be to get help. If alone, then it is their responsibility to dial 999; if the EMT is present, then the elected member should call 999 as per the EAP. CPR can now begin. This is initiated with chest compressions, followed by rescue breaths in the ratio of 30:2 and continues until the athlete starts breathing normally or the emergency medical services arrive. If the sports therapist is becoming exhausted, and no trained first aid persons are available, then a bystander should be summoned to take over; otherwise the CPR cycle should not be interrupted. Chest compressions are given at a rate of 100 per minute (a little less than two per second). With each compression the sternum in an average sized adult will be depressed approximately 4–5 cm. On return from full compression, while remaining in contact with the sternum, the pressure is released, allowing the chest to rise and heart to refill. To give chest compressions, the sports therapist will assume a kneeling position adjacent to the side of the supine-lying injured athlete. The heel of one hand will be placed in the centre of their chest, and the heel of the second hand on top of the first; fingers can now be interlocked, ensuring that shoulders are positioned vertically over the hands while keeping arms straight. To make rescue breaths it is necessary to reopen the airway. This should be done by using the head tilt chin lift method. The soft part of the athlete's nose should be pinched using the index finger and thumb of the hand supporting the forehead. The therapist should gently facilitate mouth opening with their opposite hand while maintaining the head tilt position. Taking a normal breath, the therapist should place their lips around their mouth, sealing the contact (a range of disposable resuscitation shields are available for such situations, so as to avoid cross-contamination). They should steadily blow into the mouth, ensuring the chest rises as in normal breathing, and take around one second to deliver each effective rescue breath. While still maintaining head tilt, the therapist should take their mouth away and look down the athlete's body observing for the chest to fall. The therapist will then take another normal breath and repeat the same procedure delivering another effective rescue breath. Only two rescue breaths should be attempted during each cycle. Failure to deliver effective rescue breaths may be due to airway obstructions, so if this is suspected, the airway should be re-checked and the therapist must ensure that sufficient head tilt has been applied and maintained.

Practitioner Tip Box 4.4

Ineffective rescue breaths

An effective rescue breath *will not* have been delivered if the following *have not* been observed:
- The chest has not risen when blowing into the injured athlete's mouth
- The chest has not fallen after blowing into the injured athlete's mouth

---

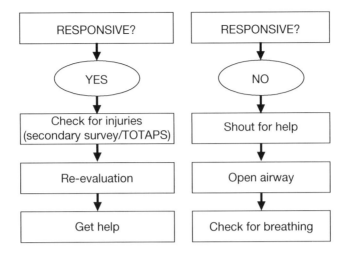

Figure 4.2   Assessment pathways for the responsive and unresponsive injured athlete.

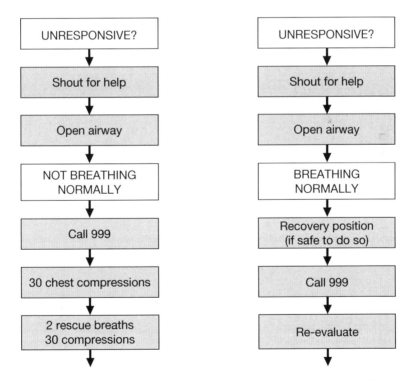

Figure 4.3   Adult basic life support: not breathing.

Figure 4.4   Adult basic life support: breathing.

If the athlete is found to be primary survey positive but breathing and a spinal injury is not suspected, the athlete can be placed in the recovery position (see Photograph 4.6). If spinal injury is suspected then this is taken into consideration and the protocol outlined later in the chapter is followed. Following either intervention, it is necessary to call 999 for the emergency medical services. A secondary survey can now be undertaken with re-evaluation at intervals.

Advanced trauma life support

Management of an airway

Airway interventions are crucial in the management of an athlete who is unconscious and not breathing as an airway compromise and hypoxia can cause irreversible brain damage and death (Brambrink and Koerner, 2004). As discussed earlier, there are several simple manual techniques that the sports therapist can use to promote an airway, two of which are the head tilt chin lift method and the jaw thrust. Following their use, other airway management protocols are available to protect the oxygen supply. These consist of simple and complex procedures which can be non-drug or drug assisted. As the administration of drugs is outside the scope of the sports therapist, only non-drug procedures will be considered. Non-drug techniques vary from the use of simple pharyngeal airway adjuncts to more advanced techniques such as endotracheal intubation and laryngeal mask airways (Lloyd, 2000). Brambrink and Koerner (2004) discuss the management of an airway using such methods, concluding that appropriate oxygenation is crucial but the means by which this is achieved should be based on the skill level of the practitioner providing the care; the resuscitation guidelines, as published by the Resuscitation Council (UK) (2010) also support this view. In light of the specialist skills and experience necessary for the use of the advanced techniques, this section will describe the use of less invasive methods such as a face mask, the provision of high-concentration oxygen and simple pharyngeal airways. Prior to the use of a mask or an airway adjunct, the airway must be clear of debris or fluids. The use of suction may help to clear the airway. There are different types of suction units available, but pitch-side a handheld suction unit will be the most likely to be available as a power source is not required. A suction unit is inadequate for removing larger debris such as teeth, foreign bodies and food, so these must be removed manually if visible, with the use of a finger sweep (Handley *et al.*, 2005). Suction is indicated when a gurgling sound is heard with artificial ventilation. Mouth masks are simple and effective adjuncts that can be used to increase the delivery of oxygen and ventilatory support to your injured athlete (Genzwuerker *et al.*, 2005). Pitch-side, these usually involve bag-valve devices or face masks (Banerjee *et al.*, 2004a).

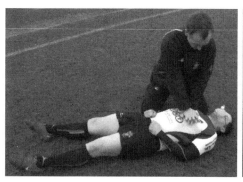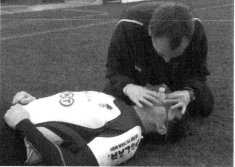

Photo 4.5   Position for chest compressions and rescue breaths.

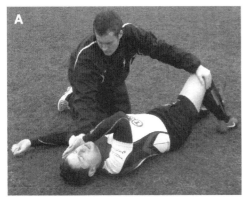
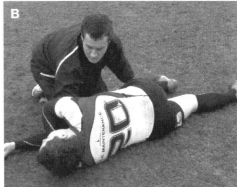
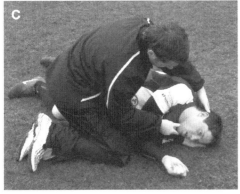

Step 1: Position the athlete's nearest arm into a right angle.

Step 2: Take the athlete's opposite arm up to their cheek, with palm facing up. Take the athlete's uppermost knee up into flexion (ensuring that their foot is flat to the floor).

Step 3: Pull the athlete's flexed knee over their lower leg towards the floor (ensuring their hand stays against their cheek). Position the flexed knee at right angles and rest it on the ground, so as to stabilize them.

Step 4: Check to ensure the airway remains open by using the head tilt chin lift method.

Step 5: Complete a secondary survey, then monitor the athlete's condition until help arrives.

Photo 4.6   The recovery position.

Pharyngeal airways are used in the injured athlete if they are found to be unresponsive or mentally impaired and prevent the closure of the oropharynx (Banerjee *et al.*, 2004a). They can be utilized either orally or nasally and selection will depend upon several factors. Oropharyngeal airways (OPA) are chosen when access is permitted to the mouth; the athlete is unresponsive, mentally impaired and does not have a gag reflex (Genzwuerker *et al.*, 2005). Nasopharyngeal airways (NPA) can be used on a responsive athlete when it is necessary to secure the airway or when access to the mouth is not permitted due to injury to the face and or mouth in an unresponsive athlete. OPAs are available in various lengths and are selected according to the size of the injured athlete. The length of the OPA is decided by measuring the distance between the angle of the jaw and the corner of the patient's mouth (see Photograph 4.7). Once the correct size has been selected the mouth is opened and the airway is inserted between the teeth in an apparent upside down position and once inserted turned 180°. This manoeuvre ensures the OPA passes the tongue (not pushing the tongue to the back of the throat), keeping the airway clear.

NPAs also vary in size and length. The appropriate size is selected by comparing the NPA diameter to the size of the athlete's fifth finger. The diameters should be of a similar size (the length of an NPA varies according to the diameter). Another method that may be used to select the appropriate sized NPA is to measure the distance from the nostrils to the ear lobe. Once the correct size of NPA is selected it may be inserted into an unobstructed nostril, ensuring sufficient lubrication is used and the tube is advanced at an angle perpendicular to the face. As the patency of an airway is vital for life (Brambrink and Koerner, 2004), the management of an airway when suspecting a cervical spine injury will not differ in approach but in the selection of techniques used, incorporating manual cervical stabilization (Banerjee *et al.*, 2004a; Crosby, 2006). Failure to appropriately manage a suspected cervical injury can worsen or cause spinal cord dysfunction and at worst further compromise the injured athlete's cardiac or respiratory system (Banerjee *et al.*, 2004a). It is essential that during airway management of a suspected cervical injury, as little motion of the cervical spine as possible occurs (Banerjee *et al.*, 2004a; Crosby, 2006). The jaw thrust technique will be utilized to cause minimal cervical spine motion in comparison with the head tilt chin lift method and therefore less likely to worsen the injured athletes' neurological status (Swartz *et al.*, 2009). A pharyngeal airway may be used to prevent closure of the oropharynx (Banerjee *et al.*, 2004a). Advanced techniques may be used in the presence of appropriately trained rescuers (Swartz *et al.*, 2009).

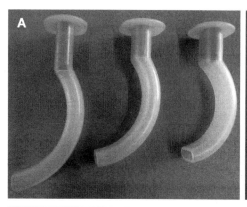
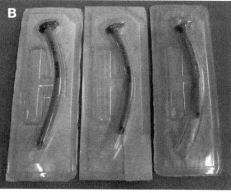
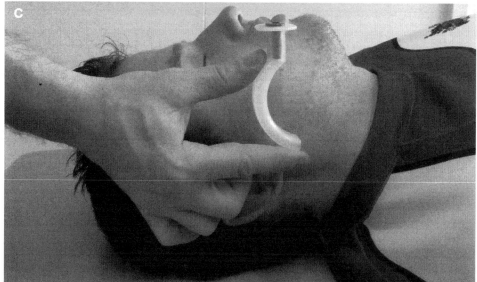

A: Oropharyngeal airways (OPA; various sizes)

B: Nasopharyngeal airways (various sizes)

C: Measurement of the victim for the section of correct sized OPA

Photo 4.7 Pharyngeal airways and measurement techniques.

Use of gases

Oxygen therapy can be considered for all trauma patients, not just airway-deficient patients, and for the majority of medical emergencies. Contraindicated medical conditions for oxygen therapy include chronic obstructive pulmonary disease (COPD), bronchitis and emphysema, as high-level oxygen concentrations are dangerous (O'Driscoll *et al.*, 2008). The use of oxygen in emergency situations is thought to be beneficial as it increases the oxygen concentration during inhalation and aids in the prevention of hypoxia and shock (Singh *et al.*, 2001). A variety of masks are used for the delivery of oxygen, but for trauma care, high-dose oxygen is being delivered therefore a high concentration reservoir mask (non-rebreathing mask) should be used (O'Driscoll *et al.*, 2008). To achieve the desired target saturation a flow rate of 5–10 l min^{-1} should be used (O'Driscoll *et al.*, 2008). Any practitioners who have undertaken recognised training in emergency oxygen use (including sports therapists) may deliver it to the ill or injured athlete as a prescription is not required. As with all interventions provided to the injured

Table 4.8 Indications for use of nitrous oxide

- To provide pain relief from musculoskeletal injuries
- To enable easier reduction of joint dislocations
- As an adjunct to other analgesia in fracture repositioning
- As an adjunct to other analgesia in wound care
- For pre-hospital analgesia

Source: adapted from O'Sullivan and Benger, 2003.

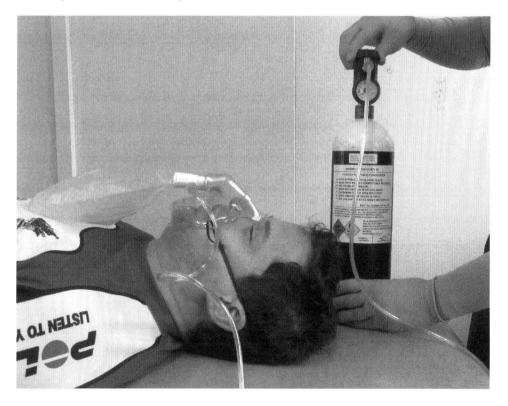

Photo 4.8   Use of oxygen with a non-rebreathe mask.

athlete, the treatment details must be recorded and given to the attending ambulance personnel on arrival (O'Driscoll *et al.*, 2008). A gaseous mixture of nitrous oxide and oxygen (trade name 'Entonox'), commonly referred to as 'gas and air', may be administered via use of either hand-held tight-fitting masks or suction on a mouthpiece, both of which are non-invasive mechanisms. Nitrous oxide can provide analgesia for the injured athlete in the pre-hospital setting. Other advantages of nitrous oxide include: a limited amount of side-effects or contraindications (however, it should not be used with suspected pneumothorax, bowel obstruction or post-scuba-diving); a rapid effect; and a rapid reversal of the effect once administration has ceased, meaning that the use of nitrous oxide is ideal in the pre-hospital setting for trained health care professionals (Faddy and Garlick, 2005; O'Sullivan and Benger, 2003).

Breathing and chest trauma

In a consensus statement by the Royal College of Surgeons of Edinburgh, Lee *et al.* (2007) describe chest injuries as being difficult to adequately assess in a pre-hospital setting as clinical signs of life-threatening injury are often absent but can cause rapid deterioration of the injured athlete. Therefore, it is necessary for the sports therapist to have the appropriate skills to be able to assess and provide immediate care, ensuring the injured athlete is transported to hospital as soon as it is safe to do so. Lee *et al.* (2007) suggest that a first aider's expected skills should be: basic airway management; positioning of the injured athlete; chest wall splinting; application of an 'Asherman' chest seal (three-sided dressing); external haemorrhage control; and, if trained and available, the administration of oxygen. Paramedics and trained care practitioners will be able to provide further care in the form of needle thoracocentesis and intravenous analgesia and fluids, and immediate care specialists will be able to add further care in the form of rapid sequence induction, thoracostomy and thoracotamy. The EMT may have such appropriately trained personnel. Assessment will begin with observing the mechanism of injury of the athlete and from this point will follow the 'DR ABCDE' protocol. The airway will be assessed with cervical spine stabilization, followed by breathing and circulation, using a look, listen and feel approach. Signs and symptoms that will be examined in each of these sections are highlighted in Table 4.9. The minimum observations that need to be recorded by the sports therapist are: the athlete's respiratory rate; peripheral (radial) pulse rate; and conscious level using the 'AVPU' scale (alert, responds to voice, responds to pain or unresponsive). If skills allow, the following can be recorded: pulse oximetry, blood pressure, conscious level using the Glasgow Coma Scale (GCS) and ECG monitoring. Observations are re-taken every ten minutes, or if there appears to be a change in the clinical status of the injured athlete or following any intervention given to the injured athlete (Lee *et al.*, 2007).

Table 4.9 Signs and symptoms that may be identified using the 'look, listen and feel' approach

LOOK	Respiratory rate and pattern. Chest wounds
Necessary exposure of the area for full assessment	or bruising
Consider: environment; cooling of the patient;	Movement of chest wall (i.e. flail segments
hypothermia	and/or abnormal movements). Reduced
	movement due to pain, pneumothorax or
	haemothorax
LISTEN	Abnormal breathing patterns
FEEL	Swelling; crepitus; tenderness; percussion.
Careful palpation	Tenderness of chest wall (fractures)

There are serious complications associated with chest injuries that may result from blunt trauma in sport (for example, as a result of a tackle in rugby or football), and the sports therapist must be aware of these. Such complications will leave the injured athlete with breathing problems and in a life-threatening state. These include:

- Pneumothorax: this occurs when a pocket of air accumulates in the pleural cavity, causing the lung to collapse due to a greater pressure on the outside of the lung.
- Tension pneumothorax: this occurs when the surrounding musculature of the pleural cavity acts as a one-way valve, allowing air into the cavity but not out. It can be associated with rib fractures.
- Open pneumothorax: this occurs as a result of air entering the pleural cavity due to an open wound in the chest wall.
- Haemothorax: this is where there is blood in the pleural cavity, often as the result of a blunt trauma; it can lead to a pneumothorax.
- Flail chest: this describes a condition in which three or more consecutive ribs on the same side are fractured in at least two places. As a result, this section of the chest wall becomes unstable (flail) and causes a paradoxical movement (i.e. the flail segment will move in the opposing direction to the rest of the chest wall during inhalation and exhalation).
- Cardiac tamponade: this occurs when the heart becomes compressed due to an increase of fluid within the pericardium.

There are certain techniques and interventions which may be provided by the sports therapist to help manage such complicated chest conditions. These include: administration of oxygen; addressing external haemorrhage; covering and dressing of open wounds (including use of an 'Asherman' chest seal); and certain positioning and manual splinting techniques for a flail chest.

Automatic external defibrillators

AEDs are computerized devices which deliver electric shocks (electro cardioversion) to treat victims of cardiac arrest caused by ventricular fibrillation (VF) or pulseless ventricular tachycardia (VT). Their use can greatly increase the survival rate from a cardiac arrest, with early intervention increasing the success rate (Resuscitation Council (UK), 2010). AEDs analyse the victim's ECG rhythm and determine the necessity for a shock. Due to the safety, simplicity and reliability of its use, the Resuscitation Council (UK) (2010) recommended that an AED can be used safely and effectively without previous training; however, it is highly recommended that if the sports therapist has access to an AED, training in its use will increase knowledge and promote confident and efficient application. An AED, as suggested by its name, is automatic in nature and requires the operator to follow its voice and visual instructions. These will guide the user to the appropriate placement of surface electrodes and prompt them to clear the victim from contact and to administer the shock. The latest guidelines from the Resuscitation Council (UK) (2010) advise that interruptions to manual chest compressions should be minimal prior to the use of an AED. These can be minimized if working as a pair, as one can perform the chest compressions as the other is preparing the AED and waiting for it to charge. Figure 4.5 illustrates the pathway for use of the AED. The effective use of an AED augments BLS; it is applied following the primary survey when the athlete is found to be unresponsive (or unconscious), when medical help has been sought and when the athlete has an abnormal breathing pattern. Once the AED is attached and a shockable rhythm is confirmed, a single shock is administered. Irrespective of the resultant rhythm chest compressions and ventilations are resumed immediately to minimize the time spent without a compression and blood flow.

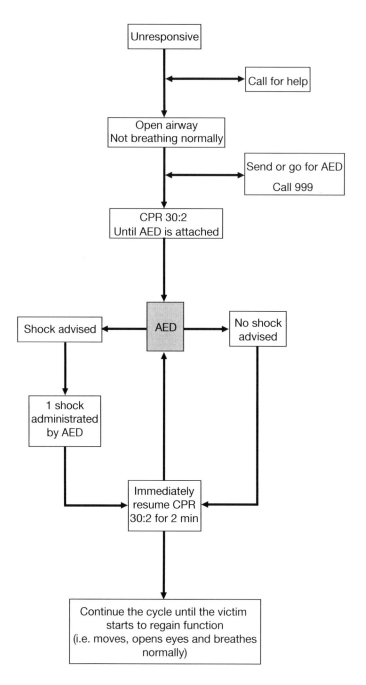

Figure 4.5 AED algorithm.

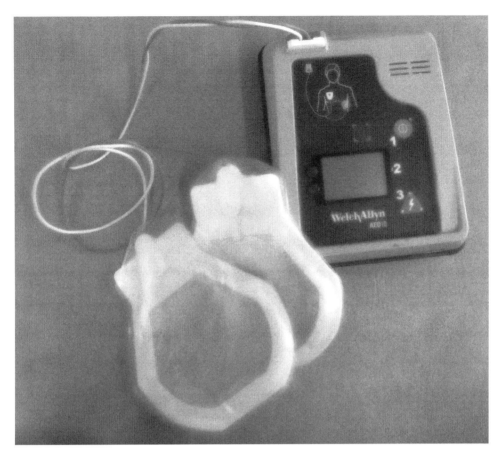

Photo 4.9 An automated external defibrillator (AED).

Emergency trauma

Pitch-side assessment (and 'TOTAPS')

Efficient and effective assessment of sports injury is an essential skill for all practitioners covering sports events (Rehberg, 2007). When assessing the conscious casualty it can be useful to follow a set procedure so as to avoid missing any aspect of the assessment in a pressurized situation. When the sports therapist has seen an incident occur and has been cleared to enter the field of play to attend to the athlete, the protocol of 'TOTAPS' can be utilized to recognize injury and make safe return-to-play (RtP) decisions. This simple on-field assessment protocol is designed to quickly ascertain the severity and nature of the injury, identifying key signs and symptoms including pain, abnormalities and loss of function, to ultimately decide whether the athlete can RtP. As with most pitch-side assessment tools, 'TOTAPS' must remain sport-specific. Some sports regulations will allow the therapist to carry out their full assessment while on the pitch; other sports regulations may force the sports therapist to make quick decisions and complete the assessment pitch-side while play continues. Such scenarios inevitably place additional pressures on the sports therapist as the coaching staff, or match officials, will require a decision on the suitability of the athlete to RtP. A decision to stop the athlete from continuing can be made at any stage of the assessment protocol.

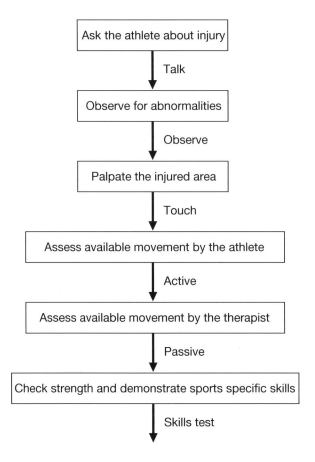

Figure 4.6 'TOTAPS' protocol.

Talking

The therapist should begin their initial on-field assessment with verbal questioning of the athlete (if possible). Careful questioning can help to clarify the mechanism, site and apparent severity of injury. Such questions as *'Can you tell me what happened?'* quickly determine the 'AVPU' state of the athlete, and providing that the response is comprehensible, allows the therapist to proceed to the musculoskeletal assessment, with an appreciation of the mechanisms, forces and body regions involved in the incident. Further questions form the basis of the initial subjective assessment. The sports therapist will need to know about the type of pain and any abnormal or altered sensations. The player's response to such questions will direct the rest of the on-field assessment.

Observation

The therapist's visual inspection of the situation and the athlete's injury will have already begun while approaching the incident, and will also be occurring in conjunction with the initial questioning of the player. The therapist must aim to identify any signs of deformity or other abnormality, and this must include observing for signs of acute injury – swelling, discolouration, bleeding or structural deformity. Affected regions should be compared with the unaffected side wherever possible. The sports therapist should also be observant to other clues to problems, such as the athlete's facial expression and body language, ability to explain how they feel, and their apprehension regarding their position or any attempted movement.

Touch

If there are no obvious signs of deformity, the area should be carefully palpated, assessing for non-visible signs of acute injury. During palpation, the athlete's response should be continually monitored through verbal and visual communication. The palpation should establish any tenderness, heat, swelling, deformity or abnormal sensation. The recognition testing, in combination with full appreciation of the regional anatomy, helps the sports therapist to form their clinical impression and decide which structures may be implicated, while also considering the severity. Up to this point, no active movement has been asked for as it may be inadvisable to ask for movement if the injury is severe. However, if the on-field assessment warrants a movement assessment, the therapist should begin by seeing what the player is willing to do unassisted.

Active

Active movements will be performed by the injured athlete as directed by the sports therapist. The athlete should be invited to carry out the major movements associated with the joint(s) or region(s) involved. The range of movement should be mentally noted by the therapist, as a loss in range of movement is an obvious sign of injury. The athlete's response should also be noted and consideration given to structures being compressed, distracted, contracted or stretched during the movements. This will provide the therapist with an indication of which structures may be damaged and causing the pain. Severe injuries will usually be indicated by a complete or near-complete loss of function, and the athlete should be removed from play for a more comprehensive assessment. In more minor injuries where the range of motion is almost or completely full, passive movements should be performed.

Passive

In passive movement testing, the therapist performs movements of the affected joints without the assistance of any muscular effort from the athlete. The therapist moves the joints, with appreciation of the active range of motion, from the start to the end of range so as to carefully stretch and compress tissues, while at the same time considering the overall quality of motion. During this process, the therapist will continue to gain the athlete's feedback on the injury. It is at this stage that any specific ligamentous or capsular stability and active resisted tests may be carried out.

Skills test

Following successful progress through each of the previous stages of assessment, and if both the therapist and athlete decide that a RtP may be feasible, sports-specific skills must be tested in order to fully assess the dynamic stability and functionality of the affected region. Basic skills testing should be both progressive and sports specific. The aim is to prevent further injury and to ensure that the demands of the sport are being re-created. A sporting example of testing the lower limb may run as follows:

- The athlete is assisted into a standing position and is tested for weight-bearing function (there should be careful progression from partial to full weight-bearing – then into unaided walking).
- Linear exercises should follow – with progressive speed increases (leading up to full-paced running with stopping and starting included).

- Multi-directional activity (such as 'zig zagging') in an effort to dynamically increase the load placed on the lower limb tissues.
- Sports skills (such as kicking a ball or bilateral and unilateral jumping and landing).

The RtP decision is often unclear and difficult to make. The therapist should be guided by their clinical reasoning, which will be informed by the assessment findings, the quality of movements observed and the athlete's opinion. Experience is obviously extremely valuable, and as the sports therapist gains experience, their confidence and efficiency will also inevitably grow. Ultimately, where there is slight uncertainty, the RtP decision may lie with the athlete, and the sports therapist can only advise on the best course of action in the given situation. One of the main responsibilities of the sports therapist is to prevent the athlete from further harm. An efficient and effective evaluation is critical to ensure the athlete receives the appropriate advice and treatment in aiding them to RtP. The RtP decision is made easier when a good level of rapport, trust and mutual respect is established between therapist and athlete, as well as with the coach. If the athlete is unable to perform the tests, or if critical symptoms are apparent, and dependant on the location of injury, then the decision should be made on how to remove the player from play. Using appropriate, safe and effective methods of handling will prevent further injury to the athlete. The athlete can be moved in either a full weight-bearing (FWB), partial (PWB) or non-weight-bearing (NWB) manner (discussed later in this chapter).

Pitch-side treatment and management
Musculoskeletal trauma

Musculoskeletal trauma is the most common type of injury occurring in sport, and frequently presents as soft tissue injuries, fractures and dislocations. Such injuries are often 'walk off injuries' (injuries where the athlete is able to leave the field of play with minimal intervention). Although minimal intervention may be provided, it may still be crucial in preventing exacerbation of the condition. Rarely does a musculoskeletal injury lead to a primary survey positive patient, unless major trauma has been sustained. When managing an athlete with musculoskeletal injury it is imperative to recognize, treat and refer any life- or limb-threatening injury as swiftly as possible. Life-threatening conditions, which may occur as a result of major musculoskeletal trauma, include: concussion; severe haemorrhage; crush syndrome; pneumothorax; and fat embolism. Limb-threatening injuries that may occur include: open fracture; joint injuries; vascular injuries (including shock); acute compartment syndrome; and neurological injuries. There are times where the athlete can present with signs and symptoms which mimic a musculoskeletal injury but are in fact signs and symptoms of a potentially life-threatening condition. Fitz-Simmons and Wardrope (2005) describe a number of conditions which could be mistaken for musculoskeletal problems (see Table 4.10). In general, an athlete with one of these conditions will present with an acute onset of pain, possibly without a history of a traumatic event, and this will be supported

Table 4.10 Conditions which may mimic musculoskeletal problems: signs and symptoms

Condition	Signs and symptoms
Leaking abdominal aortic aneurysm	Presenting as back pain
Aortic dissection	Presenting as inter-scapula pain
Perforation/peritonitis	Presenting as shoulder pain
Acute myocardial infarction	Presenting as shoulder or arm pain

with a positive assessment of their ABCs, demonstrating a primary survey positive athlete. It is important that the sports therapist gives appropriate consideration to such findings when managing any injured athlete presenting with musculoskeletal injury.

Soft tissue injuries

The types of soft tissue injury that occur when working in sport in a pitch-side environment include musculotendinous tears, contusions and sprains (Bleakley *et al.*, 2004). The initial assessment of such injuries uses the 'TOTAPS' protocol or similar strategy. From this assessment, the sports therapist will decide whether the athlete is able to play on or not. If the decision is that the athlete is unable to continue, then the correct method of removal from play will be utilized and the immediate management considered. For such injuries, the aim of immediate management will be to control swelling and bleeding, and reduce pain. To achieve this, the 'PRICE' principle provides clear, simple and effective guidance to both practitioner and player (Flegel, 2008; Russell, 2010):

- protection against further injury (via strapping, bracing and/or possible NWB);
- rest to facilitate early healing (i.e. avoiding activity likely to adversely stress the injured tissues);
- ice (cryotherapy) mainly to relieve pain – evidence is too limited to show how cryotherapy can effectively influence the metabolic inflammatory response (i.e. reduce oedema, effusion and the secondary ischaemic death of undamaged cells);
- compression (via circumferential strapping) to minimize oedema and to encourage venous return and lymphatic drainage;
- elevation (via supporting the affected limb in a position above the height of the heart) to further reduce swelling, and encourage venous return and lymphatic drainage.

Bleakley *et al.* (2012) have presented a revised acronym to support early management: 'POLICE' (protection; optimal loading; ice; compression; and elevation). They explain that optimal loading is an umbrella term for any mechanical intervention (including both active and passive movement). The use of cryotherapy in the immediate and acute management of soft tissue injury has traditionally been considered vital in order to minimize swelling, accelerate healing and control pain levels, although its efficacy at improving clinical outcomes in soft tissue injury has been questioned (Collins, 2008; Meeusen and Lievens, 1986). Practitioners and athletes should recognize that an initial balanced and incremental rehabilitation programme with early activity will, in most cases, encourage efficient recovery.

Muscle tears

Typically musculotendinous tear injuries occur during high-velocity situations, such as sprinting and jumping, and the athlete will usually 'pull-up' when the insult occurs. Upon questioning the athlete may describe a 'popping' sensation or explain that they 'felt it go', followed by a subsequent tightening of the involved area. During the on-field assessment the initial suspicions will be supported with localized tenderness on palpation, weakness and pain on resisted testing and an inability to complete sport-specific actions.

Sprains

Acute joint and ligamentous sprains occur as a result of a traumatic event where the joint is taken beyond its normal range of motion. In so doing the associated ligamentous and capsular

Table 4.11 Summary of immediate treatment strategy (first 72 hours)

	Action	Equipment
Protection	Remove the athlete from the injury-causing environment Suspected fracture: place the injured part in a splint Fracture not suspected: elastic bandage or semi-rigid brace Immobilized for 1–5 days Prevent weight-bearing	Splints (SAM splints; box splints; vacuum splints) Elastic bandage (cylindrical bandage; tubi-grip; cohesive bandage; light EAB; crepe) Semi-rigid brace (air-cast) Crutches
Cryotherapy	An intermittent protocol: apply ice for 10 minutes, remove for 10 minutes and re-apply ice for a further 10 minutes; repeated every 2 hours	Ice, bag, water (wetted ice bags), cryo-cuff
Compression	Immediately post-injury apply and maintain compression for the first 72 hours	Cylindrical bandage tubi-grip; cohesive bandage; light EAB; crepe; orthopaedic foam; felt Localize compression (see photograph showing 'horseshoe' at ankle) Cryotherapy and compression can be combined by either: soaking bandage in water and freezing it and placing an ice bag underneath an elastic wrap, or with the use of a cryo-cuff, or cling-film wrap, and ice
Elevation	The injured part should be elevated as soon as possible, above the level of the heart, fully supported Simultaneous elevation and compression is not advised, when elevation is not possible compression may be used	Pillows, towels
Therapeutic Exercise	Any movement of the injured area and surrounding musculature should be performed within a restricted range – with the onset of pain being the limit for RoM	Assisted movement with the use of towels, non-friction surfaces, dowels

tissue is stretched or torn. The athlete can present with swelling, pain, local temperature increase and skin discolouration. The therapist should remain vigilant for identifying the possibility of additional tissue involvement (in particular, muscles and tendons which cross the region; and specific ligamentous attachment sites – for avulsion fracture).

Contusions

A contusion is simply bruising resulting from internal bleeding. This commonly occurs in contact sports and may, for example, be caused by blunt trauma to a muscle and the resultant damage of the affected tissue's blood vessels. A particularly common site for contusion is the vastus lateralis muscle of the anterolateral thigh, which results from forceful contact with an opponent's knee (Mitchell, 2000). At the initial stage, it may be difficult to distinguish from a

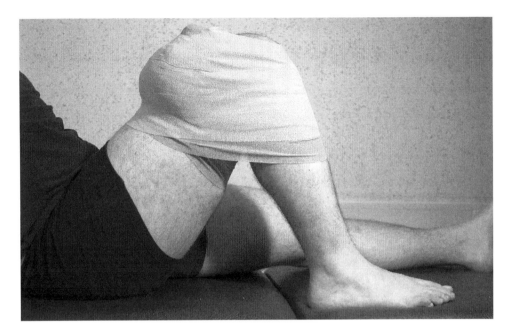

Photo 4.10   Quadriceps contusion management.

muscle tear, other than that the mechanism of injury is different. Initial management will still follow the 'PRICE' protocol so as to minimize bleeding and pain. For quadriceps contusions, La Prade *et al.* (2009) suggest that a combination of ice and compression should be applied with the knee in flexion in order to minimize future knee stiffness, and so as to enable the athlete to regain motion more quickly.

Compartment syndrome

Acute compartment syndrome (ACS) is where the development of high pressure within a muscle compartment compromises the circulation and nerve supply to a level below that which is necessary for tissue viability (Mubarak *et al.*, 1978). ACS can occur as a result of bleeding or swelling into compartmental spaces following a muscle tear, fracture, crush injury or severe contusion (Mubarak *et al.*, 1978). The most commonly affected region is the anterior compartment of the calf. With ACS of the anterior compartment, the athlete is likely to present with pain during exercise of the affected region, a sense of 'tightness' in the region, a developing weakness in the foot (particularly dorsiflexion and toe extension) and paraesthesia and numbness in the dorsal region. ACS can lead to serious complications which may be limb- or life-threatening; prevention of complications requires prompt diagnosis and referral for appropriate medical intervention (Tiwari *et al.*, 2002), which may involve a fasciotomy.

Fractures and dislocations

Fractures are commonly seen in sporting environments. There are a wide variety of fracture patterns (including: oblique; transverse; longitudinal; spiral; crush; impacted; and comminuted) which are each dependant on the athlete's age, sport, mechanism of injury and type of bone involved. Dislocations may be due to inherent static or dynamic instability, or simply due to the mechanism of injury. Some athletes experience recurrent dislocations. Appropriate management of a fracture or dislocation reduces potential morbidity and mortality of injured limbs. The sports therapist will use the 'DR ABCDE' protocol during initial assessment and management of the injured athlete. The treatment of any life-threatening condition precedes any management of a fracture or dislocation. On completion of the primary survey, the secondary survey is undertaken and follows the 'TOTAPS' regimen – also taking into consideration a 'SAMPLE' history. Any athlete who has sustained a fracture or dislocation will present with some or all of the signs and symptoms as identified in Table 4.12.

Management of fractures and dislocations

The algorithm shown in Figure 4.7 highlights the pathway for the pre-hospital management of fractures and dislocations. Open fractures and joint injuries (where bone has pierced the skin and there is open communication to the external environment) must be dressed with sterile dressings prior to the application of any splint or use of a support (such as a sling). Sufficient analgesia (such as nitrous oxide) may be administered (by trained personnel) prior to splinting the limb, and immediate transfer to an accident and emergency (A&E) department is required following the initial management. There may be an associated vascular involvement with a fracture or dislocation injury with variable presentations. To assess the vascular status of an injured limb, pulses below the injury site must be tested. Following assessment of pulses, the fractured limb, if deformed, may require realignment (reduction) with the use of a traction splint, or with the use of careful manual traction prior to repositioning (by trained personnel). Analgesia should normally be given to the injured athlete before realignment is attempted. The pulse must be immediately reassessed following any intervention. If the pulse has diminished or become abnormal then the fracture should be returned to its original position following realignment, or the splint removed if applied. The athlete must be transferred to A&E as soon as possible. Special consideration should be given to the management of an athlete with a suspected pelvic fracture, as it is a potentially life-threatening condition. High–energy, blunt trauma is the most common mechanism of injury in pelvic fractures (such as may occur in road traffic collisions or severe contact injuries in sport). Associated abdominal and additional pelvic injuries commonly occur alongside pelvic fractures, with disruption of arteries and veins resulting in major haemorrhage and decreased blood volume. Thus, it is essential that early suspicion, identification and management are applied for reducing blood loss and the risk of death (Lee and Porter, 2005). In a review of the pre-hospital management of pelvic fractures, Lee and Porter (2005) concluded that suspected pelvic fracture (pre-hospital) management should conform to the following principles:

- Knowledge and understanding of the mechanism of injury.
- Ask the alert injured athlete about the presence of pain in the pelvic, lumbar and groin regions; and routinely immobilize the pelvis if there is any positive reply.
- Examination is unreliable (especially if there is a reduced GCS or other distracting injuries), and the pelvis should not be palpated in order to avoid further internal haemorrhage.

Table 4.12 Signs and symptoms of a fracture and/or dislocation

---

- Mechanism of injury
- Gross anatomical deformity
- Pain and swelling
- Crepitus and tenderness
- Neurovascular compromise

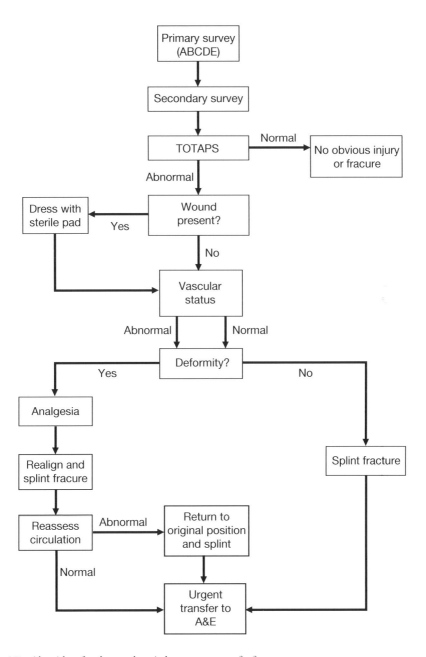

Figure 4.7 Algorithm for the pre-hospital management of a fracture.

- If there is any suspicion of fracture, the pelvis should be immobilized using an external compression splint (circumferential wrapping of a sheet around the pelvis as a sling).
- Do not 'log roll' the patient.
- Use of a 'scoop stretcher' (with a maximum 15° 'log roll' to enable positioning) to facilitate the patient's movement onto a spinal board or vacuum mattress for transport.
- The pelvic splint should not be removed when an unstable pelvic injury is suspected until it is radiologically confirmed that there is no fracture.

As in the management for any fracture, it is essential that the medical emergency services are called and that the injured athlete is transferred to A&E as soon as possible. It must be noted that the reduction of fractures or dislocations either by manual manipulation or via the use of traction splints is an advanced skill for which the sports therapist must have been trained prior to any delivery.

Foreign-body airway obstruction

An athlete's airway can become blocked due to a foreign body such as a gum shield, chewing gum or teeth that have dislodged following trauma. Blockages may be considered severe or mild, and can be identified by their signs and symptoms. For a mild obstruction, the athlete will still be able to speak, cough or breathe. A severe obstruction will be indicated by the athlete being unable to speak, cough (maybe silent attempts) or breathe (wheezy) – and unfortunately, without immediate assistance, the athlete will become unconscious (Handley *et al.*, 2005). The aim of treatment in either case is to remove the obstruction, and when necessary, transfer to hospital. If the athlete is showing signs of mild obstruction they should be encouraged to continue coughing and to remove any obvious obstructions from their mouth. If the obstruction is severe, and the athlete conscious, then the sports therapist will be required to deliver up to five back blows (slaps) to the athlete (Photograph 4.11). Following each blow the therapist must assess to see if the obstruction has been cleared and remove it from the mouth as appropriate. If the obstruction is still present following five back blows, then five abdominal thrusts must be delivered (Photograph 4.12). If the obstruction does not clear after three cycles of back blows and abdominal thrusts, medical assistance must be sought immediately (another member of the EMT should call 999) and the cycle of blows and thrusts must be continued. If the athlete becomes unconscious due to not being able to breathe, they should be supported to the floor and CPR must be commenced (Handley *et al.*, 2005).

Head injuries and neurological assessment

Head injuries are common in many sporting situations. Head injuries occur in high-risk sports (such as combat sports where the head is a legitimate target); in contact sports (particularly football, rugby, hockey and ice hockey); in non-contact sports (such as equestrian; motor sport; cycling; gymnastics; trampolining; rock climbing); and in certain sports where head injury is rare, but potentially severe (for example, golf and cricket). Although the vast majority may be minor and present with relatively short-lived symptoms, head trauma has been shown to result in more fatalities than any other sports injury (Mueller, 2001). The priority, as with all serious injuries, is to treat the greatest threat to life and avoid further harm to the athlete. Any athlete that receives a direct impact to the head, or to the body which makes the head shift rapidly in any direction, should be carefully assessed for injury to the brain. The following section will focus on the complex issue of sport-related concussion (SRC).

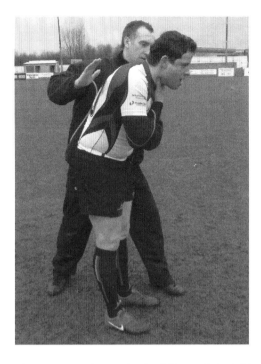

- The sports therapist will stand to the side and slightly behind the athlete.
- Support the athlete's chest with one hand and lean the athlete well forwards (to ensure that the foreign body exits the mouth if becomes dislodged following a blow).
- Using the heel of the hand make firm striking contact with the athlete, between the shoulder blades.

(Handley *et al.*, 2005)

Photo 4.11   Technique for the delivery of a back blow.

In order to appreciate the fundamental structures and basic functions of the brain, a brief review of anatomy is appropriate. The brain is the part of the central nervous system (CNS) that is contained within the cranium and consists of three main divisions: the cerebrum, cerebellum and brainstem. The cerebrum (the main structure of the brain) is recognized as the forebrain, and consists of left and right hemispheres. It is divided by a deep longitudinal fissure between each of the medial surfaces. The cerebrum coordinates voluntary muscle action, interprets the majority of sensory input and controls higher mental functions such as memory, reasoning and intelligence for complex problem solving, learning, judgement and emotions. The cerebellum, or the hindbrain, lies inferior to the posterior aspects of the cerebral hemispheres; it has a critical role in the coordination of voluntary muscle action, working unconsciously to interpret incoming messages and initiate motor output (channelled via the cerebrum) to control movement and locomotion, equilibrium and posture (Hollinshead and Rosse, 1985). The resulting motor impulses are transmitted to the appropriate muscle groups to create the desired smooth and coordinated movements; thus injury to the cerebellum will affect balance and voluntary movement. The brainstem consists of the pons and the medulla oblongata; it is situated at the base of the brain between the spinal cord and cerebrum. The brainstem receives and initiates messages which control heart rate, breathing and blood pressure. The brain and spinal cord have a multi-layered system offering some protection from external forces. The scalp (musculotendinous aponeurosis), cranium, meninges and ventricles protect the brain in various ways. Five soft tissue layers of the scalp help to dissipate forces of compression and movement about the cranium. The bones of the cranium, particularly the parietal, frontal, temporal, sphenoid and occipital, support and offer the brain hard protection from direct impact. Three meningeal membranes surround the brain and spinal cord, and their primary functions are to provide cushioning and to direct impact away from the neural tissue. They also

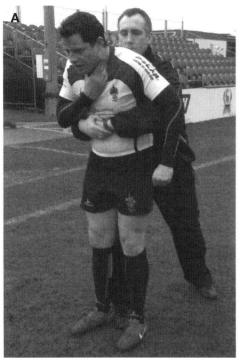

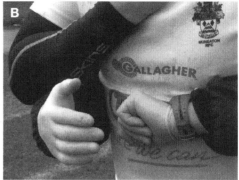

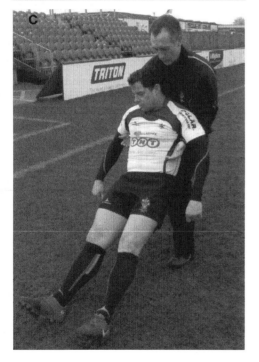

A: Delivery of an abdominal thrust

B: Hand position for delivery of an abdominal thrust

C: Catching an athlete if they have gone unconscious

- The sports therapist will stand behind the injured athlete, placing both arms around the upper portion of the abdomen.
- Lean the athlete forwards.
- Clench a fist and place between the umbilicus and xiphisternum.
- Grasp this hand with the other and pull sharply inwards and upwards.

(Handley *et al.*, 2005)

Photo 4.12   Technique for the delivery of an abdominal thrust.

provide an avenue for nerves, blood vessels and lymph vessels, and between each layer is cerebrospinal fluid (CSF), which suspends the brain, acting to cushion and diminish shock and nourish the tissues. The superficial meningeal layer is the dura mater, consisting of tough inelastic, fibrous tissue that adds to the protective quality of the meninges. Deep in the dura is the subdural space, which consists of a thin fluid layer and subdural veins. The middle layer is the arachnoid mater, which is a combination of elastic and collagenous fibres. The pia mater is the deepest meningeal layer; it is highly vascular and connects to the grey matter of the brain via its superficial fissures.

The assessment protocols used during acute SRC management aim to identify the extent and location of damage to the CNS. The sports therapist should use their knowledge of the anatomy of the CNS and surrounding structures to better understand the presenting condition and pursue appropriate lines of questioning. This should lead to a more sensitive assessment which aims to involve observation of the various subtle signs of SRC, and which should help to maximize the effectiveness of pre-hospital care.

Concussion management

The assessment and management of SRC has developed significantly over the past 20 years. There has been a renewed emphasis on this injury, which is illustrated by the amount of medical literature, as well as lay media devoted to the topic. Since 2001, an international expert committee has been established and has developed a series of consensus statements for the categorization, assessment and management of sports concussion. Central to this process has been the development of the Sports Concussion Assessment Tool ('SCAT') (McCrory et al., 2013). 'SCAT3' (the most recent version) is essentially a formal (revised) protocol for assessment and management of athletes over the age of 12 with any suspected SRC. The full 'SCAT3' was co-published in multiple journals and is widely available for free download. It incorporates pre-season screening criteria (for baseline comparison), symptom evaluation, cognitive assessment, balance and coordination assessment, and clear guidelines for a stepwise symptom-limited progressive RtP. A simplified ('pocket SCAT') Concussion Recognition Tool ('CRT') has also been developed in tandem with SCAT3 for the purpose of prompting effective pitch-side assessment (McCrory et al., 2013). The CRT simply incorporates: a symptom checklist; a memory function checklist; and a balance test checklist. A modified version of the SCAT has also recently been developed for the assessment of young athletes between the ages of five and twelve (Concussion in Sport Group, 2013). The 'Child SCAT3' includes child and parent concussion symptom rating scales, modified balance and cognitive assessment procedures and also consideration of, and criteria for, return to school and play.

Definitions of concussion have evolved and are likely to continue to do so with progressive discoveries in both sports medicine and neuroscience. The 2012 expert committee consensus maintained the basic definition of sports concussion as being *'a complex pathophysiological process affecting the brain, induced by traumatic biomechanical forces'* (McCrory et al., 2013). Although the move has been away from defining concussion as being mild or severe, the vast majority of concussive episodes resolve within seven to ten days; it is, however, important to recognize that symptoms are likely to take longer to subside in children and adolescents (McCrory et al., 2013). While it is challenging to present absolute definitions, the characteristic features for the majority of (uncomplicated) concussive episodes include the following:

- MoI – a direct blow to head, face or neck, *or* an indirect blow to another part of the body which transfers trauma to the head.
- Significant, but often transient, symptoms.

- Neuropathic changes associated with functional disturbance rather than structural change.
- SRC can occur irrespective of whether there is loss of consciousness (LoC) or not.
- Imaging (X-ray, CT and MRI) is frequently normal.

More serious or complicated concussions can present in a variety of ways. Any LoC is always an emergency (but just because a player does not lose consciousness, does not mean they are not concussed). Acute concussion can present with convulsions or tonic posturing. A concussive episode may be slow to resolve, with persistent symptoms, whether at rest or just with exertion. Obviously, intracranial haemorrhage is a major concern. MacAuley (2006) states that *'delay in recognizing and treating intracranial bleeding is the most common cause of avoidable mortality and morbidity due to head injury'*. Subdural haemorrhage can result from damage to the bridging veins between the dura and arachnoid mater – this can present as a slow bleed, which is a main reason for close monitoring of athletes for 24 hours after the event. Subarachnoid haemorrhage has been described as producing a sudden and severe 'thunderclap headache'. A range of short- and long-term complications are associated with head injury. The term 'chronic traumatic encephalopathy' (CTE) describes neurodegenerative disorder resulting from cumulative head trauma. The condition was first noticed as a 'peculiar condition' casually referred to as a 'punch-drunk' syndrome in boxers before the 1930s (McKee *et al.*, 2009). CTE may result in early dementia, amnesia, mood disorders and depression, and shares many of the defining characteristic features of Alzheimer's disease and Parkinsonism. There is evidence of significant incidence of suicide within athletic populations who have been exposed to either a single episode of severe traumatic brain injury or repeated episodes of mild traumatic brain injury (Bailes *et al.*, 2010).

When concussion is suspected, based upon the MoI and any evident features of concussion, the athlete must be immediately evaluated using standard emergency management principles (Guskiewicz *et al.*, 2004) – and with specific consideration given to the possibility of associated injuries (especially cervical spine injury; but also cranial or facial fracture, or other soft tissue injury). By using a standardized examination, supported by objective measures of concussion-related symptoms, mental status and postural control, the sports therapist can be ready to make an informed decision on continuation of play.

Once the primary survey negative has been established, concussive injury assessment protocols, such as the CRT, may be utilized. CRT is designed to help highlight a range of clinical domains to suspect concussion. The sports therapist should assess for *somatic* (LoC; headache; nausea; sensitivity to light; slurred speech; or a reported 'pressure in head'); *cognitive* (amnesia; confusion; 'not feeling right'); and *emotional* signs and symptoms (lability; irritability; sadness; anxiety). If any one or more of these is present, concussion must be suspected and the athlete removed from play and appropriate management strategies followed. Memory function should be established, observing for signs of amnesia. The following short-term memory ('Maddocks') questions should be asked: *'Who scored last in this game?'*; *'Which half are we in now?'*; *'What venue are we at today?'* Failure to answer correctly is indicative of concussion, though it should be noted that although this is a useful and necessary part of the on-field evaluation, evidence suggests that it is not a reliable indicator of injury severity (McCrory *et al.*, 2013). Eye function tests can be used at this stage, with abnormal function often relating to head

Practitioner Tip Box 4.5

Cervical spine injury must be considered due to an often similar MoI to concussion.

injury. Pupils should be assessed to see if they are equally responsive to light – looking for dilated or irregular pupils. The sports therapist should test the ability of the eyes to adapt rapidly to light variance by covering one eye with the patient's hands. The covered eye should be dilating while the open eye remains normal. When the hand is removed, the previously covered pupil should constrict to accommodate to the light. A slowly constricting pupil may indicate cerebral injury (Laio and Zagelbaum, 1999). Smooth tracking of the eyes should also be assessed; the athlete should be told to keep their head still and asked to track the movement of the therapist's finger or the end of a pen or pencil. Vertical movements up and down, and horizontal movements left and right (as in the 'H' test – see Photograph 2.39) should be assessed, observing for smooth movements or for any sign of pain. Any involuntary back and forth, up and down or rotary movements of the eyeball during this test suggests nystagmus – which may be indicative of a lesion in the posterior fossa of the brain, including the cerebellum or brainstem and cranial nerves (Hamou and Zagebaum, 1999). Blurred vision can be assessed by asking the athlete to read something – such as the time on the therapist's watch, or a similar task, to ascertain if there are any visual disturbances. A modified balance error scoring system (BESS) can then be used to gain an indication of balance problems. The athlete will be asked to stand heel-to-toe, with their non-dominant foot behind (in 'tandem stance') and with their hands on their hips and their eyes closed, attempting to maintain balance (see Photograph 2.41). Five or more errors (stumbling out of position; opening of eyes; hips ≥30° flexion; not regaining balance within five seconds) may suggest a concussion.

Table 4.13 Referral checklist for the management of concussion

Immediate referral (on the day of injury)	
Loss of consciousness on the field	Amnesia lasting longer than 15 minutes
Deterioration of neurologic function★	Decreasing level of consciousness★
Decrease or irregularity of respirations★	Decrease or irregularity in pulse★
Increase in blood pressure	Unequal, dilated or unreactive pupils★
Cranial nerve deficits	Any signs or symptoms of associated injuries, spine or skull fracture or bleeding★
Mental status change: lethargy, difficulty maintaining arousal, confusion, agitation★	Seizure activity★
Vomiting	Motor deficits subsequent to initial on-field assessment
Sensory deficits subsequent to initial on-field assessment	Balance deficits subsequent to initial on-field assessment
Cranial nerve deficits subsequent to on-field assessment	Post-concussion symptoms that worsen
Additional post-concussion symptoms as compared to those on field	Athlete still symptomatic at the end of the game (especially at adolescent level)

Delayed referral (on the next day, or days, following injury)	
Any of the findings in the above day-of-injury referral category	Post-concussion symptoms worsen or do not steadily improve over time
Increase in the number of post-concussion symptoms reported	Post-concussion symptoms begin to interfere with the athlete's daily activities (e.g. sleep disturbances; cognitive difficulties)

Source: adapted from Guskiewicz *et al.*, 2004.
Note: ★ requires immediate transport to the nearest A&E department.

When an athlete has suffered a head injury, it is the sports therapist's responsibility to consider all possibilities, and if there is any doubt as to whether the athlete is concussed, the advice must be to 'sit them out'. Table 4.13 highlights all main referral indicators. If the athlete has experienced head injury and has shown even slight signs of concussion (symptoms, memory or balance) they must be withdrawn from the game or event. Saunders and Harbough (2004) discussed the 'second impact syndrome' (SIS). Although the pathophysiology is not fully understood, this is where an athlete returns to play when not fully recovered from a first concussive episode; and where a second head injury may compound the original condition, and there can be potential for catastrophic damage. If the player's symptoms are obviously and quickly subsiding, and following ongoing assessment there are no immediate concerns for referral (as highlighted in Table 4.13) – and they appear to be recovering – the advice will generally be to send the player home to rest, to not allow them to drive and for them to be closely monitored by a family member or friend for any signs of worsening over the following 24 hours (this must include any signs of developing headache, nausea, amnesia, confusion and more). Athletes must also be restricted from alcohol, sleeping tablets or other sedatives, aspirin and NSAIDs until symptom-free for 48 hours (McCrory *et al.*, 2013). Any suspicion of more significant concussion at the time of injury (LoC; persisting or concerning symptoms – such as nausea, dizziness, blurred vision or anxiety; confusion; memory loss) must be referred immediately for medical assessment. Neural imaging technologies (such as CT or MRI) currently contribute little to the diagnosis of concussion, although they may be ordered to identify structural and vascular lesions.

The key to early concussion management must be emphasized – it is a combination of continued physical and cognitive rest until the symptoms resolve. This should be followed by a steadily graded programme of exertion prior to medical clearance and RtP (clarified in Table 4.14). Essentially, this requires that the athlete rests until they are asymptomatic. The athlete may then begin to incorporate graduated and progressively more intense activity, but there must be 24 hours before each progression. This allows for assessment of any recurrence of symptoms (symptoms can be absent with rest, but brought on by exertion). By following a monitored and progressive recovery process, the athlete may be passed fit and be able to resume

Table 4.14 Graduated return-to-play strategies

Rehabilitation stage	Functional exercise at each stage of rehabilitation	Objective
1 No activity	Complete physical and cognitive rest until asymptomatic	Recovery
2 Light aerobic exercise	Walking, swimming or stationary cycling keeping <70 per cent MPHR. No resistance training	Increase HR
3 Sports-specific exercise	Skating in ice hockey, running drills in football/ rugby	Add movement
4 Non-contact training drills	Progression to more complex training drills (e.g. passing drills). Start progressive resistance training	Exercise, coordination and cognitive load
5 Full-contact training	Following medical clearance, participate in normal training activities	Restore confidence, assessment of functional skills by coaching staff
6 Return to play	Normal game play	

Source: adapted from the 'Concussion in Sport Group' 2013.
Notes: 24 hours per step; if recurrence of symptoms at any stage, return to previous asymptomatic level and resume after further 24-hour period of rest.

full training within a week of their concussive episode. If the athlete has a recurrence of symptoms, depending upon the severity or persistence, they should either be referred, or simply rest until asymptomatic and begin the graded programme of exertion again. A more conservative RtP approach must be recommended for children (McCrory *et al.*, 2013). This may incorporate extending the symptom-free period before commencing the RtP protocol, or increasing the length of the graded exertion protocol. Certainly school attendance and activities may need to be modified, and no return to physical activities should be allowed until returned to school successfully.

Other neurological injuries

Cervico-brachial neuropraxia ('stinger')

Cervical neuropraxia has been shown to be one of the most common symptomatic upper extremity nerve injuries in athletic populations (Krivickas and Wilbourn, 2000). It involves trauma to either the brachial plexus or the cervical nerve roots. A 'stinger' may be the result of a range of mechanisms to a variety of structures, but commonly follows a blow to the head, neck or shoulders – causing downward pressure on the affected side with contralateral neck flexion or extension (Dimberg and Burns, 2005). The mechanism can include both traction and compression of the upper trunk of the brachial plexus, or traction or compressive forces at the neural foramen of cervical nerve roots (C5–6). The on-field assessment should begin by establishing the MoI, with the athlete describing the location of their symptoms, followed by clearing of the cervical spine (through palpation for tenderness and observation for oedema and muscle spasm) and immobilizing if necessary. Symptoms of 'stingers' involve a single upper extremity (bilateral or lower extremity symptoms may be more indicative of spinal cord injury), and may include a rapid onset of burning pain in the shoulder or from the neck, down the arm and possibly into the fingers. Both paraesthesia and anaesthesia may also occur throughout the upper extremity, frequently in a C5–6 dermatomal distribution pattern. The athlete may variably show signs of weakness in a myotomal pattern and may appear to shake the arm or hold it in support. Once the cervical spine has been cleared, a neurological examination should be performed, with particular attention to strength testing and sensory deficits using the contralateral side as a normal control. If symptoms resolve within minutes, and the athlete regains full strength and sensation with no neck pathologies, they may return to play in the same game. If symptoms persist past several minutes, or there is limitation in neck range of motion with associated pain, it is recommended that the athlete undergoes a cervical spine MRI before RtP (Cantu, 1997). Isolated 'stingers' are considered benign injuries – and by definition are transient injuries that usually do not require formal treatment. With the appropriate rest, rehabilitation of full neck and shoulder strength, and diagnostic neuroimaging, players may RtP. Players who remain symptomatic after a 'stinger', with persistently abnormal diagnostic results, especially after technique adjustments, should consider cessation from further participation in their contact sports.

Practitioner Tip Box 4.6

The return-to-play decision can be difficult – if in doubt always remove the athlete from play.

Seizures and epilepsy

Sports therapists should have a basic understanding of seizures and epilepsy. They should understand the relationship between exercise and such conditions, and have adequate seizure first aid management skills. A seizure is a paroxysmal stereotyped event as a result of spontaneous uncontrolled electrical activity in the brain producing a transient, hypersynchronous neuronal discharge. A seizure may produce physical convulsions, minor physical signs, thought disturbances and, commonly, a combination of symptoms. A seizure may be a result of specific insult to the brain, such as a haemorrhage or electrolyte imbalance, or may be intrinsic and unidentifiable. Epilepsy syndromes vary according to both the aetiology and the clinical and electrographic characteristics, although it is important to be aware that not all athletes who have a seizure are epileptic. The sports therapist will ideally be familiar with their athletes' seizure history, including the types of seizures and their typical manifestations (frequency; duration; severity; and after-effects), their medications and recovery characteristics. Many epileptics are aware of the catalysts that may predispose them to seizures and these should be avoided. Such information helps the therapist to prevent and deal with events as they occur. Basic first aid generally involves assisting the athlete to the ground with general convulsions, moving any potentially harmful objects and cushioning their head if possible. Restrictive clothing and any sports equipment should be loosened. The athlete should not be restrained, and only moved if they are in a potentially dangerous place. Attention must still be given to BLS principles, while those surrounding the athlete should stay calm. Once the seizure has ceased, the athlete should be placed into the recovery position in case of postictal vomiting. Dimberg and Burns (2005) presented a set of considerations and characteristics of seizures, which should be noted by sports therapists:

- activity at time of seizure;
- athlete premonition, aura or warning signs;
- time of seizure onset;
- initial clinical manifestation;
- changes in manifestation during seizure evolution;
- alteration of consciousness;
- seizure duration;
- presence of tongue biting or incontinence;
- mental state after seizure;
- duration and character of postictal state.

If it is the athlete's first known seizure, it is vital that the EAP is implemented and that safe transportation is provided to get the athlete to hospital for a full neurological evaluation, for establishing the aetiology and provision of any treatment. Medical help should also be sought if the seizure is prolonged (more than two to six minutes). The sports therapist should aim to understand the athlete's typical seizure duration. Repeated seizures are possible – this is known as 'status epilepticus' – where one seizure is followed by another without recovery to baseline mental state. This should be treated as a medical emergency, and if left untreated can lead to brain damage and possible death.

Spinal injuries

The relative incidence of catastrophic cervical spine injuries is low in comparison to other injuries. However, it is important to remember that serious spinal injuries have potentially devastating sequelae, including neurological impairment and premature mortality (Swartz *et al.*, 2009). When the sports therapist first deals with the management of a potential cervical spine injury (CSI), they will undoubtedly recognize the importance of prior preparation and a well-versed EAP. The actions of the sports medical team can mean the difference between life or death, or between an athlete walking away from a serious injury or living with a devastating disability (Cendoma and Rehberg, 2007). Consequently, the sports therapist working in a pitch-side environment must be familiar with appropriate acute management strategies for the CSI athlete. Injuries to the thoracic and lumbar spine can also be catastrophic and require appropriate management. However, this section will concentrate on the most prevalent spinal disruption; cervical spine injuries.

Mechanism

Catastrophic CSI is defined as a structural distortion of the cervical spinal column associated with actual or potential damage to the spinal cord (Banerjee *et al.*, 2004a). The most common MoI occurs when the top of the head is the point of contact or impact. Such a mechanism is referred to as 'axial load' and can occur during any sport – for example, making a tackle in rugby, falling from a horse during equestrian events, falling onto the head when being thrown in judo. During axial loading, compressive forces create a buckling effect in the cervical spine (Swartz *et al.*, 2009). The traumatic conditions that could potentially result from such a mechanism include: unstable fractures and dislocations; transient quadriplegia; and acute central disc herniations (Banerjee *et al.*, 2004a).

Prevention

NATA (the National Athletic Trainers' Association) recognize evidence for four methods of injury prevention (Swartz *et al.*, 2009). They emphasize that individuals responsible for emergency care should:

1. be familiar with sports-specific causation and understand the physiologic response to the injury;
2. have a familiarity for the safety rules of the sport relating to the prevention of CSI, taking actions to ensure that they are adhered to by players and officials;
3. be familiar with the protective equipment allowed within the rules of the sport and be aware of the manufacturers' recommendations relating to fit and maintenance;
4. educate coaches and athletes about the mechanisms of catastrophic CSI (such as the dangers of head–down contact and pertinent safety rules).

Management

Minimizing head and neck movement is the key factor in the successful management of the spine-injured athlete. Any equipment or technique that limits movement will allow for effective and safe immobilization of the injured athlete, reducing the potential for secondary injury. If the MoI is considered to be capable of causing spinal trauma, precautions must be implemented. The athlete should be stabilized and maintained until spinal injury can be excluded clinically with appropriate clinical and neurological examination. If it is difficult for the sports therapist to ascertain the MoI, and the injured athlete is unconscious or has an inability to communicate, then it is wise to institute precaution and treat as though spinal trauma has occurred. As soon as the sports therapist suspects a potential cervical spine injury, stabilization should be immediately applied to the athlete in order to minimize movement of the cervical spine during the management of the condition. Manual stabilization is offered using a firm grip of the athlete's head with both hands, ensuring ears are not covered. The hands are placed cupping the occiput, with fingertips grasping the mastoid processes (Lennarson *et al.*, 2001). This enables the sports therapist to communicate with and reassure the injured athlete (see Photograph 4.13). Once manual immobilization has been employed, clearance of CSI can begin; this will require another person in addition to the EMT. The need for further cervical spine immobilization and referral to A&E may be ruled out if the following criteria are met:

- The athlete is conscious and has a GSC score of >15.
- Upon palpation, no localized cervical pain is present.
- There are no neurological deficits (sensation or strength).
- No distracting pain is present.
- The athlete is able to move through 45° of rotation, bilaterally.

If any of the above prove positive, then it is essential that manual stabilization is converted to full spine immobilization; and the injured athlete should be transferred to A&E as soon as possible for further examination.

Primary survey considerations

The airway should be exposed immediately, with the removal of any existing barriers (such as protective face masks or gum shields). If it becomes necessary to deliver rescue breaths, the safest method should be chosen and be delivered by the most experienced member of the EMT. The jaw thrust technique is recommended over the head tilt chin lift method as the latter produces unnecessary extension at the cervical spine. Advanced airway management techniques (such as an OPA, NPA or endotracheal tube) are recommended if appropriately trained members of the EMT are present (Swartz *et al.*, 2009).

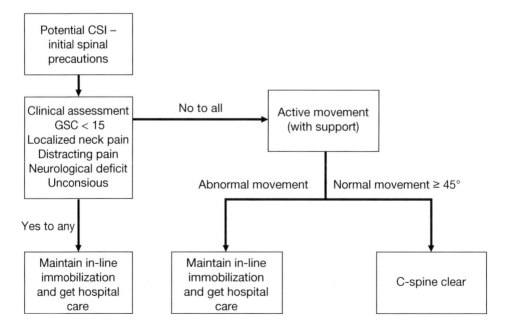

Figure 4.8 Cervical spine clearance algorithm.

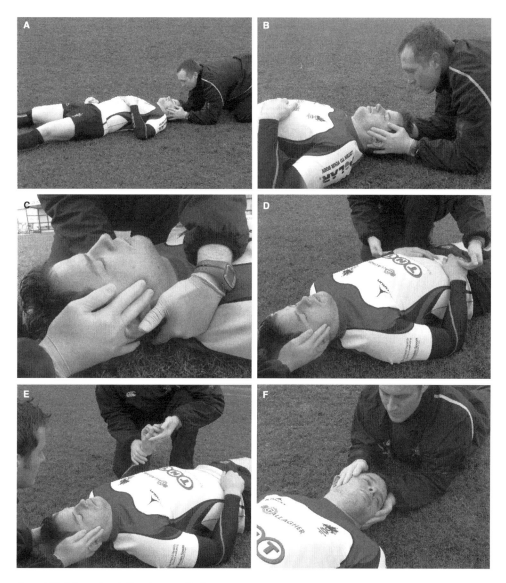

A and B: Manual stabilization applied
C: Palpation of the cervical spine
D: Sensory testing
E: Strength testing
F: Active assisted range of motion ≥45°

Photo 4.13 Management and assessment of a potential cervical spine injury.

Immobilization and transport

If upon assessment it has been decided to immobilize the spine, then the sports therapist may do so with the use of cervical collars, side head supports, a spinal board and straps. Discussion on the types of equipment that may be utilized can be found earlier in the chapter. If the spine of the injured athlete is not in a neutral position, then the sports therapist may assist realignment into neutral if the athlete is conscious, or passively realign if unconscious. This will help to minimize secondary injury to the spinal cord and allow for optimal airway management. If the injured athlete experiences any increased symptoms during this procedure, such as increased pain, neurological symptoms, muscle spasm, airway compromise or resistance, then it should be abandoned and the athlete splinted in their current position. If the athlete is found lying prone, then it may be necessary to 'log roll' into a supine position (see Photograph 4.17). To achieve immobilization of the cervical spine, a cervical collar must be fitted to the athlete. This requires two members of the EMT; one will be manually stabilizing, the other sizing and fitting the collar. It is important that the correctly sized collar is chosen to offer maximal neutral immobilization. If the collar is too short it may not provide enough support; if it is too long it may force the neck into an extended position. The measurement required for correct sizing is taken by measuring the finger distance between the top of the athlete's trapezius and the bottom of their chin. This measurement can then be transferred to the collar (see Photograph 4.14). The collar should then be assembled and fixed as necessary (depending upon type and make) and then preformed. Once this has been completed, and the injured athlete's head is in a neutral position, the collar may be fitted.

Once the collar has been fitted to the injured athlete and transportation is required, they may be placed onto a spinal board using a 'scoop stretcher' or the 'log roll' manoeuvre. A 'scoop stretcher' is designed to split into two to allow the injured athlete to be picked up and placed on the spinal board. A half 'log roll' is used to ensure the halves are in the correct place (see Photograph 4.15).

The 'log roll' is a standard manoeuvre which allows the sports therapist to move the athlete suspected of cervical spine trauma while maintaining a neutral spine alignment, and allows for further examination of the back, transfer onto a spinal board or for maintenance of a clear, viable airway (such as in the case of the athlete vomiting). The number of 'log rolls' should be kept to a minimum, and only performed as necessary. The manoeuvre requires five people to carry it out: one stabilizes and controls the head, and also coordinates the procedure; three control the chest, pelvis and lower limbs; and the final member is free to perform any further actions (for example, inserting the spinal board) (see Photographs 4.16 and 4.17). The person controlling the head of the injured athlete will instruct the other members and the commands should be clearly communicated to them prior to attempting any movement. This manoeuvre should be practised with the EMT (including the *'ready, steady, go'* command).

Once the athlete has been transferred to the spinal board, they must be secured with the use of head supports and straps. To optimize control of the injured athlete on a spinal board the body must be fixed to the board before the head. Once the body is secure, the head may be immobilized with head blocks and straps (see Photograph 4.18). There is a wide range of both equipment and techniques that may be used in immobilizing the spine-injured athlete. Selection should be made based upon skills and training, and on which the sports therapist feels most comfortable in using.

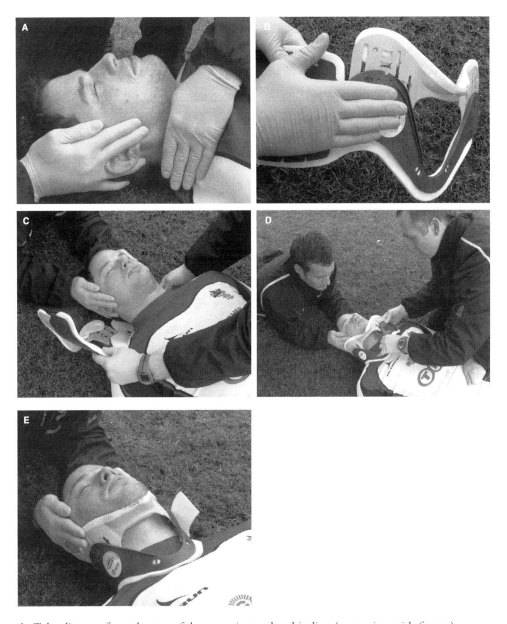

A: Take distance from the top of the trapezius to the chin line (measuring with fingers).
B: Transfer this measurement to the cervical collar to select appropriate size.
C, D, E: Preform the collar, and fit ensuring maintenance of neutral spine.

Photo 4.14 Measurement and application of a cervical collar.

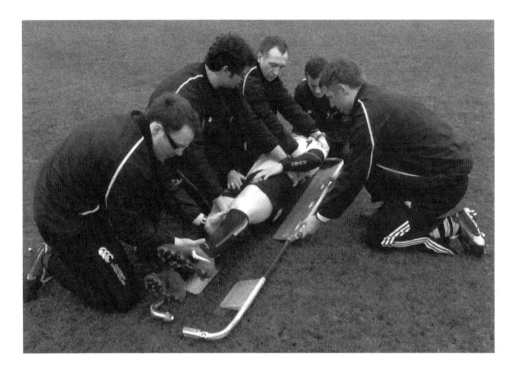

Photo 4.15   Use of a scoop stretcher.

Practitioner's Tip Box 4.7

'The log roll'

Ready-steady-go command: this must be made clear to the EMT when practising this manoeuvre; and always given by the member of the EMT stabilizing the head.

A suggested command that can be used is:

'READY – BRACE - LIFT' (when lifting)

'READY – BRACE – LOWER' (when lowering)

The final word is both an instructive and descriptive word of the action the team are about to perform.

Hand positions for the EMT:

For the three members controlling the athlete's body, this can be remembered as: '3 over and 3 under' i.e. the first three hands will be placed over the athlete's body at the shoulder, mid thorax and hip. The next three hands will be placed underneath the athlete's leg furthest from the EMT member (see Photograph 4.17). This will maximize control of the athlete during the log roll.

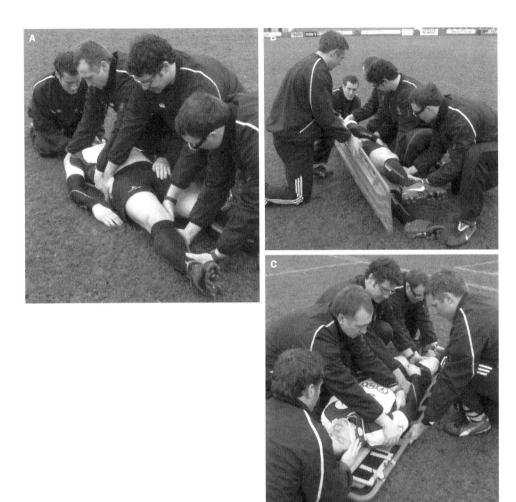

A: Start combined hand position for the log roll.
B: Insertion of spinal board by fifth member of the EMT.
C: End position with athlete on the spinal board.

Photo 4.16   Technique for 'the log roll'.

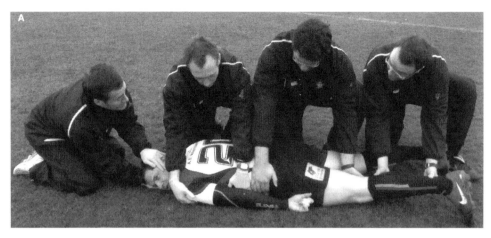

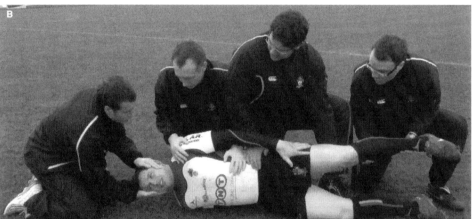

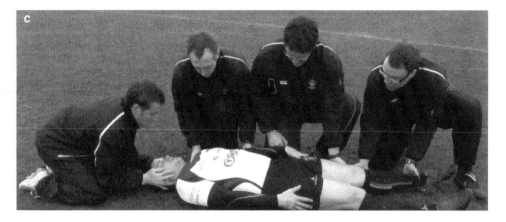

A: Start position; note crossed hands of the therapist stabilizing the head.

B: Mid–way position.

C: Finishing position with injured athlete in supine.

Photo 4.17 'The log roll' for the prone–lying injured athlete.

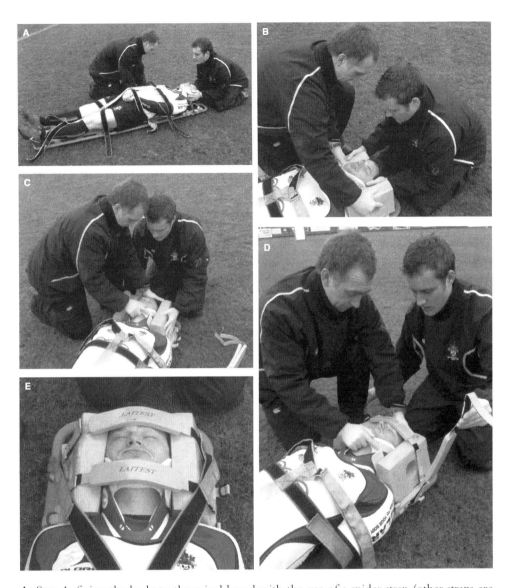

A: Step 1: fixing the body to the spinal board with the use of a spider strap (other straps are available, depending upon type and make of board).

B: Securing the head with the use of head blocks.

C: Using a changeover to secure the head with head blocks.

D: Securing the head blocks with velcro straps.

E: Completed head immobilization with cervical collar, head blocks and straps.

Photo 4.18 Immobilizing the spine and head.

Facial, dental and eye injuries

The position and anatomy of the face make it susceptible to injury and it is a frequent site of trauma in the athlete (Kaufman and Heckler, 1997). Facial injuries range from very minor to extremely complex. The majority of those experienced during athletic activities are of a minor nature, mostly affecting superficial soft tissues, and require minimal but appropriate treatment. However, some facial injuries can result in serious structural and cosmetic deformity or functional deficits. With a thorough examination and familiarity of the relevant anatomy, the sports therapist can gauge the extent of the injury and effectively treat, or refer on to a doctor or other appropriate specialist (such as a dental surgeon or maxillofacial consultant).

Facial trauma

Facial injuries often result in a large amount of bleeding – certainly in comparison to other peripheral areas, due to the high vascularity of the facial tissues. The sports therapist must approach facial injuries with an ordered and considered strategy, despite any concerns regarding cosmetic disfigurement. They must, as always, begin with a standard primary survey to rule out any life-threatening conditions.

Epistaxis

Nose bleeds can often be traumatic for the athlete; it is important to recognize that epistaxis can be a serious condition, with possible life-threatening sequelae. Appropriate first aid steps can be effective – as few as 10 per cent of individuals with nasal bleeding seek medical attention (Sparacino, 2000). Epistaxis can be classified by anterior or posterior origins. Posterior origins account for only 5–10 per cent of bleeds (Halloran, 1993). This is due to the positioning of the deep arteries supplying facial structures. Anterior epistaxis is usually the result of a direct blow to the nose, or a septal contusion. They can, however, also be the result of sinus infection, foreign bodies lodged in the nose, low environmental humidity, high altitude or allergens, as well as being related to serious other facial or head injury (Weir, 1997). Simply 'picking' or 'blowing' one's nose can cause it to bleed. Certain cardiovascular disorders can also predispose to nasal bleeding (such as arteriosclerosis, haemophilia or hypertension). Moderate to severe bleeds generally indicate a posterior epistaxis, whereas minor bleeding is usually due to an anterior bleed (Viducich *et al.*, 1995). There are several techniques which may be used in the management of epistaxis, and the decision of which to use depends upon the severity of the bleeding and the constraints of the sport, where a quick RtP is desirable. Conservative management generally consists of sitting the athlete down and asking them to tilt their head forward to allow the blood to drain from their nostrils. The athlete should be encouraged to breathe through their mouth while they apply direct thumb and finger pressure onto the bleeding nostril (i.e. pinching the soft part of their nose). A cold compress may also be applied to the area. The athlete should remain in this position for up to ten minutes, or until the bleeding subsides. During this time, the athlete should be discouraged from swallowing, coughing, sniffing or blowing their nose as this may disturb the blood–clotting process (coagulation). After ten minutes, the athlete can release the finger pressure, and if bleeding has not stopped then they should reapply for a further two periods of ten minutes. They should be transferred to A&E if the bleed is severe, or if it lasts for longer than 30 minutes. In cases where early RtP is necessary and safe for the athlete, alternative techniques may be utilized. It is essential that severe injury has not been missed and has been disregarded as a possibility. Nasal tampons may be inserted into the bleeding nostril to absorb blood and encourage clotting. It is essential that at least 1.25 cm of the tampon remains on the exterior of the nostril for ease of removal. There are limitations to this technique; the tampon is often easily disturbed or removed during contact with an opponent or simply during breathing of the athlete. Field (1997) describes an additional technique where a roll of cotton or gauze is inserted between the athlete's upper lip and gum in order to place direct pressure on the arterial supply to the anterior nasal mucosa.

Oral and dental injuries

Oral injuries can include dental avulsions, dental fractures, dental luxations, temporomandibular (TMJ) injuries as well as lacerations to the gum, cheeks, tongue or lips (O'Connor, 2005). Upon primary survey negative, the initial field examination of dental injuries begins with any external lacerations of the head, face or neck before moving to the intraoral examination. Palpations of the zygomatic arch and the angle and lower border of the mandible must be undertaken to check for tenderness, swelling and bruising and to rule out the possibility of fracture. The intraoral examination will assess the lips, tongue, cheek, palate and floor of the mouth for lacerations or disfigurement. Sterile gauze can be used to stem bleeding. If an adult tooth is knocked out, it should be replaced if possible (providing it is clean). The tooth can be gently pushed back into the socket and a sterile gauze pad placed between the top and bottom teeth to help maintain tooth position. The athlete should then go to hospital or a dentist. If the tooth cannot be replaced, the casualty should keep the tooth in his cheek, or place the tooth in milk or water to prevent it drying out. A properly fitted mouth guard will protect the teeth and may also reduce the potential for concussion from a blow to the jaw (Padilla, 2011).

Haematoma of the external ear

A forceful blow to the ear or repetitive shearing microtrauma to the ear (common in sports such as rugby, wrestling and boxing) can result in what is commonly referred to as 'cauliflower ear'. This results from tearing of the blood vessels at the perichondral level of the ear and produces a subperichondrial haematoma (Kaufman and Heckler, 1997). If early treatment is not provided, the area will begin to develop into a firm fibrotic mass with new cartilage formation and permanent deformity. Clinical diagnosis is made by noting deformity of the outer ear architecture and fluctuance on palpation. Treatment is most successful when administered early on – before fibrosis develops. Treatment, which is usually performed in hospital or GP surgery, involves needle aspiration and compressive head wrap. The condition should be monitored to ensure that re-accumulation has not occurred. When pain and swelling has subsided, the athlete may RtP; however, protective headwear should be considered for the prevention of reoccurrence.

Eye injuries

Sport is responsible for 25–40 per cent of all eye injuries severe enough to require hospital admission (MacEwen and McLatchie, 2010). The eye can be bruised or cut by direct impact, or by sharp fragments of metal, grit and glass. All eye injuries should be treated seriously due to the potential risk to the casualty's vision. Even grazes to the superficial layers of the cornea can lead to long-term visual disturbances through scarring or infection. A detailed history of the mechanism should be taken into consideration, with an estimate of visual acuity before and after the injury. Questioning should ascertain the presence of pain, photophobia, diplopia, floaters, flashing lights, tearing, headache and nausea (Martinez and Ellini, 2005). The physical examination should include checks for visual acuity using reading tests or finger counts and light perception. The pupils should be checked for reactivity to light, ensuring they are round, symmetrical and reactive. The examination should also include visual assessment of the bony orbits, eyelids, conjunctiva, cornea and iris. The extra-ocular muscles should be checked for range of movement and symmetry. The athlete should not be allowed to continue play with visual disturbances, as this may increase the chance of further injury. Transient visual disturbances will often occur with minor eye injuries, if these do not subside quickly or any corneal damage is suspected the athlete should be immediately transported to hospital. A sterile eye pad should be placed over the affected eye and secured in place; the therapist should encourage the casualty to keep the unaffected eye still as movement may cause further damage to the injured eye.

Scalp and head wounds

The MoI for an open wound to the head or scalp typically involves a direct blow, either from an opponent or via a piece of sporting equipment (such as a hockey stick or a goal post). Scalp and head wounds often lead to profuse bleeding which may make the wound appear worse than it is. Athletes should be removed from the field of play as this will allow for a careful inspection of the wound, control of haemorrhage and assessment to ensure that there are no other serious underlying head injuries (such as fracture or concussion). If a serious underlying head injury has been ruled out, the initial management begins by applying firm, direct pressure to the wound in order to help control bleeding and reduce blood loss. This can be directed by the sports therapist and administered by the injured athlete with the use of sterile gauze. Further management follows the principles and guidelines of general wound management.

Abdominal and pelvic trauma

The abdominal and pelvic region is a complex area that can produce pain sensations from a multitude of sources. It is important that the sports therapist is aware of the common injuries and illnesses involving the internal organs of the abdomen, and can recognize the extent of the injury – as blunt abdominal injury can represent an immediate threat to life (Valentino *et al.*, 2006). In the sporting environment, injuries to the abdomen usually occur as a result of blunt trauma through contact with another athlete, an immovable object (such as a goal post) or piece of equipment. During such incidents, the primary concerns must be internal bleeding from damaged solid organs such as the liver, spleen or kidneys; or damage to hollow organs such as the stomach or intestines, which can cause leakage of their contents into the abdominal cavity. In turn, this can cause peritonitis (inflammation of the serous lining – the peritoneum). Physical examination is the first step in diagnosis, but is limited due to the type and depth of structures that may be implicated in such injuries. The examination should encompass a detailed 'SAMPLE' history, relating to the injured athlete's discomfort. Treatment aims will be to relieve pain and discomfort and obtain further medical help if the MoI, onset and severity of pain indicate possible internal trauma. It is important to monitor the athlete's vital signs (pulse, blood pressure, nausea, fever and signs of shock) for any change or deterioration.

Wound management

An excessive or abnormal discharge of blood from the blood vessels is called a haemorrhage. The timing of assessment within the primary and secondary survey protocols, including the importance of early and effective wound management, is discussed in the basic and advanced life support sections of this chapter. The aims of wound management and treatment are to minimize the risk of infection, restore function and to repair tissue integrity with strength and optimum cosmesis. Haemorrhage can be venous, capillary or arterial, and may be internal or external. Venous blood flow is characteristically dark red with a continuous flow; capillary bed bleeding exudes a reddish colour from the tissue; and arterial bleeds flow in spurts with a relatively brighter red colour. External haemorrhaging can encompass simple scrapes to more serious life-threatening injuries. Open skin wounds include abrasions, lacerations, punctures, avulsions and, in rare sporting incidences, amputations.

History and examination

The most common MoI is blunt trauma; however, lacerations may occur as a result of contact with sharp equipment (such as with studs or skates). Abrasions include scrapes and scratches in which the outer layer of skin is damaged but without full penetration of all dermal layers. They may be caused as a result of friction on a playing surface or chaffing.

Management and treatment

A detailed explanation of infectious disease is beyond the remit of this chapter; nonetheless, precautions to safeguard the sports therapist from blood-borne pathogens and other diseases are of paramount importance. As the sports therapist is likely to be a primary manager of acute sports-induced wounds, it is essential to prevent contact with bodily fluids of any kind while managing wounds. This can be done via use of protective barriers such as gloves, aprons and face masks. When appropriate management has been provided, any contaminated equipment must be disposed of in the correct manner and treated as clinical waste. Initial management following identification of the wound site involves controlling the bleed (achieving haemostasis). This involves the application of direct pressure to the wound site and elevation of the limb to above the level of the heart. A contraindication to direct pressure may be the presence of an embedded body in the wound. In more serious cases of bleeding, it will be necessary to treat for shock. Once

Table 4.15 Open wound management

Wound Type	Initial care	Continued care
Abrasion	Cleanse area with mild soap and water, followed by hydrogen peroxide, debriding if necessary. Apply antibiotic ointment and cover with dressing	Change dressing daily, looking for signs of infection
Blisters (ruptured/deroofed)	Remove the overlying skin, cleanse and apply a hydroactive gel dressing	Replace gel dressing as required until healed
Laceration	Apply sterile gauze to stem bleeding, cleanse around wound. Depending on wound size, sterile strips or sutures may be necessary★	In general, staples or sutures are removed after approx. 7 days; facial sutures 3–5 days
Puncture	Apply sterile gauze to stem bleeding, cleanse around wound. Injections of a tetanus prophylaxis may be required★	In general, staples or sutures are removed after about 7 days; facial sutures 3–5 days
Avulsion	Apply direct pressure with the use of sterile gauze. Save the avulsed part by wrapping in sterile gauze dressing secured with sterile bandage. Label and keep cool (without freezing)	A&E as soon as possible
Amputation	Direct pressure at the distal edge of amputation site. Wrap the amputated part in a sterile dressing and place in a plastic bag. Label bag and keep cool on ice	A&E as soon as possible

Note: ★Doctor or hospital care may be required.

Practitioner Tip Box 4.8

Signs of wound infection

- Signs of wound infection (appearing 2–7 days after injury)
- Hot, red, swollen and tender tissue
- Swollen and painful lymph glands near the area of infection
- Mild fever and headache

---

control of bleeding is obtained, the wound surface must be cleansed and any debris removed. In the case of more serious wounds it will be necessary to decide if closure is required, and which method would be most suitable. 'Butterfly' or 'Steri-Strip' type methods may be suitable for smaller wounds or for temporary closure of larger lacerations. If a severe laceration requires closure with sutures, or an adhesive bond, the appropriately trained member of the EMT will be required to do this. If an appropriately trained practitioner is unavailable, the athlete should be transferred to A&E once control is maintained. A sterile dressing should be placed over the wound to cover and protect it, and be held in place with a bandage. Following any interventions, pulses and motor and sensory function distal to the wound should be tested. In cases where control of the bleed is not possible, immediate referral to A&E is necessary.

Blisters

Blisters occur when the skin is repeatedly rubbed against another surface, creating friction and heat. They are often associated with excessive perspiration and improperly fitted equipment or footwear. Blisters can also result following excessive exposure to UV light – i.e. sunburn. The affected area of skin gathers serosanguinous fluid or blood underneath superficial layers of the skin (epidermis) to protect the area, forming a blister. Early treatment of friction blisters with 'moleskin doughnuts', nylon foot stocking and talcum powder to absorb perspiration can be effective (Levine, 1980). Larger blisters may be drained at the edge with a small sterile needle, by appropriately trained persons, leaving the blister roof as a protective layer. Ruptured or deroofed blisters require the application of a sterile dressing as a second skin layer to reduce discomfort, reduce the chance of infection and enhance healing. Post-activity, blisters may be soothed by ice applications (keeping a barrier between the skin and ice). Primary prevention methods include wearing properly worn-in footwear, use of absorbent socks and the application of petroleum jelly over bony prominences (Batts, 2005).

Strategies for the removal of an athlete from the field of play

There are many occasions when it is necessary to remove an injured athlete from the field of play. The decision to do so will have been made following an assessment using the 'TOTAPS' protocol, taking into consideration the type and severity of the injury and necessity to do so. Once the decision has been made to move, lift or transport the injured athlete it is vital that an appropriate technique is chosen and used with correct handling, ensuring that protection to the injured athlete is offered, preventing further injury. The following section outlines strategies for the safe and effective removal of an injured athlete from the field of play.

Assisted ambulation

Following on-field assessment, if it is considered safe for the injured athlete to walk, assisted ambulation may be given. This ideally involves the assistance of two therapists of similar height. The injured athlete will be supported on both sides, placing their arms over the shoulders of the assisters, with the therapists' arms placed around the athletes back (see Photograph 4.19).

If an upper limb injury has occurred, and support is required, the athlete's playing shirt or clothing can be used as a temporary sling. This can offer sufficient support until more time can be given to assess and support accordingly (see Photograph 4.20).

Manual conveyance

Following assessment, and having made the decision to remove the athlete from the field of play, manual conveyance may be considered for an injured athlete where the distance would be too great for assisted ambulation, but where stretcher removal is not required. This can be performed with two sports therapists (see Photograph 4.21).

Stretchers

For the more seriously injured athlete it will be necessary to use a stretcher for their transportation, as this offers greater support. With a limb injury it is necessary to splint the limb prior to the injured athlete being placed on a soft stretcher (Photograph 4.22). If a spinal injury is suspected then a spinal board would be most the suitable stretcher for transportation (see Photograph 4.18).

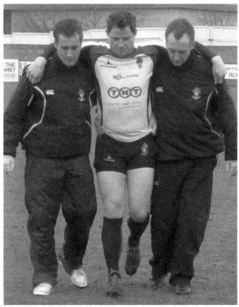 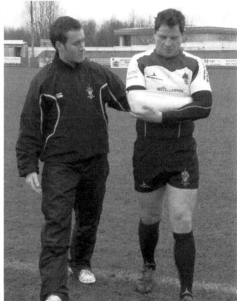

Photo 4.19   Assisted ambulation from the field of play.

Photo 4.20   Use of the shirt as a temporary sling.

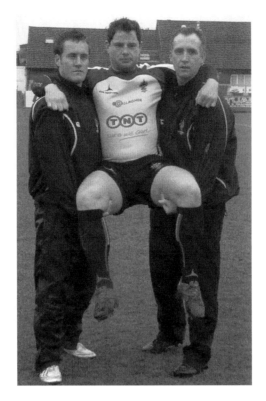

Photo 4.21   Manual conveyance of the injured athlete.

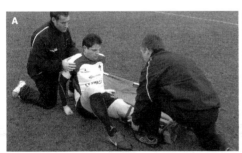

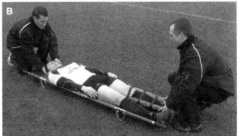

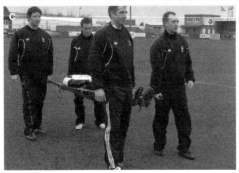

A: Splint being placed on the injured limb
B: The injured athlete placed on the stretcher
C: Carrying the seriously injured athlete on a stretcher

Photo 4.22   Use of a soft stretcher for transportation of the seriously injured athlete.

Medical emergencies

Circulation and shock

An understanding of how the body responds to intrinsic and extrinsic stress and injury through the changes in blood flow will undoubtedly help the sports therapist tend to injured athletes more effectively. Shock is a possible accompaniment to any injury and should be considered as a medical emergency, as it can leave the heart unable to circulate enough oxygenated blood to vital organs. Defined as the inadequate perfusion of tissues required to meet cellular metabolic demand, it is important that the sports therapist is able to understand the condition, recognize the early stages and apply appropriate principles of treatment. A simple understanding of the body's response to stress and how it adapts via changes in blood flow will help the emergency care provider to tend to the injured athlete more effectively (Davis, 2007). Shock is an attempt by the body to prioritize and maintain the life of the vital organs. The body will respond to an injury in one of three ways: changing the rate of blood flow by speeding up or slowing down the heart rate; controlling the flow of blood locally or systemically through vasodilation or vasoconstriction; increasing the volume of blood in the system. With a diminished blood volume available to the circulatory system, the vascular system loses its ability to retain the fluid consistency (plasma) of the blood. A quantity of blood plasma moving into surrounding tissue spaces can leave a higher proportion of solid components (red and white blood cells and platelets), causing stagnation and slowing of the blood flow. Shock can result from: damage to the heart, preventing an adequate pumping mechanism; low blood volume due to haematoma or dehydration; or vasodilatation, which leads to pooling in larger vessels, away from vital organs. The heart subsequently begins to pump more quickly, but due to reduced fluid volume, the pulse rate is weakened and the blood pressure drops. This ultimately results in insufficient oxygen being available to the tissues, particularly those of the nervous system (Prentice, 2011), leading to a general collapse of the vascular system and widespread tissue death – which may be fatal unless treated appropriately. The main types of shock and their potential causes are shown in Table 4.16.

History and examination of shock

Shock may be associated with any injury, and the sports therapist should decide if the condition is haemorrhagic or non-haemorrhagic. The essential signs of shock are seen with tachycardia hypotension, and the ensuing signs of poor organ perfusion leading to confusion or loss of consciousness. Other signs which may be present and help the sports therapist to establish the diagnosis of shock and guide effective management include, initially, a rapid and weakened pulse, and if the injured athlete deteriorates, breathing also becomes rapid and shallow, with an associated increase in sweating.

Management and treatment of shock

By correctly recognizing the signs of shock, the sports therapist's emergency management will aim to assist the athlete's natural adaptations. Depending on the cause of the shock the emergency care should be as follows:

- Do not move the athlete unless absolutely necessary to avoid further harm.
- Assess the 'ABCDE'.
- If head or neck injury is not suspected, elevate and support the legs by 10–12 inches (consideration should be made for upper limb injuries). With breathing difficulties or head injuries, the injured athlete may be more comfortable in a semi-reclined position, while reducing pressure to the brain.

Table 4.16 Types of shock

Types of shock	Definition	Possible causes
Anaphylactic	Severe allergic reaction to a foreign protein ingested, inhaled or injected	Food allergies, drugs, insect stings or inhaled pollens
Cardiogenic	The heart muscle is no longer able to sustain enough pressure to pump blood through the system	Caused by injuries to the heart or previous heart attack
Hypovolemic	Excessive blood or fluid loss leading to decrease in blood pressure and inadequate supply and oxygen perfusion to organs	Haemorrhage, dehydration, multiple trauma or severe burns
Metabolic	Severe loss of fluids due to an untreated illness that alters biochemical equilibrium	Insulin shock, diabetic coma, vomiting and diarrhoea
Neurogenic	Peripheral blood vessel dilation, causing the typical six litres of blood to no longer fill the system and adequately supply oxygen	Spinal or head injury where neural control of the vascular system is compromised
Psychogenic	Temporary dilatation of blood vessels, resulting in a drop in blood pressure to the head and pooling in the abdomen	Fainting from the sight of blood or needles
Respiratory	Insufficient alveoli capillary diffusion leading to low oxygen levels in the blood as a result of inadequate breathing	Injury to the breathing control mechanism including; spinal injury to respiratory nerves (C3–C5); airway obstruction; pneumothorax or haemothorax
Septic	Severe infection whereby toxins attack the walls of small vessels, causing dilatation and reduction in blood pressure	Usually bacterial infection through open wound, severe burns or post-surgery

Source: adapted from Anderson *et al.*, 2009.

Table 4.17 Shock: signs and symptoms

Vital sign	Signs and symptoms
Pulse rate	Rapid and weak
Blood pressure	Systolic pressure usually below 90 mmHg
Respiratory rate	Rapid and shallow
Skin colour	Cyanosis (pale blue or grey)
Skin temperature	Cool, moist and clammy
Eyes	Dull, listless
Muscle function	Decreasing ability to control
Mental status	Lightheaded, restlessness, irritability, anxiety, drowsy, loss of consciousness

- With a suspected CSI the athlete should remain flat.
- Maintain normal body temperature – if possible cover the athlete's upper and lower limbs; loosen any tight or restrictive clothing.
- Treat injuries and splint fractures.
- Continually reassure the athlete.
- Monitor vital signs and document every five minutes.
- Limit fluid and food intake.

On arrival to hospital, definitive care will be provided to treat the causative factor of the shock. Fluid therapy and transfusions may be necessary following any significant loss of blood. Medication may be given for any cardiac-related condition or to control a dilated vascular system. At this point, any associated musculoskeletal disorders will be treated.

Asthma

Asthma is a chronic inflammatory lung disease that can result in an athlete having difficulty with breathing. This may be induced through exercise, allergies, cold air, dust and respiratory infections. In an asthma attack, the smooth muscle layer of the airway spasms, narrowing the diameter, the middle layer swells and mucus may form in an attempt to plug the airway. This reduces the function of the airway, leading to difficulty in breathing. This is usually treated by the athlete using a reliever inhaler (bronchodilator), but prevention is best practice in the management of this condition. This requires the athlete to take a controlling medicine in order to prevent an attack from occurring (Hargreave *et al.*, 1979). If an attack occurs, it may be recognized with the athlete displaying some or all of the following symptoms:

- difficulty in breathing, especially on breathing out;
- wheezing as the casualty breathes out;
- difficulty speaking;
- distress and anxiety;
- features of hypoxia, such as grey-blue tinge (cyanosis) to the lips, earlobes or nailbeds.

Treatment involves encouraging the athlete to ease and control their breathing. Medical help should be sought if it is the athlete's first attack, if they do not have any medication or if the attack does not ease after a few minutes following a few doses of their inhaler. The treatment should proceed as follows:

1. Reassure the athlete and offer their reliever inhaler (usually 'the blue one').
2. Encourage slow breaths and position the athlete in sitting, slightly leaning forward (do not lie the casualty down).
3. The inhaler should take effect within a few minutes; if not, encourage the athlete to take a further dose.
4. If the inhaler has had no effect, the athlete is having further difficulty in talking or they are becoming exhausted, call 999 for emergency help.
5. Monitor and record the athlete's vital signs (level of response, breathing, pulse) until they recover, or until help arrives.
6. If the attack worsens the athlete may lose consciousness – if so, open the airway, check breathing, and prepare to begin CPR as necessary until emergency assistance arrives.

Exercise associated muscle cramps

Exercise associated muscle cramps (EAMCs) is a prevalent condition that requires medical attention during or immediately after sporting competition (Schwellnus, 2009), particularly in endurance events. Schwellnus (2009) defines EAMC as a painful, spasmodic and involuntary contraction of skeletal muscle that occurs during or immediately after exercise. The aetiology of the condition is not well understood, with theories leaning towards electrolyte depletion, dehydration and altered neuromuscular control. The current evidence favours the latter theory of altered neuromuscular control as a result of the development of fatigue being the primary factor for EAMC (Schwellnus, 2009). Initial management of EAMC should consist of rest and passive stretching of the affected area. Massage and kneading the muscle may also help to relieve the symptoms. An increase in fluid intake should be recommended. The athletes' ability to continue play will be based on a number of factors, including the length of the transient nature of the symptoms, and the athlete's pain tolerance. The athlete will likely experience some pain or discomfort post-event for up to 72 hours. The 'PRICE' protocol may be considered at this stage, followed by STT techniques and gentle pain-free stretching to the damaged muscle tissue.

Diabetes

Diabetes mellitus describes a condition in which defects in insulin secretion, insulin action or both cause disturbances of carbohydrate, fat and protein metabolism. The longer-term effects of diabetes can include damage, dysfunction and failure of body organs; however, athletes who are able to maintain their blood-glucose levels are able to participate in sport. Indeed, sport and exercise are to be recommended as a tool in the management of the condition (Sigal *et al.*, 2004). To maintain their blood-glucose levels the athlete should understand the necessary balance between diet and exercise, and regularly test their blood levels using a glucose monitor. Berger (2002) offers detailed discussion on medication adjustment to reduce the risk of hypoglycaemia, which is a condition where the blood-glucose level falls below normal. Physical activity can lead to hypoglycaemia if medication dose or carbohydrate consumption is not altered for the diabetic athlete (Sigal *et al.*, 2004). The signs and symptoms of hypoglycaemia can be found in Practitioner Tip Box 4.9. The aim of managing an athlete who is hypoglycaemic is to raise their blood-glucose levels as quickly as possible, preventing deterioration and loss of consciousness. To achieve this, the athlete should sit down and be provided with carbohydrate in the form of sugar (examples of this include sugary drinks, glucose tablets or gels) (Fowler, 2008). It should be noted that food which has a high fat content as well as sugar should be avoided as this can delay the absorption of carbohydrate (for example, ice cream and icing). Pure glucose is the preferred treatment (Fowler, 2008). If the athlete responds quickly, some more carbohydrate can be given, and they should be encouraged to rest until they feel better. The athlete should then re-test their blood-glucose (after 15 minutes) and if the glucose level is still low, consume more carbohydrate (15–20 g) (Fowler, 2008). If their condition does not improve, the therapist must seek medical help (calling 999/112) while monitoring and recording vital signs. If the athlete loses consciousness, the airway should be opened and breathing must be checked.

GP referral

A diagnosis is the use of scientific or clinical methods to establish the cause and nature of a patient's illness or injury and subsequent functional impairments caused by that pathology (Prentice, 2004). Sports therapists and other health care professionals use their clinical reasoning

---

Practitioner Tip Box 4.9

Signs and symptoms of hypoglycaemia

- History of diabetes
- Lethargy, nervousness, anxiousness, faintness, hunger
- Sweating with cold, clammy skin
- Confusion, irrational behaviour, mood changes (cognitive dysfunction)
- Seizure, loss of consciousness (late stages)

---

and assessment skills to make an informed clinical diagnosis to identify the pathology of injury; this then identifies impairments and directs the treatment and rehabilitation strategies. There will be occasions during a pitch-side assessment when the sports therapist deems the condition being assessed as outside their remit and in need of further investigation, but not necessarily in need of immediate or emergency care. In such instances, the sports therapist would seek not referral or transportation to the A&E department, but to the athlete's (or club's) medical doctor. The level of the sport at which the athlete is participating will dictate the nature of the athlete's doctor, and to where the sports therapist will refer the injured athlete. Professional-level sports generally have a club doctor to whom the athlete will be referred; at amateur level, the sports therapist is likely to be referring the athlete to their own GP. Regardless of the level, the doctor to which the sports therapist has referred will then be responsible for making a medical diagnosis – this diagnosis may be considered to be the ultimate determination of the athlete's physical condition (Prentice, 2011). The doctor may elect to refer the athlete to a suitable consultant who is specialized in an appropriate field (such as a neurologist, orthopaedic surgeon or cardiologist). Figure 4.9 demonstrates an example referral form that the sports therapist can use to provide the doctor with essential information, which in turn is highly likely to assist the process that follows.

Summary

The main role of a sports therapist working with teams and individual athletes in event and pitch-side environments is to provide effective immediate emergency aid and care. The quality of care provided has major implications for the affected athlete's health and career. The quality of care provided should be no different, whether in elite professional or enthusiastic recreational settings – the object is to deliver safe and effective, responsible and responsive on- and off-field assessment and treatment, and to ensure, if appropriate, the safe return of the athlete to play. The sports therapist is charged with minimizing the cost of life- or limb-threatening injuries, and in so doing they must be able to make educated decisions, direct an emergency medical team and liaise effectively with emergency medical services. The sports therapist must be fully prepared to undertake this role successfully (a challenge in itself); and they must be regularly updated in their skills and knowledge. It is essential that the sports therapist has the appropriate education, skills and competencies in delivering the appropriate techniques to be able to fulfil this aim. Continuous rehearsal and review of these skills are essential for the sports therapist and their team to maintain competency in delivery. The occurrence of life- and limb-threatening injuries is rare and essential skills can be easily lost as a result; the sports therapist must always be ready and able to deliver such skills, as these incidents can occur at any time.

Name of **Sports Team, Sports Therapist** *or* **Sports Therapy Clinic**		**GP Referral Form**		GP Name: Address:	
Date		Patient / Player Name		DoB	
Address			Contact Tel		
			E-mail		
Presenting Complaint					
History:			Relevant Clinical Signs:		
			Clinical Impression:		
Treatment and advice provided					
Sports therapist name:			Sports therapist contact details:		
Sports therapist signature:					

Figure 4.9 GP referral form.

Practitioner Tip Box 4.10

First aid equipment and skills: confident application

In emergency situations, it must be recommended that the sports therapist uses the first aid equipment and provides the first aid skills that they are trained in and are confident with. It is essential to recognize that the use of such specialized equipment as medical gases (e.g. oxygen, nitrous oxide), airway adjuncts, AED, fracture splints, spinal boards and collars requires appropriate (and regularly re-certificated) training, sound theoretical knowledge, and familiarity with application. For these reasons, sports therapists and their emergency medical teams working in pitch-side situations must be encouraged to regularly review, reflect upon and practise all key procedures.

Table 4.18 Short glossary of terms

Anaphylactic	A sudden, severe allergic reaction characterized by a sharp drop in blood pressure with associated breathing difficulties. May be caused by exposure to a foreign substance (such as a drug or bee venom) following a preliminary or sensitizing exposure. This may also be referred to as anaphylaxis
Cosmesis	Steps taken to improve the aesthetic appearance of the scars associated with wound management
Cyanosis	A bluish–purple discoloration of skin most commonly resulting from a deficiency of oxygen in the blood
Debridement	The surgical removal of foreign matter or dead tissue from a wound
Epistaxis	Active bleeding from the nose
Extrication	To remove from difficulty; to release from entanglement
Fissure	A long, narrow slit or groove that divides an organ into lobes. The cerebral fissure is a deep fold that involves the entire thickness of the brain wall
Haematoma	A tumour of clotted or partially clotted blood within the tissues
Hyperglycaemia	A pathologic state produced by a higher than normal level of glucose (sugar) in the blood
Hyperthermia	A condition in which a person's normal core body temperature of around 37 °C (98.6 °F) rises to, or above, the range of 37.5–38.3 °C (99.5–100.9 °F)
Hypoglycaemia	A pathologic state produced by a lower than normal level of glucose (sugar) in the blood
Hypothermia	A condition in which a person's normal core body temperature of around 37 °C (98.6 °F) drops below 35 °C (95 °F)
Perichondral membrane	A dense membrane of fibrous connective tissue that closely wraps around cartilage (with the exception of hyaline articular cartilage that is surrounded by synovial membrane)
Pneumothorax	An accumulation of air or gas in the pleural cavity, occurring as a result of disease or injury
Postictal state	The altered state of consciousness that a person enters after experiencing a seizure
Stridor	A harsh, high pitched, wheezing-type sound on inhalation or exhalation
Tachycardia	A state of abnormal rapid beating of the heart, especially over 100 beats per minute
Tachypnoea	A state of abnormal rapid breathing

References

Anderson, J.C., Courson, R.W., Kleiner, D.M. and McLoda, T.A. (2002) National Athletic Trainers' Association position statement: Emergency planning in athletics. *Journal of Athletic Training*. 37 (1): 99–104

Anderson, M., Parr, G. and Hall, S. (2009) *Foundations of athletic training, prevention, assessment and management*, 4th edition. Lippincott, Williams and Wilkins. Philadelphia, PA

Bailes, O.B.I., Hammers, J.L. and Fitzsimmons, R.P. (2010) Chronic traumatic encephalopathy, suicides and para-suicides in professional American athletes: The role of the forensic pathologist. *American Journal of Forensic Medicine and Pathology*. 31 (2):130–132

Banerjee, R., Palumbo, M. and Fadale, P. (2004a) Catastrophic cervical spine injuries in the collision sport athlete, Part 1: Epidemiology, functional anatomy and diagnosis. *American Journal of Sports Medicine*. 32 (4): 1077–1087

Banerjee, R., Palumbo, M.A. and Fadale, P.D. (2004b) Catastrophic cervical spine injuries in the collision sport athlete, Part 2. *American Journal of Sports Medicine*. 32 (7): 1760–1764

Batts, K. (2005) Dermatology. In O'Connor, F., Sallis, R., Wilder, R. and Pierre, P. (eds) *Sports medicine: Just the facts*. McGraw-Hill. New York

Berger, M. (2002) Adjustment of insulin and oral agent therapy. In Ruderman, N., Devlin, J.T., Schneider, S.H. and Kriska, A., (eds) *Handbook of exercise in diabetes*, 2nd edition. American Diabetes Association. Alexandria, VA

Bleakley, C., McDonough, S. and MacAuley, M.D. (2004) The use of ice in the treatment of acute soft-tissue injury. *American Journal of Sports Medicine*. 32 (1): 251–261

Bleakley, C.M., Glasgow, P. and MacAuley, D.C. (2012) PRICE needs updating: Should we call the POLICE? *British Journal of Sports Medicine*. 46 (4): 220–221

Brambrink, A.M. and Koerner, I.P. (2004) Pre-hospital advanced trauma life support: How should we manage the airway, and who should do it? *Critical Care*. 8: 3–5

British Trauma Society. (2003) Guidelines for initial management and assessment of spinal injury: British Trauma Society, 2002. *International Journal of the Care of the Injured*. 34: 405–425

Brooks, J.M., Fuller, C.W., Kemp, S.P.T. and Reddin, D.B. (2005) Epidemiology of injuries in English professional rugby union: Part 1. Match injuries. *British Journal of Sports Medicine*. 39: 757–766

Cantu, R. (1997) Stingers, transient quadriplegia, and cervical spinal stenosis: Return to play criteria. *Medicine and Science in Sports and Exercise*. 29 (7S): S233–S235

Cendoma, M.J. and Rehberg, R.S. (2007) Management of spinal injuries. In Rehberg, R.S. (ed.) *Sports emergency care: A team approach*. Slack Incorporated. Thorofare, NJ

Colleen, J.Y., Riemann, B.L., Munkasy, B.A. and Joyner, A.B. (2004) Comparison of cervical spine motion during application among 4 rigid immobilization collars. *Journal of Athletic Training*. 39 (2): 138–145

Collins, N.C. (2008) Is ice right? Does cryotherapy improve outcome for acute soft tissue injury? *Emergency Medicine Journal*. 25: 65–68

Concussion in Sport Group (2013) *Child-SCAT3: Sport Concussion Assessment Tool for children ages 5 to 12 years*. http://bjsm.bmj.com/content/47/5/263.full.pdf, accessed October 2013

Courson, R. and Henry, G. (2005) Communication: The critical element in emergency preparation. *Athletic Therapy Today*. 10 (2): 16–18

Courson, R., Clanton, M. and Patel, H. (2005a) Emergency assessment. *Athletic Therapy Today*. 10 (2): 19–23

Courson, R., Navtskis, L. and Patel, H. (2005b) Emergency action planning. *Athletic Therapy Today*. 10 (2): 7–15

Crosby, E.T. (2006) Airway management in adults after cervical spine trauma. *Anesthesiology*. 104 (6): 1293–1318

Davis, J.L. (2007) General medical emergencies. In Rehberg, R.S. (ed.) *Sports emergency care: A team approach*. Slack Incorporated. Thorofare, NJ

Dimberg, E. and Burns, T. (2005) Management of common neurologic conditions. *Clinics in Sports Medicine*. 24 (3): 637–662

Driscoll, P. and Houghton, L. (1999) Cervical immobilization: Are we achieving it? *Pre-hospital Immediate Care*. 3: 17–21

Driscoll, P., Laird, C. and Wardrope, J. (2004) The ABC of community emergency care. *Emergency Medicine Journal*. 21: 89–94

Faddy, S.C. and Garlick, S.R. (2005) A systematic review of the safety of analgesia with 50% nitrous oxide: Can a lay responder use analgesic gases in the pre-hospital setting? *Emergency Medical Journal*. 22: 901–906

Field, D. (1997) *Anatomy: Palpation and surface markings*, 2nd edition. Butterworth-Heinemann. Boston, MA

Fincher, L. (2001) Managing medical emergencies: Part 2. *Athletic Therapy Today*. 6 (5): 37

Fitz-Simmons, C.R. and Wardrope, J. (2005) Assessment and care of musculoskeletal problems. *Emergency Medicine Journal*. 22: 68–76

Flegel, M.J. (2008) *Sports first aid*. Human Kinetics. Champaign, IL

Fowler, M.J. (2008) Hypoglycaemia. *Clinical Diabetes*. 26 (4): 170–173

Fu, F.H., Tjoumakaris, F.P. and Buoncristani, A. (2007) Building a sports medicine team. *Clinics in Sports Medicine*. 26: 173–179

Genzwuerker, H.V., Oberkinkhaus, J., Thorsten, F., Kerger, H., Gernoth, C. and Hinkelbein, J. (2005) Emergency airway management by first responders with the laryngeal tube – intuitive and repetitive use in a manikin. *Scandinavian Journal of Trauma Resuscitation and Emergency Medicine*. 13: 212–217

Guskiewicz, K., Bruce, S. and Cantu, R. (2004) National Athletic Trainers Association position statement: Management of sport-related concussion. *Journal of Athletic Training*. 29 (3): 280–297

Halloran, T.H. (1993) Nasal packing: Stopping excessive blood loss. *Nursing*. 23 (10)

Hamou, D. and Zagebaum, B. (1999) Incidence of sports related eye injuries. *Athletic Therapy Today*. 4 (5): 27

Handley, A.J., Koster, R., Monsieurs, K., Perkins, G.D., Davies, S. and Bossaert, L. (2005) European Resuscitation Council guidelines for resuscitation 2005. Section 2. Adult basic life support and use of automated external defibrillators. *Resuscitation*. 67 (S1): S7–23

Hargreave, F.E., Cartier, A., Ryan, G., Kenworthy, M.C. and Dolovich, J. (1979) Assessment and treatment of asthma. *Canadian Family Physician*. 25: 1207–1210

Heady, J., Brooks, J.H.M. and Kemp, S.P.T. (2007) The epidemiology of shoulder injuries in English professional rugby union. *American Journal of Sports Medicine*. 35 (9): 1537–1543

Hollinshead, W. and Rosse, C. (1985) *The textbook of anatomy*. Harper and Row. Philadelphia, PA

HSE (Health and Safety Executive) (2009) *First aid training and qualifications for the purposes of the Health and Safety (First Aid) Regulations 1981: A guide for training organisations*. www.hse.gov.uk/pubns/web41.pdf, accessed April 2013

Kaufman, B. and Heckler, F. (1997) Sports-related facial injuries. *Clinics in Sports Medicine*. 16 (3): 543–562

Krivickas, L. and Wilbourn, A. (2000) Peripheral nerve injuries in athletes: A case of 200 injuries. *Seminars in Neurology*. 20 (2): 225–232

Laio, J. and Zagelbaum, B. (1999) Eye injuries in sports, *Athletic Therapy Today*. 4 (5): 36

La Prade, H.F., Wijdicks, C.A. and Griffith, C.J. (2009) Division 1 intercollegiate ice hockey team coverage. *British Journal of Sports Medicine*. 43 (13): 1000–1005

Lee, C. and Porter, K.M. (2005) Pre-hospital management of lower limb fractures. *Emergency Medicine Journal*. 22: 660–663

Lee, C., Revell, M., Porter, K. and Steyn, R. (2007) The pre-hospital management of chest injuries: a consensus statement. Faculty of pre-hospital care, Royal College of Surgeons of Edinburgh. *Emergency Medicine Journal*. 24: 220–224

Lennarson, P.J., Smith, D.W. Swain, O.D., Todd, M.M., Sato, Y. and Traynelis, V.C. (2001) Cervical spinal motion during intubation: Efficacy of stabilization manoeuvres in the setting of complete segmental instability. *Journal of Neurosurgery*. 94 (2): 265–270

Levine, N. (1980) Dermatologic aspects of sports medicine. *Journal of American Dermatology*. 3: 415

Lloyd, E.R. (2000) Upper airways obstruction. *British Journal of Sports Medicine*. 34: 69–70

Luscombe, M.D. and Williams, J.L., (2003) Comparison of a long spinal board and vacuum mattress for spinal immobilization. *Emergency Medicine Journal*. 20: 476–478

MacAuley, D. (2006) *Oxford handbook of sport and exercise medicine*. Oxford University Press. Oxford, UK

MacEwen, C. and McLatchie, G. (2010) Eye injuries in sport. *Scottish Medical Journal*. 55 (2): 22–24

Main, P.W. and Lovell, M.E. (1996) A review of seven support surfaces with emphasis on their protection of the spinally injured. *Journal of Accident and Emergency Medicine*. 13: 34–37

Martinez, R. and Ellini, K. (2005) Ophthalmology. In O'Connor, F., Sallis, R., Wilder, R. and Pierre, P. (eds) *Sports medicine: Just the facts*. McGraw-Hill. New York

McCrory, P., Meeuwisse, W.H. and Aubry, M., *et al.* (2013) Consensus statement on concussion in sport: The 4th International Conference on Concussion in Sport held in Zurich, November 2012. *British Journal of Sports Medicine*. 47: 250–258

McIntosh, A.S. and McCrory, P. (2005) Preventing head and neck injury. *British Journal of Sports Medicine*. 39: 314–318

McKee, A.C., Cantu, R.C., Nowinski, C.J., *et al.* (2009) Chronic traumatic encephalopathy in athletes: Progressive tauopathy following repetitive head injury. *Journal of Neuropathology and Experimental Neurology*. 68 (7): 709–735

Meeusen, R. and Lievens, P. (1986) The use of cryotherapy in sports injuries. *Sports Medicine*. 3 (6): 398–414

Mitchell, B. (2000) Efficacy of thigh protectors in preventing thigh haematomas. *Journal of Science and Medicine in Sport*. 3 (1): 30–34

Mubarak, S.J., Owen, C.A., Hargens, A.R., Garetto, B.S. and Akeson, W.H. (1978) Acute compartment syndromes: Diagnosis and treatment with the aid of the wick catheter. *Journal of Bone and Joint Surgery*. 60-A (8): 1091–1095

Mueller, F. (2001) Catastrophic head injuries in high school and collegiate sports. *Journal of Athletic Training*. 36 (3): 312–315

O'Connor, E. (2005) Dental. In O'Connor, F., Sallis, R., Wilder, R. and Pierre, P. (eds) *Sports medicine: Just the facts*. McGraw-Hill. New York

O'Driscoll, B.R., Howard, L.S. and Davison, A.G. (2008) BTS guideline for emergency oxygen use in adult patients. *Thorax*. 63 (Suppl. VI): vi68

Ollerton, J.E., Parr, M.J.A., Harrison, K., Hanrahan, B. and Sugrue, M. (2006) Potential cervical spine injury and difficult airway management for emergency intubation of trauma adults in the emergency department: A systematic review. *Emergency Medicine*. 23: 3–11

O'Sullivan, I. and Benger, J. (2003) Nitrous oxide in emergency medicine. *Emergency Medicine Journal*. 20: 214–217

Padilla, R. (2011) *Sports dentistry online*. www.sportsdentistry.com, accessed May 2011

Potter, B.W. and Martin, R.D. (2009) Testing the emergency action plan in athletics. *Athletic Therapy Today*. 14 (6): 29–32

Prentice, W. (2004) *Rehabilitation techniques in sports medicine and athletic training*. McGraw-Hill. St. Lucia

Prentice, W. (2011) *Principles of athletic training: A competency based approach*, 14th edition. McGraw-Hill. New York

Rehberg, R.S. (2007) Preparing for sports emergencies. In Rehberg, R.S. (ed.) *Sports emergency care: A team approach*. Slack Incorporated. Thorofare, NJ

Resuscitation Council (UK) (2010) *Resuscitation guidelines 2010*. www.resus.org.uk/pages/guide.htm, accessed July 2010

Russell, J.A. (2010) Management of acute sports injury. In Comfort, P. and Abrahamson, E. (eds) *Sports rehabilitation and injury prevention*. Wiley-Blackwell. Chichester, UK

Saunders, R. and Harbough, R. (2004) The second impact in catastrophic contact-sports head trauma. *Journal of the American Medical Association*. 252: 538–539

Schwellnus, M. (2009) Cause of exercise associated muscle cramps. *British Journal of Sports Medicine*. 43: 401–408

Sigal, R.J., Wasserman, D.H., Kenny, G.P. and Casteaneda-Sceppa, C. (2004) Physical activity/exercise and type 2 diabetes. *Diabetes Care*. 27 (10): 2518–2539

Singh, C.P., Singh, N., Singh, J., Brar, G.K. and Singh, G. (2001) Oxygen therapy. *Journal of the Indian Academy of Clinical Medicine*. 2 (3): 178–184

Sparacino, L. (2000) Epistaxis management: What's new and what's noteworthy. *Lippincotts Primary Care Practice*. 4 (5): 498–507

SST (Society of Sports Therapists) (2012) *Competencies and scope of practice for sports therapy*. www.society-of-sports-therapists.org, accessed April 2012

Swartz, E., Boden, B., Courson, R., *et al.* (2009) National Athletic Trainers' Association position statement: Acute management of the cervical spine injured athlete. *Journal of Athletic Training*. 44 (3): 306–331

Teasdale, G. and Jennet, B. (1974) Assessment of coma and impaired consciousness: A practical scale. *The Lancet*. 304 (7872): 81–84

Tiwari, A., Haq, A.I., Myint, F. and Hamilton, G. (2002) Acute compartment syndrome. *British Journal of Surgery*. 89: 397–412

Valentino, M., Serra, C., Zironi, G., De Luca, C., Pavlica, P. and Barozzi, B. (2006) Blunt abdominal trauma: Emergency contrast-enhanced sonography for detection of solid organ injuries. *American Journal of Roentgenology*. 186 (5): 1361–1367

Vickery, D. (2001) The use of the spinal board after the pre-hospital phase of trauma management. *Emergency Medicine Journal*. 18: 51–54

Viducich, R.A., Blanda, M.P. and Gerson, L.W. (1995) Posterior epistaxis: Clinical features and acute complications. *Annals of Emergency Medicine*. 25 (5): 592–596

Weir, J.D. (1997) Effective management of epistaxis in athletes. *Athletic Training*. 32: 254–255

5

THE SPINAL REGION
Anatomy, assessment and injuries

Aaron J. Caseley and Mark I. Johnson

Introduction

The prevalence of sports people with conditions related to the spinal region is high, especially in elite athletes with the increasing demands placed upon them to succeed on an international stage (Apostolos, 2013). Low back pain (LBP) is prevalent in individuals undertaking sports involving high spinal loading such as gymnastics, football, weight-lifting, ice hockey and tennis (Jonasson *et al.*, 2011); it has been suggested that LBP accounts for up to 89 per cent of musculoskeletal complaints in elite athletes participating in these sports (Jonasson *et al.*, 2011). The prevalence of conditions related to the spinal region is also high in general populations due in part to inactive lifestyles (Jackson and Simpson, 2006). According to the National Collaborating Centre for Primary Care (NCC-PC), it is estimated that about one-third of the UK adult population experience an episode of LBP each year (Savigny *et al.*, 2009); and this leads to the loss of up to 50 million working days per year and approximately 0.5 million people receiving long-term incapacity benefit.

Sports therapists need a strong working knowledge of the anatomy and physiology of the spinal region to aid assessment, treatment and rehabilitation of sports people presenting with injuries, illness and symptoms pertaining to the spine. The purpose of this chapter is to overview the functional anatomy of the spinal region and to discuss the clinical approaches used by sports therapists when assessing and managing conditions affecting the spinal region.

Functional anatomy of the spinal region

The spinal region is a broad term to describe structures related to or situated near the spine. The two main structural elements which comprise the spinal region are the spinal cord and vertebral column. The cord is made up of neural tissue, and runs through the vertebral column. The vertebral column extends from the base of the cranial occiput to the pelvis. The spinal region also includes structures that support the spine, including skin, muscles, ligaments, fascia and vascular and neural tissue (Adams *et al.*, 2006). Functions of the vertebral column include:

- protecting the spinal cord from mechanical insult;
- providing anchorage for the muscles which allow movement and support and to maintain the body for upright posture, including attachment of pectoral and pelvic girdle muscles;

- dissipating and transmitting force to and from other parts of the body via the intervertebral discs and the primary and secondary curves of the vertebral column (i.e. providing a 'shock absorbing' role);
- providing a base for rib attachment to support the thoracic cage.

Functions of the spinal cord include:

- providing neural communication between the brain and the body, and vice versa;
- generating, via neural circuitry contained therein, reflex responses associated with the autonomic and somatic nervous system.

Surface anatomy of the spinal region

At the spinal regions, there are numerous anatomical landmarks that the sports therapist must gain familiarity with. When viewed laterally, in the sagittal plane, the spinal column comprises convex and concave primary and secondary curvatures. These curvatures form as the individual develops from an embryo to an adult, a process known as ontogeny. The cervical and lumbar curvatures follow the same convex (posterior) curvature as the thoracic spine (termed kyphosis) during embryonic development, and progress to secondary concave (posterior) curvatures (termed lordoses) after birth, during the transition from crawling to standing and walking. In the adolescent and through adulthood, these kyphotic and lordotic curvatures give the spine the ability to withstand biomechanical stresses placed upon it during activities of daily living and sport (Izzo *et al.*, 2013a).

Superficially, the sports therapist must be able to appreciate key features of each spinal region and related regions (i.e. head, shoulder girdle and pelvic girdle). Posteriorly this includes ability to identify and palpate: spinous processes; transverse processes; facet joints; laminae and lamina groove; sacrum (including median crest and sacral hiatus); occipital protuberance; mastoid process; ligamentum nuchae; supraspinous ligaments; scapulae (and its various structural features); 12 pairs of ribs; the iliac crests; posterior superior iliac spine (PSIS); iliolumbar ligaments; sacroiliac joints and ligaments; greater sciatic foramen; ischial spine; sacrococcygeal junction; and, finally, the coccyx. Posteriorly the sports therapist must also appreciate location of the kidneys, which are situated superficially at either side of the posterior abdomen, adjacent to L1–3. An ability to differentiate each spinal region (cervical, thoracic, lumbar, sacral and coccygeal) is essential.

Anteriorly and superficially in the neck region, the sports therapist must appreciate the location of the following: mandible (jaw bone); submandibular and cervical lymph nodes; hyoid bone (just inferior to the mandible); thyroid cartilage (and its 'laryngeal prominence' – commonly known as 'Adam's apple') and cricoid cartilage of the larynx; thyroid gland (anterior to the cricoid cartilage) and trachea ('wind pipe'). Inferior to the anterior neck are the medial aspects of the shoulder girdle and the thoracic cage: suprasternal (jugular) notch (the uppermost aspect of the manubrium); manubrium; sternoclavicular joints; sternal body; xiphoid process (distal prominence of the sternum); the 12 pairs of ribs; intercostal spaces (between each rib); costal cartilages (of the seven pairs of 'true' and three pairs of 'false' ribs); costal notches (where the costal cartilages of ten pairs of ribs articulate with the sternal body); and costochondral joints (ten pairs of joints where the ribs join with their costal cartilage). The liver is situated underneath the right side of the lower thoracic rib cage (a region known either as the upper right abdominal quadrant, or the right hypogastrium) – if it is pathologically enlarged its lower margins can be palpable below the inferior costal cartilage (Backhouse and Hutchings, 1998).

In the abdomen, the sports therapist must particularly understand the positioning of the large intestines, which are deep to the abdominal musculature. The start of the ascending colon is located on the right side of abdomen (just superomedial to the anterior superior iliac spine – ASIS – in the lower right abdominal quadrant) and it runs upwards to the level of the ninth intercostal space. The second section of the large intestine is the transverse colon, which runs across the superior aspect of the abdomen (in the epigastric region). The final section of the large intestine is the descending colon, which runs inferiorly from approximately the level of the eighth intercostal space downwards (in the lower left abdominal quadrant) and deeply into the posterior pelvis. Another important anatomical landmark is the umbilicus, which is situated fairly centrally approximately at the level of L3–4 (its position varies depending upon spinal,

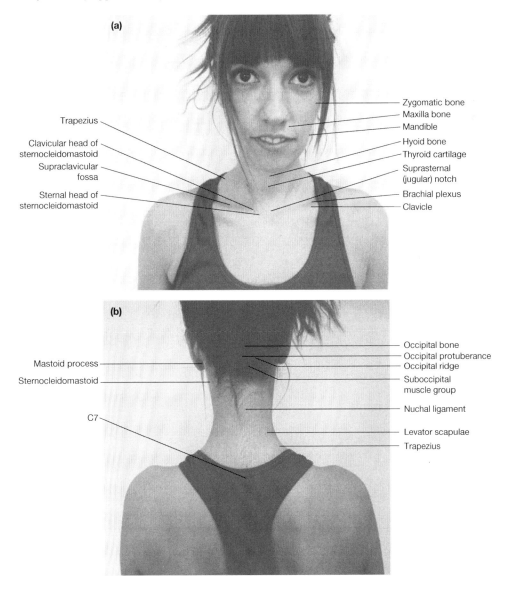

Photo 5.1 Surface anatomy of the cervical region: anterior and posterior views.

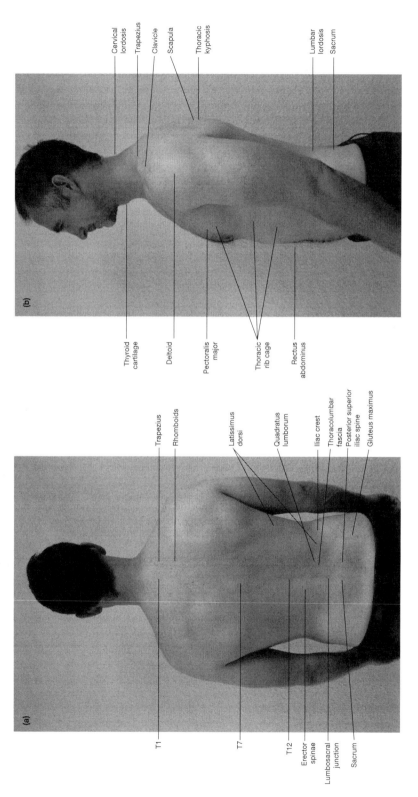

Cervical lordosis
Trapezius
Clavicle
Scapula
Thoracic kyphosis
Lumbar lordosis
Sacrum

Thyroid cartilage
Deltoid
Pectoralis major
Thoracic rib cage
Rectus abdominus

(b)

Trapezius
Rhomboids
Latissimus dorsi
Quadratus lumborum
Iliac crest
Thoracolumbar fascia
Posterior superior iliac spine
Gluteus maximus

T1
T7
T12
Erector spinae
Lumbosacral junction
Sacrum

(a)

Photo 5.2   Surface anatomy of the thoracolumbar region: posterior and lateral views.

pelvic, leg length discrepancies and abdominal distensions). The abdominal aorta lies deep to this structure. Inferiorly, the inguinal ligament, running from the ASIS to the pubic tubercle provides demarcation between the external oblique aponeurosis and the deep fascia of the upper thigh.

Skeletal anatomy of the spinal region
Vertebral column

The vertebral column (Latin: *columna vertebralis*) of the adult human has 33 bones (vertebrae), of which 24 are articulating and nine are fused. The vertebrae are irregularly shaped bones that enclose and protect the spinal cord, which lies within the vertebral foramen. The vertebrae increase in size from cephalad to caudad, and each vertebra is separated by an intervertebral disc (except the atlantoaxial C1–2 complex). The vertebrae are named according to region and position, from superior to inferior, as follows:

- Cervical: 7 vertebrae (C1–7)
- Thoracic: 12 vertebrae (T1–12)
- Lumbar: 5 vertebrae (L1–5)
- Sacral: 5 (fused) vertebrae (S1–5)
- Coccygeal: 4 (fused) vertebrae (Co).

A typical vertebra consists of two essential components: the vertebral body (anteriorly) and the neural arch (posteriorly). The vertebral body is generally cylindrical, with flattened superior and inferior surfaces for attachment to the intervertebral disc. The posterior surface is smooth and has a large foramen for the passage of the basivertebral vein. The shape and size of individual vertebral bodies depend on the location of the vertebrae in the vertebral column. The vertebral body consists of an outer dense layer of cortical bone and an inner layer of spongy cancellous bone. At the superior and inferior aspects of the cortex, there is a thickening, which forms the epiphyseal growth plate. The cancellous bone is organized into trabeculae which lie along the lines of force and run from superior to inferior and also obliquely. The orientation of these trabeculae, and a subsequent anterior 'bare' area, predisposes the vertebral body to wedge-shaped compression fractures, common in osteoporosis. An axial load of 600 kg is sufficient to cause the anterior aspect of the vertebra to fail; a load equivalent to 800 kg is required to crush the whole vertebrae (Siminoski *et al.*, 2012).

Practitioner Tip Box 5.1

Abnormal ossification and inflammation of lower thoracic and upper lumbar epiphyseal growth plates can lead to Scheuermann's disease (vertebral osteochondrosis and a characteristic wedging of adjacent vertebrae). The mechanism thought to be responsible for this is an interruption to the blood supply to the epiphysis, resulting in localized bony necrosis and then later re-growth of bone.

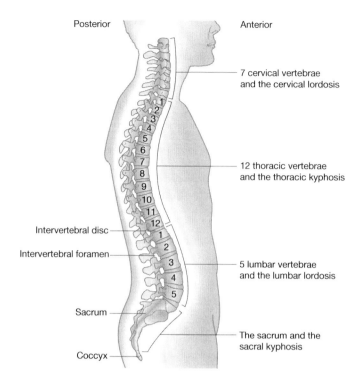

Posterior

Anterior

7 cervical vertebrae
and the cervical lordosis

12 thoracic vertebrae
and the thoracic kyphosis

Intervertebral disc

Intervertebral foramen

5 lumbar vertebrae
and the lumbar lordosis

Sacrum

The sacrum and the
sacral kyphosis

Coccyx

Figure 5.1 The vertebral column (source: adapted from Sewell *et al.*, 2013).

The neural arch consists of two pedicles, two laminae and seven processes. The pedicles and laminae form a hollow cylinder, called the vertebral foramen, which is an opening on the posterolateral aspect of the vertebral body. The vertebral foramen (also known as the vertebral canal or spinal cavity) contains the spinal cord, which is surrounded by three meningeal layers. The seven processes of the neural arch consist of four articular processes (two superior and two inferior facets), two transverse processes and one spinous process. The bony projections of the neural arch serve as attachments for muscles and ligaments to aid articulation of the adjacent vertebrae. In adjacent vertebrae, the superior and inferior articular processes form small synovial facet (zygapophyseal) joints. The shape and orientation of the articular facets determines the range and type of movement available at each spinal level. Regionally, each vertebra has specializations governed by its specific role in either movement or support (Moore and Dalley, 2006).

Cervical vertebrae

In the cervical region the first and second cervical vertebrae (C1 and C2) are atypical in structure. C1 is also known as the atlas; it has no body and no spinous process, but consists of two lateral masses connected by an anterior and posterior arch. Its concave superior articular facets receive the occipital condyles. C2 is known as the axis; it is marked by the presence of the odontoid process (also known as the 'dens') which projects upwards through the atlas, where it is attached via the apical ligament to the anterior margin of the foramen magnum at the base of the occiput. The transverse processes are small and rounded projections from the sides of the vertebral body. The spinous process of the axis is a large bifid structure. This can be easily identified on palpation when moving in a caudad direction from the occiput as it projects

---

Practitioner Tip Box 5.2

Odontoid process (dens) fractures are a serious consequence of cervical spine injury. Once called the 'hangman's fracture', these fractures are unstable and because the separated fragment of the dens no longer has a blood supply, there is a tendency for the dens to develop avascular necrosis.

---

almost 1 cm more than the posterior tubercle of C1, and covers the much thinner spine of C3 (Adams *et al.*, 2006).

Vertebrae C3–6 are similar in structure to a typical vertebra, and they present the following features: a small kidney-shaped body, with short pedicles that create a large triangular shaped vertebral canal for the cervical enlargement of the spinal cord; a short bifid spinous process, formed by the laminae as they join together and project posteriorly from the centre of the vertebral arch; and stout transverse processes that end in prominent anterior and posterior tubercles, and which also house the transverse foramen. In the upper six cervical vertebrae (excluding the atlas), the transverse foramen create a bony channel for the vertebral artery and vein, as well as a plexus of sympathetic nerves. The foramen is liable to age-related bony changes, such as osteophyte formation, and this is often a contributing factor in the development of vertebrobasilar insufficiency.

Vertebra C7 has a long, prominent spinous process (vertebrae prominens) that provides an inferior attachment for the ligamentum nuchae. Compared to other cervical vertebrae, the vertebral body of C7 is larger, the vertebral canal is smaller and the pedicles directed more posteriorly. The cervicothoracic junction between C7 and T1 (also referred to as the 'C–T junction') is a useful palpation point, a key functional junction between the cervical and thoracic regions and a common site for pain or restriction.

Thoracic vertebrae

There are 12 thoracic vertebrae, and they share common distinctive features. Each thoracic vertebra has articular (costal) facets on each side of their vertebral bodies and transverse processes; these are for articulation with the ribs, forming costovertebral and costotransverse joints, respectively. T1 has a costal facet on the superior edge of its body for the first rib and a demifacet on its inferior edge that contributes to the articular surface for the second rib. The bodies of the thoracic vertebrae are heart-shaped, with short pedicles projecting almost directly posteriorly from their vertebral body. The spinous processes are long and obliquely angled, and those in the middle of the thoracic region are almost vertical. The spinous process of T12 is horizontal and resembles those of the lumbar region. The vertebrae T9–12 have tubercles similar to the accessory and mammillary processes of lumbar vertebrae. The upper facets of T12 are oriented in the thoracic plane, while the lower facets have a tendency toward a lumbar orientation.

Lumbar vertebrae

The vertebrae L1–4 share characteristics similar to T11 and T12: large vertebral bodies, strong thick laminae and no costal facets. They have adapted to manage the weight and force of the large muscles attaching into this area. The transverse processes of lumbar vertebrae project posterolaterally, with a small accessory process on the base of the posterior surface that provides an attachment point for the medial intertransverse lumborum muscle. On the superior surface of the transverse process is the mamillary process, which gives rise to attachments for multifidus and the medial intertransverse muscles. L5 is atypical; it is characterized by a wedge-shaped body that is thinner posteriorly and largely responsible for the lumbosacral angle. The lumbosacral angle, between the long axis of the lumbar region and the superior aspect of S1, is between 130–160° in a healthy individual (Muscolino, 2012). The spinous process of L5 is smaller than typical lumbar vertebrae, and the transverse processes are thicker and elongated to provide attachment for the iliolumbar ligament that connects L5 to the ilia.

Sacrum

The sacrum is fused in adults. It is a single bone positioned between the innominate bones, with its long axis at an angle of 45°. The sacrum, in conjunction with the L5 vertebra, forms the foundation of the upright posture for the trunk and upper body (Vleeming *et al.*, 2012). The anterior surface of the sacrum is smooth and concave in shape, while the posterior surface is rough and convex and has rudimentary spinous processes along its midline. The sacral foramen and sacral foramina pass longitudinally through the sacral vertebrae, as a continuation of the lumbar vertebral foramen; these openings provide protection for the cauda equina and sacral nerve roots which pass through them (Vleeming *et al.*, 2012). The lateral aspect of the sacrum has auricle (ear) shaped articular regions creating the auricular surfaces for articulation with the ilia of the innominate bones within which it is suspended. These auricular surfaces form the synovial part of the sacroiliac joints.

Coccyx

The coccyx consists of three or four coccygeal vertebrae that are fused in adults, forming a small, triangular bone that articulates with the inferior end of the sacrum. The coccyx is characterized by its small size and the absence of vertebral arches and vertebral canal.

Thoracic cage

The thoracic cage is bounded superiorly by the anterior surface of vertebrae T1, the medial border and costal cartilage of the first rib and the anterior manubrium sterni (the upper part of the sternum). The thoracic cage itself is composed of the 12 thoracic vertebrae, 12 pairs of ribs and the sternum. The superior thoracic outlet is the superior opening of the thoracic cage and allows vital structures to enter or leave the thorax, including the oesophagus, the trachea, blood vessels and nerves. The apex of the lung is found in the lateral aspect of the thoracic inlet and is supported and covered by the suprapleural membrane. The inferior thoracic outlet is the inferior bony opening of the thoracic cavity and is larger than the thoracic inlet. The inferior thoracic outlet is bounded by the anterior surface of T12, ribs 11 and 12 and the xiphisternum (the xiphoid is the distal projection of the sternum). The inferior thoracic outlet is covered by the respiratory diaphragm. The diaphragm has tendinous structures that attach to the vertebral column called the crura of the diaphragm, within which there are specialist openings to allow passage for the aorta, vena cava and the oesophagus and vagus nerve.

The 12 pairs of ribs slope inferiorly as they pass from the costovertebral and costotransverse joints (posterolaterally). Each rib has an articulation with a thoracic vertebra, but only the costal cartilages of the upper seven ribs, known as 'true ribs', articulate with the sternum. The five pairs of ribs that do not articulate with the sternum are known as 'false ribs'. The intercostal space between each rib consists of outer, inner and innermost intercostal muscles, and a bundle of intercostal blood vessels and nerves located between the inner and innermost intercostal muscles. Ribs 3–9 have similar features, each possessing a large head and two articular facets. The larger inferior facet of the rib articulates with the superior costal facet of the vertebral body of the corresponding vertebra; and the smaller superior facet of the rib articulates with the inferior costal facet of the vertebral body above. These 'typical ribs' have a short, flattened neck with a prominent tubercle for articulation with the transverse process of the associated vertebra. More laterally, typical ribs form a thin, flat shaft. The superior aspect of a rib is smooth and rounded, and the inferior aspect is sharp, with the subcostal groove running along its length. Each rib articulates anteriorly with the corresponding costal cartilage (Drake *et al.*, 2005). There are five 'atypical ribs'. Rib 1 is almost flat when viewed horizontally, with a broad superior surface characterized by the scalene tubercle. The scalene tubercle bisects two grooves that cross the rib. The anterior groove houses the subclavian vein, and the posterior groove houses the subclavian artery. Rib 1 attaches posteriorly to T1 and slopes inferiorly to attach to the manubrium. Rib 2 is twice as long as rib 1, but has similar characteristics to rib 1, and attaches to T2. Rib 10 has a single facet for articulation and attaches to T10. Ribs 11 and 12 are short, with little curvature and have no tubercles or direct anterior articular attachment, and are often described as 'floating ribs'.

Joints of the spine

The two main types of joints involving the vertebrae are synovial joints between adjacent articular processes, and symphyses between each vertebral body. The joints in the spine are situated posteriorly to the vertebral body and allow movement to occur between adjacent vertebral segments and restrict extreme ranges of movement. Movements of the vertebral column vary according to the region of the spine. The ranges and directions of movement of the vertebral column are determined by the thickness, elasticity and compressibility of the intervertebral discs, the shape and the orientation of the joints, the degree of elasticity of the articular capsules and the resistance of the ligaments and muscles.

Synovial joints

Synovial joints (diarthroses) are the most common and moveable joints in the skeletal system. They are structurally different from cartilaginous joints and fibrous joints in that they possess a tough, fibrous capsule that surrounds the articulating surfaces of the bones and a synovial membrane which secretes synovial fluid to lubricate the joint surfaces.

Facet joints

The facet (zygapophyseal) joints give the vertebral column an ability to perform segmental and regionally specific movements. The facet joints are plane synovial joints between the superior and inferior articular processes of adjacent vertebrae. Each joint is surrounded by a thin capsule which is attached to the margins of the articular processes of adjacent vertebra. Accessory ligaments unite and help to support the laminae, transverse processes and spinous processes.

Movements of the vertebral column are greater in the cervical and lumbar regions than elsewhere (Moore and Dalley, 2006). In the cervical region, the articular capsules of the facet joints are loose and the joint planes almost horizontal, thus allowing flexion, extension, lateral flexion and rotation. In the lumbar region, the facet planes are sagitally oriented to maximize this region's ability to flex and extend; however, the interlocking articular processes here significantly reduce the rotational range. In the thoracic region, the joint planes lie on an arc centred on the vertebral body, which maximizes rotation in this region. However, this orientation, along with the ribs, limits flexion and severely restricts lateral flexion.

In the cervical region, the lateral margins of the upper surfaces of typical cervical vertebra are elevated into crests termed uncinate processes. These may articulate with the body of the vertebra above to form small 'uncovertebral' synovial joints. The upper two craniovertebral joints have no intervertebral disc and this permits a greater range of motion than in the rest of the vertebral column. These articulations consist of the occipital condyles, the atlas (C1) and the axis (C2).

Atlanto-occipital joints

The atlanto-occipital joints are condyloid type synovial joints with a thin and loose fibrous capsule which allows a greater range of movement. These joints are formed by the articulations between the lateral masses of the atlas and the two occipital condyles, and due to their facet orientation they allow flexion and extension, and some lateral flexion. The atlanto-occipital joints are supported by the anterior and posterior atlanto-occipital membranes, which extend from the anterior and posterior arches of C1 to the anterior and posterior margins of the foramen magnum. The anterior atlanto-occipital membrane is a centrally located, broad, tough band of connective tissue. The posterior atlanto-occipital membrane is weaker but has a synergistic relationship with the anterior atlanto-occipital membrane to reduce excessive movement at the atlanto-occipital joints.

Atlanto-axial joint

The atlanto-axial joint comprises three articulations; two lateral atlanto-axial joints between the superior and inferior articular facets of C2 and the lateral masses of C1 and one median atlanto-axial joint between the dens of C2 and the anterior arch of the atlas (C1). The lateral atlanto-axial joints are plane-type synovial joints, while the median atlanto-axial joint is a synovial pivot joint. Movement around all three atlanto-axial joints accounts for a significant amount of the rotatory movement available in the cervical spine. Rotation of the head occurs around the axis created by the dens. This bony axis is restrained anteriorly by the anterior arch of the vertebra C1 and posteriorly by the transverse ligament of the atlas, which extends between the tubercles of the lateral masses of the vertebra C1. Two vertical longitudinal bands also pass anteriorly and posteriorly from the transverse ligament to the occiput superiorly and vertebra C2 inferiorly. Along with the transverse ligament, these two longitudinal bands form the cruciate ligament.

The alar ligaments extend from the side of the dens to the margins of the foramen magnum and attach the occipital bone of the cranium to vertebra C1, reducing excessive rotation at these joints. The tectorial membrane is the superior continuation of the posterior longitudinal ligament; it runs in a longitudinal cephalad direction over the median atlanto-axial joint through the foramen magnum to the floor of the cranium, covering the alar and transverse ligaments.

Sacroiliac joints

The sacroiliac joint consists of an anterior synovial joint between the auricular surfaces of the sacrum and ilium and a posterior syndesmotic joint between the tuberosities of the sacrum and the ilium. Syndesmoses are slightly movable joints where the contiguous bony surfaces are united by an interosseous ligament. Unlike other synovial joints, the sacroiliac joint has limited mobility due to its role in transmitting bodyweight to the hip joints. The auricular surfaces of the ilia are lined with fibrocartilage and form ridges which articulate with the opposing auricular

---

Practitioner Tip Box 5.3

The sacroiliac joints (SIJ) are considered by many practitioners to be a potential cause of low back pain. The SIJ are dependent on a complex interplay between the articular surfaces (form closure) and the ligaments and muscles (force closure) which surround the joint. The low back pain arising from an SIJ issue is often unilateral and described as an ache around the posterior superior iliac spine. Aggravating factors include walking, sitting to standing, climbing stairs and turning over in bed. Motion testing and pain provocation testing is unreliable for SIJ pain. The current diagnostic gold standard is a fluoroscopically guided injection of lidocaine (anaesthetic) into the joint. A 'hands-on' approach is most commonly indicated when managing cases of SIJ pain, with persistent cases often treated using a rhizotomy (a procedure to block nerve activity around the joint, through a joint injection).

---

surfaces of the sacrum that are lined with hyaline cartilage. The osseous, fibrocartilage and dense support network provided by the anterior and posterior sacroiliac ligaments, sacrospinous ligament and sacrotuberous ligaments confers significant stability to the sacroiliac joints, and once in a weight bearing bipedal stance creates a form closure mechanism which increases joint stability further (Vleeming *et al.*, 2012).

Joint capsule

The joint capsule surrounds each synovial facet joint in the vertebral column and is thin, loose and attached to the margins of the articular processes of adjacent vertebrae. In high-stress areas it thickens to form capsular ligaments which vary in location on the joint capsule from one region of the vertebral column to another. The joint capsule limits end-of-range movements of the facet joints and seals the joint space to maintain negative intra-articular pressure, which increases the static stability of the joint. Additionally, the joint capsule has an abundance of proprioceptive nerve endings that provide feedback to the brain and spinal cord, contributing to the dynamic stability of each joint (Moore and Dalley, 2006).

Symphyses between vertebral bodies

Symphyses are secondary cartilaginous joints, created by a fibrocartilaginous union between two adjacent bones (Drake *et al.*, 2005). The symphysis between adjacent vertebral bodies is formed by a layer of hyaline cartilage on the superior and inferior aspect of each vertebral body and an intervertebral fibrocartilaginous disc. This intervertebral joint provides strong attachment between the inferior aspect of the vertebrae above, and the superior aspect of the vertebrae below, conferring increased weight-bearing ability and strength to the vertebral column, while also permitting a small amount of movement (Adams *et al.*, 2006).

Pubic symphysis

Anteriorly the two innominates are connected by another secondary cartilaginous joint known as the pubic symphysis. An interpubic fibrocartilaginous disc, which is wider in women, unites the bodies of the two pubic bones. Additional stability of the pubic symphysis is provided by the superior and inferior pubic ligaments and the tendinous attachments of the rectus abdominis and external oblique muscles.

Intervertebral disc

The intervertebral disc (IVD) is located between adjacent vertebrae, forming a symphysis or secondary cartilaginous joint. Each intervertebral disc is composed of two distinct layers; the annulus fibrosis and the nucleus pulposus. The annulus functions to keep the vertebral bodies bound together and to provide attachment for the ligaments and the tendons. The annulus fibrosis is the outer part of the disc and consists of type-I and type-II collagen. There is a higher concentration of type-I collagen towards the periphery because of the greater structural demands placed upon the peripheral aspect of the disc. The annulus is also strengthened by the collagen being interlaced in a network of circular, vertical and cruciate fibres that blend with tendons and ligaments, creating high tensility. This part of the disc has little or no blood vessels and depends on lymph for nourishment. Innervation of the annulus is from sympathetic trunks and sinuvertebral nerves, with a predominance of nerve fibres toward the outer part of the disc (Adams *et al.*, 2006).

The nucleus pulposus forms the central part of the disc; it keeps vertebral bodies apart and provides a strong brace for the annulus fibrosus to assist with the resistance of compressive force. The nucleus pulposus is yellow, semi-solid and consists of embryonic cells and proteoglycans (large molecules of sugar and protein). Proteoglycans have hydrophilic (water-attracting) properties and absorb and retain large amounts of water. The embryonic cells are remnants of the notochord that serves as the basis for the axial skeleton, and they enlarge and persist in the nucleus pulposus but regress in the region of the vertebral bodies. The nucleus has no blood vessels and depends on lymph derived from the vertebral blood vessels for nutrition (Drake *et al.*, 2005).

The IVDs are thicker in the lumbar and cervical regions due to the increased need to bear compressive force. Daily activities produce compressive loading of the vertebral column, and water is extruded from the discs, causing a loss of height. In non-weight-bearing (recumbent) positions water is re-absorbed and disc height restored. Claims that disc height reduces with age have limited research evidence in support (Haughton, 2011). Nevertheless, disc narrowing can occur where proteoglycans are disrupted or degraded; this is termed degenerative disc disorder.

The nucleus pulposus is under very high pressure and this intradiscal pressure can vary according to posture (see Table 5.1). If the pressure increases beyond the point of integrity, the proteoglycans may be exuded and the disc may be unable to hold water and resist compressive

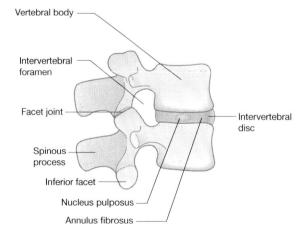

Figure 5.2   A typical vertebral segment (source: adapted from Sewell *et al.*, 2013).

Practitioner Tip Box 5.4

Intervertebral discs undergo considerable stress throughout their normal life history. Excessive strain can cause damage to the annulus fibrosis, which owing to its poor vascular supply eventually heals by laying down scar tissue. This tissue is weaker than the parent tissue, and subsequently leads to damage and dehydration in the nucleus pulposus. This leads to chronic dehydration and eventual thinning of the disc termed degenerative disc disease. It is estimated that ~30 per cent of 30–50 year olds will have some degree of disc degeneration.

Practitioner Tip Box 5.5

In-growth of new blood vessels into the outer part of the annulus fibrosis (neovascularization) has been suggested as a cause for persistent low back pain. Nociceptors are sensory receptors that detect tissue damage (or threat thereof) and their free nerve endings surround blood vessels. The repetitive loading of the disc from standing and sitting postures causes compression and, if the stimulus is sufficient, nociceptors fire to convey afferent signals to the CNS, which may then be modulated as a pain experience.

Table 5.1 In-vivo intra-discal pressure measurement in healthy individuals and in patients with ongoing back problems

	Disc pressure (kPA) via L4–L5 sensor
Prone	91
Standing upright	539
Standing flexion	1324
Standing extension	600
Sitting upright	623
Sitting flexion	1127
Sitting extension	737

Source: Sato *et al.*, 1999.

loads (prolapsed disc) (Adams *et al.*, 2006). The embryonic notochord tissue is immune discrete (i.e. never been exposed to the body's immune system) so proteoglycans are recognized as 'non-self' resulting in an immune response. The phagocytic activity of the macrophages and mast cells assist with the removal of the extruded disc material (Haughton, 2011). IVDs have long been considered a likely trigger of lower back pain and therapists often infer disc involvement if flexion and/or seated postures increase the severity of pain (Jaromi *et al.*, 2012).

Ligaments of the vertebral column

Ligaments act as (static) stabilizers to maintain the integrity of the joints they surround. The main function of the vertebral ligaments is to offer reactive forces to resist excessive spinal motion. Ligaments have a high number of proprioceptive nerve endings so they also have an important role in monitoring vertebral position and motion. While often described as inert tissues, ligaments are actually responsive to many local and systemic factors that can affect their biomechanical function. Damage to ligaments alters their histological properties due to the laying down of scar tissue, which creates a connective tissue that is biomechanically inferior to the tissue it replaces and may contribute to spinal pathology (Devin and Puttlitz, 2012).

Anterior and posterior longitudinal ligaments

The anterior and posterior longitudinal ligaments extend from the sacrum to C1–2 vertebrae. The anterior longitudinal ligament is a strong, broad, fibrous band that covers and connects the anterolateral aspects of the vertebral bodies and IVDs. The ligament extends from the pelvic surface of the sacrum to the anterior tubercle of C1. Its main function is to maintain stability of the anterior part of the motion segment, and it helps to resist hyperextension of the vertebral column. The anterior longitudinal ligament's strength has been shown to be proportional to the mineral content of the vertebral body it directly attaches to. This suggests that this ligament is capable of remodelling in response to mechanical loading in a similar manner to that seen for bone (Neumann *et al.*, 1993). The posterior longitudinal ligament is a narrower band of fibrous tissue than the anterior longitudinal ligament; it runs along the posterior surfaces of the vertebral

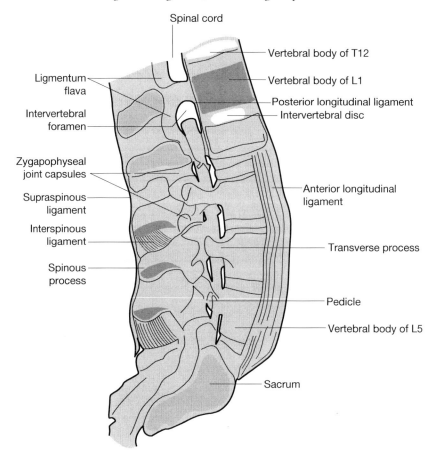

Figure 5.3   Lumbar skeletal and ligamentous anatomy: lateral view.

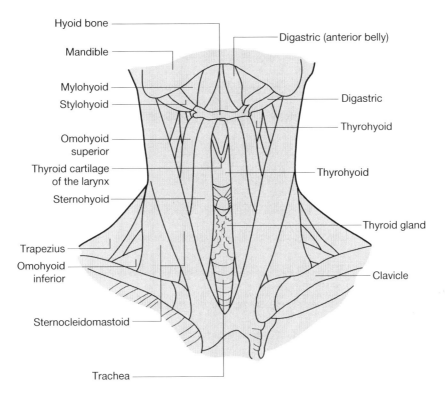

Figure 5.4 Cervical anatomy: anterior view.

bodies and intervertebral discs from the sacrum to C2. At C2, the posterior longitudinal ligament continues as the tectorial membrane, running in front of the foramen magnum and blending with the cranial dura mater. The posterior longitudinal ligament helps resist hyperflexion of the vertebral column and prevents posterior herniation or protrusions of the intervertebral disc.

Ligamentum flava

The ligamentum flava (yellow ligament) has a high proportion of elastic fibres and connects the lower portion of one lamina to the upper portion of another lamina, drawing consecutive lamina together. The high elastin content of the ligament prevents it from buckling into the spinal canal during extension, which could cause spinal canal stenosis. The main function of the ligamentum flava is to preserve the upright posture and to assist the vertebral column in returning to the anatomical position after flexion.

Interspinous ligaments

The interspinous ligaments course between the spinous processes in the posterior aspect of the vertebral column. The interspinous ligaments connect spinous processes along the length of the vertebral column and blend with the supraspinous ligament posteriorly superficially and the ligamentum flava anteriorly; they are positioned to resist hyperflexion of the spine.

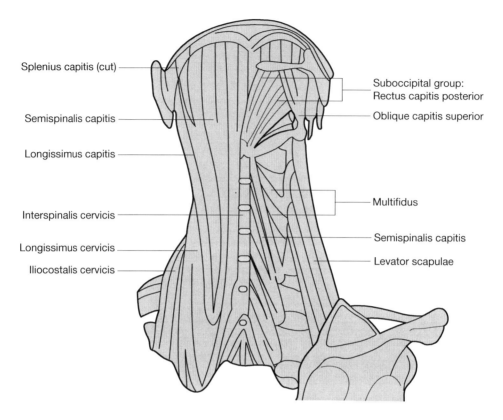

Figure 5.5 Cervical muscular anatomy: posterior view.

Supraspinous ligament and ligamentum nuchae

The supraspinous ligament connects with and passes along the tips of the vertebral spinous processes from C7 to the sacrum. The ligamentum nuchae forms from the supraspinous ligament at C7 and continues to the occiput. The ligamentum nuchae supports the head, resists flexion and its elasticity assists in returning the head to the anatomical position.

Muscular anatomy of the spinal region

The muscles and tendons of the vertebral column provide the means with which the spine generates force to create its own movement and also the means to create sufficient stability to ensure a strong base of support for movement of the limbs. Golgi tendon organs (GTOs) located at the musculotendinous junctions provide proprioceptive afferent messaging to the spinal cord, cerebral cortex and cerebellum regarding vertebral muscle tension.

Muscles of the neck

The neck is a complex musculotendinous junction, and is often divided into anterior, posterior and suboccipital triangles (Drake *et al.*, 2005).

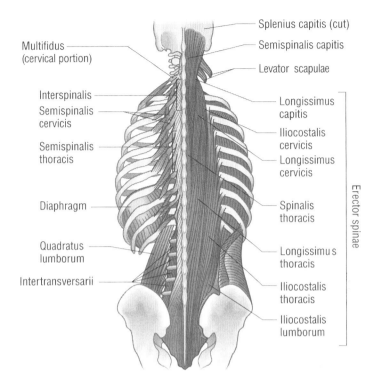

Figure 5.6   Major muscles of the posterior trunk (source: adapted from Sewell *et al.*, 2013).

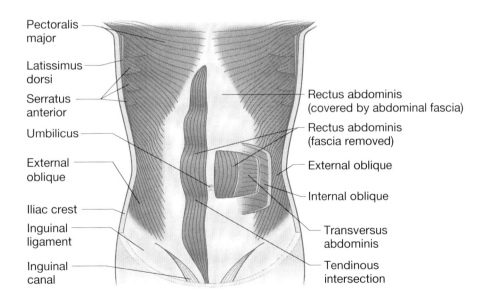

Figure 5.7   Muscles of the anterior trunk (source: adapted from Sewell *et al.*, 2013).

Anterior triangle of the neck

The anterior triangle of the neck is bounded laterally by the anterior border of the sternocleidomastoid muscle and superiorly by the inferior border of the mandible. The midline of the neck comprises the medial border. Some of the muscles within the anterior triangle of the neck are described relative to the hyoid bone. Suprahyoid muscles are superior to the hyoid bone and include the stylohyoid, digastric, mylohyoid and the geniohyoid. Hyoid fractures are becoming increasingly common in contact sports. In American football, hyoid fractures can occur due to the proximity of the helmet strap. In mixed martial arts, the triangle choke hold has also been documented as a cause of hyoid fracture (Porr *et al.*, 2012). Infrahyoid muscles lie inferior to the hyoid bone and include the omohyoid, sternohyoid, thyrohyoid and sternothyroid. The anterior triangle of the neck also contains the common carotid artery, the internal jugular vein, cranial nerves VII, IX, X, XI and XII, and the thyroid and parathyroid glands. The pre-vertebral muscles lie deeper than these structures and include longus colli and longus capitis muscles. It has been suggested that some neck pain can be caused by sustained sitting postures which leads to biological and biomechanical changes in the extensor muscles of the neck and compression of the posterior elements of the vertebrae. Longus colli and longus capitis have a role in flexion of the neck and it has been postulated that as a result of this action they are able to mechanically decompress the posterior element of the vertebrae and are consequently often the focus of neck pain management.

Longus colli

The longus colli muscle is subdivided into three portions: superior oblique, inferior oblique and vertical. The superior oblique arises from the transverse processes of C2–4 and is inserted onto the anterior arch of the atlas. The inferior oblique arises from the anterior surfaces of the vertebral bodies of T1–2/3 and is inserted into the anterior transverse processes of C5–6. The vertical portion of the longus colli muscle arises from the anterior vertebral bodies of C5–7 and T1–3 and is inserted onto the anterior vertebral bodies of C2–4. These muscles are innervated by the anterior rami of C2–6 and collectively create flexion of the cervical spine, lateral flexion and a small degree of rotation.

Longus capitis

The longus capitis muscle arises from tendinous slips attaching to the transverse processes of C3–6 and is inserted onto the inferior surface of the occipital bone. It is innervated by the anterior rami of C1–3 and produces flexion of the head.

Posterior triangle of the neck

The posterior triangle of the neck is bounded anteriorly by the posterior edge of the sternocleidomastoid muscle and posteriorly by the anterior edge of the trapezius muscle. Its base is formed by the middle third of the clavicle, while its roof is formed by the occipital bone just posterior to the mastoid process. The muscular floor of the posterior triangle is composed of the splenius capitis, levator scapulae and the posterior, middle and anterior scalenes. Other structures within the posterior triangle are the external jugular vein, the subclavian artery and its branches, the transverse cervical and suprascapular arteries, the accessory nerve (cranial nerve XI), and the cervical and brachial plexii.

Sternocleidomastoid

The sternocleidomastoid muscle occupies a significant portion of the anterolateral wall of the neck and is a large, strap-like muscle composed of two heads. The sternal head arises from the manubrium of the sternum and is inserted onto the lateral half of the superior nuchal line. The clavicular head arises from the medial clavicle and is inserted onto the mastoid process of the temporal bone. The sternocleidomastoid muscle has dual innervation from the accessory nerve and branches of the anterior rami of C2–3. The sternocleidomastoid muscle is responsible for flexion of the neck and lateral flexion and rotation of the head.

Splenius capitis
The splenius capitis muscle arises from the lower half of the ligamentum nuchae and the spinous processes of C7–T4, and is inserted onto the mastoid process of the temporal bone. It is innervated by the posterior rami of spinal nerves C3–4. Its prime role is to cause extension of the head, but it also assists in lateral flexion and rotation of the cervical spine.

Scalene muscles
The scalene muscles assist in flexion and lateral flexion of the neck and are accessory muscles of inspiration, assisting with elevation of rib 1 and 2. The group is divided into anterior, middle and posterior portions and these arise from the transverse processes of C3–6 (anterior), C2–7 (middle) and C4–6 (posterior). The anterior portion of the scalene muscles attach onto rib 1 at the scalene tubercle, and the middle portion attaches on to rib 1 posterior to the groove for the subclavian artery. The posterior portion of the scalenes attaches to the upper surface of rib 2. The anterior portion is innervated by the anterior rami of C4–7, the middle portion by the anterior rami of C3–7 and the posterior portion by the anterior rami of C5–7.

Suboccipital triangle
The suboccipital triangle is formed by the suboccipital muscle group (except rectus capitis posterior minor). The roof of the suboccipital triangle is formed by a dense fibro-fatty tissue situated beneath the semispinalis capitis muscle, while its floor is composed of the posterior atlanto-occipital membrane and the posterior arch of the atlas (C1). The vertebral artery and the suboccipital nerve arising from the nerve root of C1 make up the other important anatomical structures in this region.

Suboccipital muscles
The suboccipital group consists of four muscles at the base of the occipital bone: rectus capitis posterior major; rectus capitis posterior minor; obliquus capitis inferior; and obliquus capitis superior. Collectively they connect the atlas to the axis, and run superiorly to connect these to the occiput. Functionally, the suboccipitals serve to produce upper cervical extension at the atlanto-axial joint; they are innervated by the posterior ramus of the C1 nerve.

Muscles of the back
Muscles in the back play a vital role in the support and posture of the vertebral column due to the anterior displacement of weight in the trunk. Back musculature may be categorized as being

---

Practitioner Tip Box 5.6

The brachial plexus and subclavian artery pass between the anterior and middle scalene on their way under the clavicle into the axilla. An interscalene nerve block is typically performed at this point to provide anaesthesia or analgesia for surgery of the shoulder and upper arm.

---

superficial, intermediate (extrinsic) and deep (intrinsic) (Moore and Dalley, 2006), as well as global (i.e. latissimus dorsi; trapezius) and local (i.e. multifidus; rotatores). Despite their location, the superficial muscles are not considered true back muscles as they do not originate embryologically from the back and are innervated by the anterior rami of cervical and cranial nerves (i.e. accessory nerve). The superficial muscles consist of the trapezius, latissimus dorsi, levator scapulae and rhomboid major and minor; and these connect the upper limb to the trunk. The intermediate (extrinsic) group includes the serratus posterior superior and inferior muscles, which function as accessory muscles of respiration. The deep (intrinsic) back muscles, which extend from the pelvis to the cranium, include the erector spinae muscles, splenius cervicis and capitis, semispinalis cervicis and capitis, multifidus, rotatores, interspinales and the intertransversarii muscles. These act to control movements of the vertebrae and are innervated by the posterior rami of the adjacent spinal nerves.

Intermediate (extrinsic) muscles of the back

Serratus posterior superior

The serratus posterior superior muscle attaches to the inferior portion of the nuchal ligament and the spinous processes of C7–T3. Inferiorly it attaches to the superior borders of ribs 2–4. It is innervated by the second to fifth intercostal nerves. Its main function is elevation of the ribs, although electromyographic (EMG) studies of the serratus posterior muscle function have been inconclusive (Loukas et al., 2008).

Serratus posterior inferior

The serratus inferior muscle inserts onto spinous processes of T7–11 and runs superolaterally to attach onto the inferior borders of ribs 8–12. It receives its nerve supply from the anterior rami of thoracic nerves T9–12. The function of serratus posterior inferior is to depress the inferior ribs to which it attaches, although EMG studies have been inconclusive. Some research suggests a proprioceptive role (Loukas et al., 2008).

Deep intrinsic muscles of the back

Erector spinae

The muscles of erector spinae are the primary extensors of the vertebral column, responsible for returning the trunk to the upright position when it is flexed. They are also important muscles, when working eccentrically, in controlling trunk flexion. The erector spinae muscles, which lie adjacent to the vertebral column, vary in size and structure in different regions of the spine. The muscle group can be simply broken down to spinalis (most medial segment), longissimus (middle segment) and iliocostalis (most lateral segment). In the sacral region the muscle attaches via a broad tendon to the medial crest of the sacrum, the spinous processes of T11–L5, the supraspinous ligament, the iliac crests and the lateral crests of the sacrum, where it blends with the sacrotuberous and posterior sacroiliac ligaments. The muscle fibres arising from this tendon form a large muscular mass, which splits in the upper lumbar region into three columns. The spinalis is the most medial column and closest to the vertebral column, longissimus is situated intermediately and iliocostalis muscle forms the lateral column of the erector spinae group.

Spinalis

Spinalis is the most medial of the erector spinae muscle group and interconnects the spinous processes of adjacent vertebrae. It is absent in the lumbar spine, well developed in the thoracic spine and often absent in the cervical spine. Spinalis blends with a deeper muscle, semispinalis capitis, as the muscle approaches the skull. Spinalis thoracis originates from the spinous processes of T10–L2 and inserts into the spinous processes of T1–8. If present, spinalis cervicis originates from the lower part of the ligamentum nuchae and spinous process of C7, and inserts into the spinous process of C2 (axis). Spinalis capitis usually blends with the semispinalis muscles in the upper neck. Spinalis is innervated by the posterior rami of adjacent spinal nerves.

Longissimus

Longissimus is the intermediate portion of erector spinae muscle; it has no lumbar division, with the first tendinosus slips of this muscle forming from the common tendon of the erector spinae muscle as it divides into three columns in the upper lumbar region. Longissimus further subdivides into three distinct parts – thoracis, cervicis and capitis. Longissimus thoracis originates from the same broad tendon as the other erector spinae muscles and is attached to the transverse processes of T1–12 and ribs 1–9. Longissimus cervicis originates from the transverse processes of T1–4 and attaches onto the transverse processes of C2–6. Longissimus capitis originates from the transverse processes of T1–4 and the articular processes of C4–7 and inserts into the mastoid process of the temporal bone. Longissimus is innervated by the posterior rami of adjacent spinal nerves.

Iliocostalis

Iliocostalis is the most lateral of the three portions of the erector spinae and originates from the same broad tendon as the other two muscles comprising this muscle group. Iliocostalis is regionally subdivided into: iliocostalis lumborum (lumbar region), which inserts near the angles of ribs 6–12; iliocostalis thoracis (thoracic), which inserts near the angles of ribs 1–6 and the transverse process of C7; and iliocostalis cervicis (cervical), which arises medially from the iliocostalis thoracis division, and is inserted onto the posterior tubercles of the transverse processes of C4–7. Iliocostalis derives its nerve supply from the posterior rami of adjacent spinal nerves.

Transversospinalis muscles

The transversospinalis muscles are located deep to the erector spinae; they course in the para-spinal gutter (lamina groove), lateral to the spinous process of each vertebra. Transversospinalis muscles consist of the semispinalis, multifidus and rotatores muscles. These muscles connect each vertebra to one another through attachments from the transverse process and the superior spinous process. They provide fine segmental movement and are important in spinal stability (Kolber and Beekhuizen, 2007).

Semispinalis

Semispinalis is the most superficial of the transversospinalis muscles. The muscle arises from the transverse processes of T12–C4 and attaches onto the spinous process of the vertebra above. The semispinalis muscles are innervated by the posterior rami of adjacent spinal nerves and are responsible for postural support and extension and rotation of the spine.

Multifidus

Multifidus is a series of small segmental muscles running from the posterior sacrum, the posterior superior iliac spine, the aponeurosis of the erector spinae and the sacroiliac ligaments to the mammillary processes of the lumbar vertebra, the transverse processes of T1–3 and the articular processes of C4–7. Each muscle attaches to a lateral aspect on a vertebra such as the transverse process, and runs obliquely in a cephalad direction to a medial attachment on a vertebra such as a spinous process. The lateral attachment points vary throughout the vertebral column. The large cross-sectional area of the multifidus muscle in the lumbar region requires specialized attachment points on the transverse processes, called mammillary processes. Multifidus is innervated by the posterior rami of the adjacent spinal nerve and is responsible for postural support and assisting extension, lateral flexion and rotation of the spine. Multifidus has been implicated in recurrent episodes of back pain (Richardson *et al.*, 1999).

Rotatores
The rotatores muscles are the deepest of the transversospinalis muscle group. They are found throughout the spine and pass obliquely in a superomedial direction. The rotatores muscles are most developed in the thoracic spine and they attach from the transverse process of the vertebra below to the lamina of the vertebra above. They are innervated by the posterior rami of adjacent spinal nerves, and are responsible for postural support and extension and rotation of the spine.

Interspinales
The interspinales muscles are paired muscles situated between the spinous processes on either side of the interspinous ligament. In the cervical region they consist of six pairs, starting between C2 (axis) to C3 and running down the length of the cervical spine, with the last pair between C7 and T1. In the thoracic region they are found between T1 and T2 and are then absent until T11 and T12. There are four pairs of interspinales muscles in the lumbar region, which run between L1–5. Collectively, these muscles are too small to assist in extension of the cervical and lumbar spine, but are thought to contribute to the proprioception of each vertebral region (Hesse *et al.*, 2013). The interspinales muscle is innervated by the posterior rami of the adjacent spinal nerves.

Intertransversarii
The intertransversarii are small muscles situated between the adjacent transverse processes of the vertebra. They are well developed in the cervical region, where they consist of seven pairs of muscles running from the first pair between C1 and C2 to the last pair between C7 and T1. They attach to the anterior and posterior tubercles of the transverse processes of adjacent vertebra. The anterior rami of the cervical spinal nerves are situated between the muscles and innervate the cervical part of the intertransversarii muscles. The intertransversarii anterior muscles attach to the anterior tubercles of the cervical vertebrae; and the intertransversarii posterior muscles attach between the posterior tubercles. In the thoracic region the intertransversarii are only present between T10–11, T11–12 and T12–L1. In the lumbar region the intertransversarii are divided into a lateral division which occupies the entire interspace between transverse processes, and a medial division which passes from the accessory process of the superior vertebra to the mammillary process of the vertebra below. The intertransversarii lateral muscles are innervated by the anterior rami of the adjacent spinal nerves and the intertransversarii medial muscles are supplied by the posterior rami. Collectively, the intertransversarii are considered too weak to assist in lateral flexion of the cervical and lumbar vertebra, and their role is considered more proprioceptive (Hesse *et al.*, 2013).

Muscles of the abdomen

The abdominal cavity is bounded by the abdominal wall, which is located superior to the pelvic cavity and inferior to the thoracic cavity. The abdominal wall is covered by a fascia, the parietal peritoneum, and extra-peritoneal fat. Abdominal muscles assist in quiet and forced expiration, coughing, urination and defecation, and together with the back muscles serve an important role in postural support of the vertebral column. Muscles of the abdominal wall are sub-divided into anterolateral and posterior divisions.

Muscles of the anterolateral abdominal wall

There are five anterolateral muscles of the abdominal wall: rectus abdominus; external oblique; internal oblique; transverse abdominus; and pyramidalis. It has been suggested that weakness in the transverse abdominis may contribute to recurrent episodes of low back pain; management often involves increasing the strength and neuromuscular control of this muscle (Izzo *et al.*, 2013b).

Rectus abdominis

Rectus abdominis is a long, strap-like muscle that runs from the pubic symphysis and pubic crest inferiorly to the xiphoid process and the costal cartilages 5–7. Rectus abdominis is innervated by thoraco-abdominal nerves, which are formed by the anterior rami of T6–12. Rectus abdominis is responsible for lumbar flexion (such as during 'crunch' sit-up exercises) and compression of the abdominal viscera. Six to eight distinct muscle bellies separated by bands of connective tissue that traverse rectus abdominis (tendinous intersections) can provide the appearance of a 'six-pack' in this muscle.

External oblique

The external oblique is the largest and most superficial of the anterolateral abdominal muscles. It arises from the external surfaces of ribs 5–12 and creates the 'fleshy part' of the lateral abdominal wall. As the external oblique approaches the central linea alba, it becomes a flat, dense, fibrous, collagenous connective tissue (i.e. aponeurotic) and then decussates and becomes continuous with the tendinous fibres of the internal oblique muscle on the contralateral side. Inferiorly, the external oblique aponeurosis attaches to the medial pubic crest and the pubic tubercle. The inferior margin of the external oblique thickens and spans between the anterior superior iliac spine and the pubic tubercle, becoming the inguinal ligament. The inguinal ligament serves as a band-like structure to hold other structures in place (i.e. as a retinaculum) – such as the iliopsoas muscle and the femoral nerve, artery and vein that pass deep to enter the thigh. The external oblique is innervated by T7–12 and the sub-costal nerve.

Internal oblique

The internal oblique is a thin, muscular sheet that arises from the thoracolumbar fascia, the anterior two-thirds of the iliac crest and the lateral half of the inguinal ligament. The internal oblique forms a digastric muscle with the contralateral external oblique. The anteromedially oriented muscle fibres of the internal oblique become aponeurotic, attaching onto the inferior borders of ribs 10–12, merging with the linea alba to form the rectus sheath. The internal oblique is innervated by the anterior rami of T7–12 and L1, sharing much of its nerve supply with transverse abdominis.

Transverse abdominis

Transverse abdominis is the innermost muscle of the anterolateral abdominal wall and its transverse circumferential orientation helps to compress abdominal structures, increasing intra-abdominal pressure. The transverse fibre orientation of transverse abdominis runs from the internal surfaces of costal cartilages 7–12, the thoracolumbar fascia, the iliac crest and the lateral third of the inguinal ligament. Medially the muscle attaches to the linea alba, the pubic crest and the pecten pubis (pectilineal line) via the conjoined tendon. Transverse abdominis has intersegmental attachments to lumbar vertebrae via the thoracolumbar fascia and it is innervated by the anterior rami of T7–12 and L1.

Muscles of the posterior abdominal wall

Psoas major
Psoas major plays a role in hip flexion, spinal flexion when the hips are fixed and lateral flexion. It has been suggested that psoas major is part of the 'inner unit' muscles contributing to 'core stability' (Izzo *et al.*, 2013b). Its more medial muscle fibres are thought to contribute to spinal stability by exerting large compressive forces on the lumbar intervertebral discs (Sajko and Stuber, 2009). Proximal attachments are to the transverse processes, vertebral bodies and intervertebral discs of L1–5; and distal attachments are to the lesser trochanter of the femur, where its tendon blends with iliacus. Psoas major is innervated by the anterior rami of L1–4.

Iliacus
Iliacus is a large triangular-shaped muscle located in the superior two-thirds of the iliac fossa, extending across the sacroiliac joints via an attachment to the anterior sacroiliac ligaments. Inferiorly, most of its muscle fibres combine with the tendon of psoas major and attach into the lesser trochanter. The functional activity of iliacus is limited to hip flexion, and unlike psoas major it does not contribute to flexion or lateral flexion of the lumbar spine.

Quadratus lumborum
Quadratus lumborum forms a thick muscular layer of the posterior abdominal wall. The superior attachment of quadratus lumborum is to the inferior border of rib 12 and the medial attachment is to the transverse processes of L1–5. Inferiorly, quadratus lumborum attaches to the iliolumbar ligament and the internal aspect of the iliac crest. Quadratus lumborum is innervated by the anterior rami of T12 and L1–4 and is responsible for extension and lateral flexion of the spine and fixing rib 12 during inspiration (Kountouris *et al.*, 2012).

Muscles of the pelvic diaphragm

The pelvic diaphragm is also called the pelvic floor; it is an amalgamation of muscles with extensive anatomical attachment to form a muscular sling that supports the pelvic viscera. Two main muscles of the pelvic diaphragm separate the pelvic cavity from the perineum; the coccygeus and levator ani. The coccygeus muscle arises from the lateral sacrum and the coccyx, and lies deep to the sacrospinous ligament. The levator ani muscle is larger than the coccygeus muscle and consists of three portions: puborectalis, pubococcygeus and iliococcygeus. Anteriorly the levator ani muscle is attached to the bodies of the pubic bones and posteriorly it is attached to the ischial spines and to the obturator fascia. The urethra and the vagina in females pass through the urogenital hiatus located between the medial borders of the levator ani muscles.

Muscles of the thoracic wall
The thorax is the superior part of the trunk between the neck and abdomen. The thoracic cavity is surrounded by the thoracic wall and contains the heart, lungs, distal part of the trachea and most of the oesophagus. The thoracic wall functions to protect the thoracic and abdominal internal organs, and provides attachment for the upper limb, neck, abdomen and back muscles. The thoracic wall also provides attachment for the muscles of respiration, which assists in

inspiration and expiration by changing the dimensions of the thoracic cavity. The principal muscles of respiration are the diaphragm and the external and internal intercostals. The main muscles of the thoracic wall are the intercostals, levatores costarum, serratus posterior and transverse thoracic muscles. Some of the thoracoappendicular muscles also act as accessory muscles of respiration, assisting the elevation of the ribs during deep inspiration including pectoralis major and minor, and the inferior portion of serratus anterior.

Diaphragm

The diaphragm is a musculotendinous partition separating the thoracic and abdominal cavities and has a crucial role in the maintenance of intra-abdominal pressure, which is critical in producing spinal stiffness when load bearing, such as during the valsalva manoeuvre (Nelson, 2012). The diaphragm is the primary muscle of inspiration responsible for increasing the volume within the thoracic cavity. The peripheral aspect of the diaphragm is fixed via the xiphisternum, the costal cartilages and ribs 6–12, and L1–3 vertebrae. The oesophageal hiatus is a hole in the diaphragm that allows the oesophagus and the vagus nerve to pass between the thoracic and into the abdominal cavity. The aortic hiatus allows the aorta to pass through the diaphragm, whereas the inferior vena cava passes through the caval foramen within the central tendon of the diaphragm. The diaphragm is innervated by the phrenic nerve (C3–5) regulating motor control, and the anterior rami of T6–12, providing sensory input to the central nervous system.

Intercostal muscles

There are 11 sets of intercostal muscles on each side of the rib cage. Each set of intercostal muscles has three intercostal muscles that are situated in the intercostal space that lies between the ribs; external intercostal (superficial), internal intercostal and innermost intercostal (deep). All of these muscles arise from the inferior border of the rib above and attach onto the superior border of the inferior rib. The external intercostal muscle fibres run inferoanteriorly from attachment points on the inferior and superior ribs. The external intercostal is most active in inspiration. The internal intercostal muscle runs inferoposteriorly and is most active during expiration. The innermost intercostal muscle is the least distinct of the intercostal muscles and appears to have a very limited role in either inspiration or expiration. Between the innermost intercostal and the internal intercostal muscle are the intercostal nerves and subcostal arteries, which supply the intercostal muscles (Aleksandrova and Breslav, 2009).

Levatores costorum

There are 12 levatores costarum muscles which are attached to the transverse processes of C7–T11 and pass inferolaterally between the tubercles and the angles to the subjacent rib. The levatores costarum muscles elevate the ribs during deep inspiration; yet their role in quiet breathing is unclear (Aleksandrova and Breslav, 2009). They may also assist in lateral flexion and rotation of the thoracic spine due to their spinal attachments. They derive their innervation from the posterior rami of the adjacent thoracic nerve.

Transversus thoracic

The transversus thoracic muscle arises from the posterior surface of the xiphisternum, inferior body of the sternum and the adjacent costal cartilages. The four or five muscular slips that comprise this muscle pass superolaterally and attach to costal cartilages 2–6. This muscle is continuous inferiorly with the transverse abdominis muscle; and it comprises part of the anterolateral abdominal wall. It is innervated by the adjacent intercostal nerve. The function of the transversus thoracic muscle is to exert a weak depressive effect on the costal cartilages to which it attaches during expiration (Aleksandrova and Breslav, 2009).

Thoracolumbar fascia

Fascia invests and connects the muscles and bones of the trunk and limbs. Fascia is composed of dense and loose (areolar) connective tissue, so named due to the closely packed or sparsely arranged fibres. Together, these dense and loose connective tissues create a three-dimensional matrix which confers structural support to the muscles and bones they surround and invest. While the abdominal muscles (anteriorly) and the superficial back muscles (posteriorly) provide functional stability and support for the lumbar spine, the force transference of this arrangement is greatly increased with the support offered by the thoracolumbar fascia. The thoracolumbar fascia is a layer of tough connective tissue located in the lower spine. It is composed of three layers which collectively compartmentalize many of the important muscles in the back, such as the quadratus lumborum muscle and the erector spinae muscles (Barker *et al.*, 2007). Laterally, it is contiguous with the internal oblique and transverse abdominis muscles.

Mechanics of spinal stabilization

The vertebral column could be described as a relatively unstable collection of bones stacked up on one another, and without the dynamic interplay between the various muscles and ligaments it would fail to provide an adequate base of support (BoS) for limb movement during physical activity. Panjabi (1992) describes spinal stability as relying on the synergy of three sub-systems:

1. a passive sub-system involving the vertebrae, ligaments, fascia and discs
2. an active sub-system involving the muscles acting on the vertebral column
3. a neural sub-system involving nervous control of muscles.

Any injury involving one of the sub-systems could result in breakdown in spinal stability, resulting in spinal and/or peripheral symptoms. For example, when throwing an object, a stable spine is essential for efficient force transference from power generated through the legs and hips to the shoulder joint (Izzo *et al.*, 2013a; 2013b).

Neural anatomy
Spinal cord and spinal nerves

The spinal cord lies within the vertebral (spinal) canal. The anterior wall of the spinal canal is formed by the vertebral bodies, intervertebral discs and associated ligaments; the lateral and posterior walls are formed by the vertebral arches and ligaments. The spinal cord is surrounded by three membranes, termed meninges (Ansari *et al.*, 2012):

1. the dura mater (outermost and closest to the vertebral foramen);
2. the arachnoid mater (intermediate);
3. the pia mater (innermost and closest to the spinal cord).

The meninges envelop the brain and spinal cord and protect the central nervous system from various hazards, including microorganisms. Infection caused by bacteria and viruses can cause inflammation of the meninges, termed meningitis. The space between the arachnoid and pia maters is called the subarachnoid space, and contains cerebrospinal fluid (CSF). CSF is produced by the choroid plexus in the brain and circulates within the subarachnoid space and the central canal of the spinal cord. CSF protects the cord and brain from biological, chemical and mechanical hazards. The epidural space is located between the dura mater and the vertebral foramen and contains a network of blood vessels; it may be used as a target for administration of drugs (such as anaesthetic) into the spinal region (Ansari *et al.*, 2012).

Innervation of the head and face is derived from 12 pairs of cranial nerves that emerge through foramina in the cranium. Eleven of the cranial nerves arise from the brain, the exception being the spinal accessory nerve (cranial nerve XI), which arises from the superior portion of the spinal cord (Vilensky, 2014).

There are 31 pairs of spinal nerves which emerge from the vertebral canal between the pedicles of adjacent vertebra. There are eight pairs of cervical nerves (C1–8), 2 thoracic (T1–12), five lumbar (L1–5), five sacral (S1–5) and one coccygeal (Co). Spinal nerves are formed by the convergence of an anterior root from the anterior (ventral) horn of the spinal cord and a posterior root from the posterior (dorsal) root ganglion of the spinal cord. The anterior root contains efferent (motor) nerve fibres and the posterior root contains afferent (sensory) nerve fibres and they unite to form a mixed spinal nerve. The peripheral end of a spinal nerve divides into two primary branches called rami. The anterior primary rami supplies muscles and skin on the anterior and lateral regions of the trunk, and the upper and lower limbs, and the posterior rami innervate skin and structures of the back, including deep muscles and facet joints of the vertebral column (Farley *et al.*, 2014).

The spinal cord terminates at the conus medullaris, which lies at L1–2. Spinal nerves below L1 originate in the conus medullaris of the spinal cord and form a bundle of nerve roots called the cauda equina ('horse's tail'), still contained within the vertebral foramen. The nerve roots of L2–5 enter the sacral canal and descend with the five sacral and one coccygeal nerve roots. Termination of the nerve roots occurs at the filum terminale, which is a delicate strand of fibrous tissue with a terminal end called the coccygeal ligament (Farley *et al.*, 2014).

Dermatomes and myotomes

A dermatome is an area of skin innervated by a spinal nerve root. The location of somatosensory symptoms such as pain, numbness, paraesthesia or hyperaesthesia can be used to infer the source of a nerve root compression. Sensory testing of dermatomes can be used to evaluate the integrity of spinal nerves and spinal cord segments and is usually performed using an individual's response to somatosensory stimuli, including heat, cold, touch, pressure, and pain. A myotome is a group of muscles supplied by a spinal nerve root, and is the motor equivalent of a dermatome. The

Practitioner Tip Box 5.7

Cauda equina syndrome (CES) arises through nerve damage to the cauda equina. It is a neurological condition which is regarded as a form of spinal cord injury. Symptoms include: severe pain in a radicular pattern (i.e. back, buttock, perineum, thighs and/or legs); a loss of sensation in the saddle (perineal and groin) area; weakness in legs; and bladder, bowel and/or sexual dysfunction (incontinence and/or impotence). Although a rare combination, this combination of symptoms arising suddenly is regarded as a medical emergency and immediate medical attention should be sought.

location of weaknesses in groups of muscle can be used to evaluate the integrity of spinal nerve roots and spinal cord segments. For example, neurological testing of myotomes using isometric muscle procedures can provide information regarding the location of a lower motor neurone lesion (LMNL) in the peripheral nervous system or an upper motor neurone lesion (UMNL) in the central nervous system (Farley *et al.*, 2014).

Major nerve plexuses

Plexi are branching networks of nerves. The main spinal nerve plexii form from the nerves of the cervical, lumbar and sacral anterior rami (Farley *et al.*, 2014). The cervical (brachial) plexus provides motor and sensory innervation to the upper limb. The lumbar and sacral plexii are connected, and are often termed the lumbosacral plexus. The lumbosacral plexus provides motor and sensory innervation to the pelvis and lower limbs.

Brachial plexus

The brachial plexus is formed by the anterior rami of the nerve roots C5–T1. These pass laterally from the intervertebral foramen and converge to form the superior nerve trunk from C5–6, the middle trunk from C7 and the posterior trunk from C8 and T1 (Farley *et al.*, 2014). Each trunk divides into an anterior and posterior division which travel distally and recombine to form three cords, named according to their relative position to the brachial artery. The lateral cord lies lateral to the brachial artery, and is formed from the anterior division of the superior and middle trunks. The medial cord lies medial to the brachial artery and is formed from the anterior division of the inferior trunk. The posterior cord lies posteriorly to the brachial artery, and is formed from the posterior divisions of the superior, middle and inferior trunks. The peripheral nerves supplying some of the muscles of the thoracic wall and the upper extremity arise from these cords (Saraf-Lavi, 2014).

Brachial plexopathies are a relatively common occurrence in contact sports (Pujalte and Floranda, 2012; Rodine and Vernon, 2012). They can occur following a traction force which causes axonal shearing. Brachial plexopathy and/or neuropathy may also arise from soft tissue or bony compression of upper extremity nerve fibres as occurs in thoracic outlet syndrome (TOS) (Pujalte and Floranda, 2012; Rodine and Vernon, 2012). Clinical signs of compression of a lower cervical or upper thoracic nerve root (radiculopathy) or peripheral nerve (neuropathy) include sensory and motor disturbances in the upper limb, such as pins and needles or fasciculations (Rodine and Vernon, 2012). Thus, assessment of lower cervical and upper thoracic nerve function is performed through neurological evaluation of the upper limb.

Lumbosacral plexus

Peripheral nerves to the lower limb arise from the lumbosacral plexus formed by nerve roots T12 (subcostal nerve), L1–3 (L4) and L4–S5. The lumbar plexus forms from the lumbar nerve roots and the plexus passes through and provides motor supply to the psoas major muscle before descending through the pelvis and under the inguinal ligament to supply the lower extremity via branches of the femoral and obturator nerves (Farley *et al.*, 2014). The sacral plexus shares some of its innervation with the nerve roots of L4–5 and the anterior rami of S1–4. The largest branch of the sacral plexus is the sciatic nerve, which has a major role in supplying the innervation to the posterior thigh, lower leg and foot (Farley *et al.*, 2014). Lumbosacral plexus injuries are relatively rare in sport and rare in the general population. The integrity of lumbar and sacral neural tissue is checked by neurological assessment of the dermatomes, myotomes and reflexes of the lower limbs (Saraf-Lavi, 2014).

Circulatory anatomy

The vertebral column is well perfused with blood and supplied by the vertebral and ascending cervical arteries for the cervical region, the costocervical and posterior intercostal arteries for the thoracic region and the lumbar and iliolumbar arteries for the lumbar region (Moore and Dalley, 2006). These arteries anastomose with branches of the spinal arteries and enter the intervertebral foramen to divide into radicular arteries that supply the anterior (ventral) and posterior (dorsal) roots of the spinal nerves. Some of these arteries continue into the spinal canal and form anastomoses with anterior and posterior spinal arteries, which supply the spinal cord (Moore and Dalley, 2006).

Local venous drainage from the vertebral region is achieved through the internal and external vertebral venous plexii formed from the spinal veins (Drake *et al.*, 2005). Vertebral venous drainage may be a route for transfer of metastatic cancer cells as it is connected to the major venous systems of the head, chest and abdomen (Griessenauer *et al.*, 2014).

Assessment of the spinal region

Spinal injuries, particularly those also involving the brain and/or spinal cord, are serious consequences of sports participation and account for around 11 per cent of the annual number of traumatic spinal injuries (Benjamin and Lessman, 2013; Patel *et al.*, 2013). It is important that the sports therapist adopts a well-rehearsed assessment of the spinal region, as injury to this area of the body has the potential for serious long-term consequences and sports therapists can find themselves undertaking assessments of the injured athlete at the time of injury on the field, or in the clinical setting.

Clinical assessment of the spinal region

When assessing injuries and conditions involving the spinal region, it is important to continuously practise with vigilance – what might on first assessment appear to be an insignificant presentation could on rare occasions turn out to be something more complex or even life threatening. Being able to identify risk factors and suspicious signs associated with serious pathology is critical for the sports therapist. The autonomous sports therapist is expected to have the responsibility to make reliable and responsive decisions; this means seeking medical advice or setting up referral whenever necessary.

A variety of clinical reasoning models are available to practitioners when attempting to make sense of complex patient presentations. These range from pattern recognition models, which are relatively simple and ideal for less experienced practitioners, to illness scripts and hypothetico-deductive models which are more appropriate for the experienced practitioner (Loftus, 2012). The hypothetico–deductive model of clinical problem solving is commonly used by sports therapists, physiotherapists and osteopaths when aiming to establish and test differential diagnoses. This model involves the therapist generating several diagnostic hypotheses early in the consultation, which are then tested using subsequent information gathered as the consultation progresses (Abrahamson *et al.*, 2012). The use of objective information then assists in confirming or refuting probable causes of the patient's condition.

Subjective assessment

The initial aim of the subjective evaluation of an athlete with symptoms associated with potential problems in the spinal region is to identify any 'red flags' (signs of serious pathology). Effective communication is fundamental to obtaining the necessary information and the consultation is often prompted by thinking about what is wrong and what can be done about it (O'Sullivan and Lin, 2014).

Clinical red flags for possible serious spinal pathology

Clinical red flags are signs or symptoms that may indicate a sinister pathology and can be identified during a careful history (subjective assessment). They were developed using clinical observation and retrospective analysis (Keillar and Dunleavy, 2013) and are generally used as clinical prediction guides in combination with the practitioner's clinical experience to raise an 'index of suspicion' (Greenhalgh and Selfe, 2009). It is critical that the sports therapist is competent at screening the spinal region for red flags that may indicate the presence of pathologies such as a tumour, infection, fracture or cauda equina syndrome. It is critical that therapists are familiar with a hierarchical list of red flags to use for the spinal region (Table 5.2).

It is common for patients to present with pain in the spinal region. Only 1–2 per cent of individuals with low back pain in the general population present with serious or systemic spinal pathology (Greenhalgh and Selfe, 2009). With around 5–10 per cent of low back pain cases presenting with significant neurological deficits, the vast majority of back pain seen in a clinical presentation tends to be non-specific mechanical back pain, in which a specific patho–anatomical diagnosis cannot be made (~90 per cent of cases) (O'Sullivan and Lin, 2014). Nevertheless, the sports therapist needs to be mindful of risk factors for more sinister pathology that may affect

Table 5.2 Hierarchical list of red flags for patients presenting with spinal pain

Four flags	Three flags	Two flags	One flag
Age >50 years	Age <10 and >51	Age 11–19	Loss of mobility, difficulty with stairs, falls, trips
PMH cancer	PMH: cancer, TB, HIV/AIDS, IV drug use, osteoporosis	Weight loss 5–10% body weight (3–6 months)	Legs misbehave, odd feelings in legs, legs feeling heavy
Unexplained weight loss	Weight loss >10% body weight (3–6 months)	Constant progressive pain	Weight loss <5% body weight (3–6 months)
Failure to improve after 1/12 of EB therapy	Severe night pain precluding sleep	Band-like pain	Smoking
	Loss of sphincter tone and altered S4 sensation	Abdominal pain and changed bowel habits, but with no change in medication	Systemically unwell
	Bladder retention or bowel incontinence	Inability to lie supine	Trauma
	Positive extensor plantar response	Bizarre neurological deficit	Bilateral pins and needles in hands and/or feet
		Spasm	Previous failed treatment
		Disturbed gait	Physical appearance

Source: adapted from Greenhalgh and Selfe, 2006.

sports people. For example, hypo-calorific diets, high-intensity training and amenorrhea may increase the risk of osteoporotic fractures in female endurance athletes. Likewise, there is an increased risk of vertebral end-plate or pars interarticularis fractures in adolescent athletes involved in sports involving high impacts or high spinal loading (DeLaney *et al.*, 2013). Sports therapists should be mindful that athletes may believe that reductions in bodyweight, increased fatigue and muscle soreness may be from high training loads rather than serious spinal pathology. Therapists should also consider the possibility of age-related problems such as a traumatic spondylolisthesis in adolescents (Dimeglio and Canavese, 2012) and osteoarthritis and spinal stenosis in the elderly (Prescher, 1998). Suspicion should be aroused for younger athletes with first onset of spinal pain at <10 years old. In elderly athletes the first onset of back pain >51 years old should alert the sports therapist to the possibility of a medical cause for the patient's symptoms (Sizer *et al.*, 2007). The Royal College of General Practitioners (Savigny *et al.*, 2009) and British Orthopaedic Association (BOA, 2013) have published a diagnostic triage for individuals presenting with low back pain that can be a useful guide to the therapist when assessing spinal symptoms (Table 5.3).

Yellow flags and psychosocial influences

The subjective assessment is also used to screen for psychosocial factors (yellow flags) that are likely to increase the risk of an individual developing prolonged (chronic) symptoms, disability and reduction in the quality of life (Nicholas *et al.*, 2011). Buck *et al.* (2010) present a number of factors that may influence the development of chronic spinal pain:

- Patient attitude – for example, whether the patient believes that with appropriate help and self-management they will be able to return to normal activities.

Table 5.3 Diagnostic triage

Non-specific low back pain	Low back pain with significant neurological deficits	Serious or systemic pathology (red flags)
Aged 20–55	Unilateral leg pain worse than low back pain	Onset age <20 or >55 years
Pain in the lumbosacral region, buttocks and thighs	Pain generally radiates to foot or toes	Non-mechanical pain (unrelated to time or activity)
Pain 'mechanical' in nature	Numbness and paraesthesia in the same distribution	Thoracic pain
Varies with physical activity	Nerve irritation signs	Previous history of carcinoma, steroids or HIV
Varies with time	Reduced SLR which reproduces leg pain and motor, sensory or reflex change	Feeling unwell
Patient well	Limited to one nerve root	Weight loss
Prognosis good	Prognosis reasonable	Widespread neurological symptoms
90% recover from acute attack within six weeks	50% recover from acute attack within six weeks	Structural spinal deformity

Source: adapted from the BOA, 2013, and Savigny *et al.*, 2009.

- Misguided beliefs – for example, beliefs of the existence of serious pathology (such as cancer) despite the absence of clinical evidence; or misunderstanding of diagnosis resulting from inadequate communication from health care professionals (such as where the patient believes their 'disc has slipped' or that their 'spine is crumbling'). Misguided beliefs cause catastrophizing, where the patient describes their situation as much worse than it actually is.
- Ongoing depression and/or anxiety.
- The possibility of compensation associated with the precipitating injury, including iatrogenesis.
- Socioeconomic factors – such as relationship difficulties and low economic status.

Evidence suggests that many health care practitioners are poor at identifying the psychosocial risk factors associated with low back pain and as a result routine screening is warranted (O'Sullivan and Lin, 2014). The 'STarT Back Screening Tool' (SBST) questionnaire is useful to help identify psychosocial risk factors in low back pain populations (Hill *et al.*, 2008; O'Sullivan and Lin, 2014).

On completion of the subjective assessment the therapist needs to judge available information to make an informed clinical decision. If there is sufficient information to rule out the possibility of a serious pathology, the therapist will systematically filter the differential diagnosis and use a process of elimination to begin to make a clinical impression/working hypothesis.

Objective assessment

The use of objective information can be critical in confirming or refuting the cause of the patient/athlete's condition (Petty, 2011). Objective information is gathered to investigate the patient's symptoms using observation, movement assessment, special and functional tests and palpation. Careful consideration should be given to the rationale of any clinical tests undertaken – inappropriate choice of clinical testing may be harmful to the patient, costly to the clinic in staff time and may also produce irrelevant information that detracts from valid diagnosis (Denegar and Fraser, 2006). Therapists must also consider the validity, reliability, specificity and sensitivity of any tests chosen, as these affect the deductions made from the findings (Denegar and Fraser, 2006). The objective examination should be a systematic gathering of evidence to support or refute a specific hypothesis by observing, moving and palpating the patient. With experience, the sports therapist will clinically reason and prioritize the structure of their assessment according to their patient/athlete's subjective history, presenting symptoms and functional ability.

Observations

A significant amount of importance is placed on observation in clinical practice. Observation helps to localize gross injuries such as bruising, swelling, open wounds and anatomical spinal anomalies such as scoliosis. This may provide useful information about pathology that may be contributing to symptoms, although therapists need to be mindful that the relationship between pathology and symptoms may not be as strong as expected, especially for symptoms that have been long-standing, such as with chronic neck or low back pain (O'Sullivan, 2005). Observation begins as the patient enters the treatment room and continues throughout the consultation, with attention given to standing, walking, sitting, facial expression, fidgeting and re-positioning. More formal observation of posture remains a key component of the assessment of biomechanical status, whereby the therapist undertakes structural observations from anterior, posterior and lateral perspectives, from the head to the feet.

Postural assessment

The assessment of static and dynamic posture is integral to sports therapy and is commonly used to assess alignment of the spinal region, and its potential influence locally and globally. It is claimed that postural assessment can inform the potential for excessive mechanical stresses on joints that may contribute to symptoms (Arun *et al.*, 2014). Often, assessment of posture is made with the patient standing and comparing their posture against an imaginary 'plumb-line' that aligns a set of structural coordinates (such as, in the lateral view – the external meatus of the ear; the glenohumeral joint; the centre of the lumbar vertebrae; the greater trochanter; the centre of the knee joint; and just anterior to the lateral malleolus) (Kendall *et al.*, 2005). The concept of an 'ideal' or 'efficient' body posture against which an assessment of an individual can be made is prevalent in health care education (Lederman, 2010). It is claimed that deviation from this ideal posture may result from, or contribute to, pathology (Borghuis *et al.*, 2008). Moreover, it is claimed that deviations from an 'ideal' posture may contribute to the development of dysfunctional motor control, such as hypertonia and weakness, and chronic musculoskeletal pain in the neck and lower back (Borghuis *et al.*, 2008; O'Sullivan, 2005). The usefulness of postural assessment for individuals with neck pain has been challenged because evidence suggests that clinicians would be unable to detect differences considered clinically meaningful through observation alone (Silva *et al.*, 2009). Posture is not fixed and may alter over time. For example, it is not uncommon for the dominant arm of tennis players to be well developed in comparison to their non-dominant arm, creating potential asymmetries around the shoulder girdle. This can compound postural assessment as perceived asymmetry and deviation from the 'ideal' posture by a practitioner may be unrelated to presenting symptoms.

Clearing tests and screening of joints

Screening of the joints is used to streamline assessment routines so that practitioners do not spend inordinate amounts of time assessing several potential joints suspected of causing symptoms (Petty, 2011). Screening of the spinal region, however, is not as useful as the screening undertaken in the case of painful joints in the arms and legs, as movement in each region of the spine is interdependent, making it more difficult to rule out the contribution of an adjacent spinal region to an athlete's symptoms (Wong and Johnson, 2012). Cervical spine clearing movements may typically consist of simple (seated) rotation to the left and right with overpressure (if asymptomatic), followed by a closing quadrant position (such as a combination of extension, lateral flexion and rotation) and/or a 'Spurling's test' (see *Special tests* section). Thoracic clearing movements may typically consist of rotation to the left and right with overpressure (if asymptomatic). Lumbar clearing movements may involve flexion with overpressure, and a closing quadrant, or 'Kemp's quadrant test' (see *Special tests* section). If any clearing test produces regional pain or recreation of symptoms, then a full examination of that joint region may be warranted.

Assessment of movement of the spinal region

Movements, both active and passive, that increase or reduce symptoms provide useful information about potential causes of symptoms which can aid home care advice and specific exercise regimes (Rutledge *et al.*, 2013). The sports therapist needs to have an appreciation of average ranges of movement for each spinal region in order to identify movement dysfunctions (i.e. hypermobility or hypomobility). The athlete's willingness to move provides valuable information about the severity of the pain and the tissue irritability of that region. Tissue irritability is a spurious term and relates to how quickly symptoms in the spinal region are provoked by a particular movement and how quickly the symptoms resolve once the movement has stopped (Barakatt *et al.*, 2009). This information may be used to inform the therapist's order of active or passive movement assessment (i.e. testing the least provocative movements first) and may also be used to inform home care advice (Barakatt *et al.*, 2009). For example, if flexion of the lumbar spine reproduces symptoms and extension reduces symptoms, an athlete may be advised to perform 'McKenzie' type extension exercises and advised to reduce lumbar flexion exercises during an acute episode of low back pain.

Active range of movement assessment
Active ranges of movements are used to assess the ability and willingness to engage contractile tissues (i.e. muscles and tendons) that move a target joint. This enables the therapist to ascertain range of movement, quality of movement and any symptom response related to movement. Appreciation of average ranges of movement for each region of the spine is essential (Table 5.4).

Specific vectors of movement give potentially useful information regarding the nature of the tissues likely to be causing an athlete's symptoms (May and Aina, 2012). The use of these established vectors of movement can aid hypotheses related to tissues potentially contributing to symptoms (Berthelot *et al.*, 2007). In the lumbar spine, movements involving forward flexion and sitting produce increased intra-discal pressure, so if these manoeuvres aggravate symptoms the sports therapist may, in conjunction with other findings, be able to suspect discogenic injury, or vertebral body or epiphyseal plate fracture (May and Aina, 2012). Conversely, if extension increases symptoms, the therapist may be able to suspect facet joint or pars interarticularis involvement (May and Aina, 2012). For individuals with both low back pain and radicular leg pain, active ranges of movements that cause a distal spread of symptoms into the leg (i.e. peripheralization) suggest increased compression of the nerve roots, whereas active movements which reduce peripheral symptoms from distal to proximal (i.e. centralization) suggest decreased compression of the nerve roots (Massalski, 2011). Individuals suspected of having lumbar spine instability may have signs including segmental hinging, catching, juddering or shaking on active range of movement testing. They may complain of increased symptoms on returning from a flexed position, in some cases having to walk their hands up their thighs to support their trunk in order to return to standing (this is known as 'Gower's sign') (O'Sullivan, 2005).

Table 5.4 Cervical and lumbar spine: average ranges of movement

	Average range of movement
Cervical spine	
Flexion	40–45°
Extension	45–70°
Lateral flexion	20–45°
Rotation	50–60°
Lumbar spine	
Flexion	80–105°
Extension	25–60°
Lateral flexion	35–40°
Rotation	20–45°

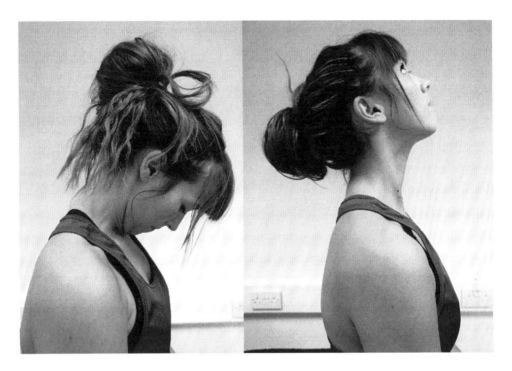

Photo 5.3   Cervical active range of movement assessment: flexion and extension.

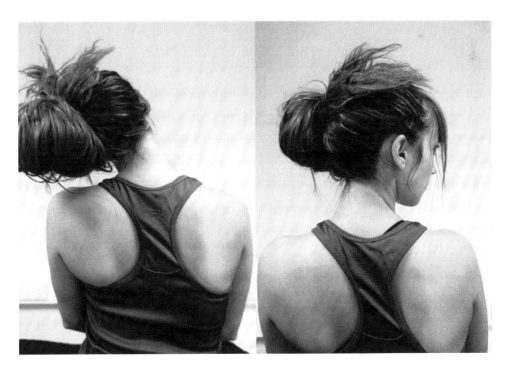

Photo 5.4   Cervical active range of movement assessment: lateral flexion and rotation.

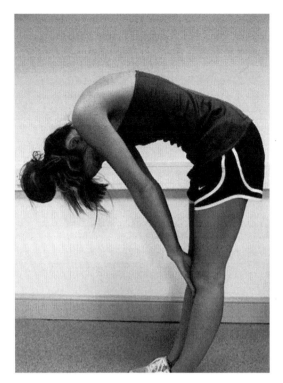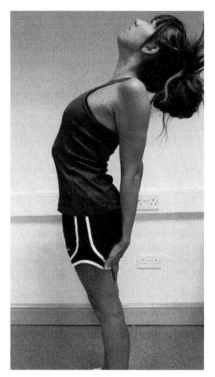

Photo 5.5   Lumbar active range of movement assessment: flexion and extension.

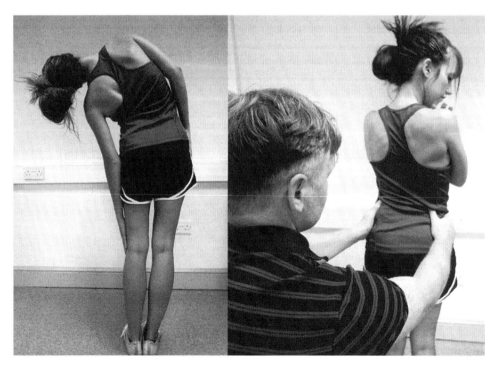

Photo 5.6   Lumbar active range of movement assessment: lateral flexion and rotation.

Passive physiological range of movement assessment

It is important that the patient/athlete is comfortable and relaxed when undertaking assessment of passive range of movement. Passive physiological intervertebral movements (PPIVM) are used to assess segmentally the regions of the spine (Petty, 2011). When undertaking PPIVM therapists need to be skilled in palpation of the vertebral bony landmarks, particularly between adjacent spinous processes and the facet joints. These anatomical structures are palpated while performing PPIVM to detect the range of motion (i.e. normal; hypermobile; or hypomobile), the quality of movement and any symptom response throughout the physiological movements tested. PPIVM can be used to corroborate any movement restrictions seen during assessment of active ranges of movement; and when the movement is taken to the end of range they can determine the end-feel of a vertebral segment (i.e. the quality and symptom response at that specific end position). PPIVM are useful in determining the nature of a movement dysfunction in the spinal region, and these findings contribute to the decisions regarding delivery of any manual therapy (Abbott *et al.*, 2005).

Passive accessory movement assessment

Assessment of passive accessory intervertebral movements (PAIVM) enables identification of segmental movement abnormalities (Abbott *et al.*, 2005). Accessory movements include spinning, rolling or gliding of the joint surfaces which are a vital part of normal physiological movement. Assessment of PAIVM requires good tactile acuity coupled with good clinical reasoning to detect segmental hypomobility, hypermobility, or to localize segmentally produced

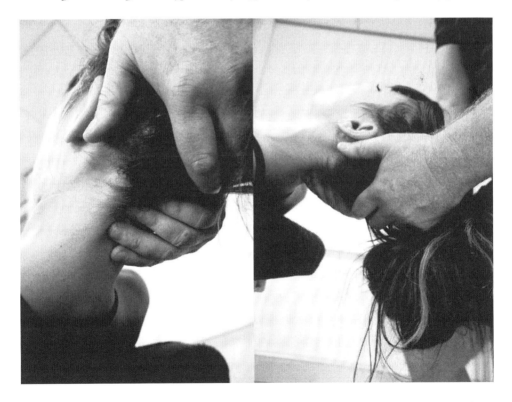

Photo 5.7   Cervical passive physiological intervertebral movement (PPIVM) assessment: flexion and extension.

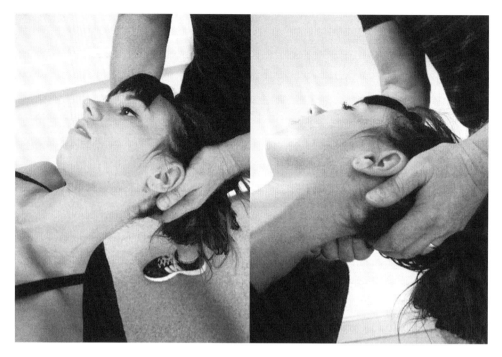

Photo 5.8 Cervical passive physiological intervertebral movement (PPIVM) assessment: lateral flexion and rotation.

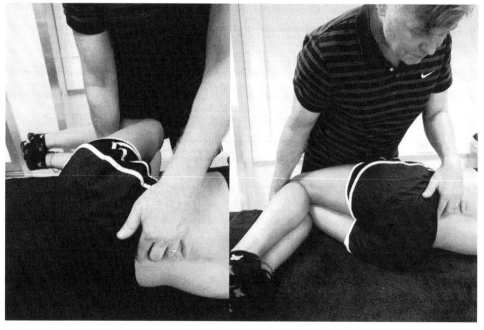

Photo 5.9 Lumbar passive physiological intervertebral movement (PPIVM) assessment: flexion and extension.

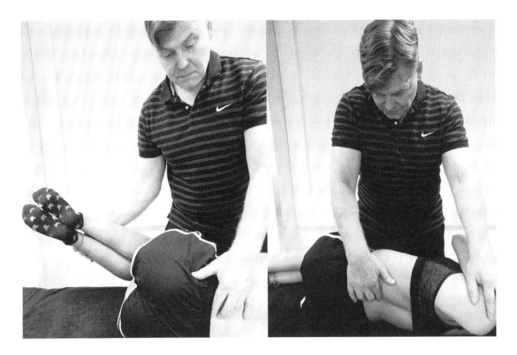

Photo 5.10 Lumbar passive physiological intervertebral movement (PPIVM) assessment: lateral flexion and rotation.

pain. In general, assessment of the spine is undertaken using central posteroanterior glides, unilateral posteroanterior glides, longitudinal caudad or cephalad glides, and transverse glides, with the direction and amplitude of these accessory movements directed by facet orientation of the region and patient morphology. The therapist attempts to detect a normal or capsular end-feel on accessory motion testing, with abnormal movements being hyper- or hypomobile. Hypermobile movements typically produce a palpatory feeling as though the joint has no definitive end of movement; and hypomobility tends to have a hard end-feel, as though blocked. The final finding is the presence of pain with the application of the posteroanterior pressure. Normal and abnormal accessory movements should be documented (Petty, 2011).

Assessment of active resisted movement

Active resisted movement testing enables the sports therapist to assess the strength and symptom response of a muscular contraction around a joint. It is normally (initially) performed using physiological movements in a mid-range of movement where the muscle is at its strongest, and in a safer position in case of the presence of an injury which may be aggravated at extremes of range. Muscle strength is usually measured using the five-point Oxford Grading Scale (OGS). Five points are allocated when the patient makes a movement against gravity and resistance through the entire range; zero points are allocated when the patient is unable to make a muscle contraction. Active resisted movement testing seems to be used more for assessment of peripheral joints than assessment of the spine because in the spine it is more difficult to differentially diagnose which tissue is potentially causing symptoms, especially as there is no identifiable cause in ~90 per cent of individuals presenting with low back pain (Mueller *et al.*, 2012). Nevertheless, performing an active resisted movement test provides the sports therapist with another layer of information to create a working hypothesis.

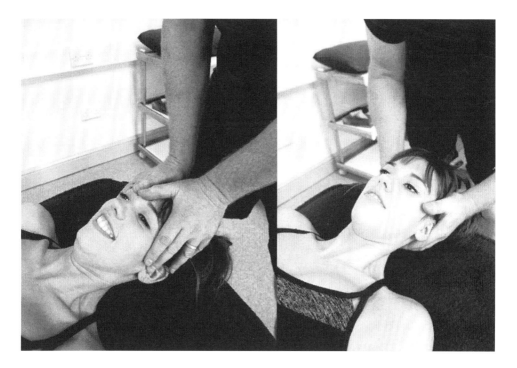

Photo 5.13   Cervical resisted range of movement assessment: flexion and extension.

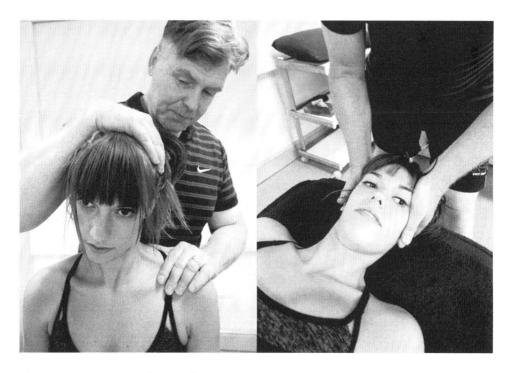

Photo 5.14   Cervical resisted range of movement assessment: lateral flexion and rotation.

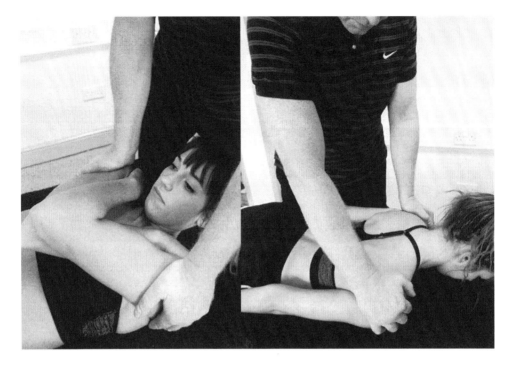

Photo 5.15 Thoracolumbar resisted range of movement assessment: flexion and extension.

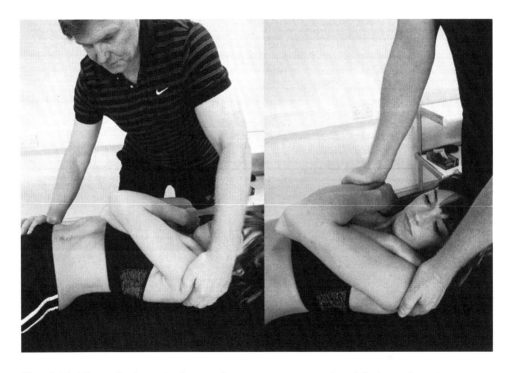

Photo 5.16 Thoracolumbar resisted range of movement assessment: lateral flexion and rotation.

Palpation of the spinal region

Palpation helps to determine the anatomical and functional state of tissue and may provide information leading to more precise diagnosis. According to Maitland *et al.* (2005), palpation enables location of tissue changes, such as:

- tightness of paravertebral muscles;
- localized thickening adjacent to a vertebral level;
- soft thickening over the facet joints;
- hard bony thickening and prominence over the facet joints.

Palpation is also used to screen specific tissues for their ability to reproduce symptoms.

In the cervical spine, C1 has no spinous process, so the first bony prominence that is palpable is C2. With careful palpation for the interspinous spaces it is possible to palpate down to C7 quite easily. Palpation for midline tenderness in the cervical spine following a cervical acceleration/deceleration (whiplash) injury may indicate ligamentum nuchae trauma (Bacchus, 2011). Palpable crepitus may be elicited with flexion or extension movements which may suggest cervical spondylosis (McDonnell and Lucas, 2012).

The thoracic spine is often divided according to the similarity of the facet orientation of the thoracic and cervical segments into upper, middle and lower. The upper region of the thoracic spine runs from C7 to T4 and the mid to lower region from T5 to T12. The spinous process of C7 is identified by locating the most prominent spinous process at the base of the neck and is confirmed by having the patient extend their neck – C6 will typically appear to 'disappear' as it glides anteriorly, while C7 remains palpable. Other bony landmarks useful for locating thoracic spinal segments are the superior angle of the scapula (approximately level with T2), the spine of the scapula (T4) and the inferior angle of the scapula (T7), although this is subject to individual anatomical variation. In the thoracic region, mechanical pain and visceral pain, due to serious pathology, can mimic each other due to the shared innervation of these structures from the sympathetic division of the autonomic nervous system, which runs from T1 to L2 (Krassioukov, 2009). Palpation for bony tenderness in the thoracic spine is important to help eliminate the possibility of visceral referred pain and to detect osteoporotic fractures, as these are common in the elderly in the thoracic spine (Siminoski *et al.*, 2012).

It is more difficult to ascertain bony levels in the lumbar spine because of the depth of the spine and variation in bony anatomy between individuals. Identification of L4 may be achieved by identifying the iliac crests and tracing across in an horizontal line medially. The posterior superior iliac spine (PSIS) aids identification of S2; and with careful palpation should allow differentiation from an area of no movement, the bony sacrum, to the L5–S1 junction. Pain on palpation over the sacroiliac joints is common with sacroiliac joint inflammation (Capra *et al.*, 2010). A palpable step between L5 and S1 may be indicative of a spondylolisthesis (Koerner and Radcliff, 2013).

Percussion of the vertebral column, on the spinous processes, or the ribs in the thoracic region, is a useful element of the palpatory assessment. Significant pain production on percussion is a possible indicator of infection, fracture or malignancy (Siminoski *et al.*, 2012). Pain provocation tests are commonly used as part of the objective examination. In the spinal region, however, their use is often limited due to the fact that despite having good sensitivity (i.e. production of pain) they often have poor specificity (i.e. they do not reliably incriminate specific structure) and consequently can lead to false positives (Denegar and Fraser, 2006).

Special tests of the spinal region

Orthopaedic special tests are commonly used in the objective assessment, often at the expense of information gleaned from other elements of the objective assessment. The sports therapist needs to be aware that some special tests have weak inter- and intra-rater reliability (Denegar and Fraser, 2006). Thus, positive findings should always be interpreted in conjunction with the rest of the objective examination. Pain provocation tests are commonly used in clinical practice to identify mechanically sensitive structures as potential sources of pain (such as Kemp's quadrant test). Neural provocation tests are also commonly used to identify mechanically sensitive neural structures as sources of pain (such as Spurling's test). Neurodynamic tests evaluate the mobility of various components of the nervous system and include the straight leg raise test (predominantly the sciatic nerve and its distributions), slump test, prone knee bend (predominantly the femoral nerve and its distributions) and the upper limb tension tests, which can be used to assess primarily the integrity of the median, ulnar and radial nerves.

Neurodynamic and neural provocation tests of the spinal region
Straight leg raise test

The straight leg raise (SLR) test is performed when the sports therapist suspects a lumbar radiculopathy as a cause of leg symptoms (Scaia *et al.*, 2012). Radiculopathy is caused by mechanical compression or irritation of the nerve roots as they exit the spine. This compression is most commonly attributed to an intervertebral disc herniation and tends to affect the L4–5 or the L5–S1 levels (Iversen *et al.*, 2013). The test is performed with the athlete supine while the therapist raises the leg with the knee fully extended, maintaining support under the popliteal fossa to prevent knee flexion. The leg is lifted until maximum hip flexion is attained or until the patient reports the onset of any symptoms. A positive test is when pain, paraesthesia or anaesthesia is reproduced – typically at <60° of hip flexion (Scaia *et al.*, 2012). To try to differentiate between hamstring muscle tension and adverse neural tension, therapists may use additional movements including passive ankle dorsiflexion and internal rotation of the femur to further test neural mobility (these are termed sensitizing movements). Reproduction of the athlete's symptoms with any sensitizing movements should lead the sports therapist to suspect a radiculopathy as a potential source of the leg symptoms (Scaia *et al.*, 2012). For further information on the SLR and other neurodynamic tests, see Chapter 2.

Crossed straight leg raise test

The crossed SLR test is often used in conjunction with the SLR test and involves the therapist flexing the uninvolved hip while maintaining the knee in full extension. A positive test is noted when the patient reports reproduction of their leg symptoms contralateral to the leg being tested. This will often occur at <40° and a positive test may be referred to as a 'crossover sign'.

Slump test

The slump test is widely used and involves sitting the patient on the edge of the treatment couch in a slumped position (with flexed thoracolumbar and cervical spine). The knee is extended and the ankle dorsiflexed to place increasing mechanical load upon the neural structures along the length of the spine; this may produce or reproduce symptoms of low back or leg pain. Following the ankle dorsiflexion movement, cervical spine extension is introduced which reduces the tension in the mechanically loaded neural system and this may reduce the patient's previous symptoms. The sports therapist should appreciate that the slump test has received criticism because non–neural structures such as subcutaneous fascia, muscle and blood vessels are also under mechanical loading during the movements, and these may contribute to false positives (Walsh *et al.*, 2007).

Upper limb neurodynamic tests

Upper limb neurodynamic testing is performed to test for the presence of cervical radiculopathy (Davis *et al.*, 2008) as well as for any irritation of the targeted nerve pathway at any of its mechanical interfaces. Further information regarding upper limb neurodynamic testing to incriminate the median, ulnar and radial nerve pathways can be found in Chapter 2.

Spurling's test

Spurling's test is a neural provocation test that involves performing cervical extension and lateral flexion to the same side as the arm symptoms (Shah and Rajshekhar, 2004). These combined movements serve to reduce the size of the intervertebral foramen, and make nerve impingement more likely. A positive test is noted with any provoked upper extremity pain and suggests that symptoms are being caused in part by cervical intervertebral disc herniation occurring most commonly in the C5–6, C6–7 and C4–5 regions (Shah and Rajshekhar, 2004). Several authors describe the addition of gradual axial compression (Cipriano, 2010). The axial compression test involves manual application of compression to the cranium, with the head and neck in the aforementioned position, and also attempts to reproduce symptoms (Ghasemi *et al.*, 2011). Another procedure which may help confirm suspicions is manual distraction of the neck, applied via the occiput while stabilizing the shoulders; if this reduces or relieves symptoms, the diagnosis of neural compression is supported (Ghasemi *et al.*, 2011).

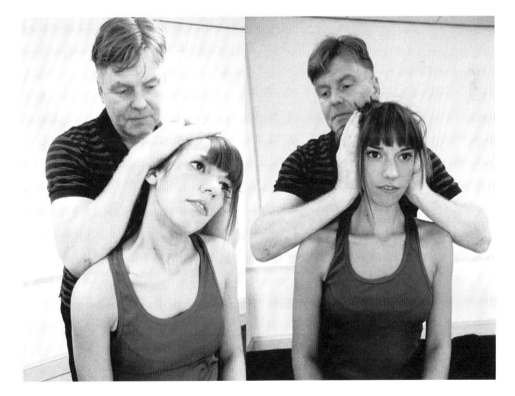

Photo 5.17   Cervical compression and distraction tests.

Kemp's quadrant test

Kemp's test, also called the lumbar quadrant test, involves loading the lumbar facet joints. A positive test is noted when a patient's low back symptoms are reproduced (Wong and Johnson, 2012). The facet joints are often implicated as a source of pain when the patient presents with unilateral low back pain and there is an exacerbation of symptoms with closing movements, such as extension or lateral flexion (Wong and Johnson, 2012). The lumbar facet joints are prone to facet joint syndrome due to the high demand on their load-bearing properties with lifting, throwing and rotational forces (Beresford *et al.*, 2010). Facet joint syndrome is defined as arthrogenic pain (originating from the lumbar or cervical facet joints), with the intra-articular structures such as the joint surfaces commonly being the tissues causing symptoms (Beresford *et al.*, 2010).

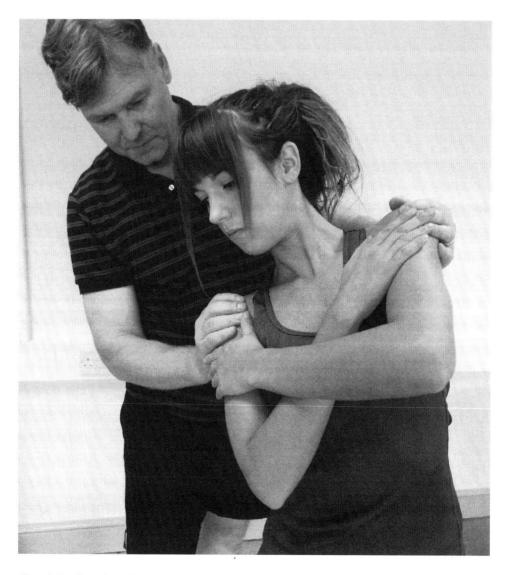

Photo 5.18 Kemp's quadrant test.

Vertebrobasilar tests

Vertebrobasilar insufficiency (VBI) may result in a transient ischaemic attack (TIA) (commonly referred to as a mini-stroke), which can be a serious predictor of an impending cerebrovascular accident (CVA) (commonly referred to as a stroke). VBI may be caused by atherosclerosis affecting the large arteries of the neck, causing narrowing and occlusion (Hutting *et al.*, 2013b). Risk factors associated with atherosclerosis leading to vertebrobasilar artery insufficiency are high-fat diets, diabetes mellitus, hypertension, smoking, obesity and chronic stress (Sweeney and Doody, 2010). Beyond this, such cervical presentations as intervertebral disc degeneration and/or spondylosis can significantly increase compression on the vasculature, particularly at the intervertebral foramen.

Vertebrobasilar artery insufficiency test (VAIT)

Traditionally, it has been recommended that therapists should test for VBI by positioning the patient supine, with their head supported (by the therapist) off the end of the couch. The patient's head should then be passively extended and held for ten seconds; then laterally flexed in the extended position and held for a further ten seconds; and finally, rotated while in the extended and laterally flexed position, and held for a further ten seconds. This should also be repeated in the opposite direction. A positive test would be identified if the patient reported dizziness, nausea, dysarthria (difficulty speaking), dysphagia (difficulty swallowing), diplopia ('double-vision'), fainting, dilated pupils, nystagmus (rapid involuntary eye movements) and/or pain. VBI is a red flag and the patient/athlete complaining or presenting with these symptoms should be referred to their GP. More recently it has been suggested that VBI testing lacks sufficient reliability and specificity and should no longer be recommended for routine testing

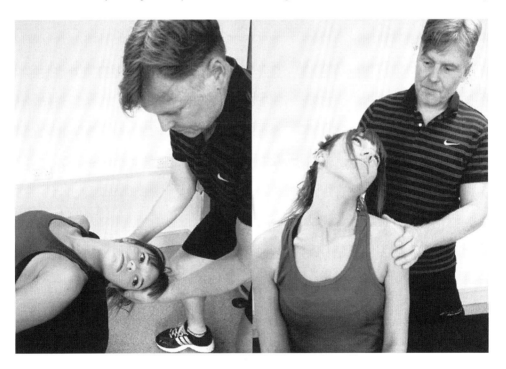

Photo 5.19 Vertebrobasilar artery insufficiency tests (supine-lying VAIT and seated Wallenberg's VAIT).

(Hutting *et al.*, 2013b). However, whenever the therapist is presented with any patient (particularly older patients) who, in subjective assessment, reveals episodes of dizziness, nausea or more (as above), especially when related to neck movements, they must still be carefully assessed and managed. As such, the VAIT – or a modified version such as Wallenberg's test – may be considered, even if seen more as a functional test. Wallenberg's test has the patient seated with shoulders gently supported; they are then asked to perform a combined active rotation and extension movement, left and right (held for 30 seconds each side) (Cook and Hegedus, 2013).

Cervical instability tests

Modified Sharp–Purser test

The Sharp–Purser test is used to help assess the possibility of myelopathic symptoms specifically related to instability in the upper neck. This is most likely related to subluxation of the axis on the atlas due to injury to the transverse ligament (which contributes stability to the odontoid process of the atlas relative to its articulation with the axis) (Magee, 2008). Such instability can occur during acceleration–deceleration (whiplash) mechanisms of injury. Although the exact procedure for the original Sharp–Purser test was not clearly described by the authors (Sharp *et al.*, 1958), a standardized description of the test has been presented by Cook and Hegedus (2013). In a seated position, the patient is simply asked to flex their cervical spine; a symptom response in this position may be considered positive. If no symptoms are reproduced, gentle overpressure into flexion is performed via the forehead of the patient. Cook and Hegedus (2013) also describe the modified version of the test (as do Magee, 2008; and Vizniak, 2012). For the modified Sharp–Purser test, the patient is seated and then supported at their forehead, with the therapist's palm of hand in a position of slight neck flexion. With their other hand, the therapist identifies and stabilizes the spinous process of C2 (axis) with a 'pincer grip' involving their thumb and index finger. With extreme care, the therapist may then, from this position, perform a very gentle anterioposterior translation movement of the head and neck via the palm of their hand on the patient's forehead. Symptom reproduction or reduction, significant displacement or 'clunking' are all considered positive signs, and referral for imaging should be considered.

Tectorial membrane test

The tectorial membrane is a continuation of the posterior longitudinal ligament above the axis – from C2 to the occiput (Loudon *et al.*, 2008). It can be damaged during rapid acceleration–deceleration (whiplash) type mechanisms, and there are several tests which aim to identify upper cervical instability attributed to its disruption. Osmotherly *et al.* (2012) present good evidence for testing using distraction for excessive vertical displacement. The patient should be supine with their head resting on a pillow (to relax suboccipital musculature and off-load the nuchal ligament); the therapist fixes C2 with one hand, and applies a distraction force via the occiput (in neutral, flexion and extension). It can be recommended for the therapist to utilize a 'pincer grip' to fix C2, and additionally use their abdomen to support the patient's forehead during this test. A positive test is indicated by displacement of more than 2 mm and/or a symptom response (such as reproduced pain, or 'clunking' sensation).

Fitness tests

Returning to sport or physical activity before an injury has healed has the potential to create further tissue damage. The athlete's suitability to undertake training can be assessed using clinical findings and a suitable fitness test (Frohm *et al.*, 2012). In many sports athletes will undertake

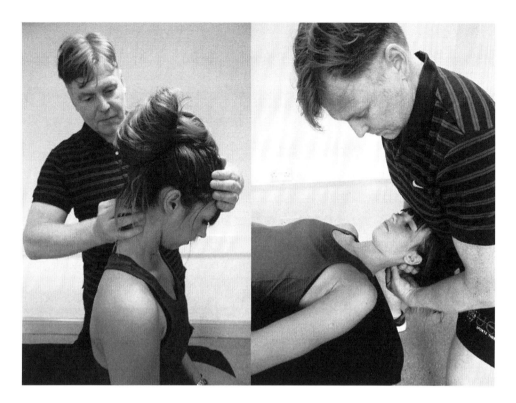

Photo 5.20   Modified Sharp–Purser and tectorial membrane tests.

fitness testing prior to pre-season training and at periods throughout the competitive period. The types of test will be determined by the sport in which the athlete is engaged. For example, in endurance athletes this may entail a maximum oxygen uptake (VO_2 maximum) test. In strength- and power-based sports it may be a vertical jump test, Wingate test or testing of an athlete's one repetition maximum (1RM) (Frohm *et al.*, 2012). The results of these fitness tests can be used to assess how closely the athlete has recovered in comparison to their pre-injury status. Other clinical criteria used to decide an athlete's readiness to return to training or competition usually include being pain free, having no swelling, having full range of movement (when compared to the uninjured side), having close to full strength (when compared to the uninjured side) and the ability to perform functional movements (including hops, multidirectional running and jumps). Psychological readiness to return to play is also an essential component of any return to play criteria (Shrier *et al.*, 2014).

Injuries of the spinal region

Around 1,000 people sustain a spinal cord injury each year in the UK, of which 11 per cent are attributable to participation in sport (Patel *et al.*, 2013). Common sporting spinal injuries include whiplash injury, brachial plexopathies (referred to as 'burner syndrome', 'burners', 'stingers' or neurapraxias) and discogenic injuries (Apostolos, 2013; Benjamin and Lessman, 2013). Less common sports-related spinal conditions include cauda equina syndrome, upper cervical instability, thoracic outlet syndrome and spondylolysis. Sports with a greater risk of cervical spine injuries include diving, rugby, football, skiing, boxing, gymnastics, ice hockey and wrestling, which can result in muscle damage, ligament sprain, intervertebral disc injuries, fractures or dislocations and nerve root, brachial plexus or peripheral nerve neurapraxias.

When working pitch-side, sports therapists should remember that neck pain in any athlete following trauma must be treated as an unstable cervical spine injury until it has been demonstrated otherwise. Fractures and dislocations, however, are rare, and many cervical injuries tend to be sprains and muscle tears (Benjamin and Lessman, 2013). Likewise, low back pain is often considered to be secondary to a muscle injury or sprain, and many episodes of low back pain are self-limiting and respond to a multi-modal, conservative approach using progressive exercise rehabilitation, manual therapy, cryotherapy, thermotherapy and/or electrotherapy (Anubhav *et al.*, 2013). Additional risk factors to the development of low back pain in athletes appear related to strength or mobility imbalances, sudden increases in training duration or intensity, poor technique or inappropriate equipment. Spondylolysis in the lumbar spine is often associated with repeated hyperextension of the spine and can be prevalent in wrestlers, dancers, gymnasts, divers, pole-vaulters and swimmers. Lumbar intervertebral disc injuries are common in contact sports where there is high spinal loading (Nandyala *et al.*, 2013).

The primary goal with an athlete presenting with an acute injury to the spinal region is to rule out the possibility of a spinal cord injury that requires immediate referral to accident and emergency (Sarhan *et al.*, 2012). All injuries affecting the spine have the potential to damage the spinal cord, resulting in spinal cord injury that may be life-threatening or career-ending. Once the nature of the injury has been established the therapist then needs to help identify interventions to modulate pain and promote recovery, and then support a progressive return to play. In non-specific low back pain, identifying specific features of an athlete's presentation (such as instability or reduced mobility), may allow the sports therapist to allocate the patient to a specific sub-group, where targeted interventions may help in reducing their symptoms (Kumar and Kumar, 2013).

Spinal cord injuries

Damage to the spinal cord resulting from trauma rather than disease is termed spinal cord injury. Sporting injuries are a common cause of spinal cord injury resulting in loss or impairment of motor and sensory function according to the level and severity of the injury (Patel *et al.*, 2013). Initially, spinal cord injury may cause a transient acute reaction with a temporary loss of spinal cord-mediated reflexes such as deep tendon reflexes, and the bulbocavernosus reflex associated with anal function. This is termed 'spinal shock' (Assenmacher *et al.*, 2013). Providing the injury is reversible there can be a gradual return of reflexes within hours, or in severe cases over a period of months. Irreversible spinal cord injury is categorized as complete where there is an absence of sensation and voluntary movement on both sides of the body, below the level of the injury, and incomplete where some function remains below the level of the injury (Patel *et al.*, 2013).

Complete cord injuries in the cervical region result in quadriplegia; and if the injury is above C3–4 tracheal intubation is needed to assist breathing. Complete injuries in the thoracic region result in paraplegia of the lower extremities but tend to spare upper extremity function. Injuries at L1 (the conus medullaris) often produce a mixed presentation of upper and lower motor neuron signs, whereas injuries below L1 produce cauda equina damage, resulting in bladder or bowel incontinence, sexual dysfunction and/or loss of motor function in the hip, knee and foot. Incomplete spinal cord injuries are sub-classified as anterior, central and posterior cord syndromes dependent upon the anatomical location of the damage to the spinal cord.

Trauma management of neck injury prioritizes the possibility of spinal cord injury until proven otherwise. This means that people are immobilized at the scene of an injury using spinal boards and semi-rigid cervical collars (Assenmacher *et al.*, 2013). Medical management of spinal cord injuries usually involves a radiographic investigation using X-ray, MRI or CT scanning to locate the level and extent of damage sustained. Surgery is often warranted to stabilize the spine, and corticosteroids prescribed to help control swelling. This is usually followed by a lengthy period of rehabilitation for the individual in an attempt to try to regain some functionality.

Vertebral fractures

Any traumatic incident involving the spine should raise the level of suspicion in the sports therapist of a fracture (Chao *et al.*, 2010; Skovrlj and Quresh, 2013). Vertebral fractures relating to sports injury commonly involve the cervical or lumbar regions of the spine. This is considered to be due to the increased load bearing and mobility of these regions (Assenmacher *et al.*, 2013; Benjamin and Lessman, 2013; Lowrie, 2013). The thoracic spine is at lower risk of fractures due to the support given from the adjacent ribs, although rib fractures are relatively common. Vertebral fractures are often described according to the area affected as follows:

- Anterior column: consisting of the anterior longitudinal ligament and the anterior half of the vertebral body and intervertebral disc.
- Middle column: consisting of the posterior half of the vertebral body and intervertebral disc and the posterior longitudinal ligament.
- Posterior column: consisting of the facet joints, ligamentum flavum, the spinous process, transverse processes and inter-connecting ligaments.

Minor fractures are classed as those affecting the spinous or transverse processes, the facet joints and the pars interarticularis. The main types of fracture of the spinal region most commonly associated with sporting participation are: compression, burst, fracture-dislocations, and flexion-distraction fractures (Assenmacher *et al.*, 2013).

Compression fractures

Compression fractures affect the anterior column and in sport usually result from a traumatic episode where the spine is put in a hyperflexed position. The most common areas for compression fractures are the middle, lower thoracic and the upper lumbar vertebrae. These fractures tend to be stable and it is unusual for there to be neurological compromise.

Burst fractures

Burst fractures affect the anterior and middle columns and typically occur from high axial loading of the spine, such as landing on the feet from a height. Burst fractures are described as stable if the posterior column remains intact on radiographic imaging, and if there is less than a 50 per cent anterior vertebral body height collapse. In these cases neurological compromise is rare.

Fracture-dislocations

Fracture-dislocation injuries tend to affect anterior, middle and posterior columns and are typically caused by direct trauma with anterior to posterior shear force or posterior to anterior shear force (such as during rugby tackles). The force displaces the superior vertebra in relation to the inferior vertebra. Fracture-dislocation injuries create highly unstable fractures in addition to neurological deficits, dural tears and intra-abdominal injuries.

Flexion-distraction fractures

Flexion-distraction fractures are often termed 'seat belt' fractures because they are a common consequence of a motor vehicle accident (MVA). They tend to affect anterior, middle and posterior columns and occur where the lumbar spine is forcibly flexed and distracted from the pelvis and lower body. The anterior column fails under a compressive load and the middle and posterior columns are forcibly pulled apart, often causing secondary damage in the interspinous, supraspinous ligaments, the joint capsule and the posterior part of the intervertebral disc. This type of fracture is usually stable and there is rarely any neurological compromise.

Up to 65 per cent of cases of vertebral fracture may be asymptomatic (Guglielmi *et al.*, 2013). Symptoms, when present, vary and may include movement impairment and constant deep pain exacerbated by coughing and sneezing (Guglielmi, *et al.*, 2013). There is often increased kyphosis in the thoracic region due to the damage to the vertebral body and there may be a local muscular spasm and midline tenderness with pain on percussion of the associated spinous process (Lowrie, 2013). Referral for radiographic (X-ray) imaging is warranted, with MRI only requested if neurological damage and/or compression are suspected. Evidence of the Female Athletic Triad (i.e. anorexia, amenorrhea and osteoporosis) needs to be sought during the subjective assessment of young female athletes with signs and symptoms of a vertebral fracture (Payne and Kirchner, 2014).

Vertebral fractures tend to be managed conservatively, with immobilization of the spine for 6–12 weeks using either a halo-thoracic jacket or, more commonly, confinement to bed with skeletal traction for cervical fractures or a pillow wedge for thoracic, lumbar and sacral fractures (Papa, 2012). Often, realignment and fixation surgery is used because it leads to fewer complications than conservative management because of the shorter immobilization period (Sinha *et al.*, 2010).

Whiplash associated disorders

A recognized definition of whiplash injury has been provided by the Quebec Task Force (QTF) (Spitzer *et al.*, 1995): '*an acceleration–deceleration mechanism of energy transfer to the neck. It may result from rear-impact or side-impact motor vehicle collisions, but can also occur with other sporting mishaps. The impact may result in bony or soft tissue injuries (whiplash injury), which in turn may lead to a variety of clinical manifestations (whiplash associated disorders).*'

Sports injuries involving the cervical spine may be caused by excessively forceful movements of the neck and are extremely common in road traffic accidents (RTA) as well as in contact sports such as football, rugby, ice hockey, skiing, snowboarding and horse riding (Benjamin and Lessman, 2013; Sharpe and Van Horne, 2011). These cervical acceleration–deceleration syndromes classically result from the lower cervical and upper thoracic spine being driven into extension while the upper cervical spine is forced into flexion, generating an 'S' shape in the neck. In RTAs, whiplash injury is believed to occur at 60–100 ms following initial impact, and since the average person's reflexes typically take about 100 ms to respond, and voluntary responses about 250 ms, the cervical spine is passively subjected to the insulting forces with no ability to actively protect itself. Active bracing prior to insult can help to reduce the severity, as can well-positioned head-rests in motor vehicles. The acceleration–deceleration mechanism most typically causes an abnormal axis of rotation at the affected spinal segments, resulting in facet joint and IVD compression and extreme physiological hyperextension, most commonly at two primary segments – C2–3 and C5–6, and can create significant soft and bony tissue damage (Benjamin and Lessman, 2013). The mechanism can cause a range of whiplash associated disorders (WAD); these include: cervical fracture; cervical vertebral dislocation; muscle tears of the neck and/or upper back; cervical ligamentous sprains; cervical nerve root and brachial plexopathy; cervical IVD injury; cervical spinal stenosis (myelopathy); sensorimotor disturbance; and acromioclavicular injury. Commonly reported symptoms of WAD include: neck and/or shoulder pain; numbness, tingling or pain into the arms and/or legs; dizziness or unsteadiness; nausea; 'ringing in the ears'; concentration problems; and low back pain (Ferrari *et al.*, 2005). A simple grading criteria for WAD has been presented by the QTF (Spitzer *et al.*, 1995):

- No WAD = no complaints or physical signs at the time of assessment.
- WAD Grade 1 = indicates neck complaints such as pain, tenderness and stiffness, but no physical signs and no or little interference with activities of daily living (ADL).
- WAD Grade 2 = indicates neck complaints and musculoskeletal signs, such as decrease in range of movement or muscle weakness. Additionally there is substantial interference with ADL.
- WAD Grade 3 = indicates neck complaints and neurological signs, such as sensorimotor deficits. Major interference with ADL.
- WAD Grade 4 = indicates major structural pathology, such as fracture or dislocation. Major interference with ADL.

The sports therapist must be especially vigilant in their assessment of patients who have experienced acceleration–deceleration injury – particularly for red flags (including: bilateral paraesthesia in upper or lower limbs; shooting pain into lower limbs or all four limbs with cervical flexion (positive L'Hermitte's sign); hyper-reflexia; nerve root signs at more than two adjacent levels; progressively worsening neurological signs (such as motor weakness or gait disturbances); and symptoms of upper cervical instability. It is essential to establish whether the patient has been medically assessed, or had fracture or dislocation ruled out via X-ray. Psychosocial yellow flags can be an issue, especially where there may be compensation claims being pursued. The sports therapist must, as always, undertake rigorous assessment and document all findings carefully. Management of WAD depends on the presenting severity and symptoms, and on what tissues are involved.

It is estimated that only 8 per cent of cervical acceleration–deceleration syndromes result in significant damage to the spinal cord, although mild traumatic brain injury (concussion) is relatively common (Broglio *et al.*, 2014; Harmon *et al.*, 2013; McKeever and Schatz, 2003). Symptoms of concussion may be subtle, presenting some time after the precipitating event and including changes in mood and/or behaviour, heightened anxiety and irritability, loss of concentration and memory, visual disturbances, feeling dazed and difficulty in word selection (Echemendia *et al.*, 2013). Concussion is a complex injury and challenging to diagnose, assess and manage. There is no gold-standard test or marker that the sports therapist can rely on to aid diagnosis (McCrory *et al.*, 2013) and symptoms can be missed by therapists assessing under high pressure training or match-play situations. Further discussion of concussion is presented in Chapter 4.

Injuries to intervertebral discs

Injuries that involve IVDs include herniation, prolapse and sequestration. Disc injuries are most commonly found at the C5–6 and C6–7 levels, and at the L4–5 and L5–S1 levels, and may be associated with age-related biochemical, morphological and degenerative changes in the IVD (Meredith *et al.*, 2013; Nandyala, *et al.*, 2013). For example, an increasing number of radial and concentric fissures in the annulus fibrosis occur with ageing and reduce the structural integrity and stability of the disc, predisposing the individual to annular tears (Stefanakis *et al.*, 2012). In addition, the loss of the proteoglycans within the nucleus reduces disc rehydration and increases the likelihood of disc desiccation (Haughton, 2011). There is a high incidence of annular tears and the potential for herniation or prolapsing of the nucleus pulposus in sports where the spine is exposed to high loads and rotational forces, such as rugby, weight lifting, cricket and athletics (particularly javelin and discus) (Nandyala *et al.*, 2013). Injuries of the IVD may sometimes be asymptomatic, but more commonly present as pain in the low back or neck and possibly altered neurological sensation (paraesthesia and/or anaesthesia) in the limb on the affected side (as a radiculopathy). These symptoms often worsen with flexion or closing movements on the affected side, and improve with opening movements of the affected side (Meredith *et al.*, 2013; Nandyala *et al.*, 2013).

The majority of disc injuries will respond to conservative management (Stefanakis *et al.*, 2012). Pain is often managed using analgesic medication and electrophysical agents, including transcutaneous electronic nerve stimulation (TENS) or interferential therapy, alongside patient education. Manual therapy may be used to help manage initial symptoms, along with exercise prescription (Anubhav *et al.*, 2013). Surgery is usually only required in around one in ten cases of disc injury, and may be considered if: there is evidence of severe nerve compression; symptoms have not resolved with conservative management; there is prolonged difficulty with activities of daily living, such as walking or standing; or if there is evidence of bowel or bladder dysfunction (cauda equina syndrome). In such cases, and depending upon the extent of damage to the IVD and the nerve/thecal compression evident on MRI, surgery may involve (micro) discectomy, laminectomy, foraminotomy or even disc replacement (Tessitore *et al.*, 2014).

Cauda equina syndrome

Cauda equina syndrome is a serious neurological condition where two or more nerve roots constituting the cauda equina have been damaged by any of the following: a traumatic event; high-grade (unstable) spondylolisthesis; spinal stenosis; or large central IVD prolapse (Kavanagh and Walker, 2013). Each nerve root in the region of the cauda equina contributes to a lower extremity or perineal dermatome and a lower extremity myotome, so presenting symptoms may include 'saddle anaesthesia' (numbness in the perineum, buttock and upper inner thigh region), bilateral radicular leg pain, bowel or bladder incontinence and sexual dysfunction (Todd, 2010). These are red flag signs and the patient needs immediate referral to an A&E department for medical assessment that may result in decompressive surgery, followed by rehabilitation (Kavanagh and Walker, 2013).

Upper cervical instability

A potentially serious consequence of traumatic injury is damage to the connective tissue and ligamentous support of the cervical region causing upper cervical instability (Hutting *et al.*, 2013a). Potential causes of upper cervical instability include cervical acceleration–deceleration (whiplash type) syndromes, forced cervical hyperflexion and cervical axial compression as may occur in a 'spear' tackle in rugby union (Hutting *et al.*, 2013a). Upper cervical instability may initially present as neck pain due to abnormal pressure on the cervical and cranial nerves, vertebral artery compromise or spinal cord compression due to laxity created in the alar ligament, transverse ligament or tectorial membrane (Nemani and Han Jo, 2014) (see Table 5.5). This laxity may also be associated with an underlying congenital condition that affects the

Table 5.5 Signs and symptoms of cervical instability

Symptoms of cervical instability	Signs of cervical instability
Head and neck pain	Worsening symptoms
Facial paraesthesia (due to trigeminal nerve and anterior/posterior ramus of C2 involvement)	Nystagmus
Drop attacks	Bilateral or quadrilateral paraesthesia or motor deficits including weakness/lack of coordination
Nausea	Cervical musculature hyperactivity
Feeling of lump in throat	

composition of collagen (such as Down's syndrome, Ehlers-Danlos syndrome or Marfan's syndrome) or a sero-positive arthropathy from the presence of rheumatoid arthritis (Slater *et al.*, 2013). The presence of gait disturbances, trips and falls, or an overtly anxious patient who has a tendency to want to support the head and neck may alert the sports therapist to upper cervical instability during the subjective assessment.

Management of suspected upper cervical instability following trauma involves immobilization of the neck and head with a collar, pending a radiological investigation. In more sub-acute or chronic clinical cases, the sports therapist should consider traditional instability tests such as the modified Sharp–Purser or tectorial membrane distraction tests. Although these tests are relatively safe to perform, the therapist needs to have sufficiently skilled palpatory awareness in order to detect an increase in motion or an empty end-feel in the upper cervical region. There is always a possibility of side-effects of testing, including lateral nystagmus, nausea or reproduction of neurological symptoms (Hutting *et al.*, 2013a). A systematic approach is needed for the assessment of cases of suspected upper cervical instability prior to any manual therapy intervention. The current approach combines active (patient generated) movements with passive movements and, where appropriate, overpressure, coupled with passive accessory movement tests. During the assessment process the sports therapist should aim to reproduce symptoms and to identify the degree of movement or restriction at each joint, which should help to identify the intactness of the ligamentous structures (Hutting *et al.*, 2013a). Positive findings require referral for orthopaedic assessment and radiographic imaging; operative treatment of cervical instability can include lateral mass fixation and use of cervical pedicle screws and facet joint wiring (Ogihara *et al.*, 2012).

Thoracic outlet syndrome

Thoracic outlet syndrome (TOS) results from compression (or traction) of the neurovascular structures in the supraclavicular fossa as they pass over the first rib; this can occur anywhere between the scalene muscles or under the clavicle. The neurovascular structures of concern include the brachial plexus (most common), subclavian artery, axillary artery, subclavian vein and axillary vein. Bayford (2009) suggests that TOS is actually a misnomer, as the scalene muscles, clavicle and first rib demarcate the thoracic inlet. The stereotypical demographic for neurogenic TOS are middle-aged females with underlying respiratory dysfunction and a forward head posture (Carnes and Vizniak, 2012; Hooks, 2012). Another cause of TOS is the presence of a 'cervical rib' – a congenital anomaly where an additional rib grows from the base of the neck above the first rib and clavicle (Laulan *et al.*, 2011). TOS may also be experienced by athletes who perform repetitive overhead movements such as swimming, volleyball, weightlifting, badminton and dance (Laulan *et al.*, 2011). However, it remains a nebulous condition as there are neither specific symptoms nor sensitive or specific investigations to confirm its presence; furthermore, symptoms vary depending on whether the condition is neurogenic, arterial or venous. Common neurogenic symptoms (relating to the brachial plexus) include pain, paraesthesia, anaesthesia, weakness and atrophy (in more established conditions) involving the intrinsic muscles of the hand (Laulan *et al.*, 2011). Arterial symptoms (following compression of the subclavian or axillary artery) can include: upper limb pain, paraesthesia and/ or claudication; pallor, cyanosis or erythema; upper limb coolness or pulselessness; cold hypersensitivity; and hypotension (Bayford, 2009). Venous symptoms (following compression of the subclavian or axillary vein) may include upper limb oedema and distension of superficial veins, in addition to symptoms mentioned above. Treatment strategies should be aimed at relieving compression (or distraction) of neurovascular structures by maximizing the potential outlet space and restoring normal movement and physiology (Bayford, 2009). Manual therapy may be used in the first instance to manage the symptoms of the neurovascular compression (Laulan *et al.*, 2011). Common techniques include Maitland (physiological and accessory) mobilizations (i.e. lower cervical, upper thoracic and upper ribs), neural mobilizations (via upper limb neurodynamic mobilization techniques) and soft tissue mobilization (targeting any involved restricted myofascia, such as scalenes or pectoralis minor). Grade III and IV Maitland mobilizations of the spine and thoracic outlet region are often used. The first rib may also be mobilized in conjunction with postural exercise (Twaij *et al.*, 2013). Advice includes avoidance of overhead activities. Excision of the cervical rib is the most common surgical approach, if necessary (Ferrante, 2012).

Spondylolysis and spondylolisthesis

Spondylolysis refers to a stress fracture or disassociation of the pars interarticularis, usually at L5. This may be unilateral, but if bilateral can lead to a spondylolisthesis, which refers to the (forward or anterior) displacement of one vertebra on another. Spondylolisthesis should not to be confused with a 'slipped disc' (which refers to herniation of an IVD) (Wright *et al.*, 2013). Spondylolysis in the cervical spine most commonly occurs at C2–3 ('hangman's fracture') and tends to result in a retrolisthesis (backward or posterior slippage), which if there is significant backward slippage can cause a myelopathy (spinal cord damage). Spondylolisthesis may be caused by congenital abnormalities, fractures (i.e. isthmic or spondylolitic spondylolisthesis) or degenerative disease (Wright *et al.*, 2013). Lumbar spondylolysis and spondylolisthesis are more common in sports involving repeated flexion or extension activities, with a high incidence in adolescent gymnasts, fast bowlers in cricket and athletes involved in contact sport (Wright *et al.*, 2013).

Spondylolisthesis also commonly presents in young adults whose symptoms are aggravated by exercise or mobilization. There is likely to be no resistance on palpation at the vertebral level of slippage, but severe stiffness at adjacent vertebral levels (Kalpakcioglu *et al.*, 2009). In severe cases a palpable step may be detected (observed or palpated) via spinous process positioning. Additional neurological signs may be present, dependent on the degree of slippage (Kalpakcioglu *et al.*, 2009). Operative management, if required, will involve stabilization of the spinal segment and prevention of neurological compromise (Aihara *et al.*, 2012). Conservative management may initially involve analgesic medication and a period of rest from aggravating activity. Grade I and II physiological and accessory mobilizations may be used to attenuate pain, and grade III and IV mobilizations to treat stiffness. Grade IV high-velocity, short-amplitude manipulations are contraindicated due to hypermobility of the vertebrae. A programme of specific exercise is recommended to improve the strength of the 'core' musculature and help stabilize the segment involved (Hardwick *et al.*, 2012; Kalichman and Hunter, 2008).

Spinal stenosis

Spinal stenosis is narrowing of the spinal canal and is categorized as primary (congenital) or secondary. Secondary spinal stenosis is more common and usually occurs as a result of degenerative processes, including degeneration of the IVD (central stenosis), osteophytic encroachment, or syndesmophytic encroachment due to hypertrophy of the posterior longitudinal ligament or ligamentum flavum (Kreiner *et al.*, 2013). Lumbar spinal stenosis results in compression of the cauda equina because the spinal cord terminates at L1 and usually presents in patients >65 years old with symptoms in the back and legs (Macedo *et al.*, 2013). There may be pain on standing, paraesthesia while walking, general complaints of heaviness in the legs, and nocturnal cramping in one or both legs. Symptoms are classically aggravated by extension and relieved by flexion and sitting, and the patient may have decreased lumbar lordosis (Macedo *et al.*, 2013). NSAIDs, opioids, GABA analogues (inhibitory neurotransmitters) or muscle relaxants may be prescribed for pain, in combination with manual therapy including grade III and IV mobilization techniques, active mobilizations (stretching of the back and hips), strengthening of the hip and core musculature and ambulation/coordination exercises (Macedo *et al.*, 2013). Patients failing to respond to conservative approaches may require surgery (May and Comer, 2013). Cervical spinal stenosis is caused by spondylosis, central herniation of IVDs, congenital stenosis and, in sport, by cervical acceleration–deceleration mechanisms (Tyrakowski *et al.*, 2013). Cervical spinal stenosis is serious because of the potential for compression of the spinal cord (cervical myelopathy) resulting in widespread symptoms such as bilateral tingling into all four limbs (Clark *et al.*, 2011). Cervical myelopathy presents earlier and is more common in men than in women. Symptoms include paraesthesia and/or anaesthesia into the limbs, heaviness in the legs, poor tolerance to activity/exercise, poor fine motor skills and intermittent electric shock-like symptoms into the extremities that are increased with neck flexion (L'Hermitte's phenomenon) (Clark *et al.*, 2011). Treatment is similar to that for lumbar spinal stenosis, and the use of a soft neck collar may prove beneficial. As cervical myelopathy progresses bowel and bladder dysfunction and quadriparesis may appear; in these cases surgical decompression is imperative (Chikuda *et al.*, 2013).

Disorders affecting the spine

Sports people may present with chronic back or neck pain owing to an underlying disorder of the spinal region (Jennings *et al.*, 2008). In older athletes this is commonly attributable to the presence of osteoarthritis, and in younger athletes can be attributable to an inflammatory arthritis (Jennings *et al.*, 2008). Inflammatory arthritides (plural of arthritis) are subdivided into sero-negative arthritis (where rheumatoid factor antibodies are not present in the bloodstream) and sero-positive arthritis (where rheumatoid factor antibodies are present in the bloodstream) (Jennings *et al.*, 2008). The four sero-negative arthritides are ankylosing spondylitis, enteropathic arthritis, psoriatic arthritis and Reiter's syndrome. Aside from ankylosing spondylitis, the other three sero-negative arthritides are usually associated with inflammatory bowel disease (such as Crohn's disease or ulcerative colitis), psoriatic skin or nail lesions, or urethral, gut or lung infections, which makes their detection easier (Jennings *et al.*, 2008).

Osteoarthritis

Osteoarthritis (degenerative joint disease) is a condition affecting the knees, hips, small joints of the hands and spine, where mechanical abnormalities of structures such as articular cartilage and subchondral bone result from degradation of joints (Friery, 2008). Common characteristic features of osteoarthritis are progressive degenerative change to articular surfaces (cartilage and subchondral), osteophyte formation (irregular bony growth on the articular margins), eburnation (smooth 'polished' subchondral bone) and mild synovitis (inflammation of joint tissue). Osteoarthritis of the spine is a common age-related condition in the vertebral column and is a common secondary consequence of prior injury (Friery, 2008). The prevalence in the general population has been estimated to be 43 per cent in individuals between 50 to 54 years, increasing to 77 per cent in individuals over 75 years of age (Arthritis Research UK, 2014). Spondylosis is the term to describe degenerative osteoarthritis of the joints between the spinal vertebrae and/or intervertebral foramina with calcification, osteophytic outgrowths and disc degeneration (Wendling *et al.*, 2013). Spondylarthrosis often occurs simultaneously with spondylosis as degenerative changes occur in the facet joints. Spondylosis and spondylarthrosis commonly occur in lumbar or cervical regions of the spine (Wendling *et al.*, 2013). The main symptoms are pain and stiffness, with reduced range of movement of the neck and back. Pain tends to worsen following periods of inactivity, especially at the beginning and end of the day (Swann, 2009). Spondylosis may cause narrowing of the spinal canal, intervertebral foramen, or osteophyte encroachment, and there may also be pressure on nerve roots. Thus, symptoms of spinal stenosis and/or nerve root involvement can present as radicular pain, paraesthesia and/or muscle weakness in limbs (Swann, 2009). Diagnosis is usually based on history and age of the patient; X-ray can usually confirm degenerative changes (Jennings *et al.*, 2008). Conservative management will normally involve prescriptive exercise. Pain-relieving treatments may be useful, including hot and cold therapies, TENS, soft tissue therapy and taping. Grade III and IV mobilizations may be used to help improve range of movement in the affected segment(s) (Wendling *et al.*, 2013).

Rheumatoid arthritis

Rheumatoid arthritis is a chronic, progressive, polyarticular, inflammatory, auto-immune disease affecting paired joints in the hand, wrist, feet, knees, shoulders and can affect the spine (Stark, 2013). Characteristics include widespread inflammation and destruction of joint synovium with unpredictable flare-ups when symptoms worsen (Stark, 2013). Periods of exacerbation and remission further characterize the condition. Rheumatoid arthritis affects over 580,000 people in the UK, affecting women more than men. Although the typical age of onset is 40–60 years, there are 12,000 children with the juvenile form of the disease. Presenting symptoms include bilateral joint swelling and pain, morning stiffness lasting >30 minutes, fatigue, weight loss and general malaise (feeling unwell) (Chamberlain, 2014). Systemic effects on the cardiovascular and respiratory systems may result in myocardial infarctions and cerebrovascular accidents (strokes) in severe cases (Stark, 2013). Involvement of the cervical spine, especially C1–2, is common and may be asymptomatic. This can have serious consequences as the disease tends to destroy joint structure, causing mild to severe instability/subluxation and cervical myelopathy in extreme cases (Stark, 2013).

Early diagnosis results in better prognosis and is made on the basis of history, joint involvement, and the presence of various biomarkers from blood tests (Chamberlain, 2014). Biomarkers include erythrocyte sedimentation rate (ESR) to differentiate rheumatoid arthritis from osteoarthritis and the presence of rheumatoid factor, an anti-citrullinated protein antibody (i.e. sero-positive) (Chamberlain, 2014). Treatment includes disease modifying anti-rheumatic drugs (DMARDs) and NSAIDs to manage inflammation (Palmer and El Miedany, 2014). Manual therapy may be useful to help reduce the effect of long-term joint destruction on mobility and includes joint mobilization, soft tissue therapy and active stretching alongside progressive rehabilitation (Iversen and Brandenstein, 2012). The use of Grade V manipulation is contraindicated due to the risk of instability, especially in the cervical spine (Slater *et al.*, 2013).

Ankylosing spondylitis

Ankylosing spondylitis is a progressive inflammatory arthritis of the spine that causes joint stiffness due to abnormal soft tissue adhesion and rigidity of bones (i.e. 'fusing together') (Bond, 2013). Bone rigidity may be caused by inflammation of soft tissues inside or outside the joint, and there may be destruction of the ligaments and tendons that attach to the bone in these spinal regions (enthesitis) (Bond, 2013). This erodes bony surfaces at these joints (enthesopathy). Repeated bouts of erosion and remodelling of bone around the joint causes restricted movement and eventual fusion of joint surfaces (Bond, 2013). Ankylosing spondylitis tends to affect the spine, although other joints can be involved. Individuals with ankylosing spondylitis are sero-negative and do not have rheumatoid factor antibodies in their blood. The condition often begins at the sacroiliac joints, and the lower back, thoracic cage and cervical region are also usually affected. The subjective assessment is used by the sports therapist to explore the possibility of this or other systemic inflammatory conditions causing the patient/athlete spinal symptoms. Symptoms associated with ankylosing spondylitis include:

- pain described as deep, gnawing or throbbing;
- pain that does not improve with rest;
- morning stiffness and pain >30 minutes;
- symptoms >3 months;
- a history of recurrent back pain;
- an onset <40 years of age;
- a family history of autoimmune conditions;
- enthesitis affecting the ankle, knees and ribs – commonly associated with inflammatory arthritis;
- the presence of a systemic condition including iritis, psoriasis, inflammatory bowel and peripheral joint involvement;
- alleviation of symptoms with NSAIDs.

Pharmacological management is aimed at reducing inflammation and symptoms using DMARDs, NSAIDs, corticosteroids and, in severe cases, anti–TNF medication (Bond, 2013). Non–pharmacological management employs active exercise and manual therapy to minimize mobility deficits and maintain muscle length and strength, improve posture and maintain lung function (Jennings *et al.*, 2008).

Principles for managing acute and subacute spinal injuries

Spinal symptoms may be managed non-conservatively (i.e. surgery), when there is an identifiable structural problem such as unstable fracture or spondylolisthesis, or where prolonged symptoms are resulting from a prolapsed IVD. Pharmacological interventions, including injection therapy, may be utilized when there is significant pain or inflammation present (Aihara *et al.*, 2012). Effective (and evidence-based) management of spinal symptoms can very often be achieved through a conservative approach by the sports therapist (Anubhav *et al.*, 2013). Early diagnosis is critical in terms of discounting red flags (Greenhalgh and Selfe, 2009); in the acute stage of an injury it may be difficult to identify vectors of movements for identifying tissues likely to be causing symptoms, so a greater reliance on thorough subjective examination is often warranted. The general principles of the conservative management of acute injuries includes protection, rest, ice, compression, elevation (PRICE). Protection involves the use of back and neck braces to reduce the mechanical load on pain-sensitive structures and the avoidance of prolonged flexion. In most situations, rest should involve remaining active but refraining from high spinal load activity that could cause further injury. Ice and cold therapies can be used to reduce pain and includes 'frozen peas' and commercially available sprays, gels and creams, with some evidence suggesting that heat may also confer similar effects. Compression and elevation are used to aid lymph drainage from limbs, although it is difficult to compress and/or elevate the back and neck without risk of serious consequence. Bleakley *et al.* (2012) recommend early inclusion of optimal loading (POLICE).

The most likely common symptom causing a sports person to seek advice from the sports therapist is pain. Pain is categorized in a number of ways. Acute pain is usually defined as the duration of an episode of pain persisting for fewer than six weeks; sub-acute pain as pain persisting 6–12 weeks; and chronic pain as pain persisting for 12 weeks or more (Ford *et al.*, 2011). Pain can also be classified according to the pathophysiological mechanisms involved; a predominantly nociceptive mechanism results from direct activation of tissue damage receptors (i.e. nociceptors) following trauma of peripheral tissues (Smart *et al.*, 2012). A predominantly neuropathic mechanism results from damage or malfunction involving neural tissue (i.e. neuropathies) (Enthoven *et al.*, 2013). Neuropathic pain can be identified by the words used by patients to describe their pain, such as burning, pins and needles, numbness and electrical shock-like. The S-LANSS ('Self-report Leeds Assessment of Neuropathic Symptoms and Signs') is a useful screening tool to identify neuropathic pain (Vining, 2012). During episodes of spinal pain, sports therapists may utilize pain-modulating techniques including hands–on treatments, cryotherapy or thermotherapy and electrotherapy (such as interferential therapy or TENS), alongside patient education. Hands–on techniques excite peripheral nerves and physiological research shows that this can inhibit onward transmission of nociceptive (pain-related) information en route to the brain, i.e. by 'closing the pain gate' (Mendell, 2014).

Principles for managing chronic spinal injuries

Acute pain is usually related to tissue damage (Darlow *et al.*, 2013). In contrast, chronic pain may result from ongoing tissue damage from underlying disease or degeneration; but it may also present without clear pathology (i.e. pain that persists beyond the expected time for healing of the original tissue damage) (O'Sullivan, 2012). Persistant pain in the absence of clear pathology has been associated with increased sensitivity of the nervous system (i.e. central sensitization) (Imamura *et al.*, 2013). Most chronic low back pain (CLBP) does not present as neuropathic and is not associated with red flags (Redwood, 2013). It is often impossible to make a specific pathophysiological diagnosis for CLBP; hence this may be described as non-specific CLBP (Redwood, 2013). Once sinister pathology has been discounted it is critical that the patient/athlete receives reassurance and education about the influence of a 'sensitized nervous system' in generating pain (Baron *et al.*, 2013). Individuals may have misguided beliefs about the cause of their pain and may begin to catastrophize about their condition, resulting in maladaptive coping strategies, including fear avoidance (Baron *et al.*, 2013). Careful attention should be paid to explaining pain mechanisms to persistent pain sufferers, which will contribute to a conducive mind-set for proactivity (Butler and Moseley, 2006).

Principles for a treatment-based classification in athletes with spinal symptoms

An alternative way of assigning athletes with spinal pain into sub-groups for the purposes of treatment is through the use of a treatment-based classification (Ford *et al.*, 2011; Apeldoorn *et al.*, 2010; O'Sullivan, 2012). Using this model, athletes are assigned to either a stabilization, mobilization or exercise category based on their presenting signs and symptoms. Research suggests that using targeted patient-centred interventions can lead to better outcomes in this population (Stanton *et al.*, 2013).

Stabilization classification approach

Patients are assigned to this intervention according to signs of segmental instability. Segmental instability is identified when an individual's symptoms vary from mild to severe, with very minimal perturbation. Athletes in this category usually have a history of mild to severe episodes of back pain with minimal perturbation. Aberrant active movements, positive active movement tests and excessive segmental mobility is noted when passive accessory movements are tested (Stanton *et al.*, 2013). Early exercise involves the athlete trying to regain motor control of the deep abdominal musculature (transverse abdominis) with co-activation of some of the deep mono-segmental spinal musculature (such as multifidus) using a pressure biofeedback unit and leg-loading exercises. Once effective motor control has been re-learnt the athlete is progressed into more dynamic exercises to replicate movement of a more functional nature (Stanton *et al.*, 2013).

Mobilization classification approach

This classification identifies a specific sub-group of individuals with spinal symptoms such as stiffness, movement restriction with or without pain, a specific movement pattern, a unilateral presentation to their symptoms and decreased specific segmental mobility (hypomobility) on passive accessory movement testing (Stanton *et al.*, 2013). Hands-on treatment involves manual therapy mobilizations. It is essential if the therapist is attempting to help make long-term tissue length changes that sustained stretching and mobilizing of soft tissues is prescribed as part of the athlete's management plan, with current evidence suggesting two minutes or more spent in each position (Seidenburg, 2014).

Exercise classification approach

Individuals in the exercise classification group will generally have progressed from stabilization or mobilization classifications and require further conditioning before being cleared to return to their normal training environment with the increased physiological demands (Ford *et al.*, 2011). Research suggests that an active lifestyle and regular exercise also reduces the re-occurrence of episodes of low back pain (Hayden *et al.*, 2005). Exercise prescription for individuals in the exercise classification group should focus on increasing physical loads and integration of a more dynamic motor control strategy, which is more akin to the demands of the athlete's chosen sport (Hides *et al.*, 2010). At this stage of the athlete's rehabilitation, closed kinetic chain multi-joint exercises (such as squats and deadlifts) should be selected, with an emphasis on dynamic trunk control and improving load tolerance (Moseley and Hodges, 2006). Nevertheless, there is insufficient good-quality evidence to support the view that specific modes of exercise consistently improve back pain when compared to other modes of exercise (O'Sullivan, 2012); exercises to strengthen 'core' musculature for prophylaxis and management of back pain have not reduced the incidence of back pain in the general population (Lederman, 2010).

Principles for use of manual therapy when treating spinal conditions

Generally, the choice of manual therapy for the spinal region is practitioner- and profession-dependent, due in part to the diversity of views about the relative merits of the different approaches (Anubhav *et al.*, 2013). Manual therapy techniques used when treating the soft tissues of the spinal region are grouped under the broad umbrellas of therapeutic massage or soft tissue therapy. These include the use of techniques such as effleurage, petrissage, tapotement, vibration, shaking, friction techniques, soft tissue release (STR), myofascial release (MFR), instrument assisted soft tissue mobilization (IASTM), manual lymphatic drainage (MLD) and neuromuscular techniques (NMT) (Fritz, 2005). Therapeutic stretching techniques aimed to lengthen soft tissues in the spinal region include active, passive, dynamic, maintenance and corrective stretching, and also include muscle energy techniques (MET) and positional release techniques (PRT) (Hammer, 2008). Manual therapy techniques used to ameliorate pain or re-establish normal range of joint movement in the spinal region include Maitland's mobilization techniques, Mulligan's mobilizations with movement (MWM) and sustained natural apophyseal glides (SNAG).

Soft tissue therapy

Soft tissue therapy involves manipulation of soft tissue and is popular both with patients and therapists. There are a wide range of methodologies, approaches and techniques. Soft tissue therapy has demonstrated reasonable effect in managing pain and disability in patients with sub-acute and CLBP, especially when combined with exercise and education (Furlan *et al.*, 2008). It has also been reported that 'trigger point therapy' appeared more effective than 'remedial massage' in these populations (Furlan *et al.*, 2008).

Therapeutic stretching

Therapeutic stretching employs techniques aimed at mechanically lengthening myofascia to achieve goals including pain relief from structural compression, joint malalignment, low-grade oedema and restriction (Lederman, 2014). It is claimed that therapeutic stretching improves soft tissue and segmental length and alignment; assists in normalizing range of joint movement; improves circulatory flow to dehydrated connective tissues; reduces low-grade interstitial oedema; improves movement control; and stimulates the production of tissue cells during repair (i.e. fibroblasts; myofibroblasts). In all of the studies to date in this area (Hayden *et al.*, 2005; Mayer *et al.*, 2005), exercise therapy with individualized regimes, including supervision, stretching and strengthening, were associated with the best outcomes.

Mobilization techniques

Mobilization techniques involve the therapist applying passive physiological intervertebral movement (PPIVM) or passive accessory intervertebral movement (PAIVM) to the structures forming joints, including the joints of the vertebral column (spinal mobilization), with an aim of producing at least short-term relief of pain and/or stiffness, and aiding the restoration of range of movement at a joint (Maitland *et al.*, 2005). The two main mobilization techniques used by therapists are Maitland's and Mulligan's techniques. The application of Maitland's mobilizations uses purely passive movements, with the patient/athlete's joints in an unloaded position (Maitland *et al.*, 2005). Mulligan's technique, on the other hand, uses combinations of active and passive movement (MWM) with the patient/athlete's joints in a loaded position (Mulligan, 1993; 2004). Maitland's mobilization techniques are most commonly used by sports therapists to re-establish motion between joint surfaces (i.e. utilizing the accessory movements of spin, glide and roll), and unlike Mulligan's technique, a grading system is used according to where in the range of movement the mobilization is applied and the amplitude of the mobilization (Maitland *et al.*, 2005). Mobilizations undertaken before the therapist encounters resistance from the ligaments, joint capsule and muscles surrounding and supporting the joint are referred to as being performed before resistance one (R1). Mobilizations undertaken from

R1 to the end of the available range of movement are described as being performed in resistance two (R2) (Maitland *et al.*, 2005). Sports therapists can be recommended to use grade I (small-amplitude mobilization before R1) and grade II (large-amplitude mobilization before R1) vertebral mobilizations to ameliorate pain, and these should be of short duration (i.e., less than two minutes), repeated once or twice in a treatment session and applied using a slow, smooth, rhythmic motion (Hengeveld and Banks, 2005). Sports therapists can use grade III (large-amplitude mobilization between R1 and R2) and grade IV (small-amplitude mobilization performed at the end of R2) vertebral mobilizations for several minutes, repeated several times within a session, using a quick, oscillating, rhythmic motion to ameliorate vertebral hypomobility (Hengeveld and Banks, 2005). A more detailed discussion of manual therapy principles is presented in Chapter 3.

Cervical spine mobilization

Any of the passive physiological or accessory intervertebral movement examination techniques described earlier (Maitland *et al.*, 2005) can be used as treatment techniques in the spinal regions (i.e. PPIVM and PAIVM). In the cervical region, longitudinal cephalad mobilizations may be considered with patients reporting radicular symptoms into their upper extremities to reduce the severity of neuropathic pain. Central posteroanterior mobilizations (CPAM) can be of most benefit to those patients whose cervical symptoms are situated either in the midline of the spine or distributed evenly to each side of the head or neck. Unilateral posteroanterior mobilizations (UPAM) can be performed on the same side of the patient's unilateral symptoms and, grade dependent, can be used to ameliorate pain or reduce stiffness. Transverse mobilizations may also be applied when dealing with unilateral symptoms of a cervical origin. When this technique is used for treating unilateral pain, the direction of pressure is often best applied from the non-painful to the painful side.

Thoracic spine mobilization

Mobilizations undertaken in the thoracic spine may be applied using similar principles and techniques to those used in the cervical spine. CPAMs are likely to produce a satisfactory outcome for symptoms arising in the midline, or when symptoms are evenly distributed to each side of the body (Maitland *et al.*, 2005). In all symptoms arising from the thoracic spine, it can be worth trying this procedure first. Transverse mobilizations can be useful for pain which is unilateral in distribution, particularly when applied from the non-painful towards the painful side. UPAMs are used almost entirely for unilaterally distributed pain arising from the thoracic spine and are applied to the painful side. Posteroanterior glides may also be applied to restricted or painful spinal segments, or costovertebral or costotransverse joints, via the involved rib (most commonly at their 'angle' – i.e. a few centimetres lateral to the spinal segment).

Lumbar spine mobilization

While there are a number of mobilization approaches for the lumbar spine, they should not be viewed as an exhaustive range of techniques to apply to any clinical encounter; they should merely form a basis from which the sports therapist can select an appropriate technique until such time as experience allows them to self-select based on the patient/athlete's symptoms, signs and pathology (Maitland *et al.*, 2005). CPAMs are often best used in the treatment of conditions of the lumbar spine that present with pain that is evenly distributed to both sides of the spine. UPAMs may be useful when there is a palpable muscle spasm identified in the deep intra-segmental muscles; and the technique is performed on the same side as the muscle spasm or pain. Transverse vertebral mobilizations can be of greatest value when dealing with unilateral symptoms, particularly when applying the transverse glide from the painless side towards the painful side. In this manner the joint of the painful side is opened.

Injuries and conditions affecting the spinal region are a common consequence of sporting participation and a common presentation amongst the general population. Sports therapists need to have a good working knowledge of the anatomy of the spinal region to aid assessment, diagnosis and management. While working in a clinical setting, sport therapists need to triage spinal symptoms to rule out the possibility of a serious pathology by identifying the presence of red flags. Sports therapists should also routinely screen for the presence of psychosocial yellow flags as these may predict the possibility of chronicity. The allocation of patients/athletes into a treatment-based classification based on their presenting signs and symptoms appears to improve outcomes in this population. Manual therapy for treatment of the spinal region may encompass soft tissue therapy and joint mobilization techniques in the early phases, alongside rehabilitation exercises designed to improve dynamic trunk control and load tolerance.

References

Abbott, J.H., McCane, B., Herbison, P., Moginie, G., Chapple, C. and Hogarty, T. (2005) Lumbar segmental instability: A criterion-related validity study of manual therapy assessment. *BMC Musculoskeletal Disorders.* 6: 56–10

Abrahamson, E., Egan, K. and West, L. (2012) Towards a conceptual model of clinical reasoning development in an undergraduate sports rehabilitation curriculum. *SportEX Medicine.* 51: 16–21

Adams, M., Bogduk, N., Burton, K. and Dolan, P. (2006) *The biomechanics of back pain,* 2nd edition. Churchill Livingstone. Edinburgh, UK

Aihara, T., Toyone, T., Aoki, Y., Ozawa, T., Inoue, G., Hatakeyama, K. and Ouchi, J. (2012) Surgical management of degenerative lumbar spondylolisthesis: A comparative study of outcomes following decompression with fusion and microendoscopic decompression. *Journal of Musculoskeletal Research.* 15 (4): 1

Aleksandrova, N.P. and Breslav, I.S. (2009) Human respiratory muscles: Three levels of control. *Human Physiology.* 35 (2): 222–229

Ansari, S., Heavner, J.E., McConnell, D.J., Azari, H. and Bosscher, H.A. (2012) The peridural membrane of the spinal canal: A critical review. *Pain Practice.* 12 (4): 315–325

Anubhav, J., Sreeharsha, V.N., Alejandro, M.L., Kern, S. and Yu-Po, L. (2013) Spinal interventions: The role in the athlete. *Operative Techniques in Sports Medicine.* 21: 185–190

Apeldoorn, A.T., Ostelo, R.W., van Helvoirt, H., Fritz, J.M., de Vet, H.C.W. and van Tulder, M.W. (2010) The cost-effectiveness of a treatment-based classification system for low back pain: Design of a randomised controlled trial and economic evaluation. *BMC Musculoskeletal Disorders.* 11: 58

Apostolos, S. (2013) Why are elite athletes suffering from low back pain? *Biology of Exercise.* 9 (2): 5–7

Arthritis Research UK (2014) *Arthritis information.* www.arthritisresearchuk.org/arthritis-information. aspx, accessed May 2014

Arun, B., Velusamy, M. and Sambandamoorthy, A.K.C. (2014) Role of myofascial release therapy on pain and lumbar range of motion in mechanical back pain: An exploratory investigation of desk job workers. *Ibnosina Journal of Medicine and Biomedical Sciences.* 6 (2): 75–80

Assenmacher, B., Schroeder, G.D. and Patel, A.A. (2013) On-field management of spine and spinal cord injuries. *Operative Techniques in Sports Medicine.* 21 (3): 152–158

Bacchus, H. (2011) Soft tissue considerations and treatment in sports-induced whiplash. *SportEX Dynamics.* 27: 17–23

Backhouse, K.M. and Hutchings, R.T. (1998) *Clinical surface anatomy,* 2nd edition. Mosby. St Louis, MO

Barakatt, E.T., Romano, P.S., Riddle, D.L., Beckett, L.A. and Kravitz, R. (2009) An exploration of Maitland's concept of pain irritability in patients with low back pain. *Journal of Manual and Manipulative Therapy.* 17 (4): 196–205

Barker, P.J., Urquhart, D.M., Story, I.H., Fahrer, M. and Briggs, C.A. (2007) The middle layer of lumbar fascia and attachments to lumbar transverse processes: Implications for segmental control and fracture. *European Spine Journal.* 16 (12): 2232–2237

Baron, R., Hans, G. and Dickenson, A.H. (2013) Peripheral input and its importance for central sensitization. *Annals of Neurology*. 74 (5): 630–636

Bayford, T. (2009). Thoracic oulet syndrome: An overview of diagnosis and treatment. *SportEx Medicine*. 44: 13–17

Benjamin, H.J. and Lessman, D.S. (2013) Sports-related cervical spine injuries. *Clinical Pediatric Emergency Medicine*. 14 (4): 255–266

Beresford, Z.M., Kendall, R.W. and Willick, S.E. (2010) Lumbar facet syndromes. *Current Sports Medicine Reports*. 9 (1): 50–56

Berthelot, J.M., Delecrin, J., Maugars, Y. and Passuti, N. (2007) Review: Contribution of centralization phenomenon to the diagnosis, prognosis, and treatment of discogenic low back pain. *Joint Bone Spine*. 74 (4): 319–323

Bleakley, C.M., Glasgow, P., and MacAuley, D.C. (2012) PRICE needs updating: Should we call the POLICE? *British Journal of Sports Medicine*. 46 (4): 220–221

BOA (British Orthopaedic Association) (2013) *Commissioning guide: low back pain – broad principles of the patient pathway*. www.boa.ac.uk/wp-content/uploads/2014/08/CCG_Low-Back-pain-final.pdf, accessed March 2015

Bond, D. (2013) Ankylosing spondylitis: Diagnosis and management. *Nursing Standard*. 28 (16): 52–59

Borghuis, J., Hof, A.L., Lemmink, K.A. (2008) The importance of sensory-motor control in providing core stability: Implications for measurement and training. *Sports Medicine*. 38 (11): 893–916

Broglio, S.P., Cantu, R.C., Gioia, G.A., Guskiewicz, K.M., Kutcher, J., Palm, M. and Valovich-McLeod, T.C. (2014) National Athletic Trainers' Association position statement: Management of sport concussion. *Journal of Athletic Training*. 49 (2): 245–265

Buck, R., Barnes, M.C., Cohen, D. and Aylward, M. (2010) Common health problems, yellow flags and functioning in a community setting. *Journal of Occupational Rehabilitation*. 20 (2): 235–246

Butler, D. and Moseley, L (2006) *Explain pain*. Noigroup Publications. Adelaide, Australia

Capra, G., Clough, A. and Clough, P.J. (2010) Clinical tests for the sacro–iliac joint: A literature review. *International Musculoskeletal Medicine*. 32 (4): 173–177

Carnes, M. and Vizniak, N. (2012) *Quick reference evidence-based conditions manual*, 3rd edition. Professional Health Systems. Canada

Chamberlain, V. (2014) Rheumatoid arthritis: Making an early diagnosis. *Practice Nursing*. 25 (2): 73–76

Chao, S., Pacella, M.J. and Torg, J.S. (2010) The pathomechanics, pathophysiology and prevention of cervical spinal cord and brachial plexus injuries in athletics. *Sports Medicine*. 40: 59–75

Chikuda, H., Ohtsu, H., Ogata, T., Sugita, S., Sumitani, M., Koyama, Y., Matsumoto, M. and Toyama, Y. (2013) Optimal treatment for spinal cord injury associated with cervical canal stenosis (OSICS): A study protocol for a randomized controlled trial comparing early versus delayed surgery. *Trials*. 14: 245

Cipriano, J.J. (2010) *Photographic manual of regional orthopaedic and neurological tests*, 5th edition. Lippincott, Williams and Wilkins. Philadelphia, PA

Clark, A.J., Auguste, K.I. and Sun, P.P. (2011) Cervical spinal stenosis and sports-related cervical cord neuropraxia. *Neurosurgical Focus*. 31 (5): E7–E7

Cook, C.E. and Hegedus, E. (2013) *Orthopaedic physical examination tests*, 2nd edition. Prentice Hall. London, UK

Darlow, B., Dowell, A., David Baxter, G., Mathieson, F., Perry, M. and Dean, S. (2013) The enduring impact of what clinicians say to people with low back pain. *Annals of Family Medicine*. 11 (6): 527–534

Davis, D.S., Anderson, I.B., Carson, M.G., Elkins, C.L. and Stuckey, L.B. (2008) Upper limb neural tension and seated slump tests: The false positive rate among healthy young adults without cervical or lumbar symptoms. *Journal of Manual and Manipulative Therapy*. 16 (3): 136–141

DeLaney, M., Booton, J. and Hernandez, D.A. (2013) Pediatric spinal trauma. *Pediatric Emergency Medicine Reports*. 18 (6): 65–75

Denegar, C.R. and Fraser, M. (2006) How useful are physical examination procedures? Understanding and applying likelihood ratios. *Journal of Athletic Training*. 41 (2): 201–206

Devin, L.P. and Puttlitz, C.M. (2012) The effects of ligamentous injury in the human lower cervical spine. *Journal of Biomechanics*. 45 (15): 2668–2672

Dimeglio, A. and Canavese, F. (2012) The growing spine: How spinal deformities influence normal spine and thoracic cage growth. *European Spine Journal*. 21 (1): 64–70

Drake, R.L., Vogl, W. and Mitchell, A.W.M. (2005) *Gray's anatomy for students*. Elsevier, Churchill Livingstone. Philadelphia, PA

Echemendia, R.J., Iverson, G.L., McCrea, M., Macciocchi, S.N., Gioia, G.A., Putukian, M. and Comper, P. (2013) Advances in neuropsychological assessment of sport-related concussion. *British Journal of Sports Medicine*. 47 (5): 1–7

Enthoven, W.T.M., Scheele, J., Bierma-Zeinstra, S.M.A., Bueving, H.J., Bohnen, A.M., Peul, W.C., Tulder, M.W., Berger, M.Y., Koes, B.W. and Luijsterburg, P.A.J. (2013) Back complaints in older adults: Prevalence of neuropathic pain and its characteristics. *Pain Medicine*. 14 (11): 1664–1672

Farley, A., McLafferty, E., Johnstone, C. and Hendry, C. (2014) Nervous system: Part 3. *Nursing Standard*. 28 (33): 46–50

Ferrante, M.A. (2012) The thoracic outlet syndromes. *Muscle and Nerve*. 45 (6): 780–795

Ferrari, R., Russell, A.S., Carroll, L.J. and Cassidy, J.D. (2005) A re-examination of the whiplash associated disorders (WAD) as a systemic illness. *Annals of the Rheumtic Diseases*. 64: 1337–1342

Ford, J.J., Thompson, S.L. and Hahne, A.J. (2011) A classification and treatment protocol for low back disorders: Part 1. Specific manual therapy. *Physical Therapy Reviews*. 16 (3): 168–177

Friery, K. (2008) Incidence of injury and disease among former athletes: A review. *Journal of Exercise Physiology Online*. 11 (2): 26–45

Fritz, S. (2005) *Sports and exercise massage: Comprehensive care in athletics, fitness and rehabilitation*. Elsevier, Mosby. Philadelphia, PA

Frohm, A., Heijne, A., Kowalski, J., Svensson, P. and Myklebust, G. (2012) A nine-test screening battery for athletes: A reliability study. *Scandanavian Journal of Medicine and Science in Sports*. 22 (3): 306–315

Furlan, A.D., Imamura, M., Dryden, T. and Irvin, E. (2008) Massage for low-back pain. *Cochrane Database of Systematic Reviews*. 8 (4):CD001929

Ghasemi, M., Golabchi, K., Mousavi, S.A., Farajzadegan, Z. and Shaygannejad, V. (2011) The value of provocative tests in diagnosis of acute and chronic cervical radiculopathy. *Journal of Isfahan Medical School*. 29 (143): 1–8

Greenhalgh, S. and Selfe, J. (2006) *Red flags: A guide to identifying serious pathology of the spine*. Churchill Livingstone, Elsevier. Edinburgh, UK

Greenhalgh, S. and Selfe, J. (2009) A qualitative investigation of red flags for serious spinal pathology. *Physiotherapy*. 95 (3): 224–227

Griessenauer, C.J., Raborn, J., Foreman, P., Shoja, M.M., Loukas, M. and Tubbs, R.S. (2014) Venous drainage of the spine and spinal cord: A comprehensive review of its history, embryology, anatomy, physiology, and pathology. *Clinical Anatomy*. doi: 10.1002/ca.22354

Guglielmi, G., di Chio, F., Delle Vergini, M.R., La Porta, M., Nasuto, M. and Di Primio, L.A. (2013) Early diagnosis of vertebral fractures. *Clinical Cases in Mineral and Bone Metabolism*. 10 (1): 15–18

Hammer, W. (2008) The effect of mechanical load on degenerative soft tissue. *Journal of Bodywork and Movement Therapies*. 12: 246–256

Hardwick, D., Tierney, D., Fein, C., Reinmann, S. and Donaldson, M. (2012) Outcomes of strengthening approaches in the treatment of low-grade spondylolisthesis. *Physical Therapy Reviews*. 17 (5): 284–291

Harmon, K.G., Drezner, J.A., Gammons, M., Guskiewicz, K.M., Halstead, M., Herring, S.A., Kutcher, J.S., Pana, A., Putukian, M. and Roberts, W.O. (2013) American Medical Society for Sports Medicine position statement: Concussion in sport. *British Journal of Sports Medicine*. 47 (1): 15–26

Haughton, V. (2011) The 'dehydrated' lumbar intervertebral disc on MR: Its anatomy, biochemistry and biomechanics (35th Annual Meeting of the European Society of Neuroradiology). *Neuroradiology*. 53: 191–194

Hayden, J.A., van Tulder, M.W., Malmivaara, A. and Koes, B.W. (2005) Exercise therapy for treatment of non-specific low back pain. *Cochrane Database Systematic Review*. 20 (3): CD000335

Hengeveld, E. and Banks, K. (2005) *Maitland's peripheral manipulation*, 4th edition. Elsevier, Butterworth Heinemann. London, UK

Hesse, B., Fröber, R., Fischer, M.S. and Schilling, N. (2013) Research article: Functional differentiation of the human lumbar perivertebral musculature revisited by means of muscle fibre type composition. *Annals of Anatomy*. 195 (6): 570–580

Hides, J.A., Stanton, W.R., Wilson, S.J., Freke, M., McMahon, S. and Sims, K. (2010) Retraining motor control of abdominal muscles among elite cricketers with low back pain. *Scandinavian Journal of Medicine and Science in Sports*. 20 (6): 834–842

Hill, J.C., Dunn, K.M., Lewis, M., Mullis, R., Main, C.J., Foster, N.E. and Hay, E.M. (2008) A primary care back pain screening tool: Identifying patient subgroups for initial treatment. *Arthritis Care and Research*. 59 (5): 632–641

Hooks, T.R. (2012) Cervical spine rehabilitation. In Andrews, J.R., Harrelson, G.L. and Wilk, K.E. (eds) *Physical rehabilitation of the injured athlete*, 4th edition. Elsevier, Saunders. Philadelphia, PA

Hutting, N., Scholten-Peeters, G.G.M., Vijverman, V., Keesenberg, M.D.M. and Verhagen, A.P. (2013a) Diagnostic accuracy of upper cervical spine instability tests: A systematic review. *Physical Therapy*. 93 (12): 1686–1695

Hutting, N., Verhagen, A.P., Vijverman, V., Keesenberg, M.D.M., Dixon, G. and Scholten-Peeters, G.G.M. (2013b) Review article: Diagnostic accuracy of premanipulative vertebrobasilar insufficiency tests: A systematic review. *Manual Therapy*. 18 (3): 177–182

Imamura, M., Chen, J., Suely Reiko, M., Targino, R.A., Alfieri, F.M., Kamura Bueno, D. and Wu Tu, H. (2013) Changes in pressure pain threshold in patients with chronic nonspecific low back pain. *Spine*. 38 (24): 2098–2107

Iversen, M.D. and Brandenstein, J.S. (2012) Do dynamic strengthening and aerobic capacity exercises reduce pain and improve functional outcomes and strength in people with established rheumatoid arthritis? *Physical Therapy*. 92 (10): 1251–1257

Iversen, T., Solberg, T.K., Romner, B., Wilsgaard, T., Nygaard, Ø., Waterloo, K., Brox, J.I. and Ingebrigtsen, T. (2013) Accuracy of physical examination for chronic lumbar radiculopathy. *BMC Musculoskeletal Disorders*. 14 (1): 1–9

Izzo, R., Guarnieri, G., Guglielmi, G. and Muto, M. (2013a) Biomechanics of the spine. Part I: Spinal stability. *European Journal of Radiology*. 82 (1): 118–126

Izzo, R., Guarnieri, G., Guglielmi, G. and Muto, M. (2013b) Biomechanics of the spine. Part II: Spinal instability. *European Journal of Radiology*. 82 (1): 127–138

Jackson, M.A. and Simpson, K.H. (2006) Continuing education in anaesthesia. *Critical Care and Pain*. 6 (4): 152–156

Jaromi, M., Nemeth, A., Kranicz, J., Laczko, T. and Betlehem, J. (2012) Treatment and ergonomics training of work-related lower back pain and body posture problems for nurses. *Journal of Clinical Nursing*. 21 (11/12): 1776–1784

Jennings, F., Lambert, E. and Fredericson, M. (2008) Rheumatic diseases presenting as sports-related injuries. *Sports Medicine*. 38 (11): 917–930

Jonasson, P., Halldin, K., Karlsson, J., Thoreson, O., Hvannberg, J., Swärd, L. and Baranto, A. (2011) Prevalence of joint-related pain in the extremities and spine in five groups of top athletes. *Knee Surgery, Sports Traumatology, Arthroscopy*. 19 (9): 1540–1546

Kalichman, L. and Hunter, D.J. (2008) Diagnosis and conservative management of degenerative lumbar spondylolisthesis. *European Spine Journal*. 17:327–335

Kalpakcioglu, B., Altınbilek, T. and Senel, K. (2009) Determination of spondylolisthesis in low back pain by clinical evaluation. *Journal of Back and Musculoskeletal Rehabilitation*. 22 (1): 27–32

Kavanagh, M. and Walker, J. (2013) Assessing and managing patients with cauda equina syndrome. *British Journal of Nursing*. 22 (3): 134–137

Keillar, E. and Dunleavy, K. (2013) Are we missing any patients with serious spinal pathology? *International Journal of Therapy and Rehabilitation*. 20 (10): 487–494

Kendall, F.P., McCreary, E.K., Provance, P.G., Rodgers, M.M. and Romani, W.A. (2005) *Muscles, testing and function with posture and pain*, 5th edition. Lippincott, Williams and Wilkins. Baltimore, MD

Koerner, J. and Radcliff, K. (2013) Spondylolysis in the athlete. *Operative Techniques in Sports Medicine*. 21 (3): 177–184

Kolber, M.J. and Beekhuizen, K. (2007) Lumbar stabilization: An evidence-based approach for the athlete with low back pain. *Strength and Conditioning Journal*. 29 (2): 26–38

Kountouris, A., Portus, M. and Cook, J. (2012) Quadratus lumborum asymmetry and lumbar spine injury in cricket fast bowlers. *Journal of Science and Medicine in Sport*. 15 (5): 393–397

Krassioukov, A. (2009) Autonomic function following cervical spinal cord injury. *Respiratory Physiology and Neurobiology*. 166 (3): 157–164

Kreiner, D.S., Shaffer, W.O., Baisden, J.L., Gilbert, T.J., Summers, J.T., Toton, J.F., Hwang, S.W., Mendel, R.C. and Reitman, C.A. (2013) An evidence-based clinical guideline for the diagnosis and treatment of degenerative lumbar spinal stenosis (update). *Spine Journal*. 13 (7): 734–743

Kumar, S.P. and Kumar, A. (2013) Treatment-based classification and low back pain-sharpening: The two-edged sword of clinical decision-making. *Journal of Physical Therapy*. 8 (1):1–4

Laulan, J., Fouquet, B., Rodaix, C., Jauffret, P., Roquelaure, Y. and Descatha, A. (2011) Thoracic outlet syndrome: Definition, aetiological factors, diagnosis, management and occupational impact. *Journal of Occupational Rehabilitation*. 21 (3): 366–373

Lederman, E. (2010) The myth of core stability. *Journal of Bodywork and Movement Therapies*. 14 (1): 84–98

Lederman, E. (2014) *Therapeutic stretching: Towards a functional approach*. Churchill Livingstone, Elsevier. London, UK

Loftus, S. (2012) Rethinking clinical reasoning: Time for a dialogical turn. *Medical Education*. 46 (12): 1174–1178

Loudon, J., Swift, M. and Bell, S. (2008) *The clinical orthopedic assessment guide*, 2nd edition. Human Kinetics. Champaign, IL

Loukas, M., Louis, R., Wartmann, C., Tubbs, R., Gupta, A., Apaydin, N. and Jordan, R. (2008) An anatomic investigation of the serratus posterior superior and serratus posterior inferior muscles. *Surgical and Radiologic Anatomy*. 30 (2): 119–123

Lowrie, M. (2013) The emergency spine: Part 2. Causes and diagnosis. *Companion Animal*. 18 (6): 288–293

Macedo, L.G., Hum, A., Kuleba, L., Mo, J., Truong, L., Yeung, M. and Battié, M.C. (2013) Physical therapy interventions for degenerative lumbar spinal stenosis: A systematic review. *Physical Therapy*. 93 (12): 1646–1660

Magee, D. (2008) *Orthopedic physical assessment*, 5th edition. Saunders. Philadelphia, PA

Maitland, G.D., Hengeveld, E., Banks, K. and English, K. (2005) *Maitland's vertebral manipulation*, 7th edition. Elsevier, Butterworth Heinemann. London, UK

Massalski, Ł. (2011) McKenzie's method of back pain classification. *Physiotherapy/Fizjoterapia*. 19 (3): 63–71

May, S. and Aina, A. (2012) Review article: Centralization and directional preference. A systematic review. *Manual Therapy*. 79 (6): 497–506

May, S. and Comer, C. (2013) Is surgery more effective than non-surgical treatment for spinal stenosis, and which non-surgical treatment is more effective? A systematic review. *Physiotherapy*. 99 (1): 12–20

Mayer, J.M., Ralph, L., Look, M., Erasala, G.N., Verna, J.L., Matheson, L.N. and Mooney, V. (2005) Treating acute low back pain with continuous low-level heat wrap therapy and/or exercise: A randomized controlled trial. *Spine*. 5 (4): 395–403

McCrory, P., Meeuwisse, W.H. and Aubry, M., *et al.* (2013) Consensus statement on concussion in sport: The 4th International Conference on concussion in sport held in Zurich, November 2012. *British Journal of Sports Medicine*. 47: 250–258

McDonnell, M. and Lucas, P. (2012) Cervical spondylosis, stenosis, and rheumatoid arthritis. *Medicine and Health*. 95 (4): 105–109

McKeever, C.K. and Schatz, P. (2003) Current issues in the identification, assessment, and management of concussions in sports-related injuries. *Applied Neuropsychology*. 10 (1): 4–11

Mendell, L.M. (2014) Constructing and deconstructing the gate theory of pain. *Pain*. 155 (2): 210–216

Meredith, D.S., Jones, K.J., Barnes, R., Rodeo, S.A., Cammisa, F.P. and Warren, R.F. (2013) Operative and nonoperative treatment of cervical disc herniation in national football league athletes. *American Journal of Sports Medicine*. 41 (9): 2054–2058

Moore, K.L. and Dalley, A.F. (2006) *Clinically oriented anatomy*, 5th edition. Lippincott Williams and Wilkins. Philadelphia, PA

Moseley, G.L. and Hodges, P.W. (2006) Reduced variability of postural strategy prevents normalization of motor changes induced by back pain: A risk factor for chronic trouble? *Behavioral Neuroscience*. 120 (2): 474–476

Mueller, S., Stoll, J., Mueller, J. and Mayer, F. (2012) Validity of isokinetic trunk measurements with respect to healthy adults, athletes and low back pain patients. *Isokinetics and Exercise Science*. 20 (4): 255–266

Mulligan, B. (1993) Mobilisations with movement (MVMs). *Journal of Manual and Manipulative Therapy*. 1: 154–156

Mulligan, B. (2004) *Manual therapy: NAGS, SNAGS, MWMs etc.*, 5th edition. Plane View Services Limited. Wellington, New Zealand

Muscolino, J. (2012) Lumbopelvic rhythm. *Journal of the Australian Traditional Medicine Society*. 18 (2): 85–87

Nandyala, S.V., Marquez-Lara, A., Frisch, N.B. and Park, D.K. (2013) The athlete's spine-lumbar herniated nucleus pulposus. *Operative Techniques in Sports Medicine*. 21 (3): 170–176

Nelson, N. (2012) Diaphragmatic breathing's influence on core stability and neck pain. *IDEA Fitness Journal*. 9 (3): 28–30

Nemani, V.M. and Han Jo, K. (2014) The management of unstable cervical spine injuries. *Clinical Medicine Insights: Trauma and Intensive Medicine*. 5: 7–13

Neumann, P., Keller, T., Ekstrom, L., *et al.* (1993) Structural properties of the anterior longitudinal ligament: Correlation with lumbar bone mineral content. *Spine*. 18: 637–645

Nicholas, M.K., Linton, S.J., Watson, P.J. and Main, C.J. (2011) Early identification and management of psychological risk factors ('yellow flags') in patients with low back pain: A reappraisal. *Physical Therapy*. 91 (5): 737–753

Ogihara, N., Takahashi, J., Hirabayashi, H., Hashidate, H., Mukaiyama, K. and Kato, H. (2012) Stable reconstruction using halo vest for unstable upper cervical spine and occipitocervical instability. *European Spine Journal*. 21 (2): 295–303

Osmotherly, P.G., Rivett, D.A. and Rowe, L.J. (2012) The anterior shear and distraction tests for craniocervical instability: An evaluation using magnetic resonance imaging. *Manual Therapy*. 17 (5): 416–421

O'Sullivan, P. (2005). Diagnosis and classification of chronic low back pain disorders: Maladaptive movement and motor control impairments as underlying mechanism. *Manual Therapy*. 10 (4): 242–255

O'Sullivan, P. (2012) It's time for change with the management of non-specific chronic low back pain. *British Journal of Sports Medicine*. 46 (4): 224–227

O'Sullivan, P. and Lin, I. (2014). Acute low back pain beyond drug therapies. *Pain Management Today*. 1 (1): 8–13

Palmer, D. and El Miedany, Y. (2014) Rheumatoid arthritis: Recommendations for treat to target. *British Journal of Nursing*. 23 (6): 310–315

Panjabi, M.M. (1992) The stabilizing system of the spine. Part I: Function, dysfunction, adaptation, and enhancement. *Journal of Spinal Disorders*. 5 (4): 383–389

Papa, J.A. (2012) Conservative management of a lumbar compression fracture in an osteoporotic patient: A case report. *Journal of the Canadian Chiropractic Association*. 56 (1): 29–39

Patel, S., Vaccaro, A.R. and Rihn, J.A. (2013) Epidemiology of spinal injuries in sports. *Operative Techniques in Sports Medicine*. 21 (3): 146–151

Payne, J.M. and Kirchner, J.T. (2014) Should you suspect the female athlete triad? *Journal of Family Practice*. 63 (4): 187–192

Petty, N.J. (2011) *Neuromusculoskeletal examination and assessment*, 4th edition. Churchill Livingstone, Elsevier. Edinburgh, UK

Porr, J., Laframboise, M. and Kazemi, M. (2012) Traumatic hyoid bone fracture: A case report and review of the literature. *Journal of the Canadian Chiropractic Association*. 56 (4): 269–274

Prescher, A. (1998) Anatomy and pathology of the aging spine. *European Journal of Radiology*. 27 (3): 181–195

Pujalte, G.G.A. and Floranda, E.E. (2012) Stingers and burners. *International Journal of Athletic Therapy and Training*. 17 (1): 24–28

Redwood, D. (2013) Chronic low-back pain. *ACA News (American Chiropractic Association)*. 9 (8): 14–18

Richardson, C., Jull, G., Hodges, P. and Hides, J. (1999) *Therapeutic exercise for spinal segmental stabilization in low back pain*. Churchill Livingstone. Sydney, Australia

Rodine, R.J. and Vernon, H. (2012) Cervical radiculopathy: A systematic review on treatment by spinal manipulation and measurement with the neck disability index. *Journal of the Canadian Chiropractic Association*. 56 (1): 18–28

Rutledge, B., Bush, T.R., Vorro, J., Mingfei, L., DeStefano, L., Gorbis, S., Francisco, T. and Seffinger, M. (2013) Differences in human cervical spine kinematics for active and passive motions of symptomatic and asymptomatic subject groups. *Journal of Applied Biomechanics*. 29 (5): 543–553

Sajko, S. and Stuber, K. (2009) Psoas major: A case report and review of its anatomy, biomechanics, and clinical implications. *Journal of the Canadian Chiropractic Association*. 53 (4): 311–318

Saraf-Lavi, E. (2014) Imaging of the brachial and sacral plexus. *Applied Radiology*. 43 (1): 5–10

Sarhan, F., Saif, D. and Saif, A. (2012) An overview of traumatic spinal cord injury: Part 1. Aetiology and pathophysiology. *British Journal of Neuroscience Nursing*. 8 (6): 319–325

Sato, K., Kikuchi, S., Yonezawa, T. (1999). *In vivo* intradiscal pressure measurement in healthy individuals and in patients with ongoing back problems. *Spine*. 24 (23): 2468–2474

Savigny, P., Kuntze, S., Watson, P., Underwood, M., Ritchie, G., Cotterell, M,. Hill, D., Browne, N., Buchanan, E., Coffey, P., Dixon, P., Drummond, C., Flanagan, M., Greenough, C., Griffiths, M., Halliday-Bell, J., Hettinga, D., Vogel, S. and Walsh, D. (2009) *Low back pain: Early management of persistent non-specific low back pain*. National Collaborating Centre for Primary Care and Royal College of General Practitioners. www.nice.org.uk/nicemedia/live/11887/44334/44334.pdf, accessed June 2014

Scaia, V., Baxter, D. and Cook, C. (2012) The pain provocation-based straight leg raise test for diagnosis of lumbar disc herniation, lumbar radiculopathy, and/or sciatica: A systematic review of clinical utility. *Journal of Back and Musculoskeletal Rehabilitation.* 25 (4): 215–223

Seidenburg, M. (2014) The role of modalities in chronic low back pain. *Rehab Management: The Interdisciplinary Journal of Rehabilitation.* 27 (2): 24–27

Sewell, D., Watkins, P. and Griffin, M. (2013) *Sport and exercise science: An introduction*, 2nd edition. Routledge. Abingdon, UK

Shah, K.C. and Rajshekhar, V. (2004) Reliability of diagnosis of soft cervical disc prolapse using Spurling's test. *British Journal of Neurosurgery.* 18 (5): 480–483

Sharp, J., Purser, D.W. and Lawrence, J.S. (1958) Rheumatoid arthritis of the cervical spine in the adult. *Annals of Rheumatic Diseases.* 17 (3): 303–313

Sharpe, L. and Van Horne, T. (2011) Cervical spine injuries in sports. *Hughston Health Alert.* 23 (1): 1–4

Shrier, I., Safai, P. and Charland, L. (2014) Return to play following injury: Whose decision should it be? *British Journal of Sports Medicine.* 48 (5): 394–401

Silva, A.G., Punt, D., Sharples, P., Vilas-Boas, J.P. and Johnson, M.I. (2009) Head posture assessment for patients with neck pain. Is it useful? *International Journal of Therapy and Rehabilitation.* 16 (1): 43–53

Siminoski, K., Lee, K.C., Jen, H., Warshawski, R., Matzinger, M., Shenouda, N., Charron, M., Coblentz, C., Dubois, J., Kloiber, R., Nadel, H., O'Brien, K., Reed, M., Sparrow, K., Webber, C., Lentle, B. and Ward, L. (2012) Anatomical distribution of vertebral fractures: Comparison of pediatric and adult spines. *Osteoporosis International.* 23 (7): 1999–2008

Sinha, P., Sedgley, L., Sutcliffe, D. and Timothy, J. (2010) Surgery for vertebral compression fractures: Understanding vertebroplasty and kyphoplasty. *British Journal of Neuroscience Nursing.* 6 (8): 377–382

Sizer, P.S., Jr., Brismée, J. and Cook, C. (2007) Medical screening for red flags in the diagnosis and management of musculoskeletal spine pain. *Pain Practice.* 7 (1): 53–71

Skovrlj, B. and Quresh, S.A. (2013) Management of cervical injuries in athletes: Timing of treatment. *Operative Techniques in Sports Medicine.* 21 (3): 164–169

Slater, H., Briggs, A.M., Fary, R.E. and Chan, M. (2013) Upper cervical instability associated with rheumatoid arthritis: What to 'know' and what to 'do'. *Manual Therapy.* 18 (6): 615–619

Smart, K.M., Blake, C., Staines, A., Thacker, M. and Doody, C. (2012) Mechanisms-based classifications of musculoskeletal pain: Part 3 of 3. Symptoms and signs of nociceptive pain in patients with low back (± leg) pain. *Manual Therapy.* 17 (4): 352–357

Spitzer, W.O., Skovron, M.L., Salmi, L.R., *et al.* (1995) Scientific monograph of the Quebec Task Force on whiplash-associated disorders: Redefining whiplash and its management. *Spine.* 20 (8 Suppl): 1S–73S

Stanton, T.R., Hancock, M.J., Apeldoorn, A.T., Wand, B.M. and Fritz, J.M. (2013) What characterizes people who have an unclear classification using a treatment-based classification algorithm for low back pain? A cross-sectional study. *Physical Therapy.* 93 (3): 344–356

Stark, S. (2013). *Rheumatoid arthritis.* Salem Press. Pasadena, CA

Stefanakis, M., Key, S. and Adams, M.A. (2012) Healing of painful intervertebral discs: Implications for physiotherapy. *Physical Therapy Reviews.* 17 (4): 234–240

Swann, J. (2009) Cervical spondylosis part 2: Coping with the condition. *British Journal of Healthcare Assistants.* 3 (3): 125–128

Sweeney, A. and Doody, C. (2010) The clinical reasoning of musculoskeletal physiotherapists in relation to the assessment of vertebrobasilar insufficiency: A qualitative study. *Manual Therapy.* 15 (4): 394–399

Tessitore, E., Molliqaj, G., Schatlo, B. and Schaller, K. (2014) Clinical evaluation and surgical decision making for patients with lumbar discogenic pain and facet syndrome. *European Journal of Radiology.* DOI: 10.1016/j.ejrad.2014.03.016

Todd, N.V. (2010) For debate: Guidelines for the management of suspected cauda equina syndrome. *British Journal of Neurosurgery.* 24 (4): 387–390

Twaij, H., Rolls, A., Sinisi, M. and Weiler, R. (2013) Thoracic outlet syndromes in sport: A practical review in the face of limited evidence – unusual pain presentation in an athlete. *British Journal of Sports Medicine.* 47 (17): 1080–1084

Tyrakowski, M., Nandyala, S.V., Marquez-Lara, A. and Siemionow, K. (2013) Congenital and developmental anomalies of the cervical spine in athletes: Current concepts. *Operative Techniques in Sports Medicine.* 21 (3): 159–163

Vilensky, J.A. (2014) The neglected cranial nerve: Nervus terminalis (Cranial Nerve N). *Clinical Anatomy.* 27 (1): 46

Vining, R.D. (2012) Is there an efficient tool to help identify neuropathic pain? *Journal of the American Chiropractic Association.* 49 (6): 7–9

Vizniak, N.A. (2012) *Quick reference, evidence-based physical assessment,* 3rd edition. Professional Health Systems. Canada

Vleeming, A., Schuenke, M.D., Masi, A.T., Carreiro, J.E., Danneels, L. and Willard, F.H. (2012) The sacroiliac joint: An overview of its anatomy, function and potential clinical implications. *Journal of Anatomy.* 221 (6): 537–567

Walsh, J., Flatley, M., Johnston, N. and Bennett, K. (2007) Slump test: Sensory responses in asymptomatic subjects. *Journal of Manual and Manipulative Therapy.* 15 (4): 231–238

Wendling, D., Claudepierre, P. and Prati, C. (2013) Early diagnosis and management are crucial in spondyloarthritis. *Joint Bone Spine.* 80 (6): 582–585

Wong, C.K. and Johnson, E.K. (2012) A narrative review of evidence-based recommendations for the physical examination of the lumbar spine, sacroiliac and hip joint complex. *Musculoskeletal Care.* 10 (3): 149–161

Wright, J., Balaji, V. and Montgomery, A.S. (2013) Spondylolysis and Spondylolisthesis. *Orthopaedics and Trauma.* 27 (4): 195–200

6

THE SHOULDER REGION

Anatomy, assessment and injuries

Anthony Bosson, Keith Ward and Ian Horsley

Functional anatomy of the shoulder region

In fit and healthy individuals the shoulder is the proximal powerhouse of the upper extremity, promoting dynamic capability and functional movement. Multi-muscular synergism, coordination and timing throughout the upper extremity facilitates lifting, lowering, pushing, pulling, twisting, turning, bending, carrying, striking and throwing movements. Connecting the sequential skeletal chain from the humeral head, scapula, clavicle and sternum, the shoulder is reinforced by the glenohumeral, acromioclavicular and sternoclavicular complexes and the unique scapulothoracic mechanism, and provides a strong foundation which supports both stabilization and movement of the head, neck, torso and arms. The dynamic shoulder enhances and facilitates effective sporting techniques and occupational movements, including: overhead reaching (e.g. volleyball; tennis; painter decorators); pushing (e.g. rugby; judo; hospital porters); pulling (e.g. swimming; rowing; trawlermen); crossing arms in front or behind the body (e.g. football; cricket; firefighters); and supporting bodyweight (e.g. weight-lifting; gymnastics; fitness instructors). Therefore, normal shoulder function is considered essential. Sports which demand optimal upper limb control expose the shoulder to extreme loading forces. The increasing demands of elite sport are exacerbated by long seasons and short rest periods (Fusco *et al.*, 2008). In order to avoid injury, all musculoligamentous structures must absorb the various forces and provide support to the shoulder; therefore recognition of these structures' individual functions and associations will assist the sports therapist to apply safe and effective management and prevention strategies in response to injury and pathological conditions so as to promote optimal performance in sport and functional activity, while enriching perception of wellness. Over 50 per cent of the human population experience at least one episode of shoulder pain on an annual basis; therefore, for the sports therapist, it is essential to develop sound anatomical knowledge and clinical skills for effective clinical assessment and management of this complex region (Lewis, 2009).

Surface anatomy of the shoulder

A number of superficial musculoskeletal structures are visible and/or palpable around the shoulder region (Backhouse and Hutchings, 1998). Anteriorly and superiorly, the horizontally oriented clavicles (collar bones) are relatively flat s-shaped bones with an anteriorly convex curve emerging from the central upper manubrium of the sternum, before posteriorly deviating to the acromion process with an anteriorly concave curve. Superior to the clavicle, anterior to the trapezius muscle belly and lateral to the neck is the supraclavicular fossa. The infraclavicular fossa is immediately below the clavicle. Located just lateral to the fossa is the coracoid process of the anterior aspect of the scapula. This process provides important, palpable attachment for the coracoclavicular, coracohumeral and coracoacromial ligaments, as well as for the pectoralis minor, coracobrachialis and biceps brachii (short head) muscles. The deltoid muscle is a prominent superficial muscle on the anterior aspect of the shoulder; it is also normally visible on the lateral and posterior aspects. The biceps brachii muscle is visible at the middle anterior aspect of the upper arm. While overlaid with breast tissue, the defined pectoralis major muscle originates from the sternum, costal cartilages and clavicle, and its tendon is predominately visible, anterior to the axilla (armpit). Jenkins (2009) highlights how the superficial fascia of the shoulder contains a variable amount of adipose (fatty) tissue, and this also encloses the glandular tissue of the breast. With regard to the shoulder region, the sports therapist must also appreciate the relationships and positioning of the sternum (particularly the central sternal body, the manubrium on the upper aspect and the distal xiphoid process), costal cartilages, thoracic rib cage, intercostal muscles and spaces, and the general relations of the shoulder girdle to the cervical and thoracic vertebrae, the local and global spinal/torso muscles and the internal organs of the chest and abdomen.

In the lateral view, the prominent acromion process (lateral lip) is visible both superiorly to the humeral head and laterally to the clavicle (at the acromioclavicular joint). The acromion provides the roof of the subacromial space and attachment for the deltoid muscle. Located centrally at the lateral aspect of the upper arm, the deltoid tuberosity may be palpated. The deltoid muscle itself possesses three heads – anterior, middle and posterior – which respectively originate from the lateral clavicle, acromion process and spine of scapula. The lateral aspect of the triceps brachii muscle is visible posteriorly on the upper arm and becomes more prominent with isometric contraction.

Posteriorly, the scapula (shoulder blade), despite its irregularities, is classified as a flat bone representing an inverted triangle on the posterior costal surface (thoracic wall). Visible posterior landmarks of the scapula include its spine, medial border, lateral border, superior angle (level approximately with T2) and inferior angle (T7). The spine of the scapula provides a pronounced inferomedial to superolateral ridge on which the attachment points for trapezius and posterior deltoid may be palpated. Above the spine is the supraspinous fossa, where the supraspinatus muscle originates; below is the infraspinous fossa, where infraspinatus originates. Posterolaterally, teres minor and major may be palpated emerging from the lateral border. The trapezius muscle is a distinctly large triangular-shaped muscle originating from the occipital protuberance and all cervical and thoracic vertebrae; it extends laterally towards the shoulder girdle to attach superficially at the spine of scapula, acromion process and lateral clavicle. Just underneath trapezius, situated between the lower cervical and upper thoracic vertebrae and the medial borders of the scapulae, are the rhomboid minor and major muscles, which may be prominent on some individuals. The large latissimus dorsi muscle is visible and bilaterally located in the mid and lower back, and gains definition at the inferolateral aspect of the axilla.

Skeletal anatomy of the shoulder

The shoulder or, more specifically, the glenohumeral joint, is a synovial ball-and-socket joint composed of a relatively spheroidal humeral head which articulates with the comparatively

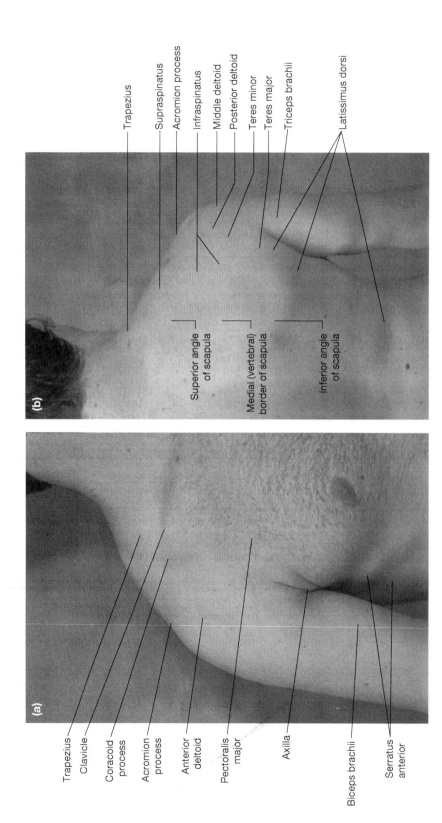

Trapezius

Supraspinatus

Acromion process

Infraspinatus

Middle deltoid

Posterior deltoid

Teres minor

Teres major

Triceps brachii

Latissimus dorsi

(b)

Superior angle
of scapula

Medial (vertebral)
border of scapula

Inferior angle
of scapula

(a)

Trapezius

Clavicle

Coracoid
process

Acromion
process

Anterior
deltoid

Pectoralis
major

Axilla

Biceps brachii

Serratus
anterior

Photo 6.1 Surface anatomy: anterior and posterior views.

shallow glenoid fossa of the scapula (Thompson, 2010). The scapula is a relatively large, flat bone resembling an inverted triangle with a prominent superior and inferior angle overlying ribs 2–7. The three finely laminated, almost translucent surfaces of the supraspinous, infraspinous and subscapular fossae are reinforced by five dense ridges located along the lateral and medial borders; the spinous (spine of scapula), coracoid and acromion processes; and the supraglenoid and infraglenoid tubercles immediately above and below the glenoid fossa, which is the articulation point for the humeral head (Gupta and van der Helm, 2004). As mentioned previously, the superior and inferior angles typically respectively align with T2 and T7. The resting position of the scapulae relative to the thoracic ribcage is approximately 30° of anteversion to the frontal plane; this is commonly referred to as 'the plane of the scapula' or as 'scaption' (Rockwood *et al.*, 2009). The acromion process is the relatively flat anterolateral extension of the spine of scapula which serves as a lever arm for the deltoid muscle and articulates with the lateral end of the clavicle to establish the acromioclavicular joint (Terry and Chopp, 2000). The acromion morphology can differ throughout the human population. Based on oblique sagittal MRI scans, type I remains flat inferiorly, compared to type II, which remains parallel to the humeral head with a convex inferior surface. A type III acromion presents as a 'hook-shaped' bone displaying up to 90° convexity at its anterior aspect, which reduces the subacromial space and can be associated with shoulder impingement (Mansur *et al.*, 2012). A type IV convex-shaped acromion (at its inferior distal end) has also been identified; however, research indicates this classification has no correlation with subacromial impingement syndrome (Chang *et al.*, 2006). The coracoid process projects anterolaterally from the superior aspect of the scapula in the infraclavicular fossa to provide the attachment for the coracoclavicular (conoid and trapezoid), coracohumeral and coracoacromial ligaments. The coracoid tip also provides origin attachment for the short head of biceps brachii and coracobrachialis, as well as insertion attachment of the pectoralis minor (Terry and Chopp, 2000).

As mentioned previously, the horizontally oriented clavicles are relatively flat s-shaped bones originating with an anteriorly convex curve from the manubrium of the sternum before posteriorly angulating to the acromion process with an anteriorly concave curve (Pansky and Gest, 2011). The clavicles act as struts supporting the anterior aspect of the shoulder girdle, maintaining space between the shoulder and thoracic ribcage, and acting as pivots for the muscles which promote lateral movement of the humerus (Rockwood *et al.*, 2009). The medial end of the clavicle has an articular facet and a small, flat, circular intra articular fibrocartilaginous disc that articulates with the clavicular notch of the manubrium (sternoclavicular joint), and inferiorly a small oval surface which articulates with the costal cartilage of the first rib (costoclavicular joint) (Johnson *et al.*, 2008). The lateral end of the clavicle also has an oval facet and small intra-articular fibrocartilaginous disc for articulating with the acromion process of the scapula. The inferior surface of the clavicle possesses two key attachment sites for the coracoclavicular ligaments. The more medial conoid ligament attaches to the conoid tubercle situated at the posteroinferior aspect of the clavicle from which the trapezoid line, an oblique anterolateral-oriented ridge, emerges to accommodate the more lateral trapezoid ligament (Johnson *et al.*, 2008). With the shoulder fully elevated, mobility at the sternoclavicular joint is exhibited by clavicular elevation to approximately 30°. In addition, the clavicle rotates approximately 50° about its longitudinal axis (Mirzayan and Itamura, 2004). Clavicular mobility at the acromioclavicular joint is restricted to approximately 5–8° rotation resulting from scapuloclavicular synchronization in which superior rotation of the clavicle is counteracted by downward rotation of the scapula (Ellenbecker, 2011). Interestingly, the clavicle is the first human bone to ossify during fetal development and is one of the most commonly fractured bones in the human population (Rockwood *et al.*, 2009).

The humerus is a long, cylindrical bone – the largest in the upper extremity. It articulates distally with the ulna and radius at the elbow joint, and proximally with the scapula at the glenoid fossa. Focusing on the middle aspect of the humerus, its compact shaft presents an abrasive attachment site on the lateral aspect where the three deltoid muscle bellies converge to insert. Ascending along the shaft, the bicipital groove emerges and eventually dissects the prominent greater and lesser tubercles which provide attachment sites for the rotator-cuff muscle complex – supraspinatus, infraspinatus and teres minor (greater tubercle), and the subscapularis (lesser tubercle). The bicipital groove also provides a protective, guiding passage through which the long head of the biceps tendon travels, while its lateral lip and medial lip provide respective attachment sites for pectoralis major and teres major. At the point where the cylindrical humeral shaft expands into the larger bony projection composed of the greater and lesser tubercles, the common fracture site known as the surgical neck is established. The relatively narrow neck is required to support upper limb activities and is frequently exposed to trauma, especially from powerful external force. The anatomical neck presents as an oblique groove which subtly divides the greater and lesser tubercles while creating an attachment site for the articular capsule and glenoid fossa. The highly vascularized humeral head posteriorly angulates 26–31° from the epicondylar plane and superomedially inclines 130–150° relative to the shaft at the anatomical neck to articulate with the shallow glenoid fossa, establishing the synovial ball and socket joint (Terry and Chopp, 2000).

Practitioner Tip Box 6.1

Skeletal landmarks of the shoulder region

Scapula

Superior angle

Inferior angle

Medial (vertebral) border

Lateral (axillary) border

Superior border

Suprascapular notch

Supraspinous fossa

Infraspinous fossa

Subscapular fossa

Glenoid fossa

Spinous process

Angle of acromion

Acromion process

Acromial articular facet

Coracoid process

Supraglenoid tubercle

Infraglenoid tubercle

Clavicle

Acromial end

Sternal end

Trapezoid line

Conoid tubercle

Humerus

Head of humerus

Articular surface

Anatomical neck

Surgical neck

Greater tubercle

Lesser tubercle

Intertubercular (bicipital) groove

Deltoid tuberosity

Table 6.1 Anatomical overview of the shoulder region

Average active ranges of movement (glenohumeral)	Flexion 160–180°
	Extension 50–60°
	Abduction 160–180°
	Adduction 35°
	Medial rotation 70–90°
	Lateral rotation 80–100°
Close-packed position	Abduction and lateral rotation (maximum range)
Loose-packed position	55–70° abduction
	40° abduction (scapula plane) (Hsu *et al.*, 2002)
	30° horizontal abduction
Capsular pattern	External rotation
	Abduction
	Internal rotation
Main ligaments	Superior glenohumeral
	Middle glenohumeral
	Inferior glenohumeral
	Coracohumeral
	Acromioclavicular
	Coracoclavicular (trapezoid and conoid)
	Coracoacromial
	Sternoclavicular
	Interclavicular
	Costoclavicular
	Transverse
Main bursae	Subacromial
	Subcoracoid
	Subscapular
Main accessory movements	Longitudinal caudad distraction of humerus
	Longitudinal cephalad compression of humerus
	Anteroposterior glide of humerus
	Posteroanterior glide of humerus
	Lateral distraction of humerus
	Anterioposterior glide of clavicle
	Posteroanterior glide of clavicle
	Cephalad glide of clavicle
	Caudad glide of clavicle

Articulations of the shoulder region

Glenohumeral joint

Located between the head of the humerus and the glenoid fossa of the scapula, this ball-and-socket joint provides exceptional ranges of motion and functional movements to suit athletes requiring extreme shoulder mobility (Hamill and Knutzen, 2009). The glenoid fossa provides an extremely shallow socket approximately 25 per cent of the size of the partially accommodated humeral head, 30 per cent of which articulates with the glenoid fossa on a continual basis to provide outstanding mobility. Excessive movement and potential dislocation is prevented by an intricate ligamentous complex and reinforced by ancillary dynamic stabilization via a unique musculotendinous mechanism which confines the humeral head to within 2 mm of the centre of the glenoid fossa (Terry and Chopp, 2000; Tovin, 2006). From a cross-sectional aspect, the fibrocartilaginous glenoid labrum exhibits triangular wedge-shaped characteristics which essentially deepens the cavity, protects the bone, assists with lubrication and provides increased articulatory capability and stability of the joint physically and also by helping to create a suction effect on the humeral head (Brukner and Khan, 2009; Johnson *et al.*, 2008; Rockwood *et al.*, 2009). Its fibrocartilaginous lip circumferentially attaches to the glenoid fossa ridge before enveloping the depth of the glenoid cavity and attaching to the articular surface to cushion the glenohumeral joint as it sustains movement forces (Thompson, 2010). Howell and Galiant (1989) identified that the labrum may increase fossa depth by 5 mm anteroposteriorly and 9 mm superoinferiorly. Anatomical variations include labral attachments which are meniscoid, with a free lip overlapping the glenoid ridge towards the articular attachment. This normal anatomical variation is occasionally misdiagnosed as a lesion during MRI. Lippitt and Matsen (1993) identified that an intact labrum will provide significantly greater protection against dislocation. Repetitive overhead sports movements or traumatic impact often predisposes the meniscoid labrum to a type III superior labral anteroposterior (SLAP) lesion (Wilk *et al.*, 2013).

The glenohumeral joint is encapsulated by a loose synovial joint capsule which originates from the glenoid neck and labrum, extending towards the anatomical neck (proximal shaft) of the humerus, coracoid process and the anteroposterior recesses of the scapular body. The capsule is reinforced by the rotator-cuff complex, except the inferior aspect which remains prone to laxity, resulting in a prevalence of inferior dislocation or subluxation (Rockwood *et al.*, 2009; Wilk *et al.*, 2006). High osmotic pressure within the interstitial tissues draws fluid from the glenohumeral joint, creating a vacuum of negative intra-articular pressure (NIP). The ensuing suction effect on the articular surfaces increases static stability and prevents displacement of the humeral head (Hurschler *et al.*, 2000). NIP has been shown to alter in relation to glenohumeral position (approximately 83 mmHg at 20° abduction, and 10 mmHg at 80°) (Inokuchi *et al.*, 1997). NIP also typically reduces in patients with severe rotator-cuff deficits (Lewis, 2006), and can become significantly ineffective when dynamic stabilization is compromised or with glenohumeral ligamentous laxity (Iannotti and Williams, 2007) as defects in the tissue surrounding the capsule allow atmospheric pressure into the joint. Originating from the supraglenoid tubercle, and protected by a synovial sheath, the long head of biceps tendon penetrates the extended joint capsule, travelling within the structure before evolving into the biceps brachii muscle (DePalma and Brand, 2008).

Reinforcement for sustaining increased forces is provided by three anterior focal thickenings, or capsular ligaments, referred to as the superior glenohumeral ligament (SGHL), middle (MGHL) and inferior (IGHL), which provide static stabilization and help to prevent excessive translation or displacement of the humeral head. While anatomical variations have been observed, the SGHL generally originates from the anterosuperior labrum, the attachment point for long head of biceps tendon, before merging with the coracohumeral ligament (CHL) and inserting onto the lesser tubercle of the humerus. The MGHL originates from the glenoid neck or anterosuperior labrum. Compared to the weak shoulder stabilization attributes of the SGHL, the MGHL predominantly acts as a secondary shoulder stabilizer but is frequently compromised following anterior glenohumeral dislocation. The most significant ligament of the capsulolabral complex is the IGHL, which originates from the entire inferior glenoid labrum before dividing into two collagenous bands which act as a supportive hammock-like sling around the anterior and posterior aspects of the humeral neck to stabilize the shoulder during abduction and external rotation (Chang *et al.*, 2008; Thompson, 2010).

The superior aspect of the glenohumeral joint is secured by the coracohumeral ligament (CHL). From the lateral base of the coracoid process, two independent bands attach superiorly to both sides of the bicipital groove, to the lesser tubercle (anterior band) and to the greater

Table 6.2 Glenohumeral ligaments and functions

Ligament	Attachments	Function
Superior (SGHL)	Anterosuperior glenoid labrum to proximal lesser tubercle	Resists anterior translation and external rotation in shoulder adduction. Resists posterior translation in 90° of forward flexion
Middle (MGHL)	Anterosuperior glenoid labrum (inferior to SGHL) to medial lesser tubercle	Resists anteroposterior translation in 45° of abduction. Secondary restraint to translation and external rotation in shoulder adduction
Inferior (IGHL)	Anterior glenoid labrum to inferior humeral neck (AIGHL)	Resists anterior and inferior translation in abduction and external rotation
	Posterior glenoid labrum to inferior humeral neck (PIGHL)	Resists posterior translation in internal rotation and 90° flexion

Source: adapted from Thompson, 2010.

tubercle (posterior band). The CHL combines with the SGHL to promote stability and resistance against inferior translation of the humeral head as the arm rests in adduction. Both ligaments also serve as a pulley system which stabilizes the biceps tendon as it negotiates the bicipital groove (Cael, 2010; Thompson, 2010). The transverse humeral ligament is simply a band of connective tissue crossing between the two tubercles of the humerus, effectively providing a restraining retinacula for the long head of biceps brachii (Johnson *et al.*, 2008).

There are a number of bursae present around the glenohumeral joint. Without bursae, many musculotendinous structures would deteriorate from continuous friction against bony surfaces. Bursae are fibrous fluid-filled sacs protected by a sheath which secretes the synovial-like fluid to promote gliding of muscles and tendons over the bony attachment sites and ligamentous surfaces (Foglia and Musarra, 2008). Numerous bursae exist proximal to the shoulder muscles. The subacromial bursa separates the glenohumeral joint capsule from the inferior aspect of the acromion process and occasionally coexists with the subdeltoid bursa interacting with the inferior surface of the coracoacromial ligament and the superior surface of the supraspinatus tendon, preventing friction of the rotator-cuff complex against the inferior aspect of the acromion process during shoulder abduction and flexion (Hutson and Speed, 2011). The subcoracoid bursa separates the glenohumeral joint capsule from the coracoid process (Cael, 2010) and is located deep to the coracohumeral ligament (Foglia and Musarra, 2008). Commonly connecting with the glenohumeral joint cavity, it can be located between the superior portion of the subscapularis muscle and the neck of glenoid as it prevents friction of the subscapularis, coracobrachialis and short head of biceps tendons (Hutson and Speed, 2011). The subscapular bursa, situated on the inferior aspect of the glenohumeral joint, is suspended from the coracoid process by a suspensory ligament which separates and protects the subscapularis tendon from the neck of scapula and prevents further friction against the glenohumeral joint capsule through which it penetrates, passing between the SGHL and MGHL. In some anatomical variations, the subscapular bursa fuses with the subcoracoid bursa, creating a significantly wider bursa (Rockwood *et al.*, 2009).

Movements of the glenohumeral joint
Similar to the femoroacetabular joint of the hip, the glenohumeral joint is a multi-axial synovial ball-and-socket joint; it is formed with the less congruent articulation of the humeral head and

the glenoid fossa. Occurring in the sagittal plane (frontal axis) shoulder flexion and extension end-range of movement parameters are considered to be 160–180° and 40–60°, respectively. Shoulder abduction and adduction occur in the frontal plane (about a sagittal axis) and reach end-range parameters of 160–180° and 30–40°, respectively (Kenyon and Kenyon, 2009; Vizniak, 2012). By maintaining a 90° flexed elbow and upper arm adjacent to the costal surface, lateral rotation draws the anterior aspect of the humerus 80–100° away from the mid-sagittal plane as internal rotation reverses the process towards end-range parameters of 70–90° – this may be achieved with the forearm behind the trunk and the shoulder in a slightly extended position. Other movements include horizontal flexion (horizontal adduction), horizontal extension (horizontal abduction) and circumduction provided by the combination of multidirectional actions commonly seen in swimming and water polo (Tovin, 2006). Virtually all glenohumeral movements require associated movement from the other joints of the shoulder girdle; and functionally, the sports therapist must appreciate the scapulohumeral rhythm (SHR) which is the relationship and ratio of movement occurring via the glenohumeral and scapulothoracic articulations in conjunction during shoulder elevation. SHR serves to preserve length–tension relationships of the glenohumeral muscles. As the arm is being elevated and the girdle muscles control scapula rotation, the GH muscles are better able to sustain their force production (Magee, 2014).

Acromioclavicular joint

Located between the lateral (acromial) end of the clavicle and the medial facet of the acromion process, the diarthrodial acromioclavicular (AC) joint accommodates the majority of scapular movements which occur on the clavicle (Hamill and Knutzen, 2009). This synovial gliding joint located superior to the humeral head has approximately 3° of freedom and is inherently protected by an incomplete fibrocartilaginous articular disc (meniscus) of varying morphology (Ellenbecker, 2006) and a joint capsule which, despite acting as a weak stabilizer, does provide sufficient support during daily activities (Thompson, 2010). The dense capsule of the AC joint is strengthened by the superior AC ligament, which is reinforced by the myofascia of the deltoid and trapezius and the inferior AC ligament, which integrates with fibres of the coracoacromial ligament (Miller and Cole, 2004) to provide dynamic stabilization capable of absorbing large contact stresses imposed by intense axial loads (Terry and Chopp, 2000) and preventing anteroposterior joint separation in the process (MacDonald and LaPointe, 2008). Although the AC joint is indirectly stabilized by the coracoclavicular ligaments comprising of the conoid and trapezoid, AC ligaments primarily support the joint during minimal low-load movements. The AC joint also provides bony restriction during overhead arm action and functions as a pivot joint assisting the clavicular strut mechanism (Hamill and Knutzen, 2009).

Preventing anteroposterior separation of the lateral clavicle and acromion process of the scapula, the horizontally flattened fibres of the AC ligament reinforce dynamic stability and offer prevention against anterior to posterior force translation and axial distraction (Ellenbecker, 2006; MacDonald and LaPointe, 2008). Two ligamentous bands encompass the AC joint, providing reinforcement of the joint and its capsule. The superior AC ligament is a quadrilateral band extending from the superior aspect of the clavicle onto the acromion process of the scapula. Its parallel fibres are interspersed with the aponeurotic fascia of the deltoid and trapezius muscles, which enhances its tensile integrity. The inferior surface retains contact with the articular disc. Despite being comparably thinner, the inferior AC ligament provides corresponding attachments on the inferior aspect of the clavicle and acromion process, with some fibres integrating with the coracoacromial ligament (Miller and Cole, 2004). During anterior rotation of the sternal end of the clavicle relative to the vertical axis of the AC joint, the posterior section of the AC ligament increases in length. In contrast, posterior clavicular rotation about the frontal axis increases laxity in the posterior section, which initiates a stretch response from the anterior section (Di Giacomo *et al.*, 2008). Functioning as indirect vertical stabilizers to the clavicle at the AC joint, the coracoid anchoring mechanism, comprising the conoid and trapezoid ligaments, forms the coracoclavicular ligament complex which adjoins the coracoid process and inferior clavicle (Palastanga and Soames, 2012). Located medial to the trapezoid, the conoid ligament possesses stronger resistance to vertical loading as its vertical fibres from the inferior clavicle to the superior base of the coracoid process prevent superior migration of the clavicle (Thompson, 2010). In contrast, the slightly oblique alignment of the trapezoid ligament fibres travelling inferiorly and medially to the superior aspect of the coracoid process contribute greater resistance against axial loading forces transmitted across the shoulder (Thompson, 2010). In the absence of AC integrity, the coracoclavicular ligaments provide support to the capsule; however, their vertical orientation does not provide substantial resistance against anteroposterior translation (Miller and Cole, 2004).

The coracoacromial arch comprising the acromion and coracoid processes is established by the distal (coracoid) to anteroinferior (acromion) attachment of the coracoacromial ligament responsible for stabilizing the humeral head within the glenoid fossa during overhead movements, particularly in abduction when supraspinatus and deltoids combine. The coracoacromial ligament also prevents humeral head migration in the rotator–cuff–deficient shoulder (Thompson, 2010). This restriction mechanism may provoke impingement of the surgical neck of the humerus on the coracoid process and anterior coracoacromial ligament or against the inferior aspect of the acromion process, resulting in a respective decrease of flexion and extension. Similarly, abduction may be compromised by impingement of the greater tubercle on the coracoacromial ligament.

Sternoclavicular joint

Located between the medial (sternal) end of the clavicle and the manubrium of the sternum, the sternoclavicular (SC) joint exists as the only true attachment between the upper extremity and the axial skeleton. The diarthrodial (double) SC joint retains rotatory freedom in the frontal plane (i.e. shoulder elevation and depression) and in the transverse plane (i.e. shoulder protraction and retraction). Possessing both the structural and functional characteristics of synovial saddle and gliding joints, the SC also demonstrates ball and socket joint characteristics by facilitating up to 50° of clavicular rotation on the fixed sternum. The SC joint capsule is reinforced by anterior, superior and posterior capsular ligaments, the latter being the strongest. Adjoining the inferior aspect of the clavicle to the first costal cartilage proximal to the SC joint, the costoclavicular ligaments emerge as the strongest SC ligament while providing additional indirect stabilization (Terry and Chopp, 2000). The anterior band fibres travel inferiorly and medially while the posterior band fibres travel inferiorly and laterally before attaching to the costal cartilage of the first rib. The SC joint is protected by a complete articular disc attached superiorly to the superior aspect of the medial end of the clavicle, inferiorly to the costal cartilage of the first rib and to the existing circumference of the joint capsule itself. This attachment allows the disc, joint capsule and posterior band of the costoclavicular ligament to strongly resist forces transmitted along the clavicle towards the axial skeleton (Thompson, 2010).

Scapulothoracic joint

The scapulothoracic (ST) joint involving the articulation of the scapula on the rib cage is one of the least congruent joints in the body and may arguably not be classified as a true joint as most joints connect directly bone to bone (Hamill and Knutzen, 2009; Paine and Voight, 2013). The ST joint provides elevation, depression, retraction, protraction, upward (lateral) rotation, downward (medial) rotation and anterior and posterior tilting – all in conjunction with varying degrees of associated girdle and glenohumeral movement. Regarded more as a functional mechanism, this unique joint requires the atypical articulation between other physiological structures including muscles, bursae and neurovascular interventions which allow the costal surface of the scapula to glide and rotate smoothly over the posterior axial ribcage (Terry and Chopp, 2000). Located between the ribcage and scapula, the serratus anterior and subscapularis muscles attach to the costal surface of the scapula. Both muscles are able to translate across each other to facilitate the functional gliding movement of the scapula (Hamill and Knutzen, 2009).

Functionally, in relation to the ribcage, the scapulothoracic articulation presents as an additional joint which enables increased humeral rotation (Gupta and van der Helm, 2004) beyond the 120° flexion and abduction initiated solely by the glenohumeral joint. During shoulder flexion or abduction, a further 60° of motion is provided (Gupta and van der Helm, 2004). The initial 30° of shoulder abduction is performed predominently by the glenohumeral joint while the scapula remains in its neutral position. Upward (or lateral) rotation of the scapula then commences to assist scapulohumeral rhythm (SHR) and, in simple terms, for every single degree of scapulothoracic elevation, two degrees of glenohumeral elevation ensues. The significant mobility provided by the AC and SC joints reinforces the scapulothoracic mechanism to enhance optimal congruency of the humeral head and glenoid fossa throughout all ranges of movement relative to the axial skeleton (Terry and Chopp, 2000).

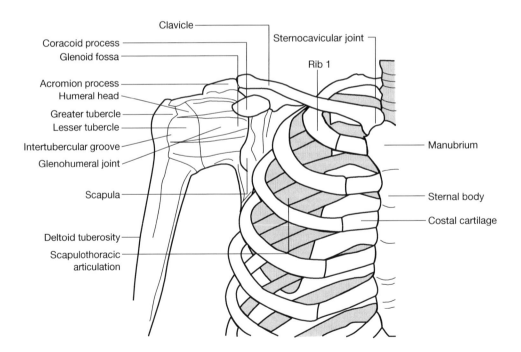

Figure 6.1   Skeletal anatomy: anterior view.

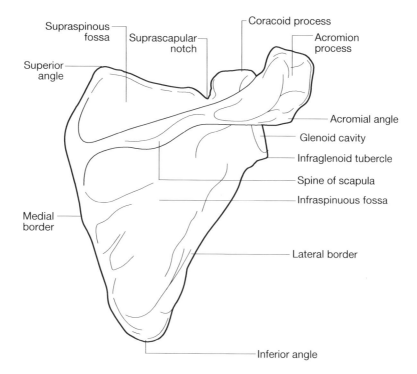

Figure 6.2 Skeletal anatomy: posterior view.

Muscular anatomy of the shoulder region

As the shoulder girdle and upper arm incorporate a number of joints (i.e. specifically the GH, AC, SC and ST joints, in addition to the related cervical, upper thoracic spinal and elbow regions) there are numerous muscles and muscle actions to consider. Seventeen muscles attach to the scapula body (Terry and Chopp, 2000). The rotator-cuff complex comprises supraspinatus, infraspinatus, teres minor and subscapularis (the 'SITS' muscles). These interdigitate and blend with the articular capsule, coracohumeral and glenohumeral ligaments to form a fascial sheet prior to their respective humeral attachment. Despite such reinforcement, dynamic shoulder stability, compression and centring of the humeral head on the glenoid is predominantly sustained by these four muscles alone, each having a specific role in positioning the humeral head in preparation for the various shoulder movements (Lewis, 2009; Matava *et al.*, 2005). Within the subacromial space, the two surfaces of the cuff are different – the deeper, bursal surface is more susceptible to irritating compression (as in subacromial impingement syndrome – [SIS]), while the superficial articular surface is more vulnerable to tears (McConnell, 2002). It is important to recognize that not all shoulder muscles attach directly to the upper arm. All main shoulder muscles will be discussed in the following section.

Supraspinatus

Originating from the supraspinous fossa of the scapula and inserting onto the greater tubercle of the humerus, the supraspinatus is innervated by the suprascapular nerve (C5–6) and contributes to the initiation of shoulder abduction. Reed *et al.* (2013) emphasize that it is misleading to state that supraspinatus is the sole initiator of shoulder abduction. Their electromyographic (EMG) study showed how supraspinatus is indeed recruited prior to movement of the humerus into abduction, but not any earlier than other shoulder muscles (including infraspinatus, deltoid and axioscapular muscles, which attach the scapula to the thorax). Reed *et al.* (2013) also identified that altering load or plane of movement made no significant change to their findings. Supraspinatus continues to assist the deltoid as it resumes abduction from 30° onwards; it is also recruited during flexion and rotation movements. Supraspinatus inferiorly stabilizes the humeral head within the glenoid fossa to prevent upward shearing forces or impingement against the inferior aspect of the acromion process, subacromial bursa and the supraspinatus tendon. Due to its exposed location, supraspinatus is predisposed to tendinopathy, impingement and potential rupture, accompanied by total incapacitation of the entire rotator-cuff complex (Palastanga and Soames, 2012).

Infraspinatus

The specific role of infraspinatus requires co-contraction with teres minor to posteriorly restrain the humeral head within the glenoid fossa to prevent anterior impingement on the coracoid process of scapula and posterior subluxation. Originating from the infraspinous fossa of the scapula and inserting onto the posterior greater tubercle of the humerus, it is acknowledged as an external rotation powerhouse receiving innervation from the suprascapular nerve (C5–6). The infraspinatus provides a crucial force-loading mechanism, while the shoulder and upper extremity is posteriorly extended with external rotation in preparation for various throwing or striking techniques (such as throwing a cricket ball from distance or a forearm return in tennis). During such explosive actions, essential deceleration is required once the projectile has been thrown or struck, therefore infraspinatus is recruited further for eccentric deceleration during the follow-through phase to alleviate the momentum distraction forces imposed on the shoulder (Houglum, 2010).

Teres minor

In addition to providing posterior restraint of the humeral head, teres minor combines with latissimus dorsi, teres major and the relatively horizontal costal fibres of pectoralis major in controlling the descent of the raised arm following overhead techniques of reaching, striking and throwing. A synergistic relationship with infraspinatus also serves to eccentrically decelerate the shoulder during the follow-through phase of striking or throwing. Despite sharing similar origins, teres minor should not be comparatively associated with teres major (inferior lateral border of scapula) as it actually performs antagonistically as an external rotator having originated from the superior lateral border of scapula prior to insertion at the greater tubercle of the humerus. The teres minor muscle is innervated by the posterior branch of the axillary nerve (C5–6).

Subscapularis

The largest rotator-cuff muscle is the subscapularis. Anteriorly, it confines the humeral head in the glenoid fossa, minimizing anterior translation and creating optimal congruency during the powerful movements initiated by pectoralis major, anterior deltoid, latissimus dorsi and teres major as they control the descending arm during pulling actions (such as during butterfly swimming or rowing). Innervated by the upper and lower subscapular nerves (C5–6), subscapularis acts as the primary medial rotator of the humerus; having originated from the subscapular fossa of scapula it inserts onto the lesser tubercle of the humerus. It synergizes further with pectoralis major to perform horizontal flexion and also force couples with infraspinatus to provide dynamic stabilization of the glenohumeral joint as its upper fibres assist the supraspinatus and deltoid muscles during abduction (Parsons *et al.*, 2002). The muscle is vulnerable to inhibition from ongoing nociception and constant pressure of the humeral head on the anterior capsule, which reduces its important stabilizing role (Cook, 2012).

Deltoid

The pennate fibres of the deltoid receive innervation from the axillary nerve (C5) and encase the inherently unstable glenohumeral joint to reinforce stability. In both the frontal and transverse planes, force coupling between the deltoid and rotator-cuff complex exerts coordinated dynamic and static contractions of opposing force direction which may be equal in magnitude, thereby creating a joint reaction force compressing the humeral into the glenoid fossa and simultaneously producing joint movement. This is reflected by force coupling between deltoid and supraspinatus during mid-range abduction in the frontal plane. Acting as the prime mover, the deltoid elevates the arm while supraspinatus contraction dynamically stabilizes the glenohumeral joint by pulling the humeral head medially into the glenoid fossa (Parsons *et al.*, 2002). Prior to their relatively slim insertion point at the deltoid tuberosity located on the middle lateral aspect of the humerus, the anterior, medial and posterior deltoids occupy a relatively large cross-sectional zone with extensive origin attachments respectively composed of the lateral aspect of the clavicle, the acromion process and the spine of scapula (Thompson, 2010). This promotes outstanding leverage and power throughout the majority of available movement on the glenohumeral joint, which establishes the deltoid as the shoulder's prime mover, particularly in shoulder abduction as we reach and lift below and above shoulder height. Co-contraction of the anterior fibres with pectoralis major produces substantial humeral flexion and internal rotation, beneficial during initial-phase throwing techniques and daily activities which demand anterior-oriented dynamism. The anterior fibres therefore become susceptible to hypertrophy as common everyday activities are performed anterior to the torso (Cael, 2010). The posterior fibres are regarded as the prime mover during external rotation and synergize with latissimus dorsi and teres major to produce powerful extension or pulling during rowing. These three components collectively combine with pectoralis major to extend the humerus from an overhead flexed position experienced by the pull-through phase in front-crawl swimming (Heinlein and Cosgarea, 2010).

Pectoralis major

Powerful punching movements including the 'hook' and 'uppercut' represent essential boxing techniques; therefore the pectoralis major promotes various movements while in shoulder flexion. Originating from the anterior sternal half of the clavicle, the superior clavicular fibres innervated by the lateral pectoral nerve (C5–7) promote humeral flexion required for maintaining guard in preparation for delivering punches. Innervated by the medial pectoral nerve (C7–T1), the sternocostal fibres, originating from the sternum and intercostal cartilages of ribs 1–6, initiate horizontal adduction effective in applying the hook technique while the most inferior costal fibres extend the humerus from an overhead or flexed position similar to dropping the arm in preparation to deliver an uppercut (Palastanga and Soames, 2012). The tripennate pectoralis major fibres possess a unique rotation located proximal to its humeral insertion on the lateral lip of the bicipital (intertubercular) groove. Assuming a humeral attachment superior to the costal fibres, the clavicular fibres anteriorly rotate over the posteriorly rotating costal fibres to establish a 180° rotational twist resulting in a humeral attachment inferior to the costal fibres. This mechanism promotes maximum leverage and is particularly advantageous during a volleyball spike as maximum shoulder flexion triggers the twist to unwind, allowing the recoiled fibres to produce powerful humeral extension and internal rotation from an overhead position (Cael, 2010).

Pectoralis minor

Originating from the anterior aspect of ribs 3–5 and inserting into the anterior aspect of the coracoid process of the scapula, the pectoralis minor muscle, innervated by the medial pectoral nerve (C7–T1), secures the scapula to the ribcage and in the process facilitates anterior scapula stabilization when forces are absorbed through the arms (such as when pectoralis minor combines with serratus anterior during press-ups). These muscles also combine with subclavius to dynamically stabilize the scapula in an optimal postural position. Synergizing with the diaphragm, pectoralis minor also functions as a secondary respiratory muscle by fixating the scapula and elevating the ribs to support thoracic expansion. This function is synergized by the external intercostals, scalenes and serratus anterior and posterior (Kendall *et al.*, 2005).

Subclavius

Ascending from the first rib and costal cartilage, the subclavius muscle inserts onto the inferior aspect of the middle-third of the clavicle and is innervated by the subclavian nerve (C5–6). It predominantly stabilizes and fixates the clavicle during glenohumeral or scapulothoracic activity. This function is reinforced by the immensely strong acromioclavicular and sternoclavicular ligaments, the joints which subclavius exerts force on, although most rotational clavicular movement during overhead movement will be available at the sternoclavicular joint due to its gliding capability (Thompson, 2010). During bodyweight-bearing activity by the arms, dynamic stabilization of the scapulothoracic joint is fortified by the subclavius as it assists pectoralis minor and serratus anterior in the process.

Trapezius

Originating at the occipital protuberance, the nuchal ligament and spinous processes of C7–T12, the traditional kite-shaped trapezius muscle attaches laterally to the lateral third of the clavicle, acromion process and spine of scapula, establishing it as one of the larger superficial muscles in the human body. The upper fibres ascend obliquely to perform scapula elevation in company with levator scapulae and are also responsible for extension, as well as contralateral flexion and rotation of the head and neck. The comparatively horizontal middle fibres synergize with the rhomboid muscles to perform scapula retraction; and the lower obliquely descending fibres produce scapula depression (Palastanga and Soames, 2012). The lower and upper fibres combine to perform upward rotation of the scapula, optimizing glenoid fossa positioning, and therefore increase the glenohumeral range of movement (RoM) required for overhead shoulder actions (Kendall *et al.*, 2005). When all trapezius fibres are simultaneously activated the scapula remains secured to the ribcage to promote strength and support during weight-bearing activity; otherwise, when the scapula is not fixated, various fibres in company with synergists have freedom to perform the scapulothoracic actions comprising protraction, retraction, elevation and depression. The trapezius is innervated by the spinal accessory nerve (CNXI) and from the ventral rami roots C3–4 via the cervical plexus (Thompson, 2010).

Levator scapulae

Requiring the synergistic recruitment of upper trapezius fibres to perform scapular elevation, the levator scapulae muscle must oppose the upper and lower trapezius fibres to perform downward (medial) rotation of the scapula. Originating from the transverse processes of vertebrae C1–4 and inserting onto the superomedial aspect of the scapula, the levator scapulae is able to create greater tension and force production with assistance from the rhomboid complex. Together with pectoralis minor and serratus anterior, co-contraction secures the scapula to the ribcage during weight-bearing activity (such as when locking onto and pushing an opponent in rugby). The levator scapulae are innervated by the dorsal scapular nerve and ventral rami of roots C3–4 (Thompson, 2010).

Rhomboid major and minor

Primarily responsible for scapular retraction and stabilization of the medial border of the scapula, the rhomboids are innervated by the dorsal scapular nerve (C5). Although synergizing with levator scapulae and trapezius to secure the scapula to the ribcage during weight-bearing activity, the rhomboid major and minor muscles may also antagonistically co-contract with serratus anterior to produce strong scapular stabilization resulting from the opposing directional force production as both simultaneously insert onto the medial border of the scapula (Cael, 2010). Rhomboid major and minor, respectively, originate from vertebrae T2–5 and C7–T1 prior to insertion onto the posteromedial border of the scapula proximal to the spinous process. A combined contraction of the inferior fibres with serratus anterior and levator scapulae facilitates the precise positioning and stabilization of the glenoid fossa, producing efficient downward rotation and retraction of the scapula (ACSM, 2014). This movement is particularly effective in rowing, where repetitive pulling actions are used, or in swimming during the recovery phase as the hand leaves the water (Paine and Voight, 2013).

Latissimus dorsi

Emerging from its wide-ranging origin composed of the posterior one-third of the iliac crest, final four ribs, through the thoracolumbar aponeurosis from lumbar and sacral vertebrae, spinous processes of vertebrae T7–12 and the inferior angle of the scapula, the latissimus dorsi attaches into the comparatively minute bicipital groove of the humerus (Kendall *et al.*, 2005). Innervated by the thoracodorsal nerve (C7–8), it establishes a strong synergistic relationship with pectoralis major when adducting the humerus and also when elevating the upper torso when the arm is positioned overhead (termed 'brachiation'), such as in rock climbing. Similarly, downward bodily displacement is prevented during weight-bearing (such as when maintaining a static position with humeral adduction on the parallel bars). Exhibiting a comparable fibrous rotation to the pectoralis major, the latissimus dorsi also possesses an evident twist close to the distal insertion point to facilitate a powerful downward motion of the humerus from an overhead position. This action is effectively intensified when synergistically assisted by pectoralis major, teres major and posterior deltoid (McCarron *et al.*, 2011).

Teres major

Possessing a strong synergistic relationship with latissimus dorsi, the teres major is innervated by the inferior subscapular nerve (C5–6) and originates from the posteroinferior angle of the scapula before inserting onto the lateral lip of the bicipital groove to produce extension, adduction and internal rotation of the shoulder. It is acknowledged that teres major only performs these actions against resistance, otherwise it is not likely to be recruited (Hamill and Knutzen, 2009). Compared to the primary rotator-cuff muscles, teres major has a significant relationship with subscapularis to promote efficient internal rotation of the shoulder. Simultaneous contraction with latissimus dorsi assists in pulling the upper torso towards the fixed arm, which is replicated during rock-climbing (Palastanga and Soames, 2012).

Serratus anterior

Originating at the anterolateral surfaces of ribs 1–8, serratus anterior inserts onto the anteromedial border of the scapula. Located between the subscapular fossa and thoracic cavity the serratus anterior lies deep to the subscapularis to facilitate the scapulothoracic gliding mechanism.

Innervated by the long thoracic nerve (C5–7), it exhibits a synergistic relationship with pectoralis minor by securing the scapula adjacent to the thoracic cavity during scapular depression (ACSM, 2014) and provides powerful scapulothoracic protraction essential for effective reaching and delivery of explosive punches by competitive boxers on whom the serratus anterior is considerably defined. Interruption to its nerve supply can cause the characteristic 'winging' of the scapula, where the medial border and anterior surface of the scapula are not dynamically secured against the posterior thoracic cage. Additional synergy with the trapezius muscle establishes optimized positioning of the glenoid fossa, resulting in effective scapulohumeral rhythm and maximum overhead range of movement and coordination of the glenohumeral and scapulothoracic joints to enhance reaching and throwing techniques (Paine and Voight, 2013; Palastanga and Soames, 2012).

Practitioner Tip Box 6.2

Primary muscle synergy of the glenohumeral joint

Flexion	Deltoid (anterior fibres)
	Pectoralis major (clavicular fibres)
	Coracobrachialis
Extension	Deltoid (posterior fibres)
	Pectoralis major (sternal fibres)
	Latissimus dorsi
	Teres major
	Infraspinatus
	Teres minor
	Triceps brachii (long head)
Abduction	Deltoid (all fibres)
	Supraspinatus
	Pectoralis major (overhead)
Adduction	Latissimus dorsi
	Teres major
	Pectoralis major (all fibres)
	Coracobrachialis
Lateral rotation (external rotation)	Deltoid (posterior fibres)
	Infraspinatus
	Teres minor
	Supraspinatus
Medial rotation (internal rotation)	Deltoid (anterior fibres)
	Pectoralis major (all fibres)
	Latissimus dorsi
	Teres major
	Subscapularis
Horizontal abduction	Deltoid (posterior fibres)
	Infraspinatus
	Teres minor
	Latissimus dorsi
Horizontal adduction	Deltoid (anterior fibres)
	Pectoralis major (clavicular fibres)

Biceps brachii

Insertion into the radial tuberosity and bicipital aponeurosis facilitates the multi-joint fusiform-shaped biceps brachii to perform its primary actions of forearm supination and elbow flexion. Innervated by the musculocutaneous nerve (C5–7), the biceps brachii remains predisposed to a decreased mechanical advantage in shoulder flexion compared to the single-joint anterior deltoid and coracobrachialis muscles. Electromyographic (EMG) research indicates that the long head of biceps displays no activation during isolated shoulder flexion and its role in shoulder flexion is perceived to be passive (Levy *et al.*, 2001). However, the bicep brachii's dual attachments originating from the supraglenoid tubercle (long head) and the coracoid process (short head) do provide dynamic shoulder stabilization (Landin *et al.*, 2008) during powerful elbow flexion and supination (Rockwood *et al.*, 2009), and resistance against anterior dislocation particularly as the shoulder engages in the cocking phase of throwing, comprising abduction and external rotation (Hammer, 2007). Its intertubercular synovial sheath also blends with the capsule of the glenohumeral joint (Jenkins, 2009). Because of its positioning, attachment site and stabilizing function, the biceps is considered part of the cuff by some.

Coracobrachialis

Innervated by the musculocutaneous nerve (C5–7) and originating at the coracoid process of the scapula, the coracobrachialis muscle combines with the short head of biceps brachii to adduct and flex the shoulder forwards similar to an under-arm crown green bowling action (Palastanga and Soames, 2012). Also functioning as a shoulder stabilizer, its medial humeral insertion is at a comparable level to the laterally attached deltoid complex and therefore performs as an antagonist to the deltoid muscle while both structures facilitate scapulohumeral rhythm. The coracobrachialis is activated in golf as the arm swings into adduction and across the body when performing drives and approach shots (Cael, 2010).

Practitioner Tip Box 6.3

Primary muscle synergy of the shoulder girdle

Elevation	Trapezius (upper fibres)
	Rhomboid major
	Rhomboid minor
	Levator scapulae
Depression	Trapezius (lower fibres)
	Serratus anterior (origin fixed)
	Pectoralis minor
Retraction (adduction)	Trapezius (middle fibres)
	Rhomboid major
	Rhomboid minor
Protraction (abduction)	Serratus anterior (origin fixed)
	Pectoralis minor
Scapula lateral (upward) rotation	Trapezius
	Serratus anterior
Scapula medial (downward) rotation	Rhomboid major
	Rhomboid minor
	Levator scapulae
	Pectoralis minor

Triceps brachii

Located on the posterior aspect of the upper arm is triceps brachii, a three-headed, multi-joint muscle which functions antagonistically with the biceps brachii to produce movements of the shoulder and elbow. Innervated by the radial nerve (C6–8, T1), its extensive origins include the infraglenoid tubercle of the scapula (long head), posterolateral proximal half of the humerus (lateral head) and posteromedial distal two-thirds of the humerus (medial head), while the olecranon process of the ulna provides its comparatively smaller insertion point (Kulkarni, 2012). The long head of triceps brachii remains extra-articular, although some fibres attach to the inferior aspect of the glenoid labrum to provide capsular reinforcement. It also provides shoulder adduction and extension from a flexed position (Palastanga and Soames, 2012).

Neural anatomy

The brachial plexus is represented by a large network of nerve fibres with five main nerve roots originating from spinal segments C5–T1 and which eventually emerge as primary peripheral nerves. These pass through the scalene muscles of the neck, run deep to the clavicle and pectoralis minor muscle, and then through the axilla (armpit) before extending distally into the lower arm. Of the five nerve roots, also referred to as the ventral rami, two superior nerve roots (C5–6) are adjoined to the two inferior nerve roots (C8–T1), while the individual C7 nerve remains centralized to form three major network trunks, each of which subdivides into an anterior and posterior division comprising superior, middle and inferior trunks (van Es, 2001). Of the three anterior divisions, the two superior divisions merge, leaving the inferior division isolated while all posterior divisions amalgamate. Collectively all divisions now establish three nerve cords which laterally, medially and posteriorly encompass the axillary artery. Division of the lateral cord proceeds to establish the musculocutaneous nerve and one half of the median

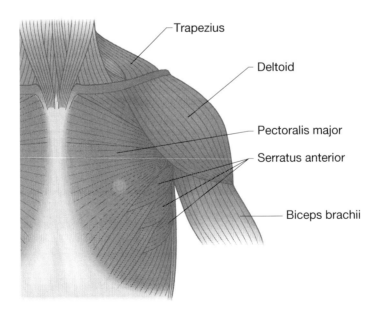

Figure 6.3   Muscular anatomy: anterior view (source: adapted from Sewell *et al.*, 2013).

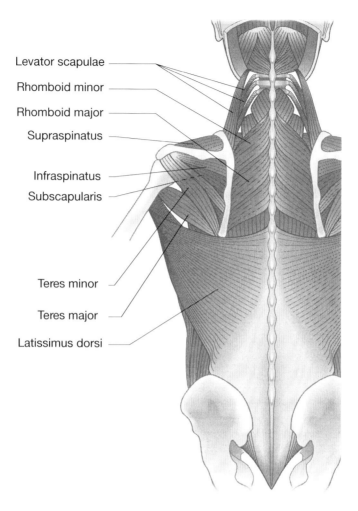

Levator scapulae

Rhomboid minor

Rhomboid major

Supraspinatus

Infraspinatus

Subscapularis

Teres minor

Teres major

Latissimus dorsi

Figure 6.4 Muscular anatomy: posterior view (source adapted from Sewell *et al.*, 2013).

nerve (Saeed and Rufai, 2003), while the medial cord establishes the ulnar nerve and the remaining median nerve (Gumusburun and Adiguzel, 2000) creating a visibly defined M-shaped neural network (Johnson *et al.*, 2008). From the posterior cord emerge the primary branches of the axillary nerve and the radial nerve (C6–T1), which innervates the triceps brachii muscle.

Focusing directly on the shoulder's neural supply the aforementioned brachial plexus cords provide neural innervation to this region. The medial cord divides into the lateral pectoral (C5–7) nerve which innervates the clavicular fibres of pectoralis major and the medial pectoral nerve (C7–T1) innervating both the superior sternal fibres of pectoralis major and the entire pectoralis minor muscles (Thompson 2010). Also emanating from the lateral cord is the musculocutaneous nerve (C5–7) which innervates coracobrachialis, biceps brachii and brachialis (Pellerin *et al.*, 2010). Four branches projecting from the posterior cord include the superior subscapular nerve (C5–6) supplying the upper portion of subscapularis and the inferior subscapular nerve (C5–6) supplying both the lower portion of subscapularis and teres major muscles (Tubbs *et al.*, 2007). The thoracodorsal nerve (C7–8), supplying latissimus dorsi, and the axillary nerve (C5–6), supplying the deltoid and teres minor muscles, jointly navigate the posterolateral humeral neck adjacent to the posterior circumflex humeral artery. The axillary nerve also conveys sensory information, including cutaneous sensation around the 'regimental badge' area of the lateral aspect of the deltoid courtesy of the superior lateral cutaneous nerve (McClelland and Paxinos, 2008). Rising from the superior trunk formed by the union of C5–6 roots ('Erb's Point'), the subclavian nerve spans the first rib (costal cartilage) and inferior clavicle to innervate the subclavius muscle. Also evolving from Erb's Point, the suprascapular nerve traverses the upper trapezius before negotiating the confined supraspinous fossa and suprascapular notch. It then travels deep to supraspinatus before entering the infraspinous fossa via the lateral border of the scapula to innervate supraspinatus and infraspinatus (Safran, 2004a; Thompson, 2010). Also ascending from the C5 root is the dorsal scapular nerve, which penetrates the medial scalene muscle before travelling deep to rhomboids and levator scapulae, which receives additional innervation from the ventral rami C3–4 roots (Kulkarni, 2012). Innervation of serratus anterior is provided by the long thoracic nerve which ascends from the anterior branches of C5–7 with C5–6 penetrating the medial scalene muscle and C7 travelling distally to the scalenes. The nerve then proceeds to travel deep to the brachial plexus and axillary tissues before attaching to the external surface of serratus anterior (Alemanno and Egarter Vigl, 2014; Safran, 2004b). Shoulder elevation or shrug is primarily initiated by the ventral rami roots C3–4 via the cervical plexus and the spinal accessory nerve, a cranial nerve (CNXI) which innervates all three sections of the trapezius including the lower trapezius where it descends into one individual branch (Kierner *et al.*, 2001; Safran, 2004b).

Circulatory anatomy

Branching off the brachiocephalic trunk of the aorta between the anterior and medial scalene muscles, the subclavian artery emerges deep to the clavicle, travelling with the brachial plexus (Netter *et al.*, 2013) to supply the upper extremity, while the subclavian vein conveys deoxygenated blood passing anteriorly to the anterior scalene. Arising from the subclavian artery, the dorsal scapular artery travels beneath the medial border of the scapula, supplying levator scapulae, rhomboids and serratus anterior muscles before it anastomoses (i.e. reforms a previously divided branch into a single source) with the subscapular artery near the inferior border of the scapula (Rockwood *et al.*, 2009). As the subclavian artery passes the lateral border of the first rib it emerges into the three-staged axillary artery which conveys fully oxygenated blood from major thoracic arteries into the upper extremity as deoxygenated blood from the upper extremity is returned via the axillary vein to other major thoracic veins and the heart (Cael, 2010). Based on the position of the pectoralis minor tendon, the first stage of the axillary artery remains proximally and possesses the superior thoracic artery which descends posterior to the axillary vein towards the first and second intercostal and serratus anterior muscles. The second axillary stage is located deep to the pectoralis minor tendon and possesses two branches, the thoracoacromial and lateral thoracic arteries (Netter *et al.*, 2013). Four additional branches emanate from the thoracoacromial artery. The anterosuperior rotator-cuff complex, particularly the supraspinatus tendon and deltoid muscles, are supplied by an acromial branch which travels laterally across the coracoid process before combining with the anterior and posterior circumflex humeral vessels to establish a vascular network onto the acromion process. Three additional thoracoacromial arterial branches vascularize pectoralis minor and major muscles (pectoral branch), the sternoclavicular joint and subclavius (clavicular branch) and the deltoid branch ascending independently as a component of the acromial branch before deviating adjacent to the cephalic vein to negotiate the channel between the deltoid and pectoral muscles to which it vascularizes (Rockwood *et al.*, 2009). The lateral thoracic artery may originate from the thoracoacromial or subscapular arteries, but predominately emerges from the axillary artery in 65 per cent of humans before descending the lateral aspect of the pectoralis minor to distribute branches to the serratus anterior and pectoral muscles (Netter *et al.*, 2013). The third stage of the axillary artery is located distal to the pectoralis minor tendon and possesses three branches comprising the subscapular, anterior circumflex humeral and posterior circumflex humeral arteries. The large subscapular artery divides into the thoracodorsal artery which predominantly supplies the latissimus dorsi muscle and the circumflex scapular artery which posteriorly negotiates the triangular space comprising of teres minor, teres major and the long head of triceps, where it distributes branches before spreading further across the infraspinous fossa and anastomoses with the dorsal scapular artery and terminals of the suprascapular artery to supply teres minor, teres major and subscapularis (Netter *et al.*, 2013). Subsequent branching of the circumflex humeral complex ensues, with an ascending curvature demonstrated by the anterior artery which supplies the humeral head and bicipital groove while the posterior artery travels posteriorly with the axillary nerve before circumnavigating the humeral neck to anastomose with the posterior circumflex humeral artery over the long head of biceps tendon (Rockwood *et al.*, 2009).

The glenohumeral joint capsule becomes a highly vascularized structure, having been continually replenished with oxygenated blood courtesy of the arterial branching network comprising the anterior circumflex, posterior circumflex, circumflex scapular and suprascapular arteries. This network produces a centripetal or pressurized blood flow throughout the natural curvature of their branches into the joint capsule. The glenoid labrum is vascularized by small periosteal and capsular vessels emanating from the suprascapular, circumflex scapular and the posterior humeral circumflex arteries; however, the innermost aspect of the labral rim is relatively avascular, similar to the menisci of the knee (Andary and Petersen, 2002).

The rotator-cuff complex is continuously vascularized by the suprascapular and the aforementioned anterior and posterior circumflex humeral arteries, all of which are partially assisted by the thoracoacromial, suprahumeral and subscapular arteries. The teres minor and infraspinatus tendons are supplied by an interwoven arterial network formed by the posterior circumflex humeral artery and suprascapular artery, which vascularizes the acromioclavicular joint and the supraspinatus and infraspinatus muscles. The suprascapular artery passes over the superior transverse scapular ligament (opposed to the suprascapular nerve, which passes underneath the ligament) before negotiating the confined supraspinous fossa deep to the supraspinatus muscle. It then diverts through the suprascapular notch towards the infraspinous fossa, where it anastomoses further with the dorsal scapular artery and circumflex scapular artery, creating a collateral circulatory network (Rockwood *et al.*, 2009).

Venous return from the hand to the shoulder is reliant on the superficial veins; however, from the shoulder the deep veins emerge as the predominant drainage system for deoxygenated blood. Emanating from the lateral aspect of the wrist, the cephalic vein ascends alongside the lateral aspect of the biceps brachii before penetrating through deep fascia level with the lower aspect of pectoralis major. The cephalic vein then enters the deltopectoral groove, forming a linkage with the deltopectoral lymph nodes before continuing towards the infraclavicular fossa where it diverts backwards, penetrating the clavipectoral fascia to enter the axilla where it terminates into the axillary vein. In comparison, the basilic vein ascends alongside the medial aspect of biceps brachii where it penetrates the brachial fascia, entering the anterior cavity at mid-arm level before uniting with the brachial veins to form the axillary vein (Kaufman and Lee, 2014; Kulkarni, 2006).

Lymphatic anatomy

The axillary vein transports deoxygenated blood from its brachial counterparts towards its destination located at the first rib, where it evolves into the subclavian vein. Lymphatic drainage from the axilla is distributed through five highly vascularized lymph nodes (Moses *et al.*, 2013).

Subscapular nodes located on the posterior wall of the axillary fossa attach to the surface of the subscapularis muscle. Located adjacent to the thoracodorsal artery, these nodes receive lymphatic flow from the posterior musculature of the back, shoulder and neck (Rockwood *et al.*, 2009) as well as the posterior walls of the chest and abdomen level with the iliac crest (Kulkarni, 2006). Pectoral nodes located deep to the pectoralis major muscle and serratus anterior fascia are located on the lateral surface of ribs 2–6 and congregate either side of the lateral thoracic artery (Rockwood *et al.*, 2009). These nodes channel all waste products from the anterolateral chest wall, upper abdominal wall and mammary glands (Moses *et al.*, 2013). Central nodes extend the lymphatic pathway as efferent vessels from these groups drain into the extensive network. Embedded within the adipose tissue of the axillary vein (Kulkarni, 2006), the central nodes are capable of receiving lymphatic flow from the lateral quadrants of the breast (Moses *et al.*, 2013) and the upper-limb courtesy of the brachial nodes which line the surfaces of the axillary vessels (Rockwood *et al.*, 2009). Apical nodes located in the axillary apex and the triangular space between the lateral aspect of the first rib, superior aspect of pectoralis minor and the axillary vein, receive lymphatic flow from the central nodes in addition to the upper arm and pectoral region. They are regarded as the terminal nodes of the upper extremity as their efferent vessels amalgamate to form the subclavian lymphatic trunk which terminates in the subclavian vein and the thoracic duct (Kulkarni, 2006). Obviously, where lymphatic nodes or channels have been removed or damaged, lymphoedema can be an ongoing issue.

Functional anatomy

The sternoclavicular articulation is the only bony link between the appendicular and the axial skeleton. The clavicle acts as a strut keeping the upper limb away from the thorax, permitting a great range of upper limb motion. Shoulder stability is the result of a complex interaction between static and dynamic shoulder restraints (Paine and Voight, 1993; Payne *et al.*, 1997). The static stabilizers of the joint consist of the labrum, capsule and ligaments, and the dynamic stabilizers of the joint are the muscles of the rotator-cuff, deltoid and scapular stabilizers (Terry and Chopp 2000; Woodward and Best, 2000). Lack of ability to maintain the humeral head centred within the glenoid fossa during movement is defined as instability (Magarey and Jones, 1992). Glenohumeral joint stability relies on the interaction between the active, passive and neural control subsystems, with the rotator-cuff muscles, activating at different positions, compressing the convex humeral head into the concave glenoid, thus resisting the shear force experienced by the humeral head (Lee *et al.*, 2000). Disruption of the delicate balance between the static and dynamic control systems can produce a varied spectrum of clinical presentations, ranging from minor instability to total shoulder dislocation (Hayes *et al.*, 2002; Horsley, 2005). This has led to the increasing diagnosis of shoulder impingement (Uhthoff and Sarkar, 1991). RoM deficits also contribute to injury, as this can produce a situation whereby some muscles become tight and some muscles become lax (Baltaci and Johnson, 2001). Pathology around the glenohumeral joint and the shoulder girdle is complex, often being multifactorial, which complicates clinical diagnosis further (Magarey *et al.*, 1996). Historically, assessment of the shoulder has been based on the premise that it is possible to isolate individual structures around the shoulder and place a mechanical stress upon it in order to elicit a response. It is unlikely that it is possible to stress one individual structure without any further stress upon adjacent structures (Lewis, 2009).

Movement patterns in swimming and throwing

As swimming and throwing are fundamental sporting functions particularly involving the shoulder region, these will be briefly discussed. Front crawl swimming demands repetitive overhead stroke techniques involving multidirectional clockwise and anti-clockwise glenohumeral circumduction, with full scapulothoracic facilitation. Front-crawl (or freestyle) involves the propulsive pull-through phase commencing with hand-entry, glide and catch, mid-pull and end pull-through; and the recovery phase as the hand leaves the water, travelling overhead to the hand-entry position to complete one single stroke – 30,000 of which are performed by competitive swimmers on a weekly basis (Heinlein and Cosgarea, 2010). As the hand enters the water, the rhomboids work to stabilize the inferior angle of the scapula as scapular protraction and upward rotation is initiated by serratus anterior and upper trapezius, providing clearance of the humeral head as the arm glides towards forward extension. As the hand catches the water, elbow flexion initiates the pulling action, which is reinforced by shoulder adduction and internal rotation courtesy of the pectoralis major and teres minor force coupling to create the effective mid-pull propulsion and progressive transition towards extension facilitated by latissimus dorsi and posterior deltoid, and abduction by supraspinatus and the middle deltoid during the end pull-through phase. The subsequent recovery phase requires the synergistic combination from the rhomboids for scapular retraction with serratus anterior and upper trapezius for upward rotation to initiate body roll in preparation to breathe during recovery as the deltoids sequentially fire to sustain optimal coordination prior to hand-entry controlled by anterior deltoid flexion (Heinlein and Cosgarea, 2010; Tovin, 2006). Pathological sequelae and injury prevention linked to swimming are demonstrated in the literature (Tovin, 2006).

With regard to throwing, baseball pitching efficiency requires precise timing and technique during the early and late cocking phase, and the subsequent acceleration and follow-through phases. Following the wind-up phase, deltoid activation increases shoulder abduction to approximately 90° abduction, with subsequent posterior rotator-cuff activation to facilitate 60° external rotation and 15° horizontal abduction throughout the preparatory early-cocking phase. A combination of excessive external rotation and insufficient horizontal abduction at this stage correlates with a significant decrease in ball velocity (Escamilla *et al.*, 2001; Stodden *et al.*, 2006). During the late-cocking phase the shoulder is momentarily subjected to approximately 170° of external rotation, with 100° abduction and 15° horizontal abduction. At this point, the rotator-cuff activity peaks as the scapula retracts to stabilize the humeral head, resisting posterior translation from the glenoid fossa; however, repetitive actions place stress on the glenohumeral ligamentous complex and anterior capsule, eventually predisposing it to laxity resulting in increased external rotation and posterosuperior humeral head translation, an advantage subsequently sacrificed by a decrease in shoulder stability (Fortenbaugh *et al.*, 2009) and posterior capsular tightness resulting in glenohumeral internal rotation deficit (GIRD) (Dwelly *et al.*, 2009; Lintner *et al.*, 2007). As the late-cocking phase terminates, the subscapularis, pectoralis major and serratus anterior muscles synergize with scapular protraction as the acceleration phase commences to propel the projectile forwards, while the deltoids sustain shoulder abduction. Stress on the anterior capsule diminishes and the humeral head restores congruity with the glenoid fossa as external rotation decreases. Early acceleration requires significant elbow extension provided by the triceps brachii muscle, while activation of the latissimus dorsi, pectoralis major and serratus anterior muscles increase during late acceleration (Beltran and Suhardja, 2007). As the projectile is released, shoulder abduction is maintained at

90° as the glenohumeral joint rapidly decelerates, utilizing extreme eccentric contractions from all muscle groups, imposing injurious compressive joint loading forces in the process (Oyama, 2012). The follow-through phase concludes as the arm crosses the chest and the glenohumeral joint decelerates to 60° horizontal flexion, with maximum internal rotation (Beltran and Suhardja, 2007; Fortenbaugh *et al.*, 2009). Pathological sequlae linked to each throwing phase (Oyama, 2012) and injury prevention focusing on GIRD (Lintner *et al.*, 2007; McClure *et al.*, 2007) are demonstrated in the literature.

Assessment of the shoulder region

It is highly recommended that all musculoskeletal assessments should follow a sequential clinical assessment protocol which promotes development of the sports therapist's theoretical underpinning knowledge, clinical reasoning skills and subsequent confidence to apply safe and effective treatment. Assessment testing protocol should also be evidence-based, reliable and valid to facilitate repeatable accuracy and consistency essential to effective interpretation of findings and safe indication of ensuing treatment protocol. Assessment may be indicated for: postural or biomechanical analysis in preparation for an injury prevention programme; evaluation of the gravity of acute or sub-acute injuries and identification of recommended treatment modalities; and for evaluation of joint RoM, strength, pain and functional fitness relating to chronic injury – throughout the rehabilitation process. Accurate recording of assessment is imperative as the collated patient-based information assists the sports therapist to implement and develop clinical reasoning skills in order to provide a working pathological hypothesis and differential diagnosis indicating the affected structure and prognosis (McFarland, 2006). The ability to recognize both musculoskeletal and non-musculoskeletal causes of pain is imperative. Musculoskeletal pain is generally influenced by movement, as opposed to non-musculoskeletal sources which may be initiated by systemic pathology, including everything from an infection to cancer. Pancoast's syndrome (an apical malignant neoplasm [carcinoma] of the lung) is an example of one such pathology which can manifest as musculoskeletal shoulder pain (Rull, 2014). Differential diagnosis of shoulder pain is therefore complicated, as any pain affecting the shoulder can cause it to act as though the pain was indeed originating from that site. As therapists, it is imperative to be aware that if patients fail to respond appropriately to treatment, the differential diagnosis needs to be reviewed and referral for further diagnostic investigation or alternative management must be considered (Arcasoy and Jett, 1997; Slaven and Mathers, 2010; Walsh and Sadowski, 2001).

Subjective assessment of the shoulder

Subjective shoulder investigation may disclose localized symptoms around a particular structure or radicular pain extending proximally to the scapula or clavicle, or distally towards the axilla, humerus or anterior chest wall. Patients may report subsequent dysfunction in normal everyday activities, including overhead reaching, lifting and associated sporting techniques. In order to facilitate deeper investigative strategies, subjective assessments should always adopt a patient-centred approach allowing the presentation of signs and symptoms to unfold, preferably devoid of pressing time constraints. The sports therapist must implement acute listening skills in order to decipher volunteered information which may appear insignificant but later transform as vital evidence exposing the underlying aetiology in the patient presenting with a shoulder complaint. It should also be observed that the glenohumeral joint sacrifices stability for mobility; therefore, glenohumeral instability or labral pathology must be investigated if the patient presents with shoulder joint laxity, especially when positioned in abduction and external rotation. Similarly, adhesive capsulitis may be indicated by an intense globalized pain accompanied by a progressive decrease in available RoM. Subacromial impingement or rotator-cuff pathology may be suspected by the patient's perception of weakness or heaviness, occasionally accompanied by pain (McFarland, 2006).

Further subjective investigation should explore the patient's daily activities, occupation(s), hobbies and sports history, including positions played. Investigation may evolve towards ascertaining the volume, time frame and intensity of such activities, and what equipment, including footwear, is used. Shoulder-focused information will identify the patient's dominant hand, their functional limitations, the mechanism of injury (MoI) which may highlight the affected structures, and the level of perceived weakness and/or pain. The patient may be able to perform the aggravating movement or technique, recreating symptoms which may highlight the affected structures. Pain may also be experienced in a dermatomal region – therefore, it is advised to ascertain whether the patient experiences neck and/or upper back pain caused by dysfunction of the cervical and thoracic spine. The majority of subjective assessments provide a clinical hypothesis indicating further recommended testing to promote a summative diagnostic confirmation. However, subjective questioning may disclose any of a range of suspicious 'red flags'. These can include bilateral pins and needles (paraesthesia) or numbness (anaesthesia), sudden unexplained weight loss or unremitting pain which prevents normal sleeping (Greenhalgh and Selfe, 2006; Ross and Boissonault, 2010). Consideration for referral to the patient's GP is essential as radiating pain originating from serious pulmonary, gastrointestinal or cardiovascular pathology can be experienced in the shoulder (Magee, 2014).

In gymnastics, the shoulder performs multiple axial-loading movements in all planes – therefore clinical assessment can be a challenging process (Caine *et al.*, 2013). Acute injury mechanisms may indicate which structure is affected; for example, a fall on to an outstretched hand ('FOOSH') may cause rupture of the AC ligament; a forceful blow to the posterior shoulder when the arm is in 90° of abduction and external rotation (running with a rugby ball tucked under the armpit) could compromise the weaker inferior glenohumeral ligament resulting in subluxation or dislocation of the glenohumeral joint. In relation to subacromial impingement syndrome (SIS), patients may be predisposed to primary or congenital aetiological factors, such as with a type III 'hook-shaped' acromion process which significantly decreases the subacromial space. In contrast, secondary or acquired dysfunction may be exposed in patients who are able to recreate their symptoms with demonstration of visibly poor and/or adapted techniques. Impingement resulting from acquired mechanical dysfunction may be instigated by adaptation to posture or technique, or as a result of capsular laxity or tightness. Patients may complain of weakness or heaviness, possibly accompanied by pain (Di Giacomo *et al.*, 2010).

Hypomobility or hypermobility within a component of the kinetic chain previously exposed to injury can also predispose acquired dysfunction. The kinetic chain is a sequential proximal-to-distal force-production linkage system. According to Kibler (1995), 54 per cent of shoulder power is transferred energy from the lower limbs and pelvis. The core of the body is attributed to robust stability, generating over 50 per cent force compared to approximately 20 per cent from the shoulder, 15 per cent from the elbow and 10 per cent from the wrist (Kibler, 2009). A tennis player experiencing chronic lumbar pain or hypomobility resulting in a 20 per cent decrease in core kinetic energy will require a 34 per cent increase in shoulder velocity or a 70 per cent increase in shoulder mass to generate the 4,000 watts of power required for each tennis serve (Kibler, 2009). The player may overcompensate for this deficit by repetitively overloading the distal chain, resulting in acute rotator-cuff strain (Elliott *et al.*, 2003). This 'catch-up' phenomenon is defined as a kinetic chain dysfunction caused by excessive overloading of the distal link, which inevitably results in scapular dyskinesis (Kibler and McMullen, 2003). In a clinical environment, the sports therapist must ascertain crucial subjective information in order to identify and treat underlying aetiology, in this case the lumbar issues, as opposed to simply treating the acute shoulder injury.

Objective assessment of the shoulder

Having ascertained a comprehensive subjective history, this framework may now facilitate an effective objective assessment involving a physical examination of the patient. Strategic testing protocol should ideally aim to confirm or eliminate the sports therapist's existing pathological hypothesis derived from the subjective assessment, while considering any differential diagnosis (Cook and Hegedus, 2013). Objective assessments are sequential and reinforced by orthopaedic principles which promote validity and reliability throughout each testing stage; however, flexibility in relation to the order, selection and application of testing protocol may vary according to the existing presentation which may be in the acute, subsequent or chronic stage of tissue-healing (Kolt and Snyder-Mackler, 2007). Development of the sports therapist's clinical reasoning skills and musculoskeletal assessment protocol may be enhanced by devising a prioritized record of the associated shoulder structures, including bone, ligament, tendon, muscle and nerve within the clinical assessment record. Such strategies facilitate identification of incriminating structures to be assessed and elimination of non-affected structures. Patients presenting with acute pathology may be examined to determine the extent of tissue trauma, but physical examination may be minimalistic to avoid exacerbating underlying inflammation. During the subsequent stage, objective examination may tolerate wide-ranging physical testing, providing a more definitive prioritized record of impairments resulting from the original injury mechanism. Effective clinical reasoning during objective assessment for chronic conditions may not only provide conclusive diagnosis of the existing condition, but expose the underlying aetiology (Kolt and Snyder-Mackler, 2007).

It is widely acknowledged that most orthopaedic physical examinations influence a dichotomous test interpretation which may be positive (pathology present) or negative (pathology not present). Physical examination may also reproduce the patient's pain and symptoms without affecting the targeted structure, thereby providing the practitioner with a false positive. A false negative will be provided as objective testing fails to identify a suspected pathology, therefore diagnostic accuracy is not always accomplished (Cook and Hegedus, 2013; Hattam and Smeatham, 2010). These two sources provide further insight into reliability of testing protocols from intra-rater and inter-rater aspects which, respectively, examine the consistency and repeatability of testing protocol for both the single practitioner and multiple practitioners.

Objective assessment for patients attending with shoulder pathology should include an upper quadrant postural analysis followed by observation assessing the quality and control of active range of movement (ARoM). Further assessment should include examination of both the static (passive) stabilizing structures during passive range of movement (PRoM) and the dynamic stabilizers, including the rotator-cuff complex during resisted strength testing. The integrity of the joint capsule, glenohumeral labrum and subacromial space should be considered throughout this process (Kolt and Snyder-Mackler, 2007). The sports therapist may consider the following:

- Postural deviation (kyphosis/lordosis): is a muscular 'upper-cross syndrome' evident?
- Poor quality of movement: is there a muscle imbalance of the shoulder's dynamic stabilizers?

- Inability to perform actions (pain or weakness): is a muscle tear or joint dysfunction present?
- Inability to perform actions (no pain): is a complete rupture or neural disruption evident?
- Pins and needles (paraesthesia): is innervation disrupted by compression?

Palpation of the shoulder region

Effective palpation skills demand an exceptional level of underpinning anatomical knowledge to facilitate precision and sensitivity throughout the systematic palpation routine of the shoulder. Palpating in an anteroposterior direction, the sports therapist should assess for and record any muscular spasm, tenderness, deformity, oedema or joint effusion around the musculoskeletal structures which may indicate the pathological source. Suspected pathological findings need to be confirmed and comparison with the contralateral shoulder is imperative in identifying the patient's condition. In addition to bony structures and muscle bellies, palpation may also incorporate assessment of the skin, subcutaneous and deep fascia, blood vessels, nerves, tendons, ligaments and joint spaces. Palpation should be sensitive during the initial objective examination to prevent exacerbating the present pathology. Progressive pressure may be applied during the ensuing passive and special testing stages as indicated by the objective process (Hertling and Kessler, 2006; Magee, 2014).

Accommodating approximately 25 per cent of the body's pacinian corpuscles, the hand is exceptionally sensitive due to the presence of these major mechanoreceptors. A key principle during the initial stage of investigating musculoskeletal dysfunction is represented by the acronym 'ART', which facilitates examination of A (asymmetry), R (restriction of mobility) and T (tissue texture abnormality). Fortunately the shoulder complex exists as a pair, providing comparison of asymmetry including misalignment of bony landmarks and muscle hypertrophy or hypotrophy. Restriction of mobility can be continually assessed, especially when palpating the various joint structures while applying overpressure in active and passive examination, or special orthopaedic testing which exposes end-feels and pathological signs. Tissue texture abnormality may be represented by tenderness within a hypertrophic muscle resulting in hyperirritable tension or trigger points detectable by applying a pincer or skin-fold grip using the pads of the thumbs and index fingers. The therapist should always apply appropriate pressure – taking into consideration the patient's medical condition, age, history and fitness level – as excessive pressure may provoke abnormal tissue responses, including dysaesthesia, often represented by an intense cutaneous burning sensation following compression of the nerve which innervates that particular area of skin. Inflammatory responses following acute trauma may produce hyperaemia and heat as opposed to decreased skin temperatures initiated by vascular deficiency, both detectable by applying light contact using the dorsal aspect of the hand (Deepak, 2005; Dvorak *et al.*, 2008; Hertling and Kessler, 2006).

Palpable bony structures of the anterior shoulder include the clavicle, the manubrium process of the sternum, the acromion process and respective sternoclavicular and acromioclavicular joints, the bicipital groove dividing the greater and lesser tubercles of the humerus, the coracoid process and the costal borders interspersed by costal cartilage. The acromion process and deltoid tuberosity may be palpated from a lateral aspect. Posterior structures of the scapula include the superior angle level with the second rib and spinous process of T2, the inferior angle level with the seventh rib and spinous process of T7, the spine of the scapula and the medial and lateral borders. Palpation of shoulder muscles should include the biceps brachii, deltoids, coracobrachialis, pectoralis major and minor, subscapularis, infraspinatus, teres major, teres minor, supraspinatus, latissimus dorsi, trapezius, rhomboid major and minor, levator scapulae, subclavius and triceps brachii (Magee, 2014).

Observations of the shoulder region

According to Kibler (1995), when one is attempting to assess the movement occurring at the glenohumeral joint, it is a prerequisite to regard the whole kinetic chain: since the power produced for overhead action (commencing with ground reaction forces – GRF) moves up, sequentially, though each body segment from the lower limbs, through the trunk and terminates in the arm (Lee, 1995).

Assessment of static posture is an important prerequisite for determining potential structures at fault during active testing. The widely accepted description of 'ideal' standing posture (lateral view) is that proposed by Kendall *et al.* (2005) as a vertical line passing through the lobe of the ear, the seventh cervical vertebra, acromion process, greater trochanter and slightly anterior to the midlines of the knee and lateral malleolus. Deviations outside this theoretical 'plumb-line' have been described (such as reduced or exaggerated kyphotic or lordotic postures) and have been linked to a range of conditions.

During the objective examination it is common to observe asymmetry in shoulder and scapular positions. Disuse atrophy in the supraspinatus or infraspinatus may indicate rotator-cuff tears, excessive scapular winging initiated by long thoracic nerve trauma affecting serratus anterior, and sagging of the shoulder may signify accessory nerve lesions (Burkhart *et al.*, 2003a; Donnelly *et al.*, 2013; Kibler *et al.*, 2002; Kibler and McMullen, 2003; Meister, 2000). The scapula generally sits between the levels of the second and seventh spinous processes of the thoracic spine with a slight upward rotation – indicated by the inferior angle of the scapula being slightly further away from the spine than the superior angle of the scapula. Many clinicians agree that asymmetric findings in shoulder posture are quite common (Kendall *et al.*, 2005), with the dominant shoulder generally being positioned lower than the non-dominant shoulder in most people. This can also be evidenced by observing anteriorly and finding that the lateral end of the clavicle is at least an inch higher than the medial end. The scapula is inclined 30° forward from the frontal plane (termed 'scaption' – the plane of the scapula) (DePalma and Johnson, 2003).

Spinal alignment has been proposed as a factor which will affect scapular position and shoulder girdle function. A common observation is that of a forward head posture, where the chin pokes forward, the upper cervical spine extends and the lower cervical spine flexes. This generally produces shortening of the posterior neck extensor muscles and tightening of the anterior neck muscles, and alters the length–tension relationship between the axio-scapular muscles, ultimately affecting scapular position and kinematics (Kebaetse *et al.*, 1999). Postural deviations observed in forward head posture involve a downwardly rotated, anteriorly tilted and protracted scapula, leading to a reduction of the subacromial space during arm elevation (Lewis *et al.*, 2005). A shortened pectoralis minor muscle is commonly identified along with this postural deviation (Ayub, 1991).

For a patient with a primary complaint of shoulder pain, observations should include:

- static postures (anterior, posterior, and left and right lateral views)
- static scapular position
- cervical spine posture
- thoracic spine posture
- dynamic movement patterns (shoulder girdle, glenohumeral and thoracic regions)
- scapulohumeral rhythm (SHR) (particularly during active flexion and abduction)
- functional tests
- hand behind neck (HBN)
- hand behind back (HBB).

Clearing tests

A key principle of neuromusculoskeletal assessment requires the screening and clearance of the proximal and distal segments; that is the joints directly above and below the target structure, as these joints may emerge as the aetiological source due to an underlying pathology which refers pain to the structure being assessed (Voight *et al.*, 2007). Any clearing tests which are symptom-producing require that the sports therapist undertakes a more detailed assessment of the identified region.

The neck and cervical spine should always be cleared due to the neural innervation to the shoulder musculature by the segmental cervical nerve roots. From the brachial plexus, five ventral rami comprising of nerve roots (C5–8, T1) commence formation of the neural network which innervates the entire shoulder, upper arm and anterior chest wall; therefore the therapist should be aware that peripheral pathologies involving pain and motor or sensory dysfunction are often diffused from the cervical spine (van Es, 2001; Wilk *et al.*, 2009). Suprascapular pain (C5–6), superior scapular pain (C6–7) and mid-scapular pain (C7, T1) can be referred from these nerve roots (Lander, 2007).

With the patient seated, the cervical quadrant test requires active cervical extension and lateral flexion followed by rotation of the cervical spine with subtle end-range overpressure applied by the therapist if previous movements are asymptomatic. Recreation of pain referral towards the aforementioned regions may indicate nerve root compression or pathology. With the patient in a supine position this test may also be adapted to assess vertebrobasilar insufficiency (VBI). Careful patient handling is imperative throughout as the therapist uses both hands to support and manoeuvre the patient's head to the end-position as it overhangs the plinth. The therapist should support the end-position for 30 seconds and observe for nystagmus or inference of dizziness, an indication of vertebral artery compression and insufficiency. Further adaptation may incorporate compression of the cervical segments – for example, the therapist may apply a downward force with the patient's head in three positions, neutral, extension and combined extension with lateral flexion. A subsequent decrease in the intervertebral foraminal space may compress any impinged or irritable nerve roots, recreating the patient's symptoms in the process (Magee, 2014; Voight *et al.*, 2007).

Simple clearing of the elbow requires active flexion and extension with overpressure, if appropriate. The patient is instructed to bend the elbow followed by end-range overpressure applied by the therapist. On straightening the arm, the therapist should support the elbow joint while applying overpressure to achieve full extension (McFarland, 2006).

Active movement assessment of the shoulder

It is recommended to assess active movements before passive, as the patient is in control. ARoM values vary among individuals due to the influence of factors such as age and specificity of movement. Ranges can be measured using standard goniometers, which have demonstrated fair to good reliability (Hayes *et al.*, 2002). Owing to the satisfactory level of intra-rater reliability, goniometry is widely recommended for recording the progression or regression of joint RoM throughout the rehabilitation process; therefore sound anatomical knowledge and palpation skills are essential during the land-marking and measurement process (Magee, 2014). The American Academy of Orthopaedic Surgeons' (AAOS) recommendations for clinical measurement of shoulder internal and external rotation is by goniometer, with the arm at 90° of humeral abduction.

Table 6.3 Recognized parameters of glenohumeral range of movement

Action	Greene and Heckman (1994)	American Medical Association (1988)	Kendall et al. (2005)	Loudon et al. (2008)	Magee (2014)
Flexion	0–180°	0–150°	0–180°	0–180°	0–160/180°
Extension	0–60°	0–50°	0–45°	0–60°	0–50/60°
Abduction	0–180°	0–180°	0–180°	0–180°	0–170/180°
Medial rotation	0–70°	0–90°	0–70°	0–70°	0–60/100°
Lateral rotation	0–90°	0–90°	0–90°	0–90°	0–80/90°

Sahrmann (2002) explains that the quality of scapulohumeral movement depends on the interaction between scapula and glenohumeral joint kinematics, and Cools *et al.* (2003) expand that stability of the scapula depends on the optimal recruitment and timing of the scapular rotators. Pathology at the glenohumeral joint can result from any small changes to these actions, which may be secondary to instability and impingement (Kuhn *et al.*, 1995; McMahon *et al.*, 1996). The interactions between upper and lower trapezius and serratus anterior are important to this functional dynamic (Ludewig and Cook, 2000; Wadsworth and Bullock-Saxon, 1997). Serratus anterior works to draw the scapula laterally around the chest wall during glenohumeral movement, and this is resisted by the action of lower trapezius; upper trapezius produces upward rotation of the scapula, while middle and lower trapezius maintain horizontal and vertical positioning of the scapula (Horsley, 2005; Wadsworth and Bullock-Saxon, 1997).

ARoM of the shoulder region should ideally be performed with the patient in a standing position, but, where the patient is tall or therapist short, or where standing is not possible, a seated position is acceptable. The normally tested standard movements are: flexion; extension; abduction; adduction; medial (internal) rotation; lateral (external) rotation. The movements produced by the patient will ideally be effortless and pain free, and it is important that the therapist is able to observe all movements from all four sides (anterior, posterior and left and right lateral views). Bilateral comparison will enable the examiner to see alterations in movement patterns and RoM. While carrying out the assessment, the sports therapist should observe and listen to the patient for indication of pain or difficulty when moving, and this should be linked into their presenting condition. Once observation of each movement has taken place, and the therapist has clarified whether there are any symptom responses, careful passive overpressure may be employed to assess for any symptom responses at the end of range.

As discussed earlier, particularly during shoulder flexion and abduction, scapulohumeral rhythm (SHR) is an important functional feature of combination shoulder joint movements. SHR should be observed during assessment of shoulder active movements. Approximately the initial 30° of shoulder flexion and abduction is performed predominently by the glenohumeral joint, while the scapula remains in a neutral position. Upward rotation of the scapula commences to assist shoulder elevation and, in simple terms, a ratio of 2:1 glenohumeral to scapulothoracic movement occurs. During active elevation the excursion of the scapula should be evaluated, particularly the movement of its inferior angle, which indicates upward rotation (typically to a point in line with the axilla). A posterior tilt of the scapula on the thorax is also a normal component of elevation (the inferior angle of the scapula moves towards the chest wall). Additionally, any excessive (or restricted) girdle elevation should be identified. Kibler (2000) highlights the importance of also observing the quality of descent (i.e. the returning control of

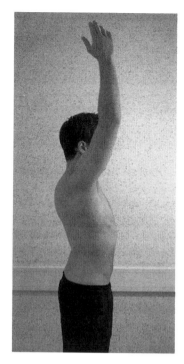
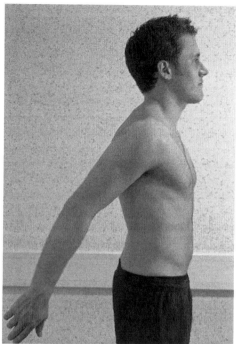

Photo 6.2   Active range of movement assessment: flexion and extension.

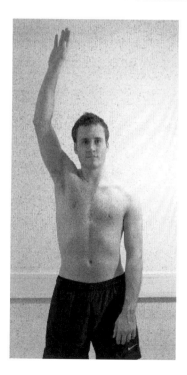

Photo 6.3   Active range of movement assessment: abduction.

adduction to neutral), which in the presence of scapular dyskinesia may show as a jerky movement. Initially a bilateral comparison will provide a general appreciation of any asymmetry. It is recommended to repeat movements eight to ten times in order to assess for any elements of fatigue responsible for any symptoms. The scapular position on the thorax, and control during motion, is a critical component of normal shoulder function. It must be remembered that virtually all movements of the shoulder complex involve movements at the four joints (McClure *et al.*, 2001), plus associated movements of the spinal region. The clavicle undergoes elevation and retraction throughout elevation, while the scapula upwardly rotates, internally rotates and posteriorly tilts. Scapulothoracic elevation also involves the SC joint (Teece *et al.*, 2008).

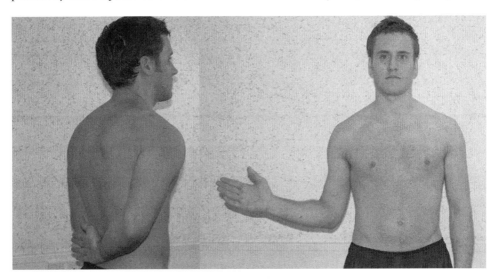

Photo 6.4   Active range of movement assessment: medial and lateral rotation.

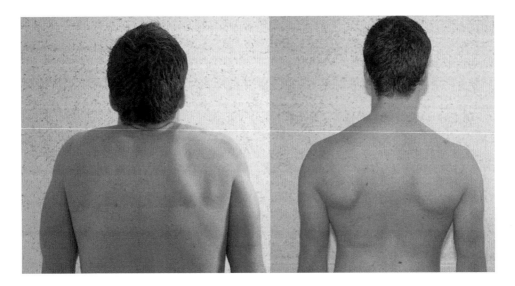

Photo 6.5   Active range of movement assessment: elevation and depression.

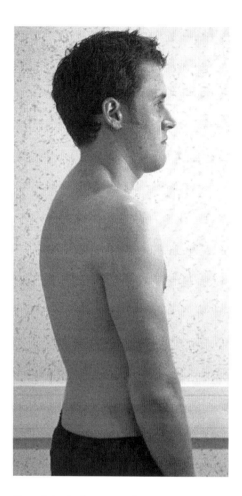 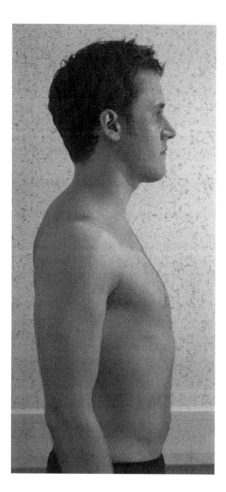

Photo 6.6   Active range of movement assessment: protraction and retraction.

Passive movement assessment of the shoulder

Performed solely by the sports therapist with the patient relaxed, passive assessment essentially verifies the available anatomical RoM, end-feels and integrity of non-contractile tissues, including the glenohumeral joint capsule, the glenoid labrum and the associated shoulder ligaments. Consideration for appropriate patient positioning is imperative and should completely facilitate the patient's available RoM without restriction. It is recommended to perform PRoM assessment with the patient supine-lying – all movements may be performed from this position and it also offers a more stable, reproducible start position. Additionally, the therapist may elect to assess movements with and without passive scapular fixation (particularly during flexion and abduction). When the scapula is fixed, the resulting glenohumeral movement is automatically made more specific; this also eliminates scapulothoracic involvement. Resistance occurring towards the end-range, or physiological barrier, provides the sports therapist with the opportunity to apply overpressure to determine the anatomical barrier while assessing the quality of the end-feel within the joint. However, abnormal end-feels may arise prior to the end-range, particularly a spasm end-feel, where a sudden resistance is initiated by musculature guarding pathological tissues (Magee, 2014). Should pain be the predominant precursor to a spasm end-feel, it may be observed that pain is experienced prior to the resistance – however, should stiffness be the underlying problem, then resistance may occur prior to any pain sensation. It is also acknowledged that spasm end-feels may occur in early and late-stage RoM, respectively indicating acute inflammation and joint instability, the latter exemplified during the apprehension test for anterior shoulder dislocation (Magee, 2014). Other pathological end-feels affecting the shoulder may include the hard capsular end-feel which produces a tight resistance in response to chronic inflammatory conditions, including adhesive capsulitis. Empty end-feels are devoid of muscle spasm and demonstrate no restriction to movement except when the patient experiences intense shoulder pain and subsequently insists on the termination of passive movement, an occurrence associated with subacromial bursitis (Hertling and Kessler, 2006; Vizniak, 2012). Differential diagnosis for shoulder joint restriction may be provided by the capsular pattern which in the glenohumeral joint usually deteriorates in the set pattern of lateral rotation, abduction and medial rotation, while both the sternoclavicular and acromioclavicular joints may induce pain in end RoM, comprising full elevation and horizontal adduction. Pathological constriction within the joint capsule may be triggered by arthritis or capsulitis (Magee, 2014).

Passive assessment should incorporate all movements performed by the glenohumeral and scapulothoracic joints, while recording any significant symptoms including the onset of pain, stiffness or tension. For example, a patient with a partial rupture of the deltoid attains 110° passive shoulder abduction and suddenly experiences a sharp pain of 7/10 on the visual (or verbal) analogue scale (VAS) in conjunction with an evident tension or spasm end-feel experienced by the practitioner. This may be recorded on the clinical record as: ABD 110° (7/10 VAS; Spasm).

End-feel sensations experienced by the practitioner are subjectively assessed, therefore intra-rater reliability may be considered good compared to the insufficient inter-rater reliability initiated by the contrasting individual perceptions of the end-feel. Both Cyriax (1982) and Kaltenborn (1999) provide extensive end-feel classifications which modern-day practitioners may implement into their own clinical practice (Peterson and Hayes, 2000). Normal shoulder end-feels are exclusively firm and elastic due to restraint induced by both the capsuloligamentous and musculotendinous structures (Berryman-Reese and Bandy, 2010).

Practitioner Tip Box 6.4

Normal end-feels of the glenohumeral joint

- Flexion: elastic, firm
- Extension: firm
- Abduction: elastic, firm
- Internal rotation: elastic, firm
- External rotation: firm
- Horizontal flexion: soft tissue
- Horizontal extension: elastic, firm

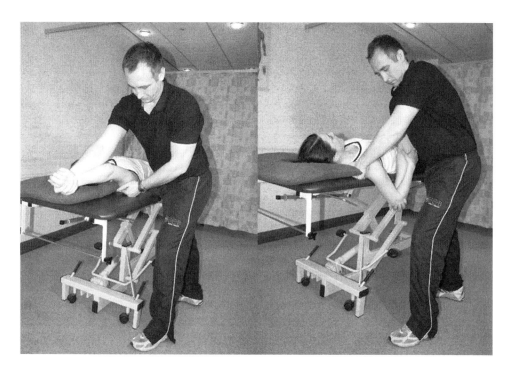

Photo 6.7 Passive range of movement assessment: flexion and extension.

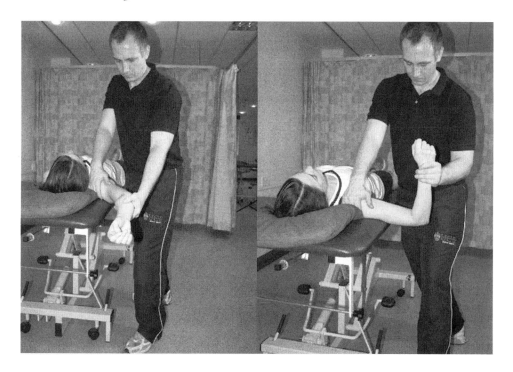

Photo 6.8 Passive range of movement assessment: abduction and medial and lateral rotation (start position).

Accessory movement assessment of the shoulder

Passive arthrokinematic or accessory movement assessment requires the sports therapist to observe the quality and RoM while recording any provocation of pain, spasm or resistance throughout the range between articulating joint surfaces (i.e. the humeral head and the glenoid fossa) (Foglia and Musarra, 2008). Accessory movements performed on the glenohumeral joint include rolling, gliding, distraction, rotation and oscillation (Donatelli, 2011); these should be applied carefully and provocatively in order to reproduce (and potentially manage) the patient's symptoms. During the application of accessory movements the patient should ideally be non-irritable, with no joint inflammation present. The shoulder joint must be fully supported by the practitioner, who should apply precise movements while observing any reproduction of symptoms (Petty, 2011). In relation to the glenohumeral joint, longitudinal caudad distraction may be progressed through an additional range of abduction to 90° and cephalad compression. Anteroposterior (AP) glides may also be progressed to include delivery in 90° abduction and also medial or lateral rotation in the presence of rotational deficits. Similarly, posteroanterior (PA) glides may be progressed with gradual addition of flexion to end of range. Lateral distraction in a neutral position is also advised (Hengeveld and Banks, 2005).

Resisted movement assessment of the shoulder

Assessment of resisted movement requires the sports therapist to apply resistance against the patient's attempt to perform specific shoulder movements. The subsequent isometric or static muscle contraction may then identify the current level of strength or weakness of the performing muscle(s) and confirm the potential presence of musculotendinous trauma or neural dysfunction without placing undue stress on the joint's non-contractile structures. Ability to generate force therefore depends on the integrity of the contractile and neural components of the target tissue. The therapist should initially apply resistance to the joint in mid-range, which is considered less injurious compared to end-range contractions. Once the isometric contraction has been initiated, the therapist should apply gradual resistance until the maximum available strength is confirmed. Resisted movements for the glenohumeral joint may include flexion, extension, abduction, adduction, lateral and medial rotation, and horizontal flexion and extension. Resisted movements for the scapulothoracic joint include protraction, retraction, elevation and depression (Magee, 2014; McFarland, 2006). Combinations of these movements may also be assessed.

Muscle length tests of the shoulder

Muscle length tests are implemented specifically to examine the functionality of individual muscles and their associated myofascia, and are either performed passively or are actively assisted; the aim is to assess the increase in distance between origin and insertion, therefore lengthening the muscle in an opposing direction to its action. Myofascial length may be normal, excessive or limited, which can be determined by comparison with the contralateral side and also against published average norms. Excessive muscle length subsequently results in weakness and dynamic instability due to elongation of the contractile sarcomeres (Allen, 2001). This predisposition may also be accompanied by compensatory shortening of the antagonist muscle, creating inadequate length–tension relationships and muscle imbalance. In contrast, limited muscle length stemming from spasm, chronic injury or biomechanical dysfunction may arguably promote greater strength production; however, the antagonist muscle will remain in a relatively elongated position (Kendall *et al.*, 2005).

The sports therapist should be aware that accuracy in testing requires fixation of the origin, while the insertion bone is moved distally to increase the muscle length (Kendall *et al.*, 2005). The pectoralis major may be assessed with the patient in a supine position with hands clasped behind the head and the lumbar spine in contact with the treatment couch. The practitioner should ensure this position is maintained with no unnecessary cervical flexion. As the shoulders relax, the elbows will move inferiorly towards the plinth, allowing the practitioner to tape-measure the distance between the olecranon process of the humerus and the couch surface. Latissimus dorsi may also be assessed in a supine position, with the patient's arms remaining at the side of the trunk with elbows extended. The therapist may then actively assist shoulder flexion towards the available end-range of movement while maintaining full elbow extension with the humerus adjacent to the head, and the lumbar spine remaining in contact with the couch. Measurement may be recorded using goniometry by applying the central axis (fulcrum) laterally to the acromion process of the scapula, the moving arm in line with the lateral epicondyle of the humerus and the stationary arm horizontally aligned to the lateral midline of the trunk (Berryman-Reese and Bandy, 2010). The local medial and lateral rotator muscle groups can be tested with the patient in a supine position with 90° shoulder abduction and 90° elbow flexion, with the forearm perpendicular to the couch. The practitioner may support the shoulder while ensuring that the patient's lumbar spine and shoulder girdle remain in contact with the couch. To assess medial rotator length, the patient may externally rotate the shoulder, moving the forearm parallel to the head, aiming to rest the forearm on the plinth and achieving the normal RoM of 90°. To assess lateral rotator length, the patient may internally rotate the shoulder, aiming to rest the forearm close to the couch; however, the normal RoM is 70° therefore the forearm may remain at a 20° angle to the couch (Kendall *et al.*, 2005). More expansive muscle length testing protocol and variations on assessment can be accessed from the aforementioned academic sources in addition to testing for optimal scapula positioning (Clarkson, 2013; Struyf *et al.*, 2012).

Special tests of the shoulder

The intricate structural anatomy of the shoulder creates a considerable diagnostic challenge, especially when confronted with the coexistence of multiple pathological presentations; therefore orthopaedic special tests for the shoulder joint provide sports therapists with an exceptionally wide-ranging choice of testing protocol for determining or eliminating the various pathologies. No individual test is exclusively sensitive or specific (Donnelly *et al.*, 2013), therefore it is imperative for therapists to examine both the reliability and validity of each special test prior to application. Indeed, there are over 120 published orthopaedic tests for the shoulder, and while the evidence-base for their use improves, a general consensus exists with regard to their having rather low diagnostic utility (Horsley, 2010). Obtaining a specific diagnosis – or at least a measured patient-specific clinical impression – in addition to determining the prognosis and appropriate treatment strategy for a patient is considered essential (van der Heijden, 1999). The resolution of shoulder conditions has historically been extremely poor, with 41 per cent of primary care patients having persistent pain 12 months after initial consultation (van der Windt *et al.*, 1996). As discussed in Chapter 2, published sensitivity ratings of special tests reflect the ability to identify patients with a given condition, while specificity ratings of tests reflect the ability to identify patients without a given condition who have a negative test. Positive and negative likelihood ratios, derived from sensitivity and specificity ratings, provide further indications of the value of a given test result. A positive likelihood ratio (+ve LR) raises the suspicion (probability) that a condition actually exists. A negative likelihood ratio (–ve LR) suggests that the condition which is being tested for probably does not exist. A +ve LR greater than 1 indicates an increased probability that the condition being tested is present (the larger the number the greater the probability); conversely, a –ve LR less than 1 indicates a decreased probability that the condition being tested is present (the smaller the number the lower the probability). The specificity and sensitivity of recommended orthopaedic tests of the shoulder has been presented in systematic reviews by Hegedus *et al.* (2008; 2012) and also in an inter-examiner assessment article by Cadogan *et al.* (2010). Sports therapists should therefore aim to identify the published reliability and validity ratings of any given test. A review of reliability ratings for a selection of commonly utilized special tests for shoulder conditions are presented in Table 6.4. Beyond this, it is often challenging to be able to make autonomous decisions pertaining to the suitability of any test in relation to the acuteness of the condition and symptom presentation, as these can cause both unnecessary aggravation, and negate the reliability of any result. Furthermore, it is the performance, positioning, handling and interpretation of any test which underpin its reliability. Below is a small selection of some of the more commonly utilized and better evidenced shoulder special tests. Because of the diagnostic challenges associated with the shoulder, a discussion on 'Shoulder Symptom Modification Procedures' (SSMP) is also presented.

Ligament stress tests of the shoulder

Piano key sign

Acromioclavicular joint instability may be assessed using the 'piano key sign test'. With the patient in a sitting position with the arm rested at the side, the therapist applies an inferiorly directed digital pressure to the lateral clavicle proximal to the AC joint. A positive test is indicated by depression and elevation of the clavicle in response to the inferiorly directed pressure and its subsequent release, which may indicate AC and/or coracoclavicular ligament sprain or separation (Schepsis and Busconi, 2006).

AC joint compression test

Acromioclavicular or coracoclavicular ligament sprains may be assessed using the 'AC joint compression test' (also known as the 'AC shear test'). The patient should be relaxed with the arm at the side in either a seated or supine position. Standing on the affected side, the therapist places one hand onto the patient's clavicle and the other on the spine of scapula before gently

Table 6.4 Reliability ratings of selected special tests

Test	Diagnosis	Sensitivity	Specificity	+ LR	– LR
Neer's test	Subacromial impingement	0.75–0.88	0.51	–	–
Hawkins–Kennedy test	Subacromial impingement	0.92	0.25–0.44	–	–
Apprehension test	Anterior GH instability	0.68	1.00	–	–
Relocation test	Anterior GH instability	0.57	1.00	–	–
Sulcus sign	Inferior GH instability	0.31	0.89	2.8	0.78
Yergason's test	Biceps tendon instability/ tendinopathy	0.12	0.86	–	–
Speed's test	Biceps tendon instability/ tendinopathy	0.90	0.14	1.1	0.72
Anterior drawer test	Anterior GH instability	0.54	0.78	2.5	0.59
O'Brien's test	Labral lesion	0.54	0.31	0.8	1.5
Crank test	Labral lesion	0.91	0.93	1.1	0.95
Lift-Off test	Subscapularis lesion	0.62	100	>25	0.38

Source: adapted from Horsley, 2010.

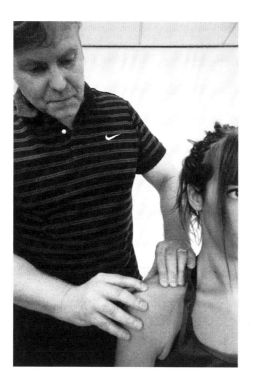

Photo 6.9   Piano key sign test.

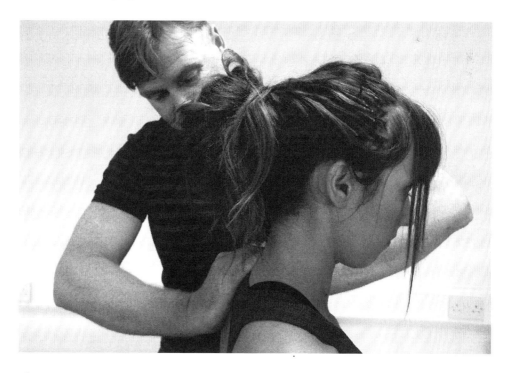

Photo 6.10   AC joint compression test.

squeezing both hands together, observing for abnormal translation of the clavicle and AC joint. This positive presentation may also be accompanied by pain (Schepsis and Busconi, 2006); the 'scarf test' may be used in conjunction.

Yergason's test

Laxity of the transverse humeral ligament may be assessed using 'Yergason's test', which aims to detect bicipital tendon subluxation (Pettitt *et al.*, 2008). The patient should be seated or standing, with the elbow flexed to 90° and the forearm in full pronation. Standing on the affected side, the therapist places one hand over the patient's bicipital groove while their other hand clasps the pronated forearm. The therapist should then instruct the patient to actively supinate the forearm while applying firm resistance. A positive test may be indicated by snapping or popping sensations proximal to the bicipital groove (Magee, 2014). Some studies have challenged the sheer existence of the transverse humeral ligament, with evidence intimating that the structure is simply a continuation of the osseous attachment of the rotator-cuff complex (Gleason *et al.*, 2006; MacDonald *et al.*, 2007). Pain in the absence of subluxation may indicate tendinopathy; pain more localized to the superior aspect of the joint may indicate labral damage.

Stress tests may be applied to assess the sternoclavicular ligament complex as the patient is seated or supine with the affected arm in a relaxed position. The therapist should place one hand on the sternal end of the clavicle and the other on the spine of the scapula before applying a moderate posteroinferior pressure to the clavicle in an attempt to elicit pain or observe excessive clavicular translation. Similarly, the acromioclavicular and coracoclavicular ligaments may be assessed, adopting the same testing protocol applying identical pressure to the acromial end of the clavicle (Amato *et al.*, 2006).

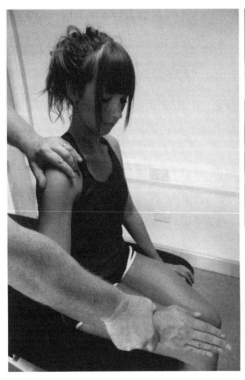
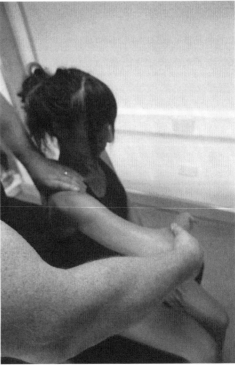

Photo 6.11   Yergason's test.   *Photo 6.12*   Hawkins–Kennedy test.

Impingement tests

Hawkins–Kennedy test

The 'Hawkins–Kennedy test' is primarily used to assess subacromial impingement of the rotator-cuff complex or subacromial bursa. Positive findings may be indicated by the reproduction of pain specifically approaching the rotational end of range manoeuvre. This test may also affect other subacromial structures, including the glenoid labrum and long head of biceps tendon (Hattam and Smeatham, 2010). The test demonstrates anatomical validity and specificity for confirming the pathology (Cadogan *et al.*, 2010); however, in the presence of subacromial inflammation, capsulitis or posterior instability this test will inevitably reproduce symptoms resulting in a false positive (Cook and Hegedus, 2013). Standing adjacent to the patient (sitting or standing) on the affected side, the therapist places one hand under the 90° flexed elbow with their other hand stabilizing the scapula as the shoulder is passively assisted to 90° flexion with the palm facing downwards. The therapist should passively assist the shoulder into internal rotation by rotating the greater tubercle under the coracoacromial arch, which may force the supraspinatus tendon against the coracoacromial ligament (Moen *et al.*, 2010).

Neer's test

Subacromial impingement, bursitis, rotator-cuff lesions and superior labral tears may also be assessed via 'Neer's test'. A positive finding may be indicated by the reproduction of pain at end-range passive flexion. The lack of specificity in this test suggests low validity in diagnosing impingement syndrome (Cook and Hegedus, 2013) implicating subacromial bursitis or rotator-cuff tears in the process (MacDonald *et al.*, 2000). Standing adjacent to patient (sitting or standing) on the affected side, the therapist will stabilize the scapula with one hand, while the

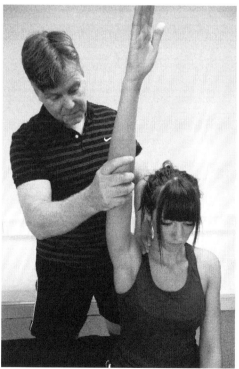
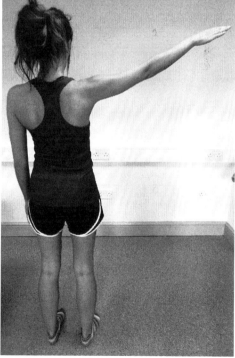

Photo 6.13   Neer's test.   *Photo 6.14*   Painful arc test.

other supports the same arm inferior to the elbow. The arm is then passively elevated into full flexion, causing potential impingement as the greater tubercle of the humerus compresses the supraspinatus tendon and subacromial bursa against the acromion process (Moen *et al.*, 2010). Several authors have described performing the test in both externally (biceps long head) and internally rotated (supraspinatus) shoulder positions, although due to the complexity of the glenohumeral anatomy the test is considered non-specific.

Painful arc test

The 'painful arc test' can help the therapist suspect subacromial impingement if pain is experienced between 60–120° (the 'painful arc') during standing active abduction; typically the pain is experienced in the anterior aspect of the shoulder. The pain may also be accompanied by compensatory hitching (elevation) of the shoulder girdle. If pain is experienced more in the outer range of abduction (around 170–180°), this may indicate pathology of the acromioclavicular joint, warranting further investigation (Magee, 2014).

Labral tests

Speed's test

Biceps tendon (long head) pathology or unstable superior labral anterior to posterior (SLAP) lesions may be suspected following a positive 'Speed's test'. Positive findings may be indicated by localized pain proximal to the bicipital groove through which the biceps tendon passes, but consideration should also be given towards a significant rupture which may produce weakness with little or no pain (Hattam and Smeatham, 2010). Deeper pain may indicate that a labral lesion is present; therefore this test is more specific for diagnosis of non-specific labral tears (Cook and Hegedus, 2013). Standing adjacent to the patient (seated or standing) on the affected side, the therapist stabilizes the patient's shoulder with one hand, while the shoulder is in 60–90° flexion with the elbow in full extension and forearm supination. The other hand is placed onto the forearm to apply downward pressure. The patient is required to resist the downward pressure applied by the therapist while maintaining the original start position.

Yergason's test may also assist in the assessment of SLAP lesions and biceps tendon pathology. Positive findings may be indicated by pain reproduction at the bicipital groove. Should the patient experience clicking sensations during this special test, the therapist may consider laxity or rupture of the transverse humeral ligament responsible for securing the biceps tendon into the bicipital groove (Hattam and Smeatham, 2010). Lacking in specificity for diagnosis of long head of biceps pathology (Cook and Hegedus, 2013), Yergason's test does provide increasing evidence for diagnosing SLAP lesions (Guanche and Jones, 2003).

Crank test

The 'crank test' investigates the presence of a SLAP lesion, with positive findings reproducing the patient's pain, commonly accompanied by a catching sensation, painful clicking or crepitus particularly during the external rotation phase of the test. Although the test is specific and demonstrates a high level of diagnostic accuracy for assessing labral lesions (Cadogan *et al.*, 2010), the therapist should also consider referral to MRI or arthroscopy for a definitive diagnosis (Hattam and Smeatham, 2010). Standing adjacent to the patient (seated or supine) on the affected side, the therapist supports their elbow in 90° flexion. The patient's arm is then passively elevated in the scapular plane until the shoulder has reached full flexion. The therapist then applies a gentle axial load through the longitudinal axis of the humerus and, using the elbow as a lever, rotates the shoulder into full external rotation immediately followed by internal rotation (Hattam and Smeatham, 2010).

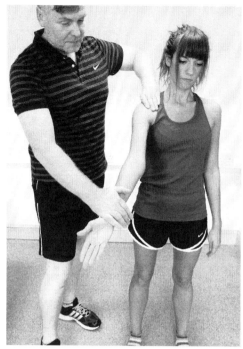 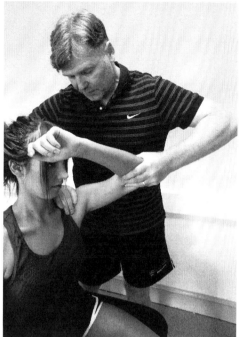

Photo 6.15 Speed's test.   *Photo 6.16* Crank test.

Clunk test

Using a similar approach to the crank test, the 'clunk test' has the patient either seated (Vizniak, 2012) or supine (Cipriano, 2010; Cook and Hegedus, 2012). The therapist applies passive external rotation in full abduction while palpating the anterior humeral head for characteristic 'clunking' or grinding that can occur with an anteriorly torn labrum in this position.

Biceps load test II

The 'biceps load test II' investigates SLAP lesions and has replaced its original prototype due to test research using 75 patients with unilateral anterior dislocations (Kim *et al.*, 1999) which exists as an indicator of SLAP lesions alone, and therefore compromised the effectiveness and validity of the original biceps load test (Cook and Hegedus, 2013). The start position of the biceps load test II reflects the cocking phase of throwing, creating an oblique angle between the long head of biceps and the posterosuperior glenoid labrum. Ensuing contraction of the tendon may recreate pain as it concurrently stresses its labral attachment during this effective test (Kim *et al.*, 2001). Positive findings for this test may be indicated by reproduction of shoulder pain as the superior labrum peels off the glenoid margin during resisted elbow flexion (Moen *et al.*, 2010). Standing adjacent to the patient (supine towards the side of the couch) on the affected side, the therapist takes the patient's elbow into 90° flexion while supporting the forearm and biceps brachii region. The shoulder is then abducted to 120° followed by full external rotation and supination of the forearm, placing maximum tension onto the long head of biceps brachii. The patient should then perform elbow flexion as an isometric contraction against the therapist's resistance (Hattam and Smeatham, 2010).

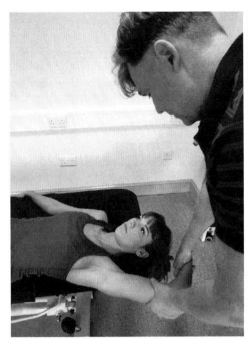 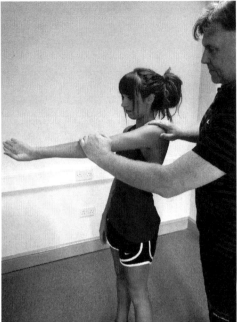

Photo 6.17 Biceps load test II.   *Photo 6.18* O'Brien's test.

O'Brien's test

The 'active compression' or 'O'Brien's test' provides considerable sensitivity when assessing SLAP lesions, and is also highly specific for assessing acromioclavicular joint pathology (Cook and Hegedus, 2013). Positive findings are indicated either by pain at the AC joint, or a deeper clicking sensation which may incriminate the labrum. The test is performed in two parts. While the patient is standing, the therapist should stand behind the patient, holding the forearm which is positioned in 90° of forward flexion, 10–15° horizontal adduction and maximal internal rotation, with the elbow in full extension. The therapist should then apply an inferiorly directed force to the patient's arm with the instruction to resist downward movement. This process is then repeated with the shoulder in full external rotation. A SLAP lesion may be suspected in the presence of deep pain (with possible clicking) during the internal rotation component, which is relieved in the external rotation component. An AC joint pathology may be suspected if pain is experienced on the superior aspect of the shoulder during the internal rotation component (and also relieved during the external rotation component). High specificity provided by O'Brien's test facilitates accurate confirmation of AC joint pathology (Moen *et al.*, 2010).

SLAP prehension test

First described by Berg and Ciullo (1998), the 'SLAP prehension test' assesses for superior labral anterior to posterior unstable lesions. It comprises two movement components. The patient may be seated or standing as they are asked to horizontally adduct (flex) their arm from a start position of 90° shoulder abduction with internal rotation, and elbow extension. The therapist notes any or pain or 'clunking' (the therapist may palpate the superior aspect of the shoulder with the palm of their hand) during the movement. The patient is then asked to repeat the movement, this time with external rotation of the shoulder. Localized anterior shoulder pain, possibly combined with a 'clunk', during the internally rotated component of the test – which is then reduced during the externally rotated component – is indicative of a SLAP lesion. The combined movements of horizontal adduction and internal rotation increases the stress on the biceps long head and its possibly loose labral attachment; this may then cause these to be displaced into the joint. Berg and Ciullo (1998) reported that the test may be helpful in differentiating patients with unstable SLAP lesions from those with impingement or acromioclavicular arthrosis.

Instability tests

Apprehension–relocation test

The 'apprehension–relocation test' implements two specific components which collaboratively assess the glenohumeral joint for anterior instability. The test has also been implemented to assess labral lesions, but research fails to support its effectiveness in diagnosing such pathology (Cook and Hegedus, 2013). Positive findings during the apprehension phase may be indicated by the patient's anxiety or resistance against the therapist's attempts to passively take the shoulder through movement into a combination of abduction and external rotation (a position likely to cause dislocation). This test provides high specificity in determining anterior instability (Lo *et al.*, 2004), especially since utilizing patient 'apprehension' as a diagnostic criterion (Duncan-Tennent *et al.*, 2003), rather than pain per se, is a reaction commonly elicited from patients who experience anterior instability (Hattam and Smeatham, 2010). If pain is the generated symptom response, other pathology should be suspected (such as a labral or rotator-cuff tear). Standing adjacent to the patient (supine) on the affected side, the therapist should support the patient's forearm (on their thigh). The shoulder is then gently abducted to 90° and passively controlled through external rotation up to 90°. Additionally, a posteroanterior glide may then be applied to the posterior humeral head. In the presence of a positive result (i.e. patient apprehension or reflexive tensing) the therapist may then apply the palmar surface of their hand to the anterior humeral head, essentially applying an anterior stabilizing force, as if relocating it into the glenoid fossa during the repeated manoeuvre. A positive result is indicated if apprehension is reduced by this component.

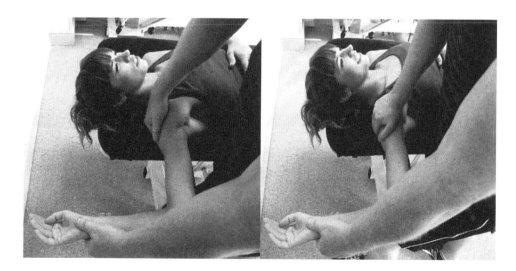

Photo 6.19   Apprehension–relocation test.

Sulcus sign

The 'sulcus sign' investigates the extent of inferior laxity of the glenohumeral joint by applying an inferior translation to the joint; it may also provide clues to a potential superior labral tear. Standing adjacent to the seated patient with an unobstructed view of the lateral shoulder, the therapist should place their middle finger and thumb onto the anterior and posterior angles of the acromion process, leaving the index finger free to palpate the sulcus region (Hattam and Smeatham, 2010). Having encouraged the patient to relax the shoulder, the therapist's remaining hand should firmly grip the arm above the elbow before applying a progressive caudad distraction of the humerus. Positive findings may be indicated by the development of a visible depression (sulcus) between the lateral border of the acromion process of scapula and the proximal humerus accompanied by tightening of the skin. Performing this test in approximately 20° abduction with minimal internal rotation promotes maximum potential for inferior humeral distraction (Helmig *et al.*, 1990). Mallon and Speer (1995) presented a grading system:

- Grade I: <1 cm distance between the inferior acromion and humeral head;
- Grade II: 1–1.5 cm;
- Grade III: >1.5 cm.

Anterior drawer test

The 'anterior drawer test' assesses the extent of anterior capsular instability of the shoulder. Positive findings may be indicated by the degree of anterior glenohumeral translation in comparison to the unaffected shoulder. The test may be performed with the patient either seated or supine-lying. Standing adjacent to the patient on the affected side, the therapist uses one hand to stabilize the lateral shoulder girdle while holding the proximal humerus with their

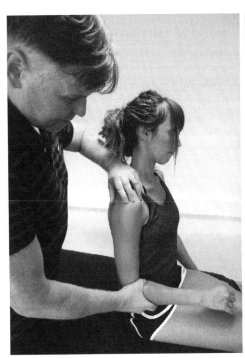

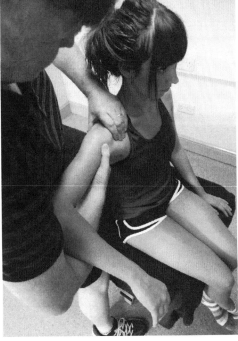

Photo 6.20 Sulcus sign.

Photo 6.21 Anterior drawer test.

other hand. The shoulder is then passively abducted to approximately 90° and a posteroanterior force is applied across the glenohumeral joint at the head of the humerus. The therapist should record the degree of anterior translation (in cm) as a marker in the rehabilitation process (Cook and Hegedus, 2013).

Rotator-cuff tests

Full can and empty can tests

The 'full can' and 'empty can' tests investigate the possible presence of tendinopathy, impingement syndrome or rupture sustained by the supraspinatus. Positive findings of supraspinatus tendinopathy or impingement syndrome may be indicated by reproduction of pain without weakness. Pain accompanied by weakness may be indicative of a partial or complete rupture. Sports therapists should also consider a differential diagnosis, where weakness in the absence of pain may reflect a suprascapular neuropathy or C5 palsy (Hattam and Smeatham, 2010). The seated patient is required to elevate both arms to 90° in the scapular plane with both thumbs pointing upwards (i.e. a 'full can' position). The therapist then applies downwards pressure through the patient's forearms as the position is maintained by the patient. The test is then repeated, still in scaption, this time with the patient's shoulder internally rotated and forearms pronated so both thumbs point downwards ('empty can'). The full can version, because of reduced potential for impingement, may be considered preferable to ascertain strength or weakness of supraspinatus.

Drop arm test

The 'drop arm test' involves the therapist passively abducting the seated patient's arm past 90° and then asking the patient to slowly lower the arm back to a neutral position. If the patient is unable to control the movement due to pain or weakness, this can indicate possible rotator-cuff tear (most likely supraspinatus) (Cipriano, 2010).

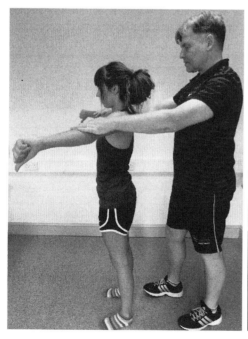
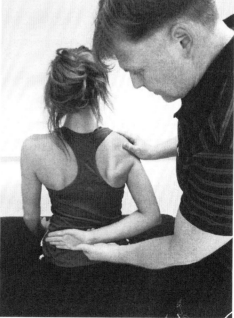

Photo 6.22   Empty can test.   *Photo 6.23*   Lift–off test.

Lift-off test

Gerber's 'lift-off test' is implemented to ascertain possible rupture of the subscapularis muscle. Positive findings may be indicated by the patient's inability (weakness or pain) to perform the movement (Gerber and Krushell, 1991). The patient is seated with the affected arm positioned behind the back (if possible) (i.e. in a position of internal rotation and slight extension) with the dorsal aspect of the hand facing the lumbar region. The patient's arm is then passively moved into further internal rotation and they are then instructed to maintain that position as the therapist's support is removed (Hattam and Smeatham, 2010). An inability to maintain this position is indicative of a subscapularis rupture. A variant of the lift-off test is the 'Gerber push-off test'. For this version, the therapist offers resistance to the patient's contraction into internal rotation, which isolates subscapularis, and if painful or weak is indicative of damage to the muscle or tendon. Patients with other pathology (such as impingement, labral or other tendon tears) may not be able to assume the start position, hence the 'abdominal compression' or 'belly-press test' version may be utilized; for this, the patient attempts to perform isometric contraction against the resistance of their abdomen (Magee, 2014).

Acromioclavicular tests

Scarf test

In addition to the previously discussed 'piano key sign' and 'AC joint compression tests', the 'scarf test' (also known as the 'cross-body [adduction] test') assesses for lesions of the acromioclavicular joint. Positive findings (for AC pathology) are indicated by localized pain over the AC joint line, or along the C4 dermatome. Further structures may be subjected to compression during this test: the subscapularis and bursa and the subacromial bursa (which may

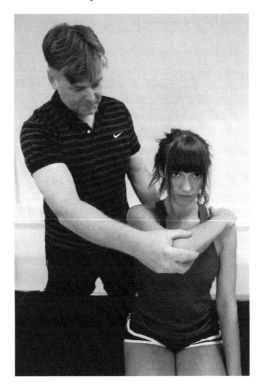

Photo 6.24   Scarf test.

be experiencing impingement); the sternoclavicular joint; and the posterior musculature (infraspinatus and teres minor) and joint capsule. Each of these may require further investigation (Atkins *et al.*, 2010). Standing adjacent to the patient (seated or standing) on the affected side, the therapist will place one hand onto the opposite unaffected shoulder to provide counter-leverage. The other hand will support 90° flexed elbow of the affected limb before passively assisting the shoulder into 90° flexion with the patient's palm facing downwards. Having established an internally rotated start position, passive horizontal adduction is applied across the patient's body to the end of available range. This test lacks specificity as apprehension or pain may be reproduced in the presence of posterior instability (Hattam and Smeatham, 2010).

Shoulder symptom modification procedures

The 'shoulder symptom modification procedure' (SSMP) was first described by Lewis (2009), and proposes that passive manual techniques may be employed by the therapist to reduce symptoms which have been previously identified; the SSMP makes no claim to confirm diagnosis or structural differentiation, but is designed to improve patient-specific management. Modification techniques may be performed to improve scapular or humeral head positioning, and/or reduce thoracic kyphosis.

Scapular assistance testing

A number of researchers have investigated the 'scapular assistance test' (SAT) (Rabin *et al.*, 2006; Seitz *et al.*, 2012). The SAT involves passive assistance or repositioning of the scapula by the therapist, most typically by increasing upward rotation and posterior tilt during shoulder abduction. For this, the therapist stands to the side of the patient and places the palms of their hands over the anterior and posterior aspects of the shoulder, stabilizing or mobilizing the scapula as the patient performs abduction. This is employed prior to active performance of previously assessed symptom-producing elevation movements and where abnormal scapular kinematics (dyskinesia) is suspected, especially in patients with impingement syndrome. Where such manual assistance provides a clear reduction in symptoms (by increasing the subacromial space), treatment and rehabilitation may then be geared towards achieving a similar response.

Positioning of the humeral head

Attention to the resting position of the humeral head within the glenoid fossa should also be a consideration, particularly in sports involving forceful overhead movements. The humeral head should ideally protrude less than one-third in front of the acromion, and there will normally be a resting position of neutral humeral internal rotation. Additionally, the proximal and distal ends of the humerus will sit within the same plane. During active elevation in the scapular plane, the movement of the humeral head should be assessed, more effectively with palpation rather than observation; and this should ideally reveal minimal humeral head movement (Graichen *et al.*, 2000; Ludewig and Cook, 2000):

- Anterior translation ~0.7–2.7 mm during the first 30–60° of scaption (abduction in the plane of the scapula);
- Posterior translation ~1.5 mm during the first 60–90° of scaption;
- Posterior translation ~4.5 mm during the first 90–120° of scaption.

To confirm the initial suspicion of excessive anterior humeral head translation, the following tests are recommended:

- Supine medial rotation: palpating for excessive humeral head translation;
- Prone medial rotation: (resisted testing) which may be weak in the inner range;
- Prone lateral rotation: palpating for anterior glide of humeral head;
- Standing shoulder abduction: palpating for anterior glide of humeral head;
- Elbow extension: palpating for anterior glide of the humeral head.

The humeral head may also appear to translate excessively superiorly, but may be due to limited inferior humeral translation, which in turn could be due to sub-optimal recruitment patterns and muscle length, such as a dominant or shortened deltoid muscle; a dominant pectoralis major or latissimus dorsi in preference to subscapularis; or a shortened or weakened infraspinatus, teres minor and/or subscapularis.

Glenohumeral internal rotation deficit

A common finding in tennis players and baseball pitchers is an alteration in the position of the total arc of humeral rotation, at 90° abduction, of the shoulder. Burkhart and co-workers (Burkhart *et al.*, 2003a) proposed the term 'GIRD' (glenohumeral internal rotation deficit) for the loss of internal rotation caused by posteroinferior capsular tightness. GIRD can be defined as the loss in degrees of glenohumeral internal rotation of the throwing shoulder compared with the non-throwing shoulder. Myers *et al.* (2005) suggested that there is an association of GIRD to the development of shoulder injuries. The important consideration with GIRD is that if the limitation of internal rotation exceeds the gain in external rotation (GERG), resulting in a decrease in rotational arc (greater than 10 per cent of the contralateral side), then the shoulder is susceptible to injury (Myers *et al.*, 2005). Posteroinferior capsular tightness can also be assessed via the method advocated by Tyler *et al.* (1999); the patient is placed in a side-lying position on the couch, with the scapula fixed in retraction and the upper arm flexed to 90°. The examiner then adducts the arm towards the couch until restriction is met. The distance from the olecranon process (point of elbow) to the couch is then measured. The amount of horizontal glenohumeral adduction indicates the amount of posterior shoulder tightness; the greater the distance measured, the greater the posterior capsular tightness.

Neural assessment

A comprehensive neurological examination may be warranted in patients presenting with a primary complaint of shoulder pain. The presence of neurological symptoms, including suspected radicular pain in the upper extremity, paraesthesia, dysaesthesia or anaesthesia, warrants such examination. Neural assessment is discussed further in Chapter 2.

Dermatomal assessment

Dermatomes are mapped sensory zones of the skin innervated by a single spinal segment. In the shoulder region, nerve root C4 innervates the clavicular and upper scapular regions, C5 innervates the 'regimental badge' zone of the deltoids and nerve roots C6 and C7, respectively, serve the anterior and lateral aspects of the upper arm, coinciding with biceps and triceps brachii muscle groups. Neural dysfunction may produce paraesthesia or altered sensations including pins and needles or numbness within the sensory zone (Magee, 2014; McClelland and Paxinos, 2008).

Sensory assessment preferably requires the patient's eyes to be closed. Initial examination may simply involve the application of light pressure from the therapist's hands on both the affected and contralateral zones while recording any abnormal sensory perception. Finer material, including cotton thread, may be used to examine response to light touch as the therapist systematically trails

---

Practitioner Tip Box 6.5

Dermatomes of the shoulder

- C4 relates to the clavicular and upper scapular region
- C5 relates to the lateral anterior and posterior upper arm
- C6 relates to the lateral anterior and posterior arm and elbow

---

the material within the targeted zone. Pain response may be examined using a sharp object, which should be used lightly to prevent injury and sporadically to prevent the patient predicting when the stimulus is applied. The therapist should be aware of sensory response which can range from an absence of sensation to hyperalgesia (Hertling and Kessler, 2006).

Myotomal assessment

Myotomes are represented by a muscle or muscle group which are innervated by a specific nerve root. Patients presenting with perceived weakness, motor dysfunction or localized muscular atrophy in the shoulder require neurological screening to assess the myotomes. Each myotome is tested by applying resistance to facilitate an isometric contraction which the patient should hold for five seconds. The sports therapist must be able to differentiate the signs and symptoms of a nerve root lesion from a peripheral nerve lesion. Nerve root lesions are invariably accompanied by paresis or partial paralysis, which may initially delay any evident weakness, hence the recommendation for a sustained isometric contraction. In contrast, a peripheral nerve lesion will result in complete muscular paralysis in the absence of neural innervation (Magee, 2014; Petty, 2011).

Focusing on the shoulder, levator scapulae and the upper trapezius fibres require innervation from nerve root C4 and cranial nerve XI to facilitate elevation and rotation of the scapulothoracic joint; therefore a resisted isometric contraction may be applied by instructing the patient to shrug their shoulders. The C5 spinal nerve innervates the supraspinatus and deltoid muscles during abduction, and infraspinatus during external rotation, therefore an isometric contraction may be imposed through a progressive RoM as the patient abducts their shoulder in conjunction with external rotation by raising the arm sideways from the trunk, while rotating their hands and corresponding forearm to face upwards (Russell, 2006). Further myotomes include the biceps brachii emanating from the musculocutaneous nerve (C5–7) and triceps brachii from the radial nerve (C6–8, T1), which can be respectively tested by applying resisted elbow flexion and extension (Rockwood *et al.*, 2009; Pellerin *et al.*, 2010).

Practitioner Tip Box 6.6

Myotomes of the shoulder

- C4 (XI) relates to shoulder elevation
- C5 (axillary) relates to shoulder abduction and external rotation
- C6 (musculocutaneous) relates to elbow flexion (connection with biceps brachii)
- C7 (radial) relates to elbow extension (connection with triceps brachii)

Practitioner Tip Box 6.7

Reflexes of the shoulder

- C5–6 Biceps brachii
- C7–8 Triceps brachii

Reflex testing

Deep tendon reflex tests assess the neural and muscular integrity which provides the specific reflex, including the associated afferent and efferent neural pathways. The therapist should be aware that early stage lower motor neuron (peripheral) lesions (LMNL) are rarely identified in response to a single reflex test; therefore, in order to promote an effective stretch reflex response of the tendon, it is recommended that six repetitive taps of a tendon hammer are performed. Reflex tests should be compared bilaterally to identify an absent, diminished (reduced) or exaggerated (brisk) reflex response. A brisk reflex (hyper-reflexia) is associated with a possible upper motor neuron lesion (UMNL), which requires further evaluation (Hertling and Kessler, 2006). The main deep tendon reflexes to test relating to the shoulder are those of the biceps and triceps. Repetitive tapping of the stimulus sites – i.e. the distal biceps tendon at the anterior elbow (C5–6) and the distal triceps tendon (C7–8) above the olecranon process, should produce a normal, visible and/or palpable muscular contraction (Magee, 2014). Absent or heightened reflexes are not in isolation a confirmatory finding.

Reassessment approaches for the shoulder

Periodic reassessment during each stage of the rehabilitation process is essential for identifying and recording progression (or possible regression) of the patient/athlete's fitness levels. A subjective review and focused objective examination should be performed each time the patient returns for treatment; an accurately recorded patient history allows the therapist to analyse previous findings and recommendations, as well as test markers (including RoM, special test and palpatory findings), and compare these against current test findings. If patient regression is evident, the therapist has the opportunity to implement new rehabilitation strategies or commence the referral process.

Return to functional training typically require the athlete to attain pre-season baseline fitness levels which demonstrate satisfactory joint RoM and strength, scapulohumeral rhythm, sensorimotor function, flexibility, aerobic capacity and a successful healing response to clinical interventions. Joint dysfunctions, including GIRD, will ideally be eliminated or reduced to within a 25° difference when compared to the contralateral side. Maximizing sensorimotor function is essential; therefore the recommended exercises to counteract the dysfunctional shoulder should be maintained throughout the functional phase in conjunction with an extensive scapulothoracic stabilization programme (Paine and Voight, 2013; Tripp, 2008). A core stability programme can also prevent excessive force on the distal kinetic segments due to the generation of increased force production at the proximal core (Cools and Fredriksen, 2012). Return to play protocols are widely reviewed in the literature (Anderson *et al.*, 2009; Beam, 2002; Brukner and Khan, 2009; Horsley, 2010; Prentice, 2011; Wilk *et al.*, 2012).

Injuries of the shoulder region

Many injury rehabilitation strategies are governed by a progressive process focusing on supporting the athlete through the acute, sub-acute, late and functional phases, and providing specific aims and interventions for each phase (Anderson *et al.*, 2009; Beam, 2002; Prentice, 2011). A common first-stage rehabilitation protocol for acute shoulder injury will often be required to help reduce immediate symptoms and prevent worsening by implementing 'PRICE' or 'POLICE' principles (Bleakley *et al.*, 2012). The typical sub-acute stage aims to reduce pain using immobilization only if necessary, otherwise early mobilization is encouraged in pain-free ranges. Glenohumeral and scapular mobility and stabilization are promoted by progressing pain-free movements through RoM, focusing on scapulohumeral rhythm and proprioceptive training (Paine and Voight, 2013). Later-stage goals aim to restore normal shoulder function, including strength and stabilization, and full RoM by progressing functional exercises contextualized to the patient's sport or activity. Functional-stage aims require the athlete to have retained pre-injury fitness levels, while demonstrating ability to recover in preparation for repeated maximum activity (Cools and Fredriksen, 2012).

Shoulder pain and dysfunction in the overhead athlete are associated with prevalent aetiological factors including intrinsic glenohumeral and capsulolabral pathologies, extrinsic rotator-cuff pathologies and also neurovascular trauma, all of which are particularly prevalent in tennis (Neuman *et al.*, 2011; van der Hoeven and Kibler, 2006), throwing sports (Seroyer *et al.*, 2009) and swimming (Heinlein and Cosgarea, 2010; Tovin, 2006). Chronic conditions attributed to repetitive overuse inevitably predispose the athlete to recurring injury, as opposed to the acute trauma sustained in direct impact mechanisms, including shoulder tackles, or via such indirect force as sustained by falling onto an outstretched hand (commonly referred to as a 'FOOSH' mechanism). The subsequent plethora of multiple pathologies and differential diagnoses arguably endorse the shoulder complex as the most challenging joint to assess (Donnelly *et al.*, 2013). A selection of the more common shoulder pathologies and recommended strategies for their management are presented here.

Glenoid labrum injuries

The glenoid labrum and its most closely associated structures, including the shoulder capsule, long head of biceps and glenohumeral ligaments are all vulnerable to injury in this complex region (Manske and Prohaskab, 2010). The most well-recognized labral pathology is the 'superior labrum anterior to posterior' ('SLAP') lesion, which occurs just anterior to the biceps attachment (at the supraglenoid tubercle). Classically, the tear terminates posterior to the tendon. Retained stability depends on the superior labrum and biceps tendon remaining secured to the glenoid attachment; unstable 'non-SLAP' lesions comprise degenerative, flap or vertical labral tears – exemplified by Bankart lesions, which occur in approximately 90 per cent of anterior glenohumeral dislocations (Donnelly *et al.*, 2013) and are occasionally accompanied by fracture of the glenoid ridge, resulting in the bony Bankart lesion (Snyder *et al.*, 1995).

The aetiology of labral injuries commonly stems from repetitive overhead actions creating excessive inferior humeral traction forces, particularly in volleyball serving or spiking, and in the cocking phase of throwing and pitching (Kuhn *et al.*, 2003). As the shoulder position acquires approximately 90° of abduction and external rotation, the cocking phase causes peel-back traction of the biceps on the glenoid labrum and posterosuperior translation of the humeral head; this is potentially initiated by glenohumeral internal rotation dysfunction and excessive scapular protraction (Burkhart *et al.*, 2003a). Common mechanisms of injury include:

Table 6.5 Types of SLAP lesions

SLAP lesion	Description
Type I (stable)	The labral attachment to the glenoid rim is firmly intact but evidence of degeneration is present
Type II (unstable)	The superior biceps–labral complex attachment is subsequently detached from the glenoid rim
Type III (stable)	The superior labral meniscoid rim sustains a bucket handle lesion with potential displacement into the joint. The long head of biceps tendon and labral attachment remain intact
Type IV (unstable)	The superior labrum sustains a bucket-handle lesion extending into the biceps tendon with potential displacement into the joint.

Source: Burkhart *et al.*, 2003b.

compressive forces sustained from falling onto an outstretched, often abducted, arm; falling directly onto an adducted shoulder; and sustaining traction forces during pulling of the shoulder (Funk and Snow, 2007; Manske and Prohaskab, 2010).

Patients may present with decreased glenohumeral internal rotation and generic shoulder pain, which is intensified by overhead or 'hand behind back' arm actions accompanied by sensations of popping, grinding or catching. On palpation, anterior shoulder tenderness is commonly evident and exacerbated during isometric activation of the biceps brachii during resisted elbow flexion or supination. Special tests include the crank test, acknowledged for its significant specificity and accuracy (Cadogan *et al.*, 2010; Cook and Hegedus, 2013), and the O'Brien (active compression) test, which is also recognized for its sensitivity and specificity (Cook and Hegedus, 2013; O'Brien *et al.*, 1998). Although moderately specific, Speed's and Yergason's tests lack consistency (Cook and Hegedus, 2013; Holtby and Razmjou, 2004); therefore referral for arthroscopy may be required for attaining a definitive diagnosis. Manske and Prohaskab (2010) undertook extensive analysis of special tests for assessing SLAP lesions. MR arthrography, considered superior to standard MRI or radiography, employs intra-articular injection of a contrast agent to emphasize the labral–bicipital complex and is able to identify labral tears and minute, detached fragments (Applegate *et al.*, 2004). The interpretation of the shoulder MR arthrogram should ideally be performed by a specialist radiologist due to the presence of normal anatomical variations within the glenoid labral–bicipital complex, which may otherwise be interpreted as abnormal by less qualified practitioners. Normal anatomical variations include the labral attachment which occasionally becomes meniscoid, presenting as a free lip which overlaps the glenoid ridge; this presentation could be misdiagnosed as a labral lesion. The mechanical irritation experienced in stable SLAP lesions (types I and III) and stable non-SLAP lesions is usually eradicated with arthroscopic debridement of the obstructive tissues. In contrast, unstable SLAP lesions (types II and IV) and unstable non-SLAP lesions (i.e. Bankart) should be respectively repaired by arthroscopic labral reattachment and fixation (Fabbriciani *et al.*, 2004).

Conservative management of SLAP lesions is unfortunately rarely successful; however, minimally invasive arthroscopic repair may facilitate significant tissue healing responses and an accelerated return to play. Arthroscopic debridement of labral degeneration and excision of abnormal tissues in types I and III SLAP lesions can restore integrity and stability to the rim, while other surgical intervention combining suturing techniques may be performed to repair the detached structures in types II and IV lesions (Chang *et al.*, 2008; Funk and Snow, 2007; Wilk *et al.*, 2013). Prescription of a safe, effective and individualized post-operative rehabilitation programme is essential and should be initially guided by the physician. SLAP lesions sustained from compressive forces, including a fall onto an outstretched hand, must initially avoid weight-bearing exercises to prevent shearing forces to the superior glenoid labrum, while peel-back lesions should avoid shoulder external rotation (Wilk *et al.*, 2013).

Non-operative rehabilitation of SLAP lesions I and III has, however, proved to improve pain relief and functional movement following the combined prescription of non-steroidal anti-inflammatory drugs, scapular stabilization and posterior capsular stretching (Edwards *et al.*, 2010). Early mobilization is indicated as anatomical repair has not been performed; therefore active-assisted internal and external rotation in the scapular plane may be commenced at 45° abduction and progressed to 90°, repeating the exercise passively after one week or so. Full passive RoM is expected following two weeks of rehabilitation (Wilk *et al.*, 2013). GIRD presentations, instigated by posterior tightness of the inferior glenohumeral ligament, prompts the posterosuperior translation of the humeral head while the shoulder is in abduction and external rotation. Hence, flexibility of the posteroinferior capsule may be promoted via implementing the 'sleeper stretch'. For this, the patient should be side-lying on the affected side; with the elbow and shoulder flexed to 90°, internal rotation of the shoulder is applied passively (by the therapist or patient). A cross-body shoulder adduction stretch can also be performed by the patient in a seated position. Using the contralateral hand, the patient supports the elbow of the affected limb, passively assisting the affected shoulder into adduction and horizontal flexion (Abrams and Safran, 2010).

Submaximal isometric strengthening exercises promoting scapular stabilization and rotator-cuff development should incorporate training elevation, depression, protraction and retraction movements, particularly targeting the scapulothoracic muscles, with additional pain-free internal and external rotation work to prevent muscular weakening and atrophy. Active elevation in the scapular plane adopting the full can position and lateral raises are observed to facilitate supraspinatus and deltoid activation for dynamic scapular stabilization, and may be progressed using light weights as tolerated from two to three weeks. Throughout this period it is advised to refrain from biceps brachii activation to prevent irritation at the debridement location. After five to six weeks, plyometric activity focusing on acceleration and deceleration can usually be introduced; this should incorporate two-handed techniques, including chest passing, horizontal side throwing and overhead passing and shooting before progressing to single-handed techniques and activity (Burkhart *et al.*, 2003b; Manske and Prohaskab, 2010; Reinhold *et al.*, 2007; Wilk *et al.*, 2013).

Return to play criteria requires full RoM, minimal pain and significant strength and dynamic stability. The rehabilitation time frame remains subject to the individual patient's tissue-healing response, which can be influenced by age, injury recurrence and existing health. Approximately 80–90 per cent of athletes successfully return to play following post-arthroscopic rehabilitation for a SLAP lesion (Funk and Snow, 2007; Park *et al.*, 2004; Wilk *et al.*, 2013).

Post-surgical prognosis for type II and IV SLAP lesions is typically six months, commencing with a six-week protective phase. Weeks 7–12 accommodate the moderate protection phase before progressing to a minimal protection phase during weeks 13–20, which concentrate on the development of dynamic stability. An advanced strengthening phase between weeks 21–26 may incorporate plyometric drills aiming to optimize scapulothoracic and rotator-cuff strength, power and endurance prior to the return to activity (Manske and Prohaskab, 2010; Wilk *et al.*, 2013).

The protective phase aims to protect the surgical repair site as inflammatory symptoms subside. A shoulder abduction sling is normally worn continuously for one week and also for sleeping up to one month. Week two may commence with passive RoM in the scapular plane, incorporating 90° glenohumeral flexion. Traditional 'Codman's pendulum' exercises provide mobilization in slight distraction (gravity-assisted) and may be applied to inhibit capsular adhesions and promote articular joint integrity and circulation (these simply involve the patient supported against a fixed surface with one hand and then leaning over to gently swing their loosely hanging arm through pain-free ranges of movement). External rotation should not exceed 10° per week or 30° following week four, while internal rotation may be tolerated up to 50°. The sports therapist may promote active movement of the distal segments while avoiding elbow flexion and supination for the first eight weeks so as to avoid excessive tensioning of the biceps attachment. Submaximal isometric contractions, combined with rhythmic stabilization drills of the scapulothoracic muscles in weeks three to four are introduced to develop dynamic stabilization, joint proprioception and neuromuscular control as pulsed non-thermal ultrasound, interferential stimulation and cryotherapy can help resolve inflammation and pain. During weeks five to six, passive glenohumeral flexion in the scapular plane can be increased to 145°, external rotation to 50° and internal rotation to 60°. ARoM may commence with 90° glenohumeral flexion in a supine position to eliminate gravitational effects. The aforementioned RoM parameters are, of course, subject to the patient's tolerance (Manske and Prohaskab, 2010; Wilk *et al.*, 2013).

The moderate protection phase aims to restore full RoM, while continuing dynamic strength and stabilization of the rotator-cuff complex and scapulothoracic muscles. Both internal and external rotation exercises may be progressed with resistance tubing using full can and lateral raise techniques (Wilk *et al.*, 2013). Posterior capsular tension remains a prevalent sequelae to post-operative intervention, therefore indicating joint mobilization techniques (Hengeveld and Banks, 2005) which may be enhanced by Mulligan's mobilizations with movement (MWM) to alleviate pain and increase RoM (Teys *et al.*, 2008). Furthermore, a randomized controlled single-blinded comparison of cross-body stretching combined with posterior joint mobilizations has provided beneficial effects for developing internal rotation RoM deficit (Manske *et al.*, 2010). Flexibility exercises should ideally restore the 90/90 position of abduction and external rotation by week nine (Wilk *et al.*, 2013), at which point provocative isotonic exercises acknowledged to produce high-level electromyographic activity in the scapulothoracic and rotator-cuff complexes, including prone rowing with horizontal abduction and side-lying external rotation, may be introduced to develop dynamic stabilization (Manske, 2006). The 'Advanced Throwers Ten Exercise Programme' is also recommended for promoting dynamic shoulder control in the overhead athlete. Wilk *et al.* (2011) explain how the programme '*bridges the gap between rehabilitation and training, facilitating a kinetic linking of the upper and lower extremities and providing a higher level of humeral head control necessary for the overhead throwing athlete's symptom-free return to sports*'. From weeks 9–12 submaximal isometric elbow flexion and supination may be commenced to restore the biceps tendon strength, while the 90/90 position is progressed with resistance tubing if the throwing shoulder is able to attain 120° external rotation (Wilk *et al.*, 2013).

Between weeks 13 and 20, the minimal protection phase aims to regain full active and passive pain-free glenohumeral RoM by continuing flexibility exercises and joint mobilizations. Isotonic resistance exercises for elbow flexion and supination may commence alongside two-handed plyometric chest-passes, chopping techniques and trampoline throw–return catches, before progressing to single-handed throwing. From around week 21, advanced strengthening exercises may be implemented using single-handed plyometric throwing while maintaining full pain-free RoM in preparation for return to play (Manske and Prohaskab, 2010; Wilk *et al.*, 2013).

Shoulder instability

Shoulder instability is a complex abnormality and provides a variety of clinical presentations, with symptoms ranging from intense pain or apprehension of displacement and signs (including subtle subluxation incurred by congenital, developmental or acquired factors) to dislocation sustained by traumatic impact (Lewis *et al.*, 2004; Wilk *et al.*, 2006). Jaggi and Lambert (2010) detail how the structures and associated functions affected by this condition may be presented individually or as a combination of the following:

- the capsulolabral complex and its proprioceptive mechanism;
- the rotator–cuff;
- the surface area of contact between the glenoid and humeral head;
- the central and peripheral nervous systems.

Poor articular congruency and capsular laxity of the shoulder prompts a significant demand for dynamic stabilization and neuromuscular innervation to sustain functional stability; therefore shoulder instability is often a complex combination of structural and neurological disturbances. The Stanmore classification system has been proposed to aid the therapist in differentiating the specific type of shoulder instability (according to aetiology – traumatic, atraumatic and/or muscle patterning) and recommended management strategies (Lewis *et al.*, 2004). The Stanmore classification is represented as a triangle and should be seen as a continuum (see Figure 6.5). Patients are classified into three polar groups (or combinations upon the continuum): Type I (TUBS – traumatic unilateral Bankart surgery); Type II (AMBRI – atraumatic multidirectional bilateral rehabilitation inferior capsular shift); and Type III (muscle patterning dysfunction – habitual non-structural). Such a classification system allows for the marked overlap between traumatic and atraumatic causes of instability and compensates for the actuality that causes change over time. Each axis between the poles acts as a spectrum of each classification and it is possible to fit patients into one of the three polar groups or somewhere along the lines which join them (Bayley, 2014). In order to classify a patient it is vital that a comprehensive history is taken and an accurate clinical examination performed (Lewis *et al.*, 2004; Jaggi and Lambert, 2010).

Recent research has highlighted that common shoulder pathologies have a commonly presenting feature: loss of translational control (Ludewig and Cook, 2000). In addition to this, there is an abundance of clinical research which has identified alterations in the dynamic and

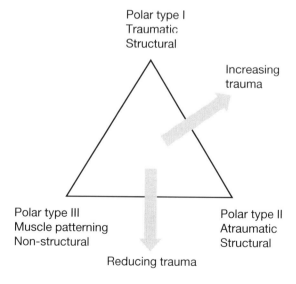

Figure 6.5 Stanmore classification of shoulder instability (source: adapted from Lewis *et al.*, 2004).

static positioning of the scapula within a cohort of individuals with shoulder pathology (Kibler, 1998; Ludewig and Cook, 2000).

Seven primary elements surrounding shoulder instability should be considered during the planning process of the rehabilitation programme. These elements are: the onset of pathology; the degree of instability; the frequency of dislocation; the direction of instability; the presence of concomitant pathologies; the level of neuromuscular control; and the activity level which the patient requires to return (Wilk *et al.*, 2006). The onset of pathology and mechanism of injury can influence the rehabilitation strategy. Asymptomatic instability involving a repetitive history of joint laxity and inability to perform specific techniques may require the therapist to implement proprioceptive shoulder stabilization exercises to increase neuromuscular control and a rotator-cuff strengthening programme to promote dynamic stability. In contrast, traumatic subluxation or dislocation requires strategies which decrease pain and inflammation and early pain-free restoration of joint mobility. The degree of instability is influenced by the severity of the trauma. Gross instability may occur following a dislocation involving a Bankart lesion where the joint capsule has avulsed from the glenoid rim, requiring early manual reduction by medical staff and potential surgical intervention. In contrast, mild subluxations with a relatively low muscle guarding reaction may tolerate early-stage neuromuscular control and strengthening exercises. A mean average of 67 per cent of athletes between the ages of 21 and 30 experience recurrent dislocations requiring a progressive rehabilitation plan which emphasizes the athlete's safety. In contrast, chronic atraumatic subluxations may be treated more provocatively due to the absence of inflammatory symptoms and muscle guarding; however, RoM exercises should still be progressive, avoiding excessive flexibility which may unduly stress the joint capsule. The direction of instability element highlights the 95 per cent prevalence of anterior instability compared to posterior or multidirectional instability. Extreme external rotation and abduction of the humeral head may result in gross instability represented by dislocation and glenoid lesions. A progressive rehabilitation protocol should focus on scapular setting, improving dynamic stability and neuromuscular control in mid-range of movement, and increasing joint force coupling using co-contraction exercises, rhythmic stabilization and proprioceptive control exercises. The sports therapist may need to consider differential diagnoses such as osseous lesions represented by a Hill–Sach's lesion or capsulolabral complex trauma represented by SLAP lesions. It is recommended to examine the athlete/patient's level of neuromuscular control, particularly at end RoM. Afferent and efferent signalling following traumatic dislocation or chronic subluxations may be compromised, resulting in impaired muscle recruitment and positioning and articulation of the humeral head; therefore neuromuscular control and proprioceptive exercises become an essential component of the rehabilitation process. Finally, the sports therapist should aim to assist the patient to return to play at optimal levels by implementing sports-specific dynamic stabilization, neuromuscular control and plyometric exercises contextualized to the overhead techniques used (Wilk *et al.*, 2006).

Traumatic shoulder instability

Adopting a progressive four-stage rehabilitation model, early-stage management goals for traumatic shoulder instability must aim to reduce joint pain and inflammation and promote healing while protecting the damaged tissues and initiating the restoration of joint mobility and dynamic stability. These goals may be achieved by initial immobilization using a simple sling, accompanied by isometric contractions of the dynamic stabilizers, especially the deltoids and scapulothoracic retractors, by applying a 'pinch and hold' technique. The therapist should be aware that there is limited evidence supporting the efficacy of specialist slings which immobilize the joint in abduction and external rotation, therefore early pain-free active RoM of the distal kinetic chain is advocated in addition to performing active-assisted pendulum exercises once the deltoids are activating independently. Passive movement may also be introduced to stimulate joint mechanoreceptors and collagen organization; however, the therapist should ensure this is applied in a pain-free range and is conducive to the patient's progression. Closed kinetic chain exercises may include weight-shifting on a ball to facilitate co-contraction of the glenohumeral stabilizers and to increase proprioception within the joint mechanoreceptors. A combination of interferential electrotherapy with isometric exercises is recommended for pain reduction, decreasing muscle guarding and promoting muscle fibre recruitment (Itoi *et al.*, 2007; Provencher and Romeo, 2012; Wilk *et al.*, 2006).

Second-stage goals focus on regaining full joint mobility and increasing glenohumeral joint strength and dynamic stability. If required, active-assisted movement may be performed with gravity eliminated – such as performing 90° abduction slides in a supine position, which may be progressed against gravity using a side-lying position while performing 90° abduction with the elbow flexed to 90° (short lever) and repeated with the elbow extended to 0° (long lever). Once the patient has achieved pain-free movement with notable dynamic strength in these positions, active movements may be progressed in a standing position. The therapist should be aware that external rotation at 90° abduction should be restricted to approximately 60–70° during the initial four to eight weeks to prevent excessive stress to the anterior capsuloligamentous complex. As this range of movement develops, the therapist may promote neuromuscular control and dynamic stability by combining manual resistive eccentric exercises of the external rotator muscles and rhythmic stabilization drills towards the end-range of external rotation. Closed kinetic chain exercises may be progressed to include hand-on-wall stabilization drills in the scapular plane, aiming to withstand shoulder height activity; push-ups may be commenced in a standing position against a wall or table – however, patients with posterior instability should be closely monitored when performing closed kinetic chain exercises during the initial six to eight weeks to ensure adequate healing and strength is attained for safe progression. End-range strengthening and rhythmic stabilization drills can be advanced against resistance from the therapist or using tubing (Itoi *et al.*, 2007; Provencher and Romeo, 2012; Wilk *et al.*, 2006).

The late stage concentrates on full restoration of strength, dynamic stability and proprioception. Prior to commencing this stage the therapist must ensure that the patient has regained full RoM with a minimum 4/5 muscle strength, and has symmetrical capsular mobility with minimal pain or tenderness. Muscle endurance is promoted using low-resistance high-repetition exercises such as internal and external rotations using a lightweight resistance band, progressing into 90° abduction with increasing resistance. Once endurance is sustained, more aggressive isotonic

---

Practitioner Tip Box 6.8

Shoulder instability exercise modifications

Instability	Positions to avoid	Exercises to be modified or avoided
Anterior	Combined abduction and external rotation	Fly, pull-down, push-up, bench-press, military-press
Posterior	Combined flexion, internal rotation and horizontal adduction	Fly, push-up, bench-press, weight-bearing exercises
Inferior	Full elevation	Shrug, elbow-curl, military-press

Source: adapted from Voight *et al.*, 2007.

exercises are recommended to develop strength. Weights should be introduced to activate rotator cuff musculature, and seated rowing, bench-press and pull-downs (in front of head) may be performed in pain-free ranges, avoiding full arm extension to minimize joint traction forces. Glenohumeral proprioception exercises remain an imperative rehabilitation component which enhances visual coordination, vestibular balance and golgi tendon organ (GTO) activation. Exercises may incorporate wall dribbling in the 90/90 position, trampoline ball–bounce–catch routines; and medicine ball chest passes, progressing with push-ups on an exercise ball or wobble board. Plyometric exercises are introduced to restore functional RoM while promoting force production and dissipation. Two-handed exercises may now progress to single-handed long-lever dynamic movements using medicine balls or weighted objects to replicate sport-specific techniques, including an overhead throw-in (Itoi *et al.*, 2007; Provencher and Romeo, 2012; Wilk *et al.*, 2006).

The final stage represents the return to functional activity phase. The predominant goal for the athlete is the ability to maintain muscular endurance, strength, dynamic stability and functional RoM while progressively increasing and reacting to the functional demands of the sporting activity. To commence this stage it is recommended that the athlete has regained full functional RoM and satisfactory levels of the aforementioned components. A full clinical examination is also recommended to ensure the joint is able to perform activities at this level. Throughout this stage the athlete should be encouraged to continue late-stage activities in order to regain and maintain optimum functionality and fitness. A full clinical examination and fitness test should be undertaken prior to approving any return to play (Reinhold *et al.*, 2002).

Atraumatic shoulder instability

Patients invariably present with several occurrences of glenohumeral instability which prevent specific task completion or movement techniques. Aetiological factors including capsular laxity, impaired joint movement and muscle weakness accompanied by neuromuscular dysfunction all contribute to pathological atraumatic instability leading to excessive migration of the humeral head. While reflecting the rehabilitation principles for traumatic instability, the main principle for atraumatic instability emphasizes a slower progression which implements earlier proprioception. Conservative rehabilitative exercise programmes have proved to deliver effective management for atraumatic instability (Misamore *et al.*, 2005).

Early-stage goals involve the minimization of muscle atrophy and reflexive inhibition prompted by dysfunction following repetitive pain-induced subluxations. Interferential muscle stimulation and cryotherapy for pain relief are therefore recommended, alongside isometric contractions using manual rhythmic stabilization drills to promote force-coupling, co-contraction and joint stability. Apprehension caused by excessive stretching of the capsuloligamentous complex should be avoided in the early stages. Progression to closed kinetic chain (CKC) exercises may incorporate axial compression, adopting quadruped and tripod positions on unstable surfaces including a foam cushion or Swiss ball to increase dynamic stability and proprioceptive awareness while activating the core stabilizers in the process. The therapist should continue to exercise caution when rehabilitating patients with posterior instability.

A progressive strengthening programme for the rotator-cuff complex and scapulothoracic stabilizers should be implemented to counteract the weakness and dysfunction commonly associated with congenital instability. Strengthening of the scapular depressors and retractors provides proximal stabilization and subsequent mobility throughout the distal segmental chain. Exercises including external rotation in side-lying and prone positions, prone rowing and extension, supine serratus punching and bilateral external rotation combining scapular retraction for lower trapezius will collectively promote dynamic stabilization and neuromuscular control using manual resistance provided by the therapist (Paine and Voight, 2013). Neuromuscular control and strengthening must be progressed and once satisfactory strength is restored the patient should be encouraged to use the shoulder in the most stable positions, such as elevation in the scapular plane, while avoiding movement in positions which create apprehension. Eventually the patient may attempt movements in intrinsically unstable positions once dynamic stability, scapular muscle strength and neuromuscular control have been optimized. If immobilization or controlled RoM is required during the return to functional play stage, the sports therapist may consider taping or bracing for the glenohumeral joint to prevent further injury (Itoi *et al.*, 2007; Provencher and Romeo, 2012; Wilk *et al.*, 2006).

Acromioclavicular joint injuries

Acromioclavicular joint separations are a common injury representing approximately 9 per cent of all shoulder girdle injuries. Despite considerable restraint provided by the acromioclavicular and coracoclavicular ligament complexes, separations predominantly occur following direct force such as by falling onto the AC joint with the arm adducted close to the trunk. Forces transmitted across the shoulder by a 'FOOSH' may result in dislocation of the AC joint as the acromion process is driven underneath the lateral aspect of the clavicle, but this is less prevalent (Cote *et al.*, 2010; Mazzocca *et al.*, 2007; Trainer *et al.*, 2008). AC joint separations are usually accompanied with ecchymosis, effusion and joint tenderness, with a localized pain over the anterosuperior aspect of the shoulder. Active shoulder movements become painful and restricted, causing the patient to maintain the arm at the side of the trunk (Robb and Howitt, 2011). Special tests include O'Brien's test, renowned for its specificity and accuracy, and the scarf test – although this test is susceptible to providing false positives (Hattam and Smeatham, 2010; Moen *et al.*, 2010). The piano key sign may detect evident superioinferior translation (MacDonald and LaPointe, 2008).

It is acknowledged that grades I, II and occasionally III tend to respond efficiently to conservative treatment, while grades IV, V and VI usually require surgical intervention. The recommended rehabilitation protocol is appropriate to both conservative and post-operative

Table 6.6 Acromioclavicular joint injury classification

Grade	Acromioclavicular joint injury classification
I	A sprain of the AC joint capsule accompanied by localized pain and tenderness on palpation and movement, especially horizontal flexion
II	Complete rupture of the AC ligament complex accompanied by a sprain of the coracoclavicular ligaments. Palpation commonly reveals AC joint step-deformity
III	Complete rupture of the AC ligament complex and the coracoclavicular ligaments, the conoid and trapezoid. Palpation may reveal an increased AC step-deformity
IV	Complete rupture of all ligaments with posterior clavicular displacement resulting in increased signs of inflammation
V	Complete rupture of all ligaments with significant superior displacement and a step-deformity of the elevated lateral clavicle compared to the acromion process. The coracoclavicular space can increase by 500 per cent compared to the 25–100 per cent increase of a type III injury
VI	Complete rupture of all ligaments and an inferior clavicular displacement into the subacromial or subcoracoid cavity

Source: Cote *et al.*, 2010; adapted from Rockwood's Classification, 1996.

care. Treatment for grades I and II in the acute stage requires the application of ice to control bleeding and inflammation. Elevation slings protect the immobilized limb but are only advised in the presence of intense localized pain, and may be discarded once the patient is able to maintain the arm adjacent to the trunk without pain. Early mobilization is advocated for alleviating pain and inflammation and is commenced alongside isometric contractions of the scapular stabilizers to inhibit weakening. Pain-free passive RoM may be performed by the sports therapist, who should apply caution during provocative movements which impose stress to the AC joint – such as internal rotation, end-range glenohumeral flexion and cross-body adduction (Buss and Watts, 2003; Cools *et al.*, 2007; Cote *et al.*, 2010). Progressive strengthening exercises implemented at the earliest opportunity should focus on closed-chain drills, with the distal segment fixed to the wall or a level surface to offload the weight of the arm and stress on the rotator-cuff complex. Recommended drills including 'scapular protraction–retraction on the wall' and 'scapular clock' facilitate high-quality pain-free movement (Burkhart *et al.*, 2003b; McMullen and Uhl, 2000). Grade II separations prone to posteroanterior clavicular translation invariably demand specific closed-chain drills with emphasis on scapular retraction to reinforce dynamic AC joint stability (Cools *et al.*, 2007). Progression to open-chain exercises for grade I and II separations should advance to long-lever drills which isolate specific muscle activation. Blackburn exercises adopting the 'T' and 'Y' position with bilateral horizontal abduction with external rotation, and prone horizontal extension to 100° are observed to produce significant electromyographic activity for middle and lower trapezius, supraspinatus and infraspinatus muscles (Reinhold *et al.*, 2004; 2007). These prone-position long-lever drills may be advanced using weights or resistance tubing, while the introduction of static rowing may reinforce scapular retraction for dynamic AC stabilization (Cote *et al.*, 2010).

Grade III separations demonstrate more effective recovery rates following conservative treatment opposed to surgical intervention, which has proved to induce extended recovery periods, absence from activity and pathological complications as highlighted by research (Ceccarelli *et al.*, 2008; Nissen and Chatterjee, 2007; Smith *et al.*, 2011; Spencer, 2007). Shoulder mobility relies on full AC joint functionality provided by acromial articulation with the clavicular strut; therefore slings should be discarded as soon as symptoms permit in favour of early mobilization. A 6–12-week conservative rehabilitation plan may conclude if the athlete can return to functional activity or, in the presence of continuing symptoms, be referred to a specialist consultant. Scapular dyskinesis is prevalent in grade III pathology; therefore sustained scapular control is imperative for effective conservative rehabilitation. Grade II rehabilitation protocol is recommended in conjunction with the 'S3 bracing system' or 'IntelliSkin' shirts which claim to promote proprioceptive and postural support by retaining the scapula in optimal retraction (Cote *et al.*, 2010; Gumina *et al.*, 2009).

Additional established early-stage management strategies for the aforementioned AC joint separations may include soft tissue therapy to attenuate muscle tension, taping techniques to reduce superior clavicular translation, interferential stimulation for pain modulation and low-amplitude passive physiological intervertebral joint mobilizations (PPIVMs) to alleviate cervical spine joint restrictions (Robb and Howitt, 2011).

Patients commencing post-operative rehabilitation for grades IV, V and VI separations are primarily supported in a 'Lerman brace', which secures the shoulder in abduction and external rotation while offloading the weight of the arm and subsequent stress to the AC joint. After 6–8 weeks of immobilization the patient is encouraged to perform closed-chain sliding exercises in contact with the flat surface of a table before progressing to inclined and vertical wall slides. In corroboration with all early-stage mobilization, the patient should apply caution with movements which impose stress to the AC joint, such as internal rotation, end-range glenohumeral flexion and cross-body adduction. The addition of supine shoulder flexion and active-assisted pulley drills are effective in developing forward elevation (Cote *et al.*, 2010). Late-stage challenges usually prevent the patient's ability to perform internal rotation, therefore stretching exercises comprising hand-behind-back towel stretches are encouraged if the patient is able to maintain scapular retraction throughout. At 12–18 weeks, isotonic strength exercises including multi-level rowing may be implemented and progressed to Blackburn exercises once scapular stabilization is restored (Cote *et al.*, 2010).

Rotator-cuff injury

More than one-third of painful shoulders are ascribed for dysfunctions of the rotator-cuff, more often than not due to subacromial impingement and other extrinsic factors including anterior shoulder instability and repetitive microtrauma (Matava *et al.*, 2005; Matsen and Arntz, 1990). The concept of rotator-cuff impingement, whereby the rotator-cuff is mechanically impinged against the inferior surface of the acromion with elevation was first introduced by Neer (1972). The rotator-cuff tendons may also be damaged by overload, compression, repetitive loading (Dillman *et al.*, 1993; Vogel, 2003) and under-loading (Thornton *et al.*, 2010). A common prevalence of partial-thickness supraspinatus ruptures in throwers is induced by inefficient technique and inability to control powerful eccentric loading during the throwing phases (Aune *et al.*, 2012). Supraspinatus tendinopathy and impingement remain highly prevalent in repetitive overhead sports, especially competitive swimming (Sein *et al.*, 2010; Tovin, 2006). Shoulder pain increases significantly with age, with the typical patient being over 45 years of age and disclosing a repeated history of over-load trauma (Aune *et al.*, 2012), while it is the most prevalent musculoskeletal complaint for patients aged over 65 (Taylor, 2005). A high prevalence of intrinsically influenced factors, including repeated microtrauma combined with degenerative tearing, poor vascularity and age-related metabolic change, may contribute to full thickness ruptures (Aune *et al.*, 2012; Matava *et al.*, 2005). Usually initiated with sudden onset and experience of a stabbing pain and limited shoulder movement, minor tears usually respond to a short rest period which allows inflammatory products to disperse. In contrast, partial or complete ruptures, common in older athletes, may reproduce symptoms both during activity and sleep, leading to disturbed sleeping patterns from lying on the affected shoulder (Brukner and Khan, 2009).

MRI scans are sensitive to all rotator-cuff ruptures and concomitant pathological lesions, including labral tears and biceps tendon lesions (Aune *et al.*, 2012; Nakagawa *et al.*, 2001). However, diagnostic arthroscopic techniques including the 'bubble sign' have provided efficacious diagnosis of intratendinous tears by probing the articular or bursal aspect of the tendon with an 18-gauge spinal needle prior to injecting saline into the incriminating structure. Ease of injection and subsequent dilation is indicative of intratendinous tearing within partial-thickness ruptures (Lo and Burkhart, 2004). Clinical examination may commence with full clearance of the cervical spine, paying attention to special tests including Spurling's test to eliminate compressive neuropathy. The therapist should be aware that tests for subacromial impingement (including Hawkins–Kennedy and Neer's tests) invariably test positive in the presence of partial-thickness ruptures. Multidirectional instability tests, including the apprehension–relocation and sulcus sign, are essential in young throwing athletes who may be predisposed to rotator-cuff pathology secondary to internal impingement. The therapist should be aware that each rotator-cuff tendon operates synergistically and not as individual components; therefore clinical assessment specificity may be compromised, given the morphology of the scapula, subacromial space and the tendinous confluence prior to the humeral insertion (Lewis, 2009; Matava *et al.*, 2005).

Conservative treatment will primarily focus on alleviating pain by avoiding any provocative movements. Administration of anti-inflammatory and/or corticosteroid medication may be employed alongside the POLICE protocol. Early mobilization should focus on restoring normal shoulder kinematics with anterior and posterior capsular tightness being, respectively, treated with arm–at–side external rotation and cross–body adduction releases. Progression to rotator–cuff and periscapular strength exercises may commence using elasticated tubing or free–weights, while scapulothoracic stabilization drills will restore optimal glenohumeral function, preventing dyskinesia and sequelae, including subacromial and rotator–cuff impingement. Research advocates full can exercises for rotator–cuff and 'Y–position' exercises for lower trapezius, to be highly effective strengthening drills as revealed by EMG studies (Fleming *et al.*, 2010). Eccentric and plyometric drills may be contextualized to reflect the follow–through and deceleration throw phases, while core stability strengthening will optimize proximal force–production while reducing primary tensile–overload to the shoulder and distal segments (Matava *et al.*, 2005; Voight *et al.*, 2007), a predisposition which may be avoided by isokinetic strength machines – which although expensive, effectively control the rotator–cuff strength ratios during the rehabilitation process (Malliou *et al.*, 2004). Efficacious shoulder rehabilitation based on EMG activity feedback is available in the literature (Escamilla *et al.*, 2009; Reinhold *et al.*, 2007). Operative treatment for both partial and full–thickness ruptures may be advised following a 3–6 month period of non–resolution, the procedures of which are highlighted with rehabilitation protocol in the literature (Ainsworth and Lewis, 2007; Littlewood *et al.*, 2012; Matava *et al.*, 2005).

Tendons are composed of densely arranged collagen fibres, elastin, proteoglycans and lipids, all surrounded by an epitendon containing the neurovascular supply. The rotator–cuff tendons have been shown to have limited vascularity proximal to their insertion (Carr and Norris, 1989), which may predispose them to degenerative microtrauma. Vascularity in this critical zone is also influenced by arm position, with a significant decrease in rotator–cuff blood supply observed during adduction (Rathbun and Macnab, 1970). It has been proposed that pain from tendinopathy is due to either inflammation or separation of the collagen fibres (Khan *et al.*, 1997). However, the issue of tendon inflammation is contentious, and the evidence for the presence of cells classically associated with inflammation is still emerging. The evidence for collagen separation is also inconclusive. Patients who have undergone tendon surgery have been shown to have minimal pain and still return to function despite abnormal collagen (Kiss *et al.*, 1998), and patients with partial rotator–cuff tears were found to have more pain than those with complete tears (Gotoh *et al.*, 1998). Shoulder injury management throughout the tendinopathy continuum is discussed further in key literature (Cook and Purdham, 2009; Lewis, 2009; 2010).

In addition to targeted optimal loading of the rotator–cuff tendon to improve tendon quality, the problem of inadequate muscle control around the shoulder girdle also needs addressing. A lack of control of the shoulder girdle can contribute to a reduction in the size of the subacromial space, leading to continued (secondary) impingement (Graichen *et al.*, 1993; Hebert *et al.*, 2000).

Shoulder impingement

Shoulder impingement symptoms are common in athletes participating in overhead activities (Tate *et al.*, 2008). Historically, shoulder impingement was described as a common pathology or diagnosis; however, recent literature considers impingement as a selection of symptoms which are associated with a variety of underlying pathological mechanisms and injuries (Cools *et al.*, 2008). These underlying pathological conditions include rotator–cuff pathology, scapular dyskinesis, shoulder instability, biceps brachii pathology and SLAP lesions (Cools *et al.*, 2008).

Shoulder impingements have been described in the literature as having two types: subacromial and internal. Neer (1972) described subacromial impingement as the impingement of the tendinous portion of the rotator-cuff, long head of biceps and subacromial bursa by the fibro-osseous arch complex composed of the coracoacromial ligament and the anterior third of the acromion. Jobe *et al.* (2000) further categorized subacromial impingement as being either primary or secondary. Primary impingement relates to the structural architecture of the region and how this can contribute to the aggravating contact and resulting degeneration of the supraspinatus tendon, subacromial bursa and/or long head of biceps (Neer, 1972). Structural factors include: acromial shape (which may be abnormally curved or angled downward, as in a 'hooked' acromion); os acromiale (an unfused centre of acromial ossification); degenerative spurs; calcification of the coracoacromial ligament; the superior aspect of the glenoid fossa; glenohumeral capsular contraction; hypermobility and static instability of the glenohumeral joint; and rotator-cuff tendinopathy (which may increase the thickness of the tendon) (Bedi and Rodeo, 2009; Edelson and Teitz, 2000; Jobe *et al.*, 2000).

With secondary impingement it is proposed that dynamic instability is the cause (Jobe *et al.*, 2000). This relates to poor recruitment, weakness, inhibition or imbalance of the primary stabilizers of the glenohumeral joint and/or scapulothoracic articulation. The deeper, internal impingement pathology has been described as the friction and mechanical abrasion of the rotator-cuff tendons between the humeral head and the anterior or posterior glenoid rim, which is most likely to occur during the abducted and externally rotated position of the cocking phase of throwing (Walch *et al.*, 1992). Predisposing postures, particularly a forward head posture, associated with increased thoracic kyphosis and a downwardly rotated, anteriorly tilted and protracted scapula, are also considered to be a predominant aetiological factor in the pathogenesis of subacromial impingement syndrome due to the increased compressive forces exerted onto the subacromial space (Lewis *et al.*, 2005). Neer (1983) actually described three stages of impingement syndrome, which was elaborated upon by Wilk *et al.* (2012):

- Stage 1: a reversible lesion, most commonly seen in young adult athletes, which is characterized by the oedema and haemorrhage of tendinous irritation (supraspinatus and/or biceps long head).
- Stage 2: a fibrotic presentation of either of the tendons or subacromial bursa, most commonly seen in athletes aged between 24–40 years of age, which is characterized by recurrent pain with overhead activity. May require operative intervention (such as bursectomy or coracoacromial ligament division).
- Stage 3: osteophytic bone spurs and possible tendon partial or full-thickness tear, most commonly seen in older athletes who demonstrate progressive painful disability. This presentation tends to respond less well to conservative management.

Management, as always, must be focused on managing symptoms while effectively addressing the individual causative factors. Wilk *et al.* (2012) present a four-stage return-to-sport rehabilitation protocol which progresses from symptom management, restoration of movement (avoiding any activities which cause an increase in symptoms) and patient education, through normalization of shoulder arthrokinematics and advanced strengthening, to a return phase which incorporates sport-specific drills (especially for throwing or racquet sports).

This chapter has presented a foundation set of functional anatomical information designed to support the sports therapist's working appreciation of this relatively complex region. Principles and recommended techniques for clinically assessing the shoulder have been presented. Finally, a selection of common shoulder pathologies have been discussed; and for each of these, characteristic aetiological features, typical presenting signs and symptoms, and evidence-based rehabilitation strategies have been provided. As always, the sports therapist must be recommended to evaluate further the presented recommendations, and recognize that all assessment and management must remain patient-focused and specific.

References

Abrams, G.D. and Safran, M.R. (2010) Diagnosis and management of superior labrum anterior posterior lesions in overhead athletes. *British Journal of Sports Medicine*. 44: 311–318

ACSM (American College of Sports Medicine) (2014) *ACSM's Resources for the Personal Trainer*, 4th edition. Lippincott, Williams and Wilkins. New York

Ainsworth, R. and Lewis, J.S. (2007) Exercise therapy for the conservative management of full thickness tears of the rotator cuff: A systematic review. *British Journal of Sports Medicine*. 41: 200–210

Alemanno, F. and Egarter Vigl, E. (2014) Anatomy of the brachial plexus. *Anesthesia of the Upper Limb*. 1 (1): 1–17

Allen, D.G. (2001) Eccentric muscle damage: Mechanisms of early reduction of force. *Acta Physiologica Scandinavica*. 171 (3): 311–319

Amato, H., Hawkins, C.D. and Cole, S.L. (2006) *Clinical skills documentation guide for athletic training*, 2nd edition. SLACK Incorporated. Thorofare, NJ

American Medical Association (1988) *Guide to the evaluation of permanent impairment*. AMA. Chicago, IL

Andary, J.L. and Petersen, S.A. (2002) The vascular anatomy of the glenohumeral capsule and ligaments: An anatomic study. *Journal of Bone and Joint Surgery*. 84 (12): 2258–2265

Anderson, M., Parr, G. and Hall, S. (2009) *Foundations of athletic training, prevention, assessment and management*, 4th edition. Lippincott, Williams and Wilkins. Philadelphia, PA

Applegate, G.R., Hewitt, M. and Snyder, S.J., *et al.* (2004) Chronic labral tears: Value of magnetic resonance arthrography in evaluating the glenoid labrum and labral–bicipital complex. *Arthroscopy*. 20 (9): 959–963

Arcasoy, M.D. and Jett, J.R. (1997) Superior pulmonary sulcus tumors and Pancoast's syndrome. *New England Journal of Medicine*. 337: 1370–1376

Atkins, E., Kerr, E. and Goodlad, J. (2010) *A practical approach to orthopaedic medicine*, 3rd edition. Churchill Livingstone. Edinburgh, UK

Aune, A.K., Cools, A. and Fredriksen, H., *et al.* (2012) Acute shoulder injuries. In Bahr, R., McCrory, P. and Laprade, R.F., *et al.* (eds) *The IOC manual of sports injuries: An illustrated guide to the management of injuries in physical activity*. Wiley-Blackwell. Chichester, UK

Ayub, E. (1991) Posture and the upper quarter. In Donatelli, R. (ed.) *Physical therapy of the shoulder*, 2nd edition. Churchill Livingstone. Melbourne, Australia

Backhouse, K.M. and Hutchings, R.T. (1998) *Clinical surface anatomy*, 2nd edition. Mosby. St Louis, MO

Baltaci, G. and Johnson, R. (2001) Shoulder range of motion characteristics in collegiate baseball players. *Journal of Sports Medicine and Physical Fitness*. 41: 236–242

Bayley, I. (2014) The classification of shoulder instability: New light through old windows. Lecture presentation. www.shoulderdoc.co.uk/article.asp?article=647, accessed July 2014

Beam, J. (2002) Rehabilitation including sports-specific functional progression for the competitive athlete. *Journal of Bodywork and Movement Therapies*. 6 (4): 205–219

Bedi, A. and Rodeo, S.A. (2009) Os acromiale as a cause for shoulder pain in a competitive swimmer: A case report. *Sports Health: A Multidisciplinary Approach*.1 (2): 120–124

Beltran, J. and Suhardja, A. (2007) Shoulder instability. In Vanhoenacker, F.M., Maas, M. and Gielen, J.L. (eds) *Imaging of orthopedic sports injuries*. Springer-Verlag. Berlin, Germany

Berg, E.E. and Ciullo, J.V. (1998) A clinical test for superior glenoid labral or 'SLAP' lesions. *Clinical Journal of Sports Medicine*. 8 (2): 121–123

Berryman-Reese, N.B. and Bandy, W.D. (2010) *Joint range of motion and muscle length testing*, 2nd edition. Elsevier Saunders. St. Louis, MO

Bleakley, C.M., Glasgow, P. and MacAuley, D.C. (2012) PRICE needs updating: Should we call the POLICE? *British Journal of Sports Medicine*. 46 (4): 220–221

Brukner, P. and Khan, K. (2009) *Clinical sports medicine*, 3rd edition. McGraw-Hill. Sydney, Australia

Burkhart, S.S., Morgan, C.D. and Kibler, W.B. (2003a) The disabled throwing shoulder: Spectrum of pathology. Part I: Pathoanatomy and biomechanics. *Arthroscopy*. 19 (4): 404–420

Burkhart, S.S., Morgan, C.D. and Kibler, W.B. (2003b) The disabled throwing shoulder: Spectrum of pathology. Part II: Evaluation and treatment of SLAP lesions in throwers. *Arthroscopy*. 19 (5): 531–539

Buss, D.D. and Watts, J.D. (2003) Acromioclavicular injuries in the throwing athlete. *Clinical Journal of Sports Medicine*. 22 (2): 327–341

Cadogan, A., Laslett, M., Hing, W., *et al*. (2010) Interexaminer reliability of orthopaedic special tests used in the assessment of shoulder pain. *Manual Therapy*. 16 (2):131–135

Cael, C. (2010) *Functional anatomy: Musculoskeletal anatomy, kinesiology, and palpation for manual therapists*. Lippincott, Williams and Wilkins. Baltimore, MD

Caine, D.J., Russell, K. and Lim, L. (2013) *Handbook of sports medicine and science: Gymnastics*. Wiley and Sons. Chichester, UK

Carr, A.J. and Norris, S.H. (1989) The blood supply of the calcaneal tendon. *Journal of Bone and Joint Surgery*. 71: 100–101

Ceccarelli, E., Bondi, R., Alviti, F., *et al*. (2008) Treatment of acute grade III acromioclavicular dislocation: A lack of evidence. *Journal of Orthopaedics and Traumatology*. 9 (2): 105–108

Chang, D., Mohana-Borges, A., Borso, M., *et al*. (2008) SLAP lesions: Anatomy, clinical presentation, MR imaging diagnosis and characterization. *European Journal of Radiology*. 68: 72–87

Chang, E.Y., Moses, D.A., Babb, J.S., *et al*. (2006) Shoulder impingement: Objective 3D shape analysis of acromial morphological features. *Radiology*. 239 (2): 497–505

Cipriano, J.J. (2010) *Photographic manual of regional orthopaedic and neurological tests*, 5th edition. Lippincott, Williams and Wilkins. Philadelphia, PA

Clarkson, H.M. (2013). *Musculoskeletal assessment: Joint range of motion and manual muscle strength*, 3rd edition. Lippincott Williams and Wilkins. Baltimore, MD

Cook, C.E. (2012) *Orthopedic manual therapy: An evidence-based approach*, 2nd edition. Pearson Education. Upper Saddle River, NJ

Cook, C.E. and Hegedus, E.J. (2013) *Orthopedic physical examination tests: An evidence-based approach*, 2nd edition. Pearson Education. Upper Saddle River, NJ

Cook, J.L. and Purdham, C.R. (2009). Is tendon pathology a continuum? A pathology model to explain the clinical presentation of load-induced tendinopathy. *British Journal of Sports Medicine*. 43: 409–416

Cools, A. and Fredriksen, H. (2012) Rehabilitation of shoulder injuries. In Bahr, R., McCrory, P., Laprade, R.F., *et al*. (eds) *The IOC manual of sports injuries: An illustrated guide to the management of injuries in physical activity*. Wiley-Blackwell. Chichester, UK

Cools, A.M., Dewitte, V., Lanszweert, F., *et al*. (2007) Rehabilitation of scapular muscle balance: Which exercises to prescribe? *American Journal of Sports Medicine*. 35: 1744–1751

Cools, A.M., Cambier, D. and Witvrouw, E.E. (2008) Screening the athlete's shoulder for impingement: A clinical reasoning algorithm for early detection of shoulder pathology. *British Journal of Sports Medicine*. 42: 628–635

Cools, A.M., Witvrouw, E.E., Declercq, G.A., Danneels, L.A. and Cambier, D.C. (2003) Scapular muscle recruitment patterns: Trapezius muscle latency with and without impingement symptoms. *American Journal of Sports Medicine*. 31 (4): 542–549

Cote, M.P., Wojcik, K.E., Gomlinski, G., *et al*. (2010) Rehabilitation of acromioclavicular joint separations: Operative and non-operative considerations. *Clinical Journal of Sports Medicine*. 29: 213–228

Cyriax, J. (1982) *Textbook of orthopaedic medicine. Volume I: Diagnosis of soft tissue lesions*, 8th edition. Balliere Tindall. London, UK

Deepak, S. (2005) *Principles of manual therapy: Manual therapy approach to musculoskeletal dysfunction*. Jaypee Brothers Medical Publishers. New Delhi, India

DePalma, A.F. and Brand, R.A. (2008) Surgical anatomy of the rotator cuff and the natural history of degenerative periarthritis. *Clinical Orthopaedics and Related Research*. 466 (3): 543–551

DePalma, M.J. and Johnson, E.W. (2003) Detecting and treating shoulder impingement syndrome: The role of scapulothoracic dyskinesis. *The Physician and Sports Medicine*. 31 (7): 25–32

Di Giacomo, G., Pouliart, N., Costantini, A., *et al*. (2008) *Atlas of functional shoulder anatomy*. Springer. Rome, Italy

Di Giacomo, G., Costantini, A. and DeVita, A. (2010) Shoulder disorder: From dysfunction to the lesion. In Angelo, R.L., Esch, J.C. and Ryu, R.K. (eds) *The shoulder*. Elsevier, Saunders. Philadelphia, PA

Dillman, C.J., Fleisig, G.S. and Andrews, J.R. (1993) Biomechanics of pitching with emphasis upon shoulder kinematics. *Journal of Orthopaedic and Sports Physical Therapy*. 12: 402–408

Donatelli, R.A. (2011) *Physical therapy of the shoulder*, 5th edition. Churchill Livingstone. St. Louis, MO

Donnelly, T.D., Ashwin, S. and Waseem, M. (2013) Clinical assessment of the shoulder. *Open Orthopaedics Journal.* 7: 310–315

Duncan-Tennent, T., Beach, W.R. and Meyers, J.F. (2003) A review of the special tests associated with shoulder examination. Part II: Laxity, instability, and superior labral anterior to posterior (SLAP) lesions. *American Journal of Sports Medicine.* 31 (2): 301–307

Dvorak, J., Dvorak, V., Gilliar, W., *et al.* (2008) *Musculoskeletal manual medicine: Diagnosis and treatment.* Thieme Medical Publishers. New York

Dwelly, P.M., Tripp, B.L and Gorin, S. (2009) Glenohumeral rotational range of motion in collegiate overhead-throwing athletes during an athletic season. *Journal of Athletic Training.* 44 (6): 611–616

Edelson, J. and Teitz, C. (2000) Internal impingement of the shoulder. *Journal of Shoulder and Elbow Surgery.* 9: 308–315

Edwards, S.L., Lee, J.A., Bell, J.E., *et al.* (2010) Non-operative treatment of superior labrum anterior posterior tears: Improvements in pain, function and quality of life. *American Journal of Sports Medicine.* 38 (7): 1456–1461

Ellenbecker, T.S. (2006) *Shoulder rehabilitation: Non-operative treatment.* Thieme Medical Publishers. New York

Ellenbecker, T.S. (2011) *Shoulder rehabilitation: Non-operative treatment.* Thieme Medical Publishers. New York

Elliott, B.C., Fleisig, G., Nicholls, R., *et al.* (2003) Technique effects on upper limb loading in the tennis serve. *Journal of Medicine and Science in Sports.* 6: 76–87

Escamilla, R.F., Fleisig, G.S., Zheng, N., *et al.* (2001) Kinematics comparisons of 1996 Olympic baseball pitchers. *Journal of Sports Science.* 19: 665–676

Escamilla, R.F., Yamashiro, K., Paulos, L., *et al.* (2009) Shoulder muscle activity and function in common shoulder exercises. *Sports Medicine.* 39 (8): 663–685

Fabbriciani, C., Milano, G., Demontis, A., *et al.* (2004) Arthroscopic versus open treatment of Bankart lesion in the shoulder: A randomized study. *Arthroscopy.* 20 (5): 456–462

Fleming, J.A., Seitz, A.L. and Ebaugh, D.D. (2010) Exercise protocol for the treatment of rotator cuff impingement syndrome. *Journal of Athletic Training.* 45 (5): 483–485

Foglia, A. and Musarra, F. (2008) *The shoulder in sport: Management, rehabilitation and prevention.* Churchill Livingstone. Philadelphia, PA

Fortenbaugh, D., Glenn, S., Fleisig, G.S., *et al.* (2009) Baseball pitching biomechanics in relation to injury risk and performance. *Sports Health.* 1 (4): 314–320

Funk, L. and Snow, M. (2007) SLAP tears of the glenoid labrum in contact athletes. *Clinical Journal of Sports Medicine.* 17 (1): 1–4

Fusco, A., Foglia, A., Musarra, F., *et al.* (2008) *The shoulder in sport.* Elsevier. Milan, Italy

Gerber, C. and Krushell, R.J. (1991) Isolated rupture of the tendon of the subscapularis muscle: Clinical features in 16 cases. *Journal of Bone and Joint Surgery.* 73 (3): 389–394

Gleason, P.D., Beall, D.P., Sanders, T.G., *et al.* (2006) The transverse humeral ligament: A separate anatomical structure or a continuation of the osseous attachment of the rotator cuff? *American Journal of Sports Medicine.* 34 (1): 72–77

Gotoh, M., Hamada, K., Yamakawa, H., *et al.* (1998). Increased substance P in subacromial bursa and shoulder pain in rotator cuff diseases. *Journal of Orthopaedic Research.* 16: 618–621

Graichen, H., Bonel, H., Stammberger, T., *et al.* (1993) Three-dimensional analysis of the width of the subacromial space in healthy subjects and patients with impingement syndrome. *American Journal of Roentgenology.* 172: 1081–1086

Graichen, H., Stammberger, T. and Bonel, H. (2000) Glenohumeral translation during active and passive elevation of the shoulder. *Journal of Biomechanics.* 33: 609–613

Greene, W.B. and Heckman, J.D. (1994) *The clinical measurement of joint motion.* American Academy of Orthopaedic Surgeons. Rosemont, IL

Greenhalgh, S. and Selfe, J. (2006) *Red flags: A guide to identifying serious pathology of the spine.* Churchill Livingstone, Elsevier. London, UK

Guanche, C.A. and Jones, D.C. (2003) Clinical testing for tears of the glenoid labrum. *Arthroscopy.* 19 (5): 517–523

Gumina, S., Carbone, S. and Postacchini, F. (2009) Scapular dyskinesis and SICK scapula syndrome in patients with chronic type III acromioclavicular dislocation. *Arthroscopy.* 25 (1): 40–45

Gumusburun, E. and Adiguzel, E. (2000) A variation of the brachial plexus characterized by the absence of the musculocutaneous nerve: A case report. *Surgical and Radiologic Anatomy*. 22 (1): 63–65

Gupta, S. and van der Helm, F.C.T. (2004) Load transfer across the scapula during humeral abduction. *Journal of Biomechanics*. 37: 1001–1009

Hamill, J. and Knutzen, K.M. (2009) *Biomechanical basis of human movement*, 3rd edition. Lippincott, Williams and Wilkins. Baltimore, MD

Hammer, W.I. (2007) *Functional soft-tissue examination and treatment by manual methods*, 3rd edition. Jones and Bartlett Publishers. Sudbury, MA

Hattam, P. and Smeatham, A. (2010) *Special tests in musculoskeletal examination: An evidence-based guide for clinicians*. Churchill Livingstone. London, UK

Hayes, K., Walton, J.R., Szomor, Z.L., *et al.* (2002) Reliability of five methods for assessing shoulder range of motion. *Australian Journal of Physiotherapy*. 47: 289–294

Hebert, L.J., Moffet, H., McFadyen, B.J., *et al.* (2000). A method of measuring three-dimensional scapular attitudes using the Optotrak probing system. *Clinical Biomechanics*. 15 (1): 1–8

Hegedus, E.J., Goode, A., Campbell, S., *et al.* (2008) Physical examination tests of the shoulder: A systematic review with meta-analysis of individual tests. *British Journal of Sports Medicine*. 42 (2): 80–92

Hegedus, E.J., Goode, A., Cook, C.E., *et al.* (2012) Which physical examination tests provide clinicians with the most value when examining the shoulder? Update of a systematic review with meta-analysis of individual tests. *British Journal of Sports Medicine*. 46: 964–978

Heinlein, S.A. and Cosgarea, A.J. (2010) Biomechanical considerations in the competitive swimmer's shoulder. *Sports Health*. 2 (6): 519–525

Helmig, P., Sojbjerg, J.O., Kjaersgaard-Andersen, P., *et al.* (1990) Distal humeral migration as a component of multidirectional shoulder instability: An anatomical study in autopsy specimens. *Clinical Orthopaedics and Related Research*. 252: 139–143

Hengeveld, E. and Banks, K. (2005) *Maitland's peripheral manipulation*, 4th edition. Elsevier, Butterworth-Heinmann. London, UK

Hertling, D. and Kessler, R. (2006) *Management of common musculoskeletal disorders: Physical therapy principles and methods*, 4th edition. Lippincott, Williams and Wilkins. Philadelphia, PA

Holtby, R. and Razmjou, H. (2004) Accuracy of Speed's and Yergason's tests in detecting biceps pathology and SLAP lesions: Comparison with arthroscopic findings. *Arthroscopy*. 20 (3): 231–236

Horsley, I. (2005) Assessment of shoulders with pain of a non-traumatic origin. *Physical Therapy in Sport*. 6: 6–14

Horsley, I. (2010) Shoulder injuries in sport. In Comfort, P. and Abrahamson, E. (eds) *Sports rehabilitation and injury prevention*. Wiley-Blackwell. London, UK

Houglum, P. (2010) *Therapeutic exercise for musculoskeletal injuries*, 3rd edition. Human Kinetics. Champaign, IL

Howell, S.M. and Galiant, B.J. (1989) The glenoid labral socket: A constrained articular surface. *Clinical Orthopaedics and Related Research*. 243: 122–125

Hsu, A.T., Chang, J.H. and Chang, C.H. (2002) Determining the resting position of the glenohumeral joint: A cadaver study. *Journal of Orthopaedic and Sports Physical Therapy*. 32 (12): 605–612

Hurschler, C., Wulker, N. and Mendila, M. (2000) The effect of negative intraarticular pressure and rotator cuff force on glenohumeral translation during simulated active elevation. *Clinical Biomechanics*. 15 (5): 306–314

Hutson, M. and Speed, C. (2011) *Sports injuries*. Oxford University Press. Oxford, UK

Iannotti, J.P. and Williams, G.R. (2007) *Disorders of the shoulder: Diagnosis and management, Volume I*, 2nd edition. Lippincott, Williams and Wilkins. Philadelphia, PA

Inokuchi, W., Sanderhoff Olsen, B., Søjbjerg, J. and Sneppen, O. (1997) The relation between the position of the glenohumeral joint and the intraarticular pressure: An experimental study. *Journal of Shoulder and Elbow Surgery*. 6 (2): 144–149

Itoi, E., Hatakeyama, M.D., Sato, T., *et al.* (2007) Immobilization in external rotation after shoulder dislocation reduces the risk of recurrence: A randomized controlled trial. *Journal of Bone and Joint Surgery*. 89 (10): 2124–2131

Jaggi, A. and Lambert, S. (2010) Rehabilitation for shoulder instability. *British Journal of Sports Medicine*. 44: 333–340

Jenkins, D.B. (2009) *Hollinshead's functional anatomy of the limbs and back*, 9th edition. Saunders, Elsevier. St. Louis, MO

Jobe, C.M., Coen, M.J. and Screnar, P. (2000) Evaluation of impingement syndromes in the overhead-throwing athlete. *Journal of Athletic Training*. 35 (3): 293–299

Johnson, D., Lee, J. and Tytherleigh-Strong, G. (2008) Pectoral girdle and upper limb. In Standring, S. *Gray's anatomy: The anatomical basis of clinical practice*, 40th edition. Elsevier, Churchill Livingstone. London, UK

Kaltenborn, F.M. (1999) *Manual mobilization of the extremity joints*. Olaf Norlis Bokhandel. Oslo, Norway

Kaufman, J. and Lee, M. (2014) *Vascular and interventional radiology*, 2nd edition. Elsevier Saunders. Philadelphia, PA

Kebaetse, M., McClure, P. and Pratt, N.A. (1999) Thoracic position effect on shoulder range of motion, strength, and three dimensional scapular kinematics. *Archives of Physical Medicine and Rehabilitation*. 80: 945–950

Kendall, F.P., McCreary, E.K., Provance, P.G., *et al.* (2005) *Muscles: Testing and function with posture and pain*, 5th edition. Lippincott, Williams and Wilkins. Baltimore, MD

Kenyon, K. and Kenyon, J. (2009) *The physiotherapist's pocketbook: Essential facts at your fingertips*, 2nd edition. Churchill Livingstone. London, UK

Khan, K.M., Cook, J.L., Bonar, F., *et al.* (1997) Histopathology of common tendinopathies: Update and implications for clinical management. *Sports Medicine*. 27 (6): 393–408

Kibler, W.B. (1995) Biomechanical analysis of the shoulder during tennis activities. *Clinical Sports Medicine*. 14: 79–85

Kibler, W.B. (1998) The role of the scapula in athletic shoulder function. *American Journal of Sports Medicine*. 26: 325–337

Kibler, W.B. (2000) Evaluation and diagnosis of scapulothoracic problems in the athlete. *Sports Medicine and Arthroscopy Review*. 8: 192–202

Kibler, W.B. (2009) The 4000-watt tennis player: Power development for tennis. *Medicine and Science in Tennis*. 14 (1): 5–8

Kibler, W.B. and McMullen J. (2003) Scapular dyskinesis and its relation to shoulder pain. *Journal of the American Academy of Orthopaedic Surgeons*. 11 (2): 142–151

Kibler, W.B., Uhl T.L., Maddux, J.W., *et al.* (2002) Qualitative clinical evaluation of scapular dysfunction: A reliability study. *Journal of Shoulder and Elbow Surgery*. 11 (6): 550–556

Kierner, C., Zelenka, I. and Burian, M. (2001) How do the cervical plexus and the spinal accessory nerve contribute to the innervation of the trapezius muscle? As seen from within using Sihler's Stain. *Archives of Otolaryngology: Head and Neck Surgery*. 127 (10): 1230–1232

Kim, S.H., Ha, K.I. and Han, K.Y. (1999) Biceps load test: A clinical test for superior labrum anterior and posterior lesions in shoulders with recurrent anterior dislocations. *American Journal of Sports Medicine*. 27 (3): 300–303

Kim, S.H., Ha, K.I., Ahn, J.H., *et al.* (2001) Biceps load test II: A clinical test for SLAP lesions of the shoulder. *Arthroscopy*. 17 (2): 160–164

Kiss, Z.S., Kellaway, D.P. and Cook, J.L. (1998). Post-operative patellar tendon healing: An ultrasound study. *Australasian Radiology*. 42 (1): 28–32

Kolt, G.S. and Snyder-Mackler, L. (2007) *Physical therapies in sport and exercise*, 2nd edition. Churchill Livingstone. Philadelphia, PA

Kuhn, J.E., Plancher, K.D. and Hawkins, R.J. (1995) Scapular winging. *Journal of American Academy of Orthopaedic Surgery*. 3: 319–325

Kuhn, J.E., Lindholm, S.R., Huston, L.J., *et al.* (2003) Failure of the biceps superior labral complex: A cadaveric biomechanical investigation comparing the late cocking and early deceleration positions of throwing. *Arthroscopy*. 19: 373–379

Kulkarni, N.V. (2006) *Clinical anatomy for students: Problem solving approach*. Jaypee Brothers Medical Publishers. New Delhi, India

Kulkarni, N.V. (2012) *Clinical anatomy: A problem solving approach*, 2nd edition. Jaypee Brothers Medical Publishers. New Delhi, India

Lander, P. (2007) Selective cervical nerve blocks. In Schweitzer, M.E. and Laredo, J.D. (eds) *New techniques in interventional musculoskeletal radiology*. Informa Healthcare Inc. New York

Landin, D., Myers, J., Thompson, M., *et al.* (2008) The role of the biceps brachii in shoulder elevation. *Journal of Electromyography and Kinesiology*. 18 (2): 270–275

Lee, S.B., Kim, K.J., O'Driscoll, *et al.* (2000) Dynamic glenohumeral stability provided by the rotator cuff muscles in the mid-range and end-range of motion: A study in cadavera. *Journal of Bone and Joint Surgery*. 82: 849–857

Lee, H.W. (1995) Mechanics of neck and shoulder injuries in tennis players. *Journal of Orthopaedics and Sports Physical Therapy*. 21 (1): 28–37

Levy, A.S., Kelly, B.T., Lintner, S.A., *et al.* (2001) Function of the long head of biceps at the shoulder: Electromyographic analysis. *Journal of Shoulder and Elbow Surgery*. 10 (3): 250–255

Lewis, A., Kitamura, T. and Bayley, J.I. (2004) Mini symposium: Shoulder instability (ii). The classification of shoulder instability: New light through old windows! *Current Orthopaedics*. 18 (2): 97–108

Lewis, J.S. (2006) *The shoulder: Theory and practice*, 4th edition. Course manual. London, UK

Lewis, J.S. (2009) Rotator cuff tendinopathy/subacromial impingement syndrome: Is it time for a new method of assessment? *British Journal of Sports Medicine*. 43: 259–264

Lewis, J.S. (2010) Rotator cuff tendinopathy: A model for the continuum of pathology and related management. *British Journal of Sports Medicine*. 44: 918–923

Lewis, J.S., Green, A. and Wright, C. (2005) Subacromial impingement syndrome: The role of posture and muscle imbalance. *Journal of Shoulder and Elbow Surgery*. 14: 385–392

Lintner, D., Mayol, M. and Uzodinma, O. (2007) Glenohumeral internal deficit in professional pitchers enrolled in an internal rotation stretching program. *American Journal of Sports Medicine*. 35 (4): 617–621

Lippitt, S. and Matsen, F. (1993) Mechanisms of glenohumeral joint stability. *Clinical Orthopaedics and Related Research*. 291: 20–28

Littlewood, C., Ashton, J., Chance-Larsen, K., *et al.* (2012) Exercise for rotator cuff tendinopathy: A systematic review. *Physiotherapy*. 98: 101–109

Lo, I.K. and Burkhart, S.S. (2004) Transtendon arthroscopic repair of partial-thickness, articular surface tears of the rotator cuff. *Arthroscopy*. 20: 214–220

Lo, I.K., Nonweiler, B. and Woolfrey, M. (2004) An evaluation of the apprehension, relocation, and surprise tests for anterior shoulder instability. *American Journal of Sports Medicine*. 31: 301–307

Loudon, J., Swift, M. and Bell, S. (2008) *The clinical orthopedic assessment guide*, 2nd edition. Human Kinetics. Champaign, IL

Ludewig, P.M. and Cook, T.M. (2000). Alterations in shoulder kinematics and associated muscle activity in people with symptoms of shoulder impingement. *Physical Therapy*. 80 (3): 267–291

MacDonald, K., Bridger, J., Cash, C., *et al.* (2007) Transverse humeral ligament: Does it exist? *Clinical Anatomy*. 20 (6): 663–667

MacDonald, P.B. and LaPointe, P. (2008) Acromioclavicular and sternoclavicular joint injuries. *Orthopedic Clinics of North America*. 39: 535–545

MacDonald, P.B., Clark, P. and Sutherland, K. (2000) An analysis of the diagnostic accuracy of the Hawkins and Neer subacromial impingement signs. *Journal of Shoulder and Elbow Surgery*. 9 (4): 299–301

Magarey, M.E. and Jones, A. (1992) Clinical diagnosis and management of minor shoulder instability. *Australian Journal of Physiotherapy*. 38: 269–279

Magarey, M.E., Jones, M.A. and Grant, E.R. (1996) Biomedical considerations and clinical patterns related to disorders of the glenoid labrum in the predominantly stable glenohumeral joint. *Manual Therapy*. 1 (5): 242–249

Magee, D.J. (2014) *Orthopedic physical assessment*, 6th edition. Elsevier Saunders. St. Louis, MO

Malliou, P.C., Giannakopoulos, K., Beneka, A.G., *et al.* (2004) Effective ways of restoring muscular imbalances of the rotator cuff muscle group: A comparative study of various training methods. *British Journal of Sports Medicine*. 38: 766–772

Mallon, W.J. and Speer, K.P. (1995) Multidirectional instability: Current concepts. *Journal of Shoulder and Elbow Surgery*. 4 (1): 54–64

Manske, R. (2006) Electromyographically assessed exercises for the scapular muscles. *Athletic Therapy Today*. 11 (5): 19–23

Manske, R. and Prohaskab, D. (2010) Superior labrum anterior to posterior (SLAP) rehabilitation in the overhead athlete. *Physical Therapy in Sport*. doi:10.1016/j.ptsp.2010.06.004

Manske, R., Meschke, M., Porter, A., *et al.* (2010) A randomized controlled single-blinded comparison of stretching versus stretching and joint mobilization for posterior shoulder tightness measured by internal rotation motion loss. *Sports Health*. 2 (2): 94–100

Mansur, D.I., Khanal, K., Haque, M.K., *et al.* (2012) Morphometry of acromion process of human scapulae and its clinical importance amongst Nepalese population. *Kathmandu University Medical Journal*. 10 (2): 33–36

Matava, M.J., Purcell, D.B. and Rudzki, J.R. (2005) Partial-thickness rotator cuff tears. *American Journal of Sports Medicine*. 33 (9): 1405–1417

Matsen, F.A. and Arntz, C.T. (1990). Subacromial impingement. In Rockwood, C.A. and Matsen, F.A. (eds) *The shoulder*, 9th edition. Saunders. Philadelphia, PA

Mazzocca, A.D., Arciero, R.A. and Bicos, J. (2007) Evaluation and treatment of acromioclavicular joint injuries. *American Journal of Sports Medicine*. 18: 316–329

McCarron, J.A., Codsi, M.J. and Iannotti, J.P. (2011) Latissimus transfer for irreparable posterosuperior rotator cuff tear. In Williams, G.R., Ramsey, M.L. and Wiesel, S.W. (eds) *Operative techniques in shoulder and elbow surgery*. Lippincott, Williams and Wilkins. Philadelphia, PA

McClelland, D. and Paxinos, A. (2008) The anatomy of the quadrilateral space with reference to quadrilateral space syndrome. *Journal of Shoulder and Elbow Surgery*. 17 (1): 162–164

McClure, P.W., Michener, L.A. and Sennett B.J. (2001) Direct 3-dimensional measurement of scapular kinematics during dynamic movements in vivo. *Journal of Shoulder and Elbow Surgery*. 10: 269–277

McClure, P., Balaicuis, J., Heiland, D. *et al*. (2007) A randomized controlled comparison of stretching procedures for posterior shoulder tightness. *Journal of Orthopaedic and Sports Physical Therapy*.37: 108–114

McConnell, J. (2002) *The McConnell approach to the problem shoulder*. Course manual. McConnell Institute, UK

McFarland, E.G. (2006) *Examination of the shoulder: The complete guide*. Thieme Medical Publishers. New York

McMahon, P.J., Jobe, F.W., Pink, M.M., *et al*. (1996) Comparative electromyographic analysis of shoulder muscles during planar motions: Anterior glenohumeral instability versus normal. *Journal Shoulder and Elbow Surgery*. 5: 118–123

McMullen, J. and Uhl, T.L. (2000) A kinetic chain approach for shoulder rehabilitation. *Journal of Athletic Training*. 35: 329–337

Meister, K. (2000) Injuries to the shoulder in the throwing athlete part two: Evaluation and treatment. *American Journal of Sports Medicine*. 28 (4): 587–601

Miller, M.D. and Cole, B.J. (2004) *Textbook of arthroscopy, Volume 355*. Elsevier Saunders. Philadelphia, PA

Mirzayan, R. and Itamura, J. (2004) *Shoulder and elbow trauma*. Thieme Medical Publishers. New York

Misamore, G.W., Sallay, P.I. and Didelot, W. (2005) A longitudinal study of patients with multidirectional instability of the shoulder with 7 to 10 year follow-up. *Journal of Shoulder and Elbow Surgery*. 14: 466–470

Moen, M.H., de Vos, R.J., Ellenbecker, T.S., *et al*. (2010) Clinical tests in shoulder examination: How to perform them. *British Journal of Sports Medicine*. 44: 370–375

Moses, K.P., Banks, J.C., Nava, P.B., *et al*. (2013) *Atlas of clinical gross anatomy*, 2nd edition. Elsevier Saunders. Philadelphia, PA

Myers, J.B, Laudner K.G., Pasquale M.R., *et al*. (2005) Posterior capsular tightness in throwers with internal impingement. *Presentation at the Annual Meeting of Orthopaedic Surgeons 51st Annual Meeting*. Washington, DC

Nakagawa, S., Yoneda, M., Hayashida, K., *et al*. (2001) Greater tuberosity notch: An important indicator of articular-side partial rotator cuff tears in the shoulders of throwing athletes. *American Journal of Sports Medicine*. 29: 762–770

Neer, C.S. (1972) Anterior acromioplasty for chronic impingement syndrome in the shoulder: A preliminary report. *Journal of Bone and Joint Surgery*. 54 (1): 41–50

Neer, C.S. (1983) Impingement lesions. *Clinical Orthopaedics and Related Research*. 173: 70–77

Netter, F.H., Iannotti, J.P. and Parker, R.D. (2013) *The Netter collection of medical illustrations: Musculoskeletal system. Part I: Upper limb*, 2nd edition. Elsevier, Saunders. Philadelphia, PA

Neuman, B.J., Boisvert, C.B., Reiter, B., *et al*. (2011) Results of arthroscopic repair of type II superior labral anterior posterior lesions in overhead athletes: Assessment of return to preinjury playing level and satisfaction. *American Journal of Sports Medicine*. 39: 1883–1888

Nissen, C.W. and Chatterjee, A. (2007) Type III acromioclavicular separation: Results of a recent survey on its management. *American Journal of Orthopedics*. 36 (2): 89–93

O'Brien, S.J., Pagnani, M.J. and Fealy, S. (1998) The active compression test: A new and effective test for diagnosing labral tears and acromioclavicular abnormality. *American Journal of Sports Medicine*. 26 (5): 610–613

Oyama, S. (2012) Baseball pitching kinematics, joint loads, and injury prevention. *Journal of Sport and Health Science*. 1: 80–91

Paine, R.M. and Voight, M. (2013). The role of the scapula. *International Journal of Sports Physical Therapy.* 8(5): 617–629

Palastanga, N. and Soames, R. (2012) *Anatomy and human movement: Structure and function,* 6th edition. Churchill Livingstone. Philadelphia, PA

Pansky, B. and Gest, T. (2011) *Lippincott's concise illustrated anatomy: Back, upper limb and lower limb.* Lippincott, Williams and Wilkins. Philadelphia, PA

Park, H.B., Lin, S.K., Yokota, A., *et al.* (2004) Return to play for rotator cuff injuries and superior labrum anterior posterior (SLAP) lesions. *Clinical Journal of Sports Medicine.* 23 (3): 321–334

Parsons, I.M., Apreleva, M., Fu, F.H., *et al.* (2002) The effect of rotator cuff tears on reaction forces at the glenohumeral joint. *Journal of Orthopaedic Research.* 20 (3): 439–446

Payne, L.Z., Deng, X.H., Craig, E.V., *et al.* (1997) The combined dynamic and static contributions to subacromial impingement: A biomechanical analysis. *American Journal of Sports Medicine.* 25: 801–808

Pellerin, M., Kimball, Z., Tubbs, R.S., *et al.* (2010) The prefixed and postfixed brachial plexus: A review with surgical implications. *Surgical and Radiologic Anatomy.* 32 (3): 251–260

Peterson, C.M. and Hayes, K. (2000) Construct validity of Cyriax's selective tension examination: Association of end-feels with pin in the knee and shoulder. *Journal of Orthopaedic and Sports Physical Therapy.* 30: 512–527

Pettitt, R.W., Sailor, R.S., Lentell, G., *et al.* (2008) Yergason's test: Discrepancies in description and implications for diagnosing biceps subluxation. *Athletic Training Education Journal.* 3 (4): 143–147

Petty, N.J. (2011) *Neuromuscular examination and assessment: A handbook for therapists,* 4th edition. Elsevier. Edinburgh, UK

Prentice, W. (2011) *Principles of athletic training: A competency-based approach,* 14th edition. McGraw-Hill. New York

Provencher, M.T. and Romeo, A.A. (2012) *Shoulder instability: A comprehensive approach.* Elsevier Saunders. Philadelphia, PA

Rabin, A., Irrgang, J.J., Fitzgerald, G.K. and Eubanks, A. (2006) The intertester reliability of the scapular assistance test. *Journal of Orthopaedic and Sports Physical Therapy.* 36 (9): 653–660

Rathbun, J.B and Macnab, I. (1970) The microvascular pattern of the rotator cuff. *Journal of Bone and Joint Surgery.* 72: 181–185

Reed, D., Cathers, I., Halaki, M. and Ginn, K. (2013) Does supraspinatus initiate shoulder abduction? *Journal of Electromyography and Kinesiology.* 23: 425–429

Reinhold, M.M., Wilk, K.E. and Reed, J. (2002) Interval sport programs: Guidelines for baseball, tennis and golf. *Journal of Orthopaedic and Sports Physical Therapy.* 32: 293–298

Reinhold, M.M., Wilk, K.E., Fleisig, G.S., *et al.* (2004) Electromyographic analysis of the rotator cuff and deltoid musculature during common shoulder external rotation exercises. *Journal of Orthopaedic and Sports Physical Therapy.* 34: 384–395

Reinhold, M.M., Macrina, L.C., Wilk, K.E., *et al.* (2007) Electromyographic analysis of the supraspinatus and deltoid muscles during three common rehabilitation exercises. *Journal of Athletic Training.* 42: 464–469

Robb, A.J. and Howitt, S. (2011) Conservative management of a type III acromioclavicular separation: A case report and 10-year follow-up. *Journal of Chiropractic Medicine.* 10: 261–271

Rockwood, C.A., Matsen, F.A., Wirth, M.A., *et al.* (2009) *The shoulder,* 4th edition. Saunders, Elsevier. Philadelphia, PA

Ross, M.D. and Boissonault, W.G. (2010) Red flags: To screen or not to screen? *Journal of Orthopaedic and Sports Physical Therapy.* 40 (11): 682–684

Rull, G. (2014) *Pancoast's syndrome.* www.patient.co.uk/doctor/pancoasts-syndrome, accessed July 2014

Russell, S.M. (2006) *Examination of peripheral nerve injuries: An anatomical approach.* Thieme Medical Publishers. New York

Saeed, M. and Rufai, A.A. (2003) Median and musculocutaneous nerves: Variant formation and distribution. *Clinical Anatomy.* 16 (5): 453–457

Safran, M.R. (2004a) Nerve injury about the shoulder in athletes. Part 1: Suprascapular nerve and axillary nerve. *American Journal of Sports Medicine.* 32 (3): 803–819

Safran, M.R. (2004b) Nerve injury about the shoulder in athletes. Part 2: Long thoracic nerve, spinal accessory nerve, burners/stingers, thoracic outlet syndrome. *American Journal of Sports Medicine.* 32 (4): 1063–1076

Sahrmann, S.A. (2002). *Diagnosis and treatment of movement impairment syndromes.* Mosby. St. Louis, MO

Schepsis, A.A. and Busconi, B.D. (2006) *Sports Medicine*. Lippincott, Williams and Wilkins. Philadelphia, PA

Sein, M.L., Walton, J., Linklater, J., *et al.* (2010) Shoulder pain in elite swimmers: Primarily due to swim-volume-induced supraspinatus tendinopathy. *British Journal of Sports Medicine*. 44: 105–113

Seitz, A.L., McClure, P.W., Finucane, S., *et al.* (2012) The scapular assistance test results in changes in scapular position and subacromial space but not rotator cuff strength in subacromial impingement. *Journal of Orthopaedic and Sports Physical Therapy*. 42 (5): 400–412

Seroyer, S.T., Nho, S.J. and Romeo, A.A. (2009) Shoulder pain in the overhead throwing athlete. *Sports Health*. 1 (2): 108–120

Sewell, D., Watkins, P. and Griffin, M. (2013) *Sport and exercise science: An introduction*, 2nd edition. Routledge. Abingdon, UK

Slaven, E.J. and Mathers, J. (2010) Differential diagnosis of shoulder and cervical pain: A case report. *Journal of Manual and Manipulative Therapy*. 18 (4): 191–196

Smith, T.O., Chester, R., Pearse, E., *et al.* (2011) Operative versus non-operative management following Rockwood grade III acromioclavicular separation: A meta-analysis of the current evidence base. *Journal of Orthopaedics and Traumatology*. 12 (1): 19–27

Snyder, S.B., Banas, M.P. and Karzel, R.P. (1995) An analysis of 140 injuries to the superior glenoid labrum. *Journal of Shoulder and Elbow Surgery*. 4 (4): 243–248

Spencer, E.E. (2007) Treatment of grade III acromioclavicular joint injuries: A systematic review. *Clinical Orthopaedics and Related Research*. 455: 38–44

Stodden, D.F., Langendorfer, S.J., Fleisig, G.S., *et al.* (2006) Kinematic constraints associated with the acquisition of overarm throwing. Part II: Upper extremity actions. *Research Quarterly for Exercise and Sport*. 77 (4): 428–436

Struyf, F., Nijs, J. and Mottram, S. (2012) Clinical assessment of the scapula: A review of the literature. *British Journal of Sports Medicine*. 48 (11): 883–890

Tate, A.R., McClure, P., Kareha, S., *et al.* (2008) Effect of the scapula reposition test on shoulder impingement symptoms and elevation strength in overhead athletes. *Journal of Orthopaedic and Sports Physical Therapy*. 38 (1): 4–11

Taylor, W. (2005) Musculoskeletal pain in the adult New Zealand population: Prevalence and impact. *New Zealand Medical Journal*. 118 (1221): U1629

Teece, R.M., Lunden, J.B., Lloyd, A.S., *et al.* (2008) Three-dimensional acromioclavicular joint motions during elevation of the arm. *Journal of Orthopaedic and Sports Physical Therapy*. 38: 181–190

Terry G.C. and Chopp T.M. (2000) Functional anatomy of the shoulder. *Journal of Athletic Training*. 35 (3): 248–255

Teys, P., Bisset, L. and Vicenzino, B. (2008) The initial effects of a Mulligan's mobilization with movement technique on range of movement and pressure pain threshold in pain-limited shoulders. *Manual Therapy*. 13: 37–42

Thompson, J.C. (2010) *Netter's concise orthopaedic anatomy*, 2nd edition. Saunders, Elsevier. Philadelphia, PA

Thornton, G.M., Shoa, X., Chung, M., *et al.* (2010) Changes in mechanical loading lead to tendon-specific alterations in MMP and TIMP expression: Influence of stress deprivation and intermittent cyclic hydrostatic compression on rat supraspinatus and Achilles tendons. *British Journal of Sports Medicine*. 44 (10): 698–703

Tovin, B.J. (2006) Prevention and treatment of swimmer's shoulder. *North American Journal of Sports Physical Therapy*. 1 (4): 166–175

Trainer, G., Arciero, R.A. and Mazzocca, A.D. (2008) Practical management of grade III acromioclavicular separations. *Clinical Journal of Sports Medicine*. 18 (2): 162–166

Tripp, B.L. (2008) Principles of restoring function and sensorimotor control in patients with shoulder dysfunction. *Clinics in Sports Medicine*. 27: 507–519

Tubbs, R.S., Loukas, M. and Shahid, K., *et al.* (2007) Anatomy and quantitation of the subscapular nerves. *Clinical Anatomy*. 20 (6): 656–659

Tyler, T.F., Roy, T. and Nicholas, S.J. (1999) Reliability and validity of a new method of measuring posterior shoulder tightness. *Journal of Orthopaedic and Sports Physical Therapy*. 29 (5): 262–274

Uhthoff, H.K. and Sarkar, K. (1991) Surgical repair of rotator cuff ruptures: The importance of the subacromial bursa. *Journal of Bone and Joint Surgery*. 73: 399–401

van der Heijden, G.J. (1999) Shoulder disorders: A state-of-the-art review. *Baillieres Best Practice and Research: Clinical Rheumatology*. 13 (2): 287–309 van der Hoeven, H. and Kibler, W.B. (2006) Shoulder injuries in tennis players. *British Journal of Sports Medicine.* 40: 435–440

van der Windt, D., Koes, B., Boeke, A., *et al.* (1996) Shoulder disorders in general practice: Prognostic indicators of outcome. *British Journal of General Practice.* 46: 519–523

van Es, H. (2001) MRI of the brachial plexus. *Journal of European Radiology.* 11 (2): 325–336

Vizniak, N.A. (2012) *Quick reference evidence-based physical assessment,* 3rd edition. Professional Health Systems. Canada

Vogel, K.G. (2003) Tendon structure and response to changing mechanical load. *Journal of Musculoskeletal and Neuronal Interactions.* 3: 323–325

Voight, M.L., Hoogenboom, B.J. and Prentice, W.E. (2007) *Musculoskeletal interventions: Techniques for therapeutic exercise.* McGraw-Hill Medical. New York

Wadsworth, D.J. and Bullock-Saxton, J.E. (1997). Recruitment patterns of the scapular rotator muscles in freestyle swimmers with subacromial impingement. *International Journal of Sports Medicine.* 18: 618–624

Walch, G., Boileau, P., Noel, E. and Donell, T. (1992) Impingement of the deep surface of the supraspinatus tendon on the glenoid rim. *Journal of Shoulder and Elbow Surgery.* 1: 239–245

Walsh, R.W. and Sadowski, G.E. (2001) Systemic disease mimicking musculoskeletal dysfunction: A case report involving referred shoulder pain. *Journal of Orthopaedic and Sports Physical Therapy.* 31 (12): 696–701

Wilk, K.E., Macrina, L.C. and Reinold, M.M. (2006) Non-operative rehabilitation for traumatic and atraumatic glenohumeral instability. *North American Journal of Sports Physical Therapy.* 1 (1): 16–31

Wilk, K.E., Reinold, M.M. and Andrews, J.R. (2009) *The athlete's shoulder,* 2nd edition. Churchill Livingstone. Philadelphia, PA

Wilk, K.E., Yenchak, A.J., Arrigo, C.A., *et al.* (2011) The Advanced Throwers Ten Exercise Program: A new exercise series for enhanced dynamic shoulder control in the overhead throwing athlete. *The Physician and Sports Medicine.* 39 (4): 90–97

Wilk, K.E., Macrina, L.C. and Arrigo, C. (2012) Shoulder rehabilitation. In Andrews, J.R., Harrelson, G.L. and Wilk, K.E. *Physical rehabilitation of the injured athlete,* 4th edition. Saunders, Elsevier. Philadelphia, PA

Wilk, K.E., Macrina, L.C., Cain, E., *et al.* (2013) The recognition and treatment of superior labral (SLAP) lesions in the overhead athlete. *International Journal of Sports Physical Therapy.* 8 (5): 579–600

Woodward, T.W. and Best, T.M. (2000) The painful shoulder. Part I: Clinical evaluation. *American Family Physician.* 61: 3079–3088

7

THE ELBOW REGION

Anatomy, assessment and injuries

Keith Ward

Functional anatomy of the elbow region

The elbow, or cubital region, has direct relationships with the shoulder, upper arm, forearm, wrist and hand. The function of the elbow is to enable fundamental activities such as putting hand to mouth, transmitting force from the shoulder to the hand and gross positioning of the hands. The elbow provides both hinged and rotational open and closed chain leverage for upper limb movement. As a central component of the upper limb, the elbow presents itself as a more inherently stable region when compared to the shoulder or wrist, due to both the firm articular congruency of the humeroulnar joint and to the strong static stability provided by its collateral ligaments and interosseous membrane of the forearm. Although relatively stable, the elbow is still vulnerable to contact injuries due to the fact that it is typically unprotected in sporting activities. As the elbow is involved in the majority of forceful and repetitive upper limb movements of exercise, sport and work, it is also prone as a site for overuse problems such as wrist flexor or extensor tendinopathy, or valgus extension overload syndrome. The elbow is also associated with a range of other traumatic injuries, including musculotendinous ruptures of the biceps or triceps, which are common in weight-lifters. Sprains, dislocations and fractures are notably associated with fall mechanisms. Elbow injuries are becoming more prevalent as more athletes participate in throwing and racquet sports (Antuna and Barco Laakso, 2010).

Surface anatomy of the elbow

Close visual inspection and palpation of the elbow region reveals aspects of its skin, superficial and deep bony landmarks, ligamentous tissue, musculotendinous tissue, fascia, blood vessels and nerves.

Skeletal anatomy of the elbow

Johnson (2008) presents a comprehensive overview of the upper limb. The bones forming the elbow complex are the humerus, ulna and radius. The main structural landmarks of the humerus at the elbow are the distal shaft, medial and lateral epicondyles, medial and lateral supracondylar ridges, trochlea, radial fossa, coronoid fossa, olecranon fossa, capitulum (or capitellum) and the

442

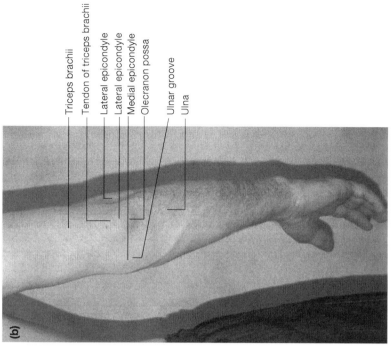

Triceps brachii
Tendon of triceps brachii
Lateral epicondyle
Lateral epicondyle
Medial epicondyle
Olecranon possa
Ulnar groove
Ulna

(b)

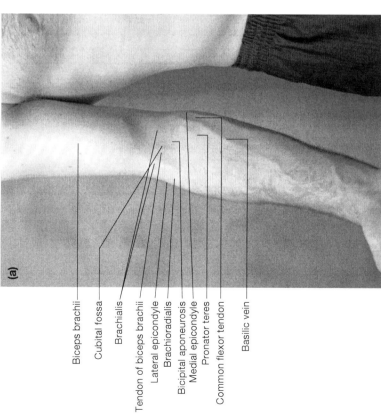

Biceps brachii
Cubital fossa
Brachialis
Tendon of biceps brachii
Lateral epicondyle
Brachioradialis
Bicipital aponeurosis
Medial epicondyle
Pronator teres
Common flexor tendon
Basilic vein

(a)

Photo 7.1   Surface anatomy: anterior and posterior views.

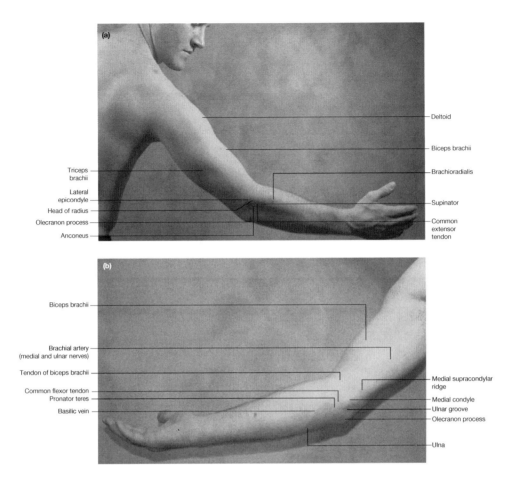

Photo 7.2   Surface anatomy: lateral and medial views.

Practitioner Tip Box 7.1

Skeletal landmarks of the elbow region

Humerus

Radial groove

Medial supracondylar ridge

Lateral supracondylar ridge

Medial epicondyle

Lateral epicondyle

Trochlea

Radial fossa

Coronoid fossa

Olecranon fossa

Capitulum

Ulnar groove

Ulna

Olecranon process

Trochlear notch

Coronoid process

Radial notch

Supinator crest

Ulnar tuberosity

Radius

Radial head

Radial neck

Radial tuberosity

ulnar groove, or sulcus, for the ulnar nerve. The skeletal landmarks on the proximal ulna are the olecranon process, trochlear notch, coronoid process, radial notch, supinator crest and tuberosity. The proximal radius has its head, neck, tuberosity and shaft.

Movements of the elbow

The elbow is a uniaxial synovial joint formed by the humeroulnar and the radiohumeral joints, allowing for flexion and extension. In close association for the function of forearm pronation and supination, is the proximal (or superior) radioulnar joint. The humeroulnar hinge joint is one of the more congruent in the body, and the snug fit of the humeral trochlea with the ulnar trochlear notch provides the foundation for its static stability. At end-range flexion the coronoid process of the ulna approximates with the coronoid fossa of the humerus. At end-range extension the olecranon process of the ulna approximates with the olecranon fossa of the humerus and provides a distinct bone-to-bone end-feel. At the gliding radiohumeral joint, the rounded and concave radial head communicates with the spherical capitulum. The radial fossa, just superior to the capitulum, provides a bony end-point to radiohumeral flexion. The movements of the radiohumeral joint are limited to flexion and extension due to its association and fixation at the proximal radioulnar joint. The proximal radioulnar joint works with the distal (or inferior) radioulnar joint to provide rotation of the radius about the ulna. The head of the radius communicates with the radial notch on the proximal lateral aspect of the ulna, just adjacent to the trochlear notch. In the anatomical supinated position, the radius and ulna are uncrossed, and in pronation the radius crosses over the ulna diagonally (Johnson, 2008; Tortora and Derrickson, 2008).

Flexion and extension movements occur in the sagittal plane about a mediolateral axis. Pronation and supination movements occur in the transverse plane about a longitudinal axis. Normal active ranges of movement at the elbow are considered to be: flexion 0–140°; extension 0–10°; pronation 80–90°; supination 80–90° (Aviles *et al.*, 2009; Hamill and Knutson, 2009). For normal daily activities, movement ranges significantly less than these will suffice, but there are differences in what could be considered functionally acceptable for certain sports, such as gymnastics and weight-lifting. Additionally, there are individual factors and variations to consider, for example an increase in end-range elbow extension, termed cubitus recurvatus, is where around 10° extension may still be considered within the realms of normal, particularly for females. Hypermobile patients or those with localized hypomobility associated with previous structural injury or arthritic degeneration will present with alterations in range. Normal constraints to any joint movement include those structures which are being stretched or tensioned and those which are being compressed or approximated. Joint movements may also be affected by articular abnormalities (capsular inflammation; arthritic degeneration; mechanical derangement or intra-articular loose bodies; soft tissue impingement). Additionally, one or more of the joint's accessory movements may be restricted to some degree. Regardless of the cause, pain, swelling, spasm, stiffness or mechanical blockage will limit movement. The normal constraints to elbow flexion are posterior joint capsule and triceps tension and anterior soft tissue approximation (muscle and fat); these factors lead to the normal yielding soft end-feel. The normal constraint to elbow extension is felt as a distinct but painless bone-to-bone end-feel where the olecranon process of the ulna meets the olecranon fossa of the humerus. Additionally, there may be tensioning of the anterior joint capsule, biceps or brachialis or other anterior elbow soft tissues.

Table 7.1 presents an anatomical summary of the elbow region and offers a set of comparisons for the three joints. The close-packed position of a joint is where the joint in question is said to

Table 7.1 Anatomical overview of the elbow

	Humeroulnar joint	Radiohumeral joint	Proximal radioulnar joint
Active range of movement norms	Flexion 140° Extension 0–10°	Flexion 140° Extension 0–10°	Pronation 80–90° Supination 80–90°
Close-packed position	Extension and supination	90° flexion 5° supination	5° supination
Loose-packed position	70° flexion 10° supination	Extension and supination	70° flexion 35° supination
Capsular pattern	Flexion and extension	Flexion and extension	Equal limitation of supination and pronation
Ligaments	Ulnar collateral ligament (UCL – anterior oblique bundle; posterior oblique bundle; intermediate bundle; transverse ligament) Lateral ulnar collateral ligament (LUCL)	Radial collateral ligament (RCL)	Annular ligament Quadrate ligament Oblique cord Interosseous membrane
Bursae	Olecranon (subcutaneous; intratendinous; subtendinous)	Cubital (radiohumeral)	
Accessory movements	Longitudinal caudad glide of ulna Longitudinal cephalad compression of ulna Lateral and medial glide of ulna	Longitudinal caudad glide of radius Longitudinal cephalad compression of the radius	Anteroposterior glide to radial head Posteroanterior glide to radial head

be most stable: for the humeroulnar joint, this is a position of full extension and supination. Conversely, the loose- or open-packed position of a joint is where it is considered to be most unstable, or movable, which, for the humeroulnar joint, is flexion. The close-packed position is likely to be the position where the articular surfaces are most congruent and tightly compressed and where the joint capsule and associated ligaments are taut. In the close-packed position, little or no discernible accessory movements are available and it is therefore not the position to attempt accessory mobilization therapy. The three joints of the elbow each have their own set of associated accessory movements, which are discussed in the assessment section of this chapter.

Joint capsule of the elbow

One single, continuous fibrous capsule, extending from the deeper fascial tissues above and below, and lined by synovial membrane, surrounds the elbow and is attached proximally around the humerus at a level above the coronoid fossa anteriorly, trochlea medially, olecranon fossa posteriorly and capitulum laterally. Distally, the capsule extends over the proximal radius and ulna to cover the three joints. It is a fairly loose capsule, relatively weaker anteriorly and posteriorly, and stronger medially and laterally. The capsule blends with the ulnar and radial collateral ligaments and is additionally reinforced by deeper fibres from brachialis and triceps (Johnson, 2008). The muscular involvement also helps keep the capsule from being impinged during movement. The capsule is richly innervated and provides a key proprioceptive function, particularly in relation to the coordination of the upper limb as a whole. Overlying the olecranon process and the joint capsule, but underneath the triceps tendon, is the subcutaneous olecranon bursa (there may also be subtendinous or infratendinous components). Another bursa, the radiohumeral (cubital) bursa, may be present, located underneath the common wrist extensor sheath, overlying the radial head.

Cubital fossa of the elbow

The anteriorly situated cubital fossa is a triangular space through which pass the biceps tendon, the median and radial nerves, the brachial artery and the cephalic, basilic and cubital veins. The cubital fossa is formed superiorly by the distal humeral bony structures, inferiorly by medial and lateral tendinous borders (pronator teres and brachioradialis), deeply by the brachialis muscle and superficially by fascia which is reinforced by the bicipital aponeurosis (Palastanga *et al.*, 2006).

Ligaments of the elbow

There are three main ligaments at the elbow specifically, plus additional restraining soft tissue structures between the radius and ulna. The ulnar (or medial) collateral ligament (UCL) is roughly triangular in shape and has four ligamentous bands (bundles). Three of these bands run from the medial epicondyle of the humerus: the anterior oblique bundle attaches at the medial aspect of the coronoid process; the posterior oblique bundle attaches at the medial aspect of the olecranon process; and the weaker intermediate bundle attaches to the medial ulna between the anterior and posterior attachments. The fourth and slightly more superficial transverse band of the UCL, also known as Cooper's ligament, runs from the medial olecranon process to the medial coronoid process and hence provides slight reinforcement to the anterior and posterior segments. The UCL is the primary ligamentous stabilizing component of the elbow, and in particular its anterior oblique band has been shown to be the most important constraint to valgus instability (Eygendaal and Safran 2006; Kaminski *et al.*, 2000). The humeroulnar joint also has an important narrow lateral ulnar collateral ligament complex: the LUCL. This attaches at the lateral epicondyle, blends with the base of the annular ligament of the radioulnar joint and inserts to the supinator crest of the ulna. The other ligament stabilizing the lateral elbow complex is the radial collateral ligament (RCL). The RCL is a single band running from the lateral epicondyle of the humerus to the radial notch of the ulna as it too blends with the annular ligament. Together, the UCL, LUCL and RCL provide the major ligamentous contribution to stability of the elbow, helping prevent joint displacement caused by excessive or forceful rotation, valgus or varus stress and anterior or posterior distraction. The UCL specifically contributes to prevent excessive valgus stress and the LUCL and RCL varus stress. All become taut in the close-packed position of extension. The annular ligament and radial notch of the ulna together form the circular fibro-osseous ring that straps the radial head against the radial notch at the proximal radioulnar joint. It is reinforced, as previously mentioned, by the LUCL, the RCL and the continuous fibrous capsule of the elbow. Additionally, the short quadrate ligament, attaching between the radial neck and radial notch, offers further stability to the proximal radioulnar joint. The radial and ulnar shafts are primarily stabilized by a syndesmosis. The strong and fibrous interosseous membrane, which begins approximately 2–3 cm distal to the radial tuberosity and ends just proximal to the distal radioulnar joint, also provides attachment for the deep forearm (wrist and hand) musculature. The membrane is somewhat slackened in positions of full pronation and supination, but tensioned in neutral. The oblique cord is a short, narrow band of thickened fascia running obliquely from the lateral proximal ulna to just distal to the radial tuberosity, above the level of origin of the interosseous membrane. It provides slight additional reinforcement to the radioulnar complex (Johnson, 2008; Morrey and An 1983; Palastanga *et al.*, 2006)

Carrying angle of the elbow

The 'carrying angle' of the elbow is the angle created between the midline of the humerus and the midline of the forearm. It can be observed (or measured with a goniometer) when the arm is in its fully extended, supinated anatomical position, with the shoulder externally rotated. The angle does vary among individuals: the male norm, which is referred to as normal cubitus valgus, has been described as being 5–10°. Females tend to demonstrate a slightly greater angle of 10–15° (Magee, 2008). The reason for this increase is likely to relate to the difference in general skeletal structure (narrower shoulder breadth; wider pelvis). The carrying angle, which has been shown often to be greater in the dominant arm of throwing athletes, allows the elbow to tuck into the waist area above the iliac crests and for the lower arm to clear the hip during the arm swing of gait. It does tend to increase when a heavy object is being lifted. Alterations in the carrying angle, whether increased or decreased, bilateral or unilateral, can be indicative of underlying structural abnormality such as joint instability, arthrosis or malunion following fracture, and may predispose athletes to chronic injury. The dominant arm in the throwing athlete is prone to osseous deformation leading to increases in the angle by 2–3°. The other variant of carrying angle is cubitus varus, or 'gunstock deformity', where the angle is significantly less than the normal valgus (Andrews *et al.*, 1993; Morrey, 2010; Shultz *et al.*, 2000; Starkey and Ryan, 2003).

Muscles of the elbow

It is important to recognize that the majority of wrist and long hand flexors and extensors originate proximal to the elbow at the medial and lateral epicondylar regions, and although this may suggest that they contribute to strength and stability in the region, their role in movement

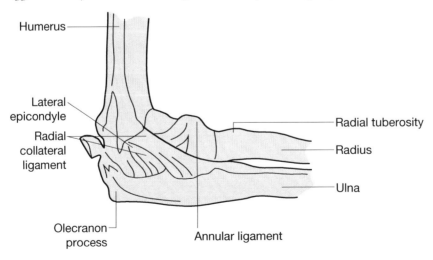

Figure 7.1   Skeletal and ligamentous anatomy: lateral view.

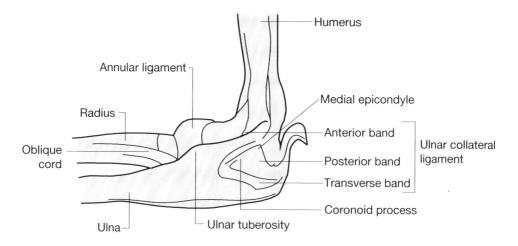

Figure 7.2 Skeletal and ligamentous anatomy: medial view.

of the elbow is minimal. However, Udall *et al.* (2009) identified that flexor digitorum superficialis, palmaris longus and flexor carpi ulnaris, originating at the medial epicondyle, do provide dynamic stability against valgus stress.

The prime mover for elbow flexion is the uniarticular brachialis muscle, running from the lower anterior humerus, underneath the biceps, to the coronoid process and tuberosity of the ulna. The larger and more superficial two-headed biceps brachii originates at the supraglenoid tubercle and the coracoid process and crosses the glenohumeral and all three elbow joints. It inserts distinctly at the radial tuberosity and also onto the ulnar side of the elbow via the bicipital aponeurosis, which blends into the common wrist flexor sheath. Its primary functions are elbow flexion and forearm supination, but it also contributes to glenohumeral flexion. The laterally positioned brachioradialis assists elbow flexion when the forearm is in a neutral position and also contributes to pronation and supination. It runs from the lateral humeral supracondylar ridge down via a long tendon, from mid-forearm, to the distal radius proximal to the styloid process. One further muscle, pronator teres, assists elbow flexion and is described with the other pronators, below. The three-headed triceps brachii is the principle elbow extensor. Although having its long head originate at the infraglenoid tubercle of the scapula, influencing glenohumeral extension and adduction, its two humeral attachments (lateral and medial heads) either side of the radial groove, provide the basis for elbow extension. Triceps inserts onto the upper surface of the olecranon process, with some fibres blending laterally with anconeus and the common wrist extensor sheath. Anconeus itself is a short, triangular muscle arising at the lateral epicondyle and inserting at the lateral olecranon and proximal posterior ulnar shaft. Anconeus weakly assists triceps in elbow extension and has a subtle stabilizing role against ulnar abduction during pronation movements. Forearm supination at the proximal and distal radioulnar joints is performed, as discussed, by biceps brachii and assisted by the supinator and brachioradialis muscles. Supinator is a short muscle, but with a rather broad origin, situated around the radial side of the elbow. It arises from the lateral epicondyle, the radial collateral and annular ligaments and the supinator crest of the ulna and inserts onto the proximal radius posteriorly, laterally and anteriorly. Supinator contributes to supination from any given position, unlike the biceps, which does not in full elbow extension. Pronation is performed by pronator teres, pronator quadratus and brachioradialis. As mentioned, the pronator teres is also a weak elbow flexor synergist. Pronator teres has two bands; its upper band originates alongside the main wrist flexor muscles at the medial epicondyle, and its lower band at the medial edge of the trochlear notch. It inserts midway down the radius on its lateral aspect. However, its partner, pronator quadratus, is the primary pronator. Pronator quadratus is a quadrilateral muscle situated just proximal to the distal radioulnar joint, transversely crossing the anterior surfaces of radius and ulna (Johnson, 2008; Tortora and Derrickson, 2008).

Practitioner Tip Box 7.2

Muscle synergy of the elbow

Flexion	Biceps brachii
	Brachialis
	Brachioradialis
	Pronator teres
Extension	Triceps brachii
	Anconeus
Pronation	Pronator teres
	Pronator quadratus
	Brachioradialis
Supination	Biceps brachii
	Supinator
	Brachioradialis

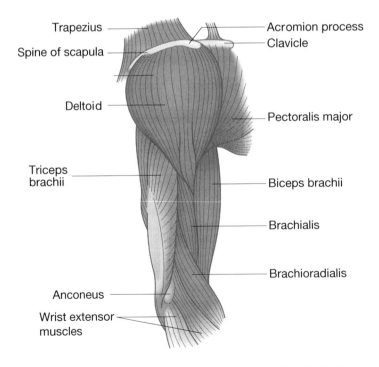

Figure 7.3 Muscular anatomy: lateral view (source: adapted from Sewell *et al.*, 2013).

Neural anatomy of the elbow

The elbow is served by the brachial plexus, which originates from the lower cervical and upper thoracic vertebral segments (C5–TI). Branching from the nerve roots of the brachial plexus arise the major peripheral nerves of the upper limb. The musculocutaneous, radial, median and ulnar nerves supply the elbow region. The musculocutaneous nerve originates at C5, C6 and C7, passes behind the clavicle and coracobrachialis muscle and continues to the elbow on the lateral aspect of biceps brachii. It continues superficially around the lateral aspect of the elbow to become the lateral cutaneous nerve of the forearm. It supplies biceps, brachialis and coracobrachialis (the BBC nerve!) and provides the sensory innervation for the anterolateral aspect of the forearm. The radial nerve originates from C5 to T1. It runs underneath the clavicle, but from the axilla continues around the posterior aspect of the humerus, along the radial (or spiral) groove from medial to lateral. It traverses between brachialis and brachioradialis and emerges over the anterolateral aspect of the cubital fossa. From the elbow, the radial nerve divides into a superficial branch and the posterior interosseous nerve. The radial nerve supplies triceps, anconeus, brachialis and extensor carpi radialis longus. The posterior interosseous branch supplies supinator and all other extensor muscles of the wrist and hand. The radial nerve is notable in that it provides all innervation for the extensors of the elbow and wrist, and sensory distribution to the posterior aspects of the upper arm, forearm, wrist and lateral dorsum of the hand. The median nerve also originates from C5–T1. From the axilla, it runs underneath biceps on the anterior upper arm, through the cubital fossa, and passes, underneath flexor digitorum superficialis, between the two heads of pronator teres. At the proximal anterior forearm a branch emerges to become the anterior interosseous nerve, as the median nerve continues distally to the hand. In the forearm, the median nerve supplies pronator teres, flexor carpi radialis and palmaris longus. It also supplies the intrinsic muscles of the hand. The anterior interosseous nerve supplies pronator quadratus and flexor digitorum profundus, plus flexor pollicis longus. The primary sensory distribution of the median nerve is on the lateral palm of the hand (thumb, index, middle and ring finger). The ulnar nerve originates from C8–T1. It runs from under the clavicle and through the axilla, to the anterior medial upper arm. It is exposed superficially at the groove for the ulnar nerve on the inferior aspect of the medial epicondyle, an area more specifically referred to as the cubital tunnel (and commonly known as the 'funny bone' area). From the elbow, it passes between the heads of flexor carpi ulnaris and flexor digitorum profundus and continues along the anterior medial forearm to the medial aspect of the hand. It provides nerve supply to the remaining wrist flexors and a number of intrinsic hand muscles. Its sensory distribution is the lateral aspect, anteriorly and posteriorly, of the wrist and hand (fourth and fifth fingers) (Johnson, 2008; Palastanga *et al.*, 2006).

Circulatory anatomy of the elbow

The main artery supplying the arm is the axillary artery, which is a continuation of the subclavian artery. The axillary artery becomes the brachial artery midway down the upper medial arm. It travels anteriorly over the medial epicondyle to run centrally through the cubital fossa and then divides below the elbow, on the proximal anterior forearm, to become the radial and ulnar arteries. The muscles involved with the elbow and the elbow joint itself are specifically served by a number of smaller arterial branches off the brachial artery. The brachial pulse, which is commonly used to assess blood pressure, may be palpated against the upper medial humerus or further down just medial to the biceps tendon.

The veins of the arm originate in the hand, with the dorsal venous arch and the anterior median vein, which then feed into the basilic (ulnar border) and cephalic (radial side) veins of the forearm. These are the relatively superficial but major veins and are joined by the deeper commitante veins in the upper medial arm. The cephalic vein links to the basilic vein just distal to the cubital fossa via the median cubital vein, but the two veins continue separately to become the main axillary vein at the infraclavicular fossa which empties into the subclavian vein and finally the superior vena cava.

In the arm, there are superficial lymphatic vessels which are closely associated with the superficial veins, and deeper lymphatic vessels which are closer to the major arteries. At the elbow are a collection of lymph nodes – the supratrochlear nodes, which lie over the medial aspect of the cubital fossa and just proximal to the medial epicondyle. The lymphatic vessels continue up through the axillary region and drain via the right lymphatic duct and the thoracic duct into the subclavian veins (Johnson, 2008; Palastanga *et al.*, 2006).

Functional anatomy of the elbow

The sports therapist must appreciate the functional relationships of the upper extremity. The upper extremity, when compared with the lower extremity, is generally less involved in closed-chain kinematic activity in normal daily functioning – humans stand, walk, run and jump on their legs. 'Load-bearing' rather than 'weight-bearing' is the preferred terminology for describing any closed-chain load-bearing function of the upper extremity. Additionally, the level of the load depends on the position of the involved limbs and what activity is being undertaken (Frostick *et al.*, 1999). The majority of functional sports movements involving the elbow also involve the hand, shoulder and trunk. The elbow is a centrally stabilized but mobile structure for all throwing, striking, catching, pulling, stroking, punching and reaching, and the majority of upper extremity weight-lifting patterns. Sports movements and loads may be variously low or high repetition, low or high intensity, fast or slow speed, partial or full range, open or closed chain, single or multi-planar, depending on the sport or training techniques undertaken. Muscular synergy provides the contractile pull for movement and incorporates the uniarticular, biarticular, agonist, antagonist and fixator muscles of the kinetic chain. The performance or execution of any sport or exercise movement is something that can always be improved, and relates to all intrinsic and extrinsic factors associated with the individual athlete. Any kinetic chain activity powerfully culminating through the upper extremity, such as with the tennis serve or shot, baseball pitch, golf swing, javelin throw or boxing punch, begins from the base of support (BoS) (usually at the feet) and transmits through the knees, hips, trunk, shoulder, elbow to the wrist and hand to create the complete and final release of power. In such activities, the elbow functions as a biomechanical link transmitting the required force, or kinetic energy, from the whole of the body to the ball, club, javelin or opponent. Not only is movement and force required to release power, it is also required to react and absorb energy, to retract the upper extremity when necessary and to reposition the arm in preparation for the next explosive movement. The well-documented four-stage throwing movement sequence (Glousman *et al.*, 1992) begins with the preparatory wind-up stage. The cocking stage opens up the main involved joints and muscles to create the optimum lever arm and positioning to facilitate the force and momentum for the acceleration (power) stage and planned release of energy. The acceleration stage is characterized by the initiation of elbow extension. Post-release, the deceleration and follow-through stages are controlled predominantly by antagonistic eccentric muscle activity (Hamill and Knutzen, 2009). The elbow is vulnerable to the excessive forces exerted on it during both explosive and repetitive movements. Explosive upper extremity movements do commonly lead to injury problems at the elbow: the overhead tennis serve or forearm smash, the baseball pitch or any other forceful throwing action tend to leave the athlete vulnerable to varying combinations of valgus (tensile), varus (compression) and posterior (shear) stresses as the elbow moves rapidly from flexion to full extension. With explosive power, specific mechanical stress is imparted onto the joint structures, as stated, and it is the articulatory surfaces, joint capsule, ligaments and tendons particularly that can suffer acute or chronic damage as result (Eygendaal *et al.*, 2007). As the elbow needs to function correctly and smoothly in harmony with the rest of the body, it is essential to analyse and train to perform sports skills carefully. Elbow injuries often occur because of faulty shoulder biomechanics proximally and poor wrist positioning distally. Postural dysfunctions, including core instability and limitations in range, glenohumeral instability, scapular dyskinesis, restricted accessory or physiological movements and muscular imbalances can easily contribute to unwanted compensatory stress at the elbow. Additionally, the athlete needs speed, agility and presence of mind to position their base of support, lower extremity and trunk to facilitate the ideal upper limb movements. Studies on athletes who perform powerful overhead movements have shown increases in external rotation of the shoulder, at the expense of internal rotation, a situation which can lead to the elbow being exposed to increased compensatory torsional demands as it is required to contribute to internal rotation of the upper limb during the later stages (acceleration, deceleration and follow-through) of the stroke or throw (Elliot, 2006). Recommendations for improving both internal rotation of the shoulder and forearm pronation have been made to offset valgus extension overload (Pluim and Safran, 2004). Additionally, preventative strengthening of the wrist flexors and extensors must be undertaken.

Assessment of the elbow region

The effective assessment of all patients, whether elite athlete, young amateur, keen enthusiast or novice exerciser requires a systematic approach, a solid theoretical underpinning, a keen focus and a practically developed confidence. Sports therapists must be confident in the practical performance of each of their selected assessment techniques. Confidence occurs when a technique is approached, delivered and interpreted correctly. Each of the assessment techniques selected should be recognized and reliable as clinical indicators and they must be reproducible (Palmer and Epler, 1998). Assessment is the basis for therapy and management, and may need to be performed in a variety of settings (clinic; changing room; gym; pitch-side) and for a variety of reasons (fitness screening; health monitoring; new injury; chronic injury; reassessment following treatment; and during stages of rehabilitation). Assessment takes place to evaluate function, fitness, performance, speed, power, strength and flexibility. Assessment takes place to evaluate problems, injuries, tissues, structures and pain. Patients are assessed each time they attend for sports therapy. Each time a patient is assessed, the information (findings) are recorded clearly, succinctly and correctly. The standardized approach to assessment incorporates the SOAP model: subjective, objective, assessment (summary and analysis of findings) and plan (of action) (Magee, 2008; Petty, 2011). The process for effective assessment is challenging; it must be clinically reasoned, and must aim to produce a working hypothesis of affected tissues and of the aetiology of the main complaint. Further, the sports therapist must produce a problem list and formulate a set of SMART goals (specific, measurable, achievable, realistic and timed).

Subjective assessment of the elbow

The standard approach for assessing a patient begins with a detailed subjective-based consultation. When exploring the patient's main complaint, the focus of subjective assessment should be on their perception of the cause, pain, weakness and sensory abnormalities. The subjective assessment should clarify the appropriateness of continuing onto objective assessment – or whether referral would be the appropriate course of action. Subjective assessment should also provide the therapist with a working clinical impression of the presenting problem and a plan for which practical tests need to be performed. Of particular relevance for the subjective assessment of the elbow is to recognize the role the elbow has in all upper limb movements and particularly in any speed-based, power-based or repetitive or skill-based activities, and the therapist must explore the sport and position that the athlete performs in (particularly: racquet sports; throwing sports; bowling sports; lifting sports; rowing; swimming). Additionally, contact sports (boxing; martial arts; rugby; football; hockey) bring a vulnerability to direct and indirect traumatic elbow injuries, as do sports where falls or other impacts are a feature (cycling; running; equestrian sports). Elbow injuries are often categorized in terms of chronic overuse type injuries (for example, lateral and medial tendinopathies; neural entrapment injuries; medial tension syndrome; posterolateral rotatory instability syndrome) and acute traumatic type injuries (contusions; bursitis; skeletal or joint injury; musculotendinous tear). It is particularly important to establish the patient's onset of symptoms – an immediate onset of pain following trauma to the elbow occurs with fracture, severe haemarthrosis, dislocation or subluxation (most common are those affecting the radial head, or less common, posterior dislocation of the ulna), muscle tear or ligamentous sprain. A more gradual, even insidious onset of pain is far more typical of an overuse, chronic type problem. Clinical impressions must build from the subjective assessment. The sports therapist should have appreciation of the common injury problems associated with any particular body region, sport and occupation (manual or sedentary work). Both Safran (1985) and Whiteside and Andrews (1989) performed reviews of athletic elbow injuries, and Brukner and Khan (2009) present common elbow injuries associated with sports.

Practitioner Tip Box 7.3

Typical aggravating and relieving factors of elbow injuries

Aggravating factors

Gripping – especially for lateral tendinopathies

Throwing – especially for medial tension syndrome and posterolateral instability syndrome

Repeated or full range movement – for all joint injuries

Stretching – especially for muscle tears and sprained ligaments

Contraction – especially for muscle tears and tendons

Compression – especially for bursitis and neural irritation

Continued activity – for most acute injuries

Relieving factors

Protection – for all acute and post-acute injuries

Rest – especially for all acute injuries

Ice – for all injuries where inflammation is a feature

Careful movements – especially for chronic injuries

Positions of ease – especially for all acute injuries

Heat – especially for chronic injuries

Practitioner Tip Box 7.4

Common sports-related elbow injuries

Sport	Injury
American football	Valgus and hyperextension stress; dislocation; olecranon bursitis
Archery	Extensor tendinopathy
Baseball	Valgus extension overload syndrome; medial traction, lateral compression and posterior shear
Basketball	Posterior forearm compartment syndrome
Golf	Flexor tendinopathy; extensor tendinopathy
Gymnastics	HR joint compression; posterior impingement; dislocation; olecranon bursitis
Tennis	Extensor tendinopathy; flexor tendinopathy
Javelin	Valgus extension overload syndrome; medial traction, lateral compression and posterior shear
Rock climbing	Elbow flexor tendinopathy
Shot-put	Posterior impingement
Volleyball	Valgus stress
Weight-training	UCL sprain; ulnar nerve irritation; muscle tears; tendinopathy

Objective assessment of the elbow

The objective assessment is the physical examination of the patient. It is based on orthopaedic principles using a set of recognized, repeatable and valid test procedures, the results of which are clearly documented on the patient's record form and are referred to in any follow-up sessions or communications. Although there is a routine approach to be followed for any objective assessment, there must be flexibility to the order of the routine, which will depend upon the patient's presenting signs and symptoms and level of function, and the therapist's rationale and ability to decide which particular tests are to be included or excluded. It is the therapist's responsibility to perform the objective assessment thoroughly and correctly, eliciting all the necessary clinical findings to enable a firm decision on the suitability of the patient to receive sports therapy intervention, or alternatively to make recommendations for referral for further investigation or intervention from another health care professional. The subjective and objective assessment will ideally facilitate a working diagnosis of the injury or problem, although this is not always clear, and the sports therapist must aim to incriminate specific tissues and reproduce the patient's symptoms. Objective test findings are said to be negative (non-incriminating) or positive (incriminating) relating to the tissues or structures that are being assessed. There will, however, be a degree of flexibility in terms of interpretation of test findings as few objective tests are absolutely conclusive, and additionally, it should be recognized that, in some instances, certain tests will provoke pain or discomfort but not in the target structures of the test. Hattam and Smeatham (2010) make useful recommendations to facilitate reliability in testing. These include: developing proficiency in test techniques (i.e. practise); making sure the patient is comfortable for each technique; recognizing what is 'normal' for each patient; being selective in tests performed (i.e. aiming for quality of test performance rather than performing an unnecessary quantity of tests); carefully modifying techniques depending on the condition presented and the tissues involved; interpreting test findings correctly; recognizing that some patients will present with co-morbidities that mimic the target condition. Practitioners must aim to achieve a high level of comparable intra-tester reliability and for efficiency in their practice.

During, and in light of, the subjective assessment, the efficient sports therapist will be thinking ahead to which tests are going to be important to investigate the patient's presenting problem. For a new patient attending with an injured elbow, the therapist should be considering the relationship of the elbow to the rest of the body. Which other regions could potentially be the cause of symptoms at the elbow? What structures and tissues are involved directly with the elbow? What movements will they need to test – including functional and sports-related movements? What special tests are indicated for this patient? Clinical reasoning is essential as the therapist assesses the gathered subjective information and the findings from their observations, movement testing, palpation and special tests. The clinical reasoning process in physical therapy settings, as presented by Jones *et al.* (2008), involves hypothesis generation, collaboration with the patient and metacognition in terms of reflective self-awareness.

Observation of the elbow

Observation begins as soon as the patient is in the view of the therapist – initial impressions can be made on the patient's stance, posture, body type, attitude and approach to movement, gait (including quality of arm swing) and general body language. Essentially, the patient is being observed throughout the whole of the assessment process, not least for their facial expressions and the way in which they remove clothing, but specifically how they respond to all tests. Once subjective assessment has been completed, observation of posture, skin and musculoskeletal contours can begin. Observations should be performed with the patient in both static and dynamic positions. Postural assessment, with regard to the elbow, should include the spine, particularly the cervical and thoracic regions and the pectoral girdle, left and right. These can each have significant influence on elbow positioning and function. Anterior, posterior and left and right lateral views should be taken. The bilateral resting positioning of the shoulder girdle (including scapulae), glenohumeral joints, elbow joints, forearms and hands must be assessed. This may give clues to such factors as previous injury, excessive muscular tension, soft tissue shortening, joint arthrosis or mechanical derangement. Decisions on whether any abnormalities are of a functional, structural or pathological nature should be left until further tests have been performed. As always, any asymmetry or abnormality must be noted. The therapist can ask the patient to assume the anatomical position to assess their carrying angle (normal valgus; excessive valgus; or varus), at the same time observing for any cubitus recurvatus (hyperextending elbow). When the elbow is extended, a posterior view should reveal a straight line between medial and lateral epicondyles and the olecranon process. When flexed, the same coordinates should form an isosceles triangle. During observation, the patient's skin and superficial tissues are inspected for any abnormal signs (discolouration – redness or ecchymosis; inter- or intramuscular haematoma; scarring; skin conditions – for example, excema; psoriasis; bursitis; swollen lymph nodes). Muscular contours can also be observed (general tone; symmetry/asymmetry; atrophy; imbalance between regions). Imbalances of muscle bulk can relate to either unilateral hypertrophy of the larger limb or the atrophy on the smaller limb that occurs following a prolonged period of immobilization or interruption of nerve supply. A number of neurological and muscular pathological conditions can also lead to muscle atrophy, and this may require consideration. Where muscle bulk imbalance is suspected, a girth measurement can be carefully taken by measuring a line from a structural landmark (for example, anterior elbow crease) and then encircling the limb with a tape measure, comparing left with right. Bony prominences and joint lines should be inspected for signs of deformity (dislocation; subluxation; fracture; malunion), asymmetry, thickening or localized intra-articular swelling (moderate to severe articular, capsular or ligamentous injury) or a more diffuse joint effusion (capsular irritation; osteochondroses), where again a local circular joint girth measurement can be taken.

Clearing tests for the elbow

When assessing problems affecting the elbow, it is important to establish whether the problem is due to a local injury or if structures above or below the region are involved. Hence, the cervical, glenohumeral, acromioclavicular, sternoclavicular, radioulnar and radiocarpal joints are routinely assessed. These elbow–related regions are either cleared (shown to be uninvolved) or implicated as being a contributor to elbow dysfunction or pain by way of assessing the main active movements with overpressure (if appropriate). These are assessed for symptom response and compared contralaterally. If symptomatic, then full examination is required.

The brachial plexus serves the arm, and the ulnar, median, radial and posterior interosseous nerves pass through the elbow region. Additionally, the musculocutaneous nerve, which although not passing through to the elbow, does supply the biceps and brachialis. Problems affecting the nerve roots or peripheral nerves of the brachial plexus (impingement at the cervical intervertebral foramen; adverse neural tension; irritation at mechanical interfaces; neuropraxia; neurotemesis) can lead to symptoms such as diffuse aching pain and motor and sensory deficits, which can present through the upper extremity as well as more locally at the elbow. Injured biarticular muscles crossing the shoulder or wrist as well as the elbow also need to be considered. Myofascial conditions may have somatic pain referral; specific muscles which could potentially affect the elbow region include scalenes, pectoralis minor, supraspinatus, infraspinatus and subscapularis. Radicular symptoms and those emanating from 'trigger points' are typically referred distally. Distal joint conditions can also be the cause of mechanically referred symptoms to a proximal joint (Loudon *et al.*, 2008; Magee, 2008; Petty, 2011).

Active movement assessment of the elbow

Active or physiological movement testing is performed to assess the patient's functional ability or apprehension to move affected joints. It is usually the first set of movements to be assessed and should be performed with caution where there is potential for aggravation of newly injured or repairing tissues. During any of the movements, a set of tissues and structures are potentially indicated as being problematic. Active movements should be briefly explained and demonstrated by the therapist and then performed by the patient without assistance from the therapist. They are undertaken initially to assess the patient's willingness to perform the movement, to observe for unwanted or compensatory movements occurring, appropriate movement at associated joints, and to clarify where in the range any onset of pain occurs, and whether the particular movement alters the intensity or quality of any pain or other symptoms. Active movements should inform the therapist of the possibility of muscle injury, nerve impairment or joint dysfunction, but they are rarely confirmative. At the elbow, full available range flexion, extension, pronation and supination are performed, with overpressure if there is low irritability. Pronation and supination are performed from a position of 90° elbow flexion and neutral or mid-pronation and supination. Overpressure is used to further stress the affected joint at the end of its range; it is only used where symptom response has been low to the active movement. If overpressure does not provoke an increase in symptoms, the movement may be considered normal. Movements of the affected limb should be compared against the contralateral limb and against published norms. Range and quality of movement should be assessed. Range may be measured by way of goniometry, inclinometry, tape measurement or, once the therapist is experienced and confident, simple visual estimation of degrees of movement ('eye-balling'). The patient should be asked to identify exactly where any pain or tightness is felt. Muscle injury, nerve impairment, joint dysfunction (impingement, mechanical derangement, capsule damage, ligamentous damage), pain and swelling can all limit joint range of movement (RoM). Therapists must also recognize the possibility of excessive movement (hypermobility and joint laxity). Standard active movements tend to be performed unilaterally in a single plane; however, the therapist may decide to ask the patient to repeat movements, to perform them bilaterally, at different speeds, observe sustained end-of-range positions or combine particular movements so as to ascertain which specific movements and combinations are most problematic (Loudon *et al.*, 2008; Magee, 2008; Petty, 2011).

Practitioner Tip Box 7.5

Active ranges of elbow movement

- Flexion 0–140°
- Extension 0–10°
- Pronation 80–90°
- Supination 80–90°

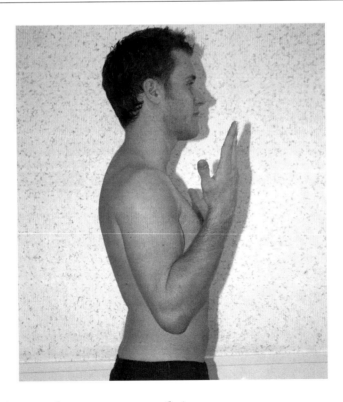

Photo 7.3   Active range of movement assessment: flexion.

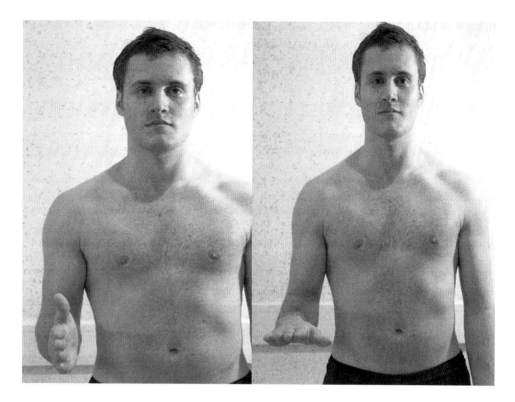

Photo 7.4   Active range of movement assessment: pronation.

Passive movement assessment of the elbow

Passive physiological movements are where the therapist performs the particular anatomical movement with the patient comfortably and appropriately positioned (i.e. fully relaxed), where they do not assist with the movement. Passive movements can be likened to palpating the joint's movement; as it is passively taken from its start to end position the therapist feels the quality and range of movement, which will normally be greater than the available active range. It is a common misconception that passive movements test simply non-contractile or inert structures, which is true: the joint's ligaments, joint capsule and intra-articular tissue are all potentially incriminated by passively taking the movement to its full available end of range, without active contraction; however, the presence of muscle spasm or extra-articular swelling, for example, are also likely to reduce the RoM. Injured contractile tissues may legitimately contribute to a symptom response during passive movement as it can be painful to stretch or compress an injured muscle–tendon unit.

The therapist should perform each movement (flexion; extension; pronation; supination) several times in an attempt to feel the quality and identify where any dysfunction is occurring, for example restriction, pain, tension, crepitus or referred pain. It is recommended to initially move the joint back and forth through its mid-range prior to proceeding to move towards the point of bind and eventual end-feel. The point of bind is the therapist's first sense of soft tissue tension occurring over the joint, which can provide clues to the presence of muscle spasm or straightforward muscle tightness. The end-feel, as presented by a range of authors, including Cyriax (1982), Kaltenborn (1999) and Magee (2008), is the 'feel at end-point' as the joint

---

Practitioner Tip Box 7.6

Normal end-feels of the elbow

- Flexion: soft tissue approximation
- Extension: bone to bone
- Pronation: tissue stretch
- Supination: tissue stretch

---

passively reaches its end of range. At the elbow, flexion has been described as having a normal soft tissue approximation end-feel (where the muscular and fatty flesh of the anterior forearm and forearm approximate, or come together). Extension has a relatively hard, bone-to-bone end-feel, (olecranon process to olecranon fossa). Pronation and supination have a soft tissue stretch end-feel. Any abnormal end-feel at the elbow will depend on what is causing it, for example, a mechanical derangement can cause a 'springy block', arthritic degeneration can cause a hard bone-to-bone sensation with possible crepitus, muscular spasm can lead to a tight end-feel, and a swollen joint will present with a soft but tight end-feel. These abnormal end-feels are likely to present with an associated reduction in range and varying degrees of pain. An 'empty' end-feel can be associated with joint laxity, reduced muscle tone or atrophy, or low body fat. The empty end-feel is likely to present as hypermobile, unless pain and a resultant patient apprehension to the movement is a factor (Gross *et al.*, 2009). There are natural or normal constraints to all physiological movements and these directly relate to the state and structure of the joint and associated muscle and other soft tissues. One further consideration to restricted joint movement is that of the capsular pattern, or pattern of limitation, first presented by Cyriax (1982) and expanded by others. Essentially, this is where the joint capsule is primarily involved in the presenting condition and most commonly can result in a capsular contraction leading to a total joint reaction. This can follow such mechanical insults as acute or chronic muscle spasm or arthritic degeneration. Hayes *et al.* (1994) described the capsular pattern as '*a joint specific pattern of restriction that indicates involvement of the entire joint capsule*'. Magee (2008) summarizes the capsular patterns associated with each moving joint. For the humeroulnar and radiohumeral joints of the elbow, the capsular pattern is considered to be restriction more in flexion than extension. Proximal radioulnar joint end-range supination and pronation are considered to be equally limited in the capsular pattern. As with active movements, range may be measured by goniometry or other methods, and movements should be compared contralaterally and against published norms. Passive movements must be performed slowly with correct positioning and handling, and awareness of the potential for symptom response.

Accessory movement assessment of the elbow

Accessory, or joint play, movements are the subtle additional specific joint movements that occur (or should occur) during any gross active or passive physiological movements. Generally classified as being a rolling, spinning or gliding of one bone on another, accessory movements allow for normal arthrokinematics. Accessory movements cannot be actively performed in isolation, but the therapist is able to passively test their range and quality, essentially attempting to identify the presence of normal accessory motion, restriction (stiffness or resistance through range), pain or provocation of muscle spasm or any other symptom response. Testing of

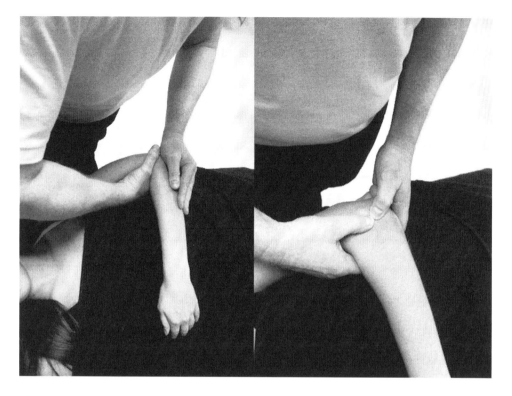

Photo 7.5 Accessory movement assessment: longitudinal caudad glide to ulna and PA glide to radial head.

accessory movements requires precise handling and communication. Petty (2011) reminds us that with any particular accessory movement of any one of the elbow joints, there is likely to be concomitant affectation at one or both of the other joints. At the humeroulnar joint, the main accessory movements to test are: longitudinal caudad glide of the ulna; longitudinal cephalad compression of the ulna; and lateral and medial glides of the ulna. At the radiohumeral joint: longitudinal caudad glide of the radius; and longitudinal cephalad compression of the radius. At the proximal radioulnar joint: anteroposterior and posteroanterior glides to the radial head (Hengeveld and Banks, 2005; Sexton, 2006).

Resisted movement assessment of the elbow

Resistance tests are performed to assess the patient's ability to generate force against the therapist's resistance, identify any pain or other symptom response and to gauge the strength or weakness of the working muscles. Isometric resistance tests help to identify the possibility of muscle or tendon injury or nerve impairment and are less likely to incriminate inert joint structures as the involved joint is not moving during the test. The therapist instructs the patient and offers specific resistance to their isometric contractile force, initially in a resting or mid-range position. Sexton (2006) recommends the instruction to the patient to be *'Don't let me move you'*, thus enabling a progressive incremental resistance to be administered if the patient can tolerate it to test full strength. For the elbow, flexion, extension, pronation and supination are performed, which assesses the muscle synergy associated with each movement. Therapists

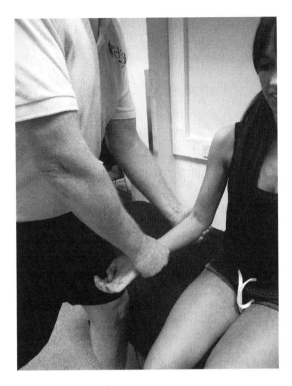

Photo 7.6   Resisted range of movement assessment: flexion and extension.

may choose to localize positioning to assess specific muscles, and isotonic resistance may also be used to further evaluate. Additional resistance tests are performed as special tests relating to particular injuries, such as extensor tendinopathy. The therapist should be able to recognize when muscle injury should be suspected by the positive finding of pain on contraction; however, a complete rupture of muscle may not be painful. Weakness is likely to be associated with muscle injury (especially with more severe injury) and nerve involvement, which in turn will be proximal to the affected region. While a number of authors (Cyriax, 1982; Magee, 2008; Medical Research Council, 1976) have presented grading systems of muscle strength, Gross *et al.* (2009) discuss the importance of the pain–strength relationship, and explain that this provides the clinician with clear insight into which structures are responsible for the problem.

Muscle length tests of the elbow

Muscle length tests are myofascial lengthening movements performed either passively or actively with an aim to specifically assess for local tightness or symptom response. They are different to the other standard active or passive RoM tests. Muscle length tests offer additional information regarding myofascial movement, tension and imbalances left to right (comparing contralateral agonists) and the therapist can also assess for antagonist muscle imbalance. Test movements aim to factor in associated attachment sites; and where the targeted muscle(s) are biarticular, will incorporate multiple joint movements. Excessive myofascial tension identified during a length test may result for a number of reasons (such as: tear; spasm; joint injury or arthritic degeneration; muscle soreness) and will influence the range and direction of movement of its joint(s) in certain positions; it may also present adverse postural and biomechanical influence. Where muscles are excessively lengthened there is likely to be dynamic instability, insufficient length–tension relationships and functional weakness. By assessing for muscle length, the sports therapist is able to understand more about the functional relationships of structures and tissues involved in the athlete's presenting complaint. Measurements may be ascertained by use of a goniometer or by careful observation. Biceps brachii may be assessed by first extending the glenohumeral joint and then extending the elbow. The triceps can be assessed by flexing the elbow in glenohumeral flexion. Assessment of muscle length is also used in the special tests for flexor and extensor tendinopathy – which involves the wrist muscles, but manifests at the elbow.

Ligament stress tests of the elbow

Several variations of standard ligament stress or instability tests are presented in the literature (Magee, 2008; Morrey and An, 1983). Valgus instability and injury to the UCL is tested with an abduction force applied to the medial elbow. This should be performed in slight elbow flexion and full supination; additionally, Morrey and An (1983) recommend full lateral rotation of the humerus. Varus instability of the LUCL and RCL is assessed, again in slight flexion, with an adduction force. Morrey and An (1983) advocate full medial rotation of the humerus for testing the lateral ligament complex. Positive findings for both tests include slight or gross gapping or laxity or loss of normal ligamentous tension and pain. Posterolateral rotatory instability (PLRI) is a not uncommon pattern of instability of the elbow, a complication associated with post-reduction dislocation. The condition most commonly involves rotational displacement of the ulna from the trochlea alongside radial displacement from the capitulum. The proximal radioulnar joint generally remains intact, with the classic posterior dislocation mechanism of axial (cephalad) compression, valgus stress and supination of the forearm, hence this injury tends to mainly involve the LUCL, although the RCL may also be involved (Aviles *et al.*, 2009; Magee, 2008). PLRI can be assessed with the PLRI stress test, which has the patient supine, shoulder flexed and elbow flexed to approximately 40°. The therapist delivers axial compression through the elbow via the forearm with their upper hand in combination with a valgus stress applied to the elbow and observes for laxity, apprehension or other symptom response. Variants of this test do exist: Magee (2008) and Hattam and Smeatham (2010) present

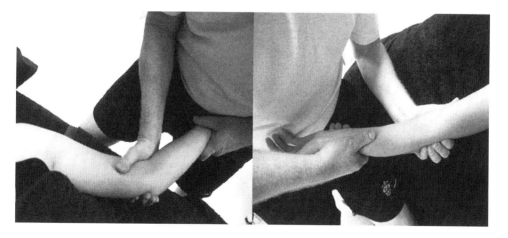

Photo 7.7   Valgus and varus stress tests.

the PLRI apprehension test, which involves a similar set-up to the PLRI stress test, but where the therapist performs movement from 20° to 70° of elbow flexion while under axial compression and valgus stress so as to assess for the specific instability. However, these authors suggest that full-range assessment is only likely under anaesthetic. The PRLI drawer test has the patient supine or seated, with shoulder in neutral and elbow flexed to 90° with the forearm in neutral pronation-supination. The therapist stabilizes the humerus with their upper hand while performing an inferior drawer of the elbow with their other hand. The therapist observes for excessive displacement, apprehension or pain. With all ligamentous and joint stress tests, the therapist must compare left and right and should attempt to palpate the affected joint line and specific ligaments at the same time as performing each stress test. The tests are not performed in isolation, as other movement tests and careful palpation are also essential.

Extensor tendinopathy tests

The classic test for lateral epicondyle (wrist extensor) tendinopathy (tennis elbow) involves resisted isometric contraction of the wrist extensors with the elbow fully extended, forearm pronated and wrist extended (Hattam and Smeatham, 2010; Konin *et al.*, 2006). A positive test result is pain reproduction over the common extensor origin at the lateral epicondyle. Variations of this test include the Cozen's test, which incorporates a closed fist, forearm pronation, radial deviation and resisted wrist extension. Mill's test is a passive muscle lengthening test which also assesses the extensor musculo-tendinous unit. The start position is 45° shoulder abduction, 90° elbow flexion, forearm pronation and wrist flexion. The therapist then further abducts the shoulder (to around 70°), maintains pronation and wrist flexion, and then slowly extends the elbow, observing for when pain occurs (Hattam and Smeatham, 2010). Extensor carpi radialis brevis, the most commonly affected muscle–tendon unit in extensor tendinopathy, is specifically tested by resisting third finger extension. All resistance and lengthening tests must be combined with careful palpation of tendinous insertions and muscle bellies.

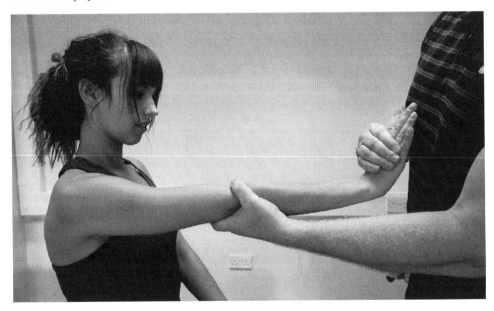

Photo 7.8   Isometric resistance test (extensor tendinopathy test).

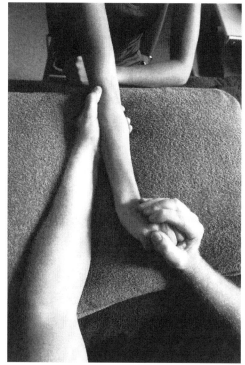

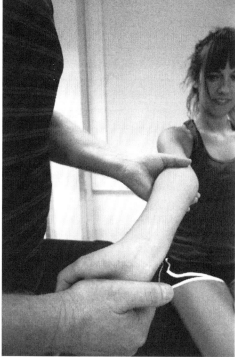

Photo 7.9   Cozen's test.

Photo 7.10   Passive flexor muscle length test (flexor tendinopathy test).

Flexor tendinopathy tests

Medial epicondyle (wrist flexor) tendinopathy (golfer's elbow) is assessed with resistance applied to wrist flexion, with the elbow in full extension and the forearm in pronation. Pain over the medial epicondyle implicates the common flexor origin. Hattam and Smeatham (2010) and Konin *et al.* (2006) also present the passive flexor muscle lengthening test, where the elbow is extended, forearm supinated, hand made into a fist and the wrist moved into extension. The anterior forearm region and the common wrist flexor origins must all be fully palpated.

Upper limb neurodynamic tests

There are four standard upper limb neurodynamic tests (ULNT). These tests are used to identify any adverse limitations in neural tissue length, or for any apparent irritation at mechanical interfaces (assessing both nerve roots and main peripheral nerves). The ulnar, median and radial nerves may be assessed, as adverse neural tension or mechanical irritation may be the cause of local symptoms at the elbow region. Positive signs from these tests are present when neurological symptoms occur, or are reproduced, along the course of the neural tissue. ULNTs should be performed whenever there is suggestion in the patient's history or other objective test findings that adverse neural tension could be a factor.

Ulnar nerve tests

Tinel's 'tap' or percussion test for the elbow involves tapping on the superficially presented ulnar nerve as it passes through the elbow region in a groove on the posterior underside of the medial epicondyle. This test is indicated to assess the possibility of compression of the ulnar nerve at the elbow, which leads to 'cubital tunnel syndrome'. Once palpated and identified, the therapist taps the nerve several times with their index finger or reflex hammer. A positive test reproduces the symptoms of paraesthesia in the ulnar nerve distribution (along the ulnar aspect of forearm and into fourth and fifth fingers). The other main symptoms tend to show as medial elbow pain and weak grip (Antuna and Barco Laakso, 2010). An additional test for cubital tunnel syndrome is the elbow flexion test, where sustained elbow flexion with forearm supination, held for around one minute, positively reproduces symptoms (Hattam and Smeatham, 2010).

Median nerve tests

Several tests have been published to assess for dysfunction of the median nerve as it passes through the elbow anteriorly to the distal extremity (Hattam and Smeatham, 2010; Konin *et al.*, 2006; Magee, 2008). The anterior interosseous nerve is a branch of the median nerve which, as it exits the elbow, runs between the two heads of the pronator teres, and when subjected to compression from muscle tension, fascial thickening, swelling or trauma can result in weakening of associated muscles (pronator quadratus, flexor pollicis longus and flexor digitorum profundus). The well-recognized 'pinch grip' test involves the patient performing an active precision grip between the thumb and index finger tips. A positive test finding is where the patient cannot approximate the

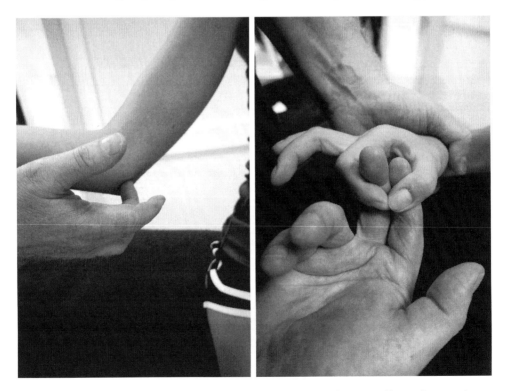

Photo 7.11   Tinel's tap test (for ulnar nerve).   *Photo 7.12*   Pinch grip test (for median nerve).

thumb and finger tips (it is a positive test even if the patient can only approximate their finger pads) (Hattam and Smeatham, 2010). The median nerve can also be compressed directly and proximal to its interosseous division, leading to a condition known as 'pronator syndrome'. Motor weakness is likely to be evident in the muscles of the median nerve distribution (except notably the pronator teres), this is in conjunction with sensory abnormality. The pronator syndrome test has the elbow flexed to 90° and the therapist offers resistance to pronation as elbow extension is performed (Petty, 2011). The pronator compression test involves up to ten seconds of local thumb pressure to the median nerve where it passes between the pronator heads. Positive test findings for these two tests will be reproduction of patient symptoms.

Radial nerve tests

The radial nerve runs posteriorly down the humerus, and from the radial groove travels over the lateral aspect of the elbow to supply the supinator and extensor muscles of the wrist and hand. Proximal to the elbow and anterior to the lateral epicondyle, the posterior interosseous nerve branches off to pass between the two heads of the supinator muscle. At this section the nerve has vulnerability to a condition known as 'radial tunnel syndrome', where local compression, adverse neural tension or cervical involvement can lead to motor and sensory deficits and pain which may be easily confused with lateral epicondylar tendinopathy (Antuna and Barco Laakso, 2010; Magee, 2008). To test for this, the therapist should apply up to ten seconds of localized thumb pressure to the nerve (approximately 3 cm distal to the lateral epicondyle). A positive test will show tenderness and a reproduction of symptoms.

Dermatome testing of the elbow

Dermatomes are the areas of skin innervated by a single spinal segment, and are 'mapped' on the body accordingly. Dermatomes relating to the elbow are assessed by gauging the patient's response to light or sharp touch. The patient is seated, preferably with eyes closed, as the therapist traces circumferentially and systematically around the upper arm, elbow and forearm. The method must compare left with right and allow opportunity for the patient to report any abnormal sensation.

Practitioner Tip Box 7.7

Dermatomes of the Elbow

- C5 relates to the lateral anterior and posterior upper arm and elbow
- C6 relates to the lateral anterior and posterior elbow, forearm and hand
- C7 relates to the midline of the anterior and posterior forearm
- C8 relates to the medial anterior and posterior forearm and hand
- T1 relates to the medial aspect of the elbow

Myotome testing of the elbow

Myotomes are the groups of muscles innervated by a specific spinal nerve root. Any presenting weakness (motor loss) of the elbow muscles must be explored by way of resisted movement assessment, held for at least five seconds (Magee, 2008). Knowledge of myotomes provides the information to recognize the possibility of neural compromise at a segmental level, where all the muscles supplied by an affected nerve root will be affected. The therapist should bear in mind that the assessment picture alters with a lesion involving a peripheral nerve, where only the muscles innervated by that nerve will be affected. The sports therapist should be able to differentiate between weakness due to motor loss or that due to muscle injury. With prolonged motor loss, muscular atrophy will be observed (Petty, 2011).

Reflex tests of the elbow

Reflex tests provide further information regarding the functional innervation of the elbow region. Deep tendon, or spinal, reflexes assess the integrity of the sensory (muscle spindles and afferent fibres) and motor (efferent) nerve pathways involved in the reflex arc, essentially checking the response of a muscle to being stretched (a stretch reflex). The patient must be relaxed and the muscle placed in a position of slight stretch. The tendon is lightly tapped five or six times. By tapping a number of times, the practitioner may observe an increase or reduction in reflex activity, which can indicate the possibility of upper motor neuron lesion (increased: UMNL) or signs of nerve root involvement, or lower motor neuron lesion (reduced: LMNL). A normal response is an observable or palpable contraction of the tested muscle and slight joint movement. Abnormal reflexes include clonus (very brisk, spasmodic) or exaggerated responses, possibly indicative of UMNL, or diminished or absent responses, which are the more likely presentations in patients attending a sports therapy clinic, indicative of LMNL. Reflexes are not always easy to elicit and can produce false positives. Reflexes are always tested bilaterally, and on their own are not conclusive (Magee 2008).

Practitioner Tip Box 7.8

Myotomes of the elbow

- C6 relates to elbow flexion
- C7 relates to elbow extension

Practitioner Tip Box 7.9

Reflexes of the elbow

- C5–6 Biceps brachii
- C5–6 Brachioradialis
- C7–8 Triceps brachii

Functional tests of the elbow

Functional tests for the elbow may simply involve basic activities of daily living (ADL), such as assessing the patient's ability to bring hand to mouth, to bear weight against a wall with arms outstretched, to open or close a door or lift a chair. These simple tests may also be graded according to repetitions achieved or resistance incorporated (Palmer and Epler, 1998). In essence, the therapist will be interested in observing the kinds of movements that the patient needs to be able to perform. If the patient has greater functional capacity, specific work, exercise or sports-related movement patterns will be assessed. These tests allow for general observation of combined elbow movements and a whole-body working relationship, as well as specific technique inspection, potentially incorporating mobility, coordination, proprioception, strength and power. Such tests may include everything from a standard push-up or lift to a plyometric medicine ball throw or golf swing, depending on the patient's ability and confidence in using the affected region. As well as assessing current ability, functional tests provide additional clues to the causes of injury problems, areas of weakness and errors in usual movement patterns.

Palpation of the elbow

Palpation is an essential assessment skill that requires sensitivity, strong anatomical knowledge, careful positioning of the patient, good communication between therapist and patient and a systematic approach. Palpatory findings can be produced by using palm of hand (for general identification of structures), dorsum of hand (for surface temperature assessment), finger and thumb pads and tips (for specific tissue exploration). Clearly, palpation requires an awareness of what could be considered as normal for the patient, and with this in mind the therapist must be mindful of the patient's age, body type, fitness, medical condition, injury history, limb dominance, occupation and sports that they are involved in. Additionally, the therapist should be sensitive to the patient's presenting condition and likelihood of causing discomfort or even aggravation during palpatory assessment. The therapist must compare palpatory findings contralaterally. Palpation is a part of all the stages of practical examination, as whenever there is contact there is palpation. Palpation may be used initially to gauge the possibility or extent of sensitivity, tenderness or pain. It can offer initial impressions of bony contours and superficial soft tissue density, over or under activity of autonomic nervous system (excess or reduced sweat gland activity), circulatory integrity and inflammation (areas of heat or cold) and oedema. Superficial muscular contours may also be assessed in the early part of the objective assessment for signs of abnormality. More comprehensive palpation of deeper and localized problem areas is left until the therapist has performed all indicated movement and special tests, as deep palpation in the early part of the objective assessment could aggravate irritable tissues and hence cloud the findings of any subsequent tests. The therapist may choose to perform initial palpation of deeper tissues during the passive and accessory movement assessment. Palpation of soft tissues may reveal such presentations as muscle spasm, atrophy, hypersensitivity, fibrous adhesions and scar tissue. The completion of palpatory assessment is usually best left until all other tests have been performed, by which time the therapist should have a much clearer clinical impression. All pertinent palpatory findings must be recorded, and it is recommended to identify and mark on the body diagrams on the assessment form all areas of dysfunction. The therapist will recognize that palpatory assessment continues during delivery of any subsequent soft tissue or manual therapy – extensive contact occurs during treatment and tissues change, to some degree, during treatment (Biel, 2005; Magee, 2008; Petty, 2011; Shultz *et al.*, 2000).

Palpatory assessment of the elbow incorporates assessment of musculoskeletal integrity and aims to identify any abnormality or unwarranted discomfort. It must also include assessment of the cervical, shoulder, wrist and hand when indicated. A comprehensive palpatory assessment of the elbow will include: the skin and subcutaneous fascial tissue; all accessible bony structures and joint lines; ligament attachments and structure (UCL; LUCL; RCL; AL); muscle bellies and their tendon attachments (biceps; brachialis; brachioradialis; pronator teres; triceps; anconeus; supinator; wrist flexors; wrist extensors); and superficial vascular, lymphatic and neural structures. Palpation of the elbow should begin with assessment of the unaffected limb, for comparison. When palpating the affected limb, the patient may be seated and the arm supported by the therapist. Palpation should commence superficially before probing the deeper tissues, and should also begin with structures above and below the affected locality of symptoms. It is important to recognize that palpation can be performed in different joint positions, and also in combination with active, passive and resisted movement, which can allow for different tissues and structures to become more prominent and readily accessible. Soft tissue lesions will be localized, and only identifiable with care and specificity.

Reassessment and fitness test approaches for the elbow

During the course of sports therapy treatment and rehabilitation, periodic reassessment of the region is required to gauge the response of the affected tissues to such interventions, to enable ongoing and appropriate progressions and, in the final stages of rehabilitation, to return to full training and eventually full normal activity and competition. Decisions on when to make rehabilitation progressions or to recommend return to training should be made on the basis of improved functional ability and clear improved responses to clinical and fitness-related tests. These decisions will additionally be guided by the type of injury or problem, the tissues involved, the severity and stage of healing. In simple terms, as patients return for each of their follow-up treatment or exercise sessions, the therapist will run through the key physical movements and special tests that relate to the presenting problem. Such test results can easily be compared to previous test findings and therapy provided accordingly. Numerous authors present guidelines on functional injury progression and return to play guidelines (Anderson *et al.*, 2009; Beam, 2002; Brukner and Khan, 2009; Comfort and Abrahamson, 2010; Prentice, 2011) and most advocate a four-stage model, which relates directly to the stages of healing, the signs, symptoms and functional capacity presented. Obviously, there are times when rehabilitation does not go to plan or where complications are present and where slow progress, no progress or even worsening will be evident. In such cases, the therapist must be able to make appropriate decisions and recommendations – this may involve adaptation of current plans or referral for a second opinion, for further medical tests or for other interventions. It is important to avoid the potential for re-injury relating to poor management of the original injury.

Injuries of the elbow region

Although less prevalent than knee, ankle and shoulder injuries, acute and chronic elbow injuries are common in athletes and the general population (Kaminski *et al.*, 2000). Typical mechanisms for acute injuries include simple overstretch or overload and impact from forceful contact or collision, which in turn may be direct or indirect, as in a 'FOOSH' (fall onto an outstretched hand), leading to all manner of fractures, dislocations or soft tissue damage. Chronic or overuse injury problems may present as a sequelae from acute injury, as a result of poor sports preparation (equipment; fitness for activity; training; technique), inherent biomechanics, related to underlying pathology (osteoarthritis; hypermobility) or, in the case of adolescents, musculoskeletal immaturity. The following section presents an overview of some of the most common conditions affecting the elbow: overuse injuries including extensor and flexor tendinopathy; ligamentous and joint injuries; dislocations; muscular injuries; adolescent osteochondroses; nerve injuries; and olecranon bursitis.

Extensor and flexor tendinopathies

Tendinopathies of the elbow have been variously described in published literature as elbow tendonitis, lateral and medial epicondylitis and epicondylalgia, extensor tendinopathy, flexor-pronator tendinopathy, insertional tendinopathy, lateral and medial elbow tendinosis, and tennis and golfer's elbow. Tendonitis and epicondylitis are terms which indicate inflammation of the tendon insertion, and where inflammation is a normal response to acute injury, which when resolving normally, gives way to the proliferation phase within a few days. These terms are, however, frequently and incorrectly used to describe the common chronic condition of tendinosis. Ochiai and Nirschl (2005) present elbow tendinosis as a tendon overuse injury where poor resolution (failure of healing) is the characteristic feature. Brukner and Khan (2009) explain that tendinosis presents with collagen disarray and neovascularization (chronic angiogenesis); there is only a minimal inflammatory response (Rees *et al.*, 2013). The abnormal tissue is locally painful due to the additional presence of increased numbers of nociceptive nerve fibres. Renstrom and Hach (2005) identify that the lateral aspect of the elbow is one of the four most common sites for insertional tendinopathy and, in fact, one of the most common clinical problems in sports medicine. Furthermore, Anderson *et al.* (2009) state that extensor tendinopathy is the most common overuse injury affecting the elbow; Prentice (2011) summarizes that the lateral elbow is particularly vulnerable to intrinsic mechanical trauma from throwing and striking activities. Extensor tendinopathy is a prevalent tennis injury, hence the term 'tennis elbow', but is also common in other sports involving repetitive or forceful upper extremity movements (squash; baseball; golf; javelin) and in physically demanding occupations where wrist and elbow actions are routinely involved. In racquet sports, this condition most commonly relates to poor positioning and backhand technique with wrist overextension (Prentice, 2011), but also the usual additional intrinsic and extrinsic factors including sudden increases in the duration or frequency of play, racquet weight, handle size, string tension and poor fitness for the sport or activity. The condition is more common in middle-aged patients and may also develop from one single trauma, such as a mis-hit shot or a hard direct blow to the epicondylar region (Corrigan and Maitland, 2004). Imbalances between the forearm musculature, such as where extensor weakness and inflexibility is an underlying biomechanical feature, can be a contributory factor. There have also been a number of studies presenting the relationship of extensor tendinopathy, or more correctly lateral epicondylalgia (pain at the lateral epicondyle region), to dysfunction of the cervical (Cleland *et al.*, 2004), shoulder (Abbot, 2001) and wrist regions (Struijs *et al.*, 2003). A number of authors have discussed the role of the CNS in the development of lateral epicondylalgia, the aetiology of which may combine local tissue pathology with peripheral and central neural adaptations resulting in mechanical hyperalgesia and associated motor control deficits (Coombes *et al.*, 2009; Scott *et al.*, 2013).

True extensor tendinopathy involves some form of lesioning of the common extensor tendon, with the tendon of extensor carpi radialis brevis being most frequently affected, although extensor carpi radialis longus and extensor digitorum can also be involved. The lesion may result primarily from pathological tendinosis, as described above, or from the development of a critical zone of vascular compromise in extensor carpi radialis brevis relating to shearing forces created during excessive or forceful wrist extension and to compression from the radial head during forearm pronation. The patient with extensor tendinopathy will present with either an acute onset following a single trauma or bout of exertion, or with the more common gradual or insidious onset associated with overuse. The acute onset is likely to show some clear signs of inflammation and have macroscopic damage. The generic process for degenerative tendinopathy follows a progressive pattern as summarized in the three-stage tendinopathy continuum (Cook and Purdam, 2009). This incorporates an initial acute reactive tendinopathy, typically with homogeneous swelling and mild pain during or after activity. If the reactive phase is poorly managed, a mid-stage tendon disrepair process may ensue, which may progress to a chronic degenerative tendinopathy. Whether acute or chronic, the patient will complain of pain around the lateral epicondyle, especially at the tenoperiosteal junction, which is likely to extend along the tendon towards the musculotendinous junction and will be confirmed and exacerbated by palpation, stretching and resisted activities. Indeed, in established conditions it is common for patients to complain of distinct pain during the most basic of functional activities, such as picking up a cup or turning a door handle. The acute (reactive) presentation is likely to be locally swollen, whereas the chronic tendinosis is likely to show focal thickening and crepitus on movement. Whether acute or chronic, objective physical tests are likely to show similar findings. Active and passive movement tests typically produce discomfort or pain at the extremes of range. As pain increases during stretching movements, Mill's test is likely to be positive. Resisted movements will show pain and associated strength reductions, hence the resisted extensor tendinopathy test and Cozen's test are also likely to be positive. Accessory movements of the elbow may show pain, restriction or laxity, indicative of their contribution to the condition. Functional tests can be used to gauge which additional, combined or loaded movements produce a symptom response. The differential diagnosis to consider around the lateral epicondylar region includes referred pain from the cervical or thoracic spine or shoulder region, posterior interosseous nerve compression, lateral collateral ligamentous injury and, in younger athletes, osteochondritis dissicans.

Management for extensor tendinopathy follows the standard progressive approach to rehabilitation, which relates directly to presenting symptoms, functional capacity and stage of healing. Although most authors indicate a return to full activity is likely within 4–6 weeks from the onset of a true extensor tendinopathy injury, chronic degenerative overuse injuries notoriously take longer to fully repair conservatively, and there is always potential for aggravation with overenthusiastic or inappropriate activity. During all stages of rehabilitation, it is important to help the athlete maintain fitness without aggravating the condition. Acute stage management is aimed at ameliorating symptoms and protecting the injury from further damage. Therefore, conservative acute stage management should include optimal loading regimes (i.e. short of bringing on symptoms) and possibly ice applications for pain relief. If the patient has to continue with activities involving the arm, protection of the common extensor origin in the form of a counterforce brace can be applied just distal to the origin (Ochiai and Nirschl, 2005; Regan *et al.*, 2010). Taping techniques to offload the common extensor origin may offer similar protection. Additional pain relief may be provided by interferential application (typically with a beat frequency sweep of 90–120 Hz). As acute symptoms fade, the next stage of management incorporates early strength restoration, initially focusing on wrist flexion and extension, radial and ulnar deviation and grip strength (typically with a period of isometrics before progressing to isotonics). Soft tissue therapy techniques can be useful (including transverse frictions, instrument-assisted techniques, myofascial release and neuromuscular therapy). Where the presenting condition is a chronic tendinosis, five minutes of transverse friction massage applied to the affected tendon for up to five treatments over a period of ten days has been recommended

(Prentice, 2004), alongside graded and specifically assessed joint mobilization therapy to restricted accessory movements. Later-stage rehabilitation may involve continued soft tissue and mobilization therapy, but the emphasis needs to be on active interventions, including progressive flexibility and muscular strength and endurance (incorporating slow and controlled eccentric loading of wrist extensors) (Ochiai and Nirschl, 2005), as well as closed-chain and proprioceptive work. The return-to-sport stage typically includes progression to full function involving plyometrics, agility and sports skills practice. Full return to activity should be approached with care and should incorporate any necessary changes to technique and equipment.

Regan *et al.* (2010) emphasize the efficacy of a conservative approach in conjunction with physical therapy, where patient education and avoidance of aggravating activities are paramount. With careful conservative management, symptoms are likely to have resolved in 80 per cent of cases within six months. For patients resistant to standard conservative approaches and where ongoing localized pain is evident, there is the option for corticosteroid or combined anaesthetic injection. However, evidence to support such intervention is limited, and at best it is likely to offer only short-term pain relief (Regan *et al.*, 2010). Risks such as injecting directly into the tendon (must be avoided), subcutaneous atrophy and tendon weakening are associated with injection therapy (MacAuley, 2007). Bruggeman *et al.* (2003) recommend injection under the tendon to avoid subcutaneous atrophy. More recent developments in conservative tendinopathy management include the use of nitric oxide donor therapy (glyceryl trinitrate [GTN] patches), extracorporeal shock wave therapy (ESWT) and botox injections. However, these techniques are not widely available and evidence to support their use is limited, with some studies showing encouraging results and others showing no more effectiveness than placebo. Other conventional interventions such as non-steroidal anti-inflammatory drugs (NSAIDs) and dry needling have limited evidence to support their use (Regan *et al.*, 2010). Surgery may be offered for patients who fail to respond to conservative management and who experience disabling symptoms for over a year. Patients who experience extreme symptoms even with correct management and adherence to advice may be indicated for earlier surgery. Objectives of surgery may include arthroscopic excision of any aberrant tissue (scar tissue; calcific deposits; bony spurs) or debridement and repair (open release and resection) of the extensor origin or fasciotomy. Scott *et al.* (2013) explain, however, how evidence is limited regarding consistent successful operative outcomes for epicondylalgia.

Medial or flexor tendinopathy relates to the common flexor origin at the medial epicondyle and, although less common than extensor tendinopathy, occurs in sports and activities involving single forceful or repeated wrist flexions or excessive valgus stress. Where extreme or repetitive valgus stress is a factor, the diagnosis may relate less to the tendons and more to the involved joint (synovitis; impingement; fragmentation) or UCL injury and resultant medial instability. Another differential diagnosis is degenerative change to the posterior medial aspect of the olecranon (Regan *et al.*, 2010). Whether acute or chronic, flexor tendinopathy is commonly associated with such sports movement patterns as the golf-swing follow-through, the baseball pitch and the javelin throw. The condition is also prevalent in manual occupations. Assessment follows a similar approach as for extensor tendinopathy, but will incorporate the flexor tendinopathy test. The therapist may additionally identify, via Tinel's sign and the elbow flexion test, ulnar nerve involvement where the nerve may be undergoing compression from local inflammatory oedema just distal to the medial epicondyle at the cubital tunnel. The patient may also exhibit weakness in grip strength. Management follows a progressive rehabilitation strategy, a similar approach to the management of extensor tendinopathy, but with emphasis on the common flexor muscle–tendon unit, and identification and correction of contributing factors.

Ligamentous and joint injuries

The ligamentous complex of the medial elbow is the UCL. The lateral elbow is stabilized primarily by the LUCL, RCL and AL. The RCL, AL, QL, oblique cord and interosseous membrane contribute to the stability of the forearm joints. Ligament injuries are generally classified in grades (I–III) of sprain and these injuries follow acute forceful injury. Numerous authors identify a chronic cause of medial elbow sprain resulting from forceful repetitive valgus and extension stress (commonly referred to as 'valgus extension overload syndrome' or 'thrower's elbow') as may occur in baseball pitching or other sports involving overhead throwing or striking. Valgus extension overload syndrome is a chronic condition associated with throwing athletes and a possible gradual development of osteophytes at the HU joint. Many authors have identified that the common mechanism for this particular injury is related to both the repetitive stress as well as faulty mechanics of the throw during the final stages of the movement sequence (acceleration, deceleration and follow-through), which can lead to damaging stress, with gapping occurring medially, compression laterally and shearing posteriorly. Additionally, the player is often too far forward early in the throwing sequence, forcing an excessive gapping of the joint with repeating stress to the UCL. Initially, the problem features localized inflammation of the ligament, but can lead to chronic scarring, calcification and greatly increased potential for complete rupture or avulsion. In the chronic presentation, there is likely to be osteophyte development at the medial epicondyle, coronoid process or most commonly the posteromedial aspect of the olecranon process. In long-standing throwers there may also be observable cubitus valgus or flexion contracture (MacAuley, 2007). The presence of osteophytes may be identified during the valgus extension overload test, which has the patient supine as the therapist offers careful passive rhythmic end-range extension in an effort to observe the crepitus, restriction and irritation of such a condition. The acute traumatic medial (UCL) injury is much more common than the lateral (RCL) and occurs with the forced valgus or abduction stress from contact or a fall. RCL injuries occur with varus or adduction stress and with complete dislocation and subluxation. The majority of grade III UCL sprains (complete ruptures), as highlighted by Aviles *et al.* (2009), occur mid-substance. Avulsion fractures are also a possibility.

Assessment for ligamentous injuries incorporates standard observations, range of movement assessment and palpation. The injury is likely to present with local swelling, reduced active and passive ranges of movement and show tenderness and defects on palpation. The special tests are the valgus and varus stress tests, which, if positive, will range from mild pain and laxity to gross instability, depending on the grade. Functional tests may include lifting or throwing pattern movements or push-up positions. Any dislocation or suspected avulsion fracture requires urgent medical assessment and X-ray. Ideally, stress radiographs are performed to demonstrate ligamentous insufficiency with the elbow in a slightly flexed position while undergoing valgus or varus stress. MRI is used to identify specific soft tissue damage and can help to identify involvement of deeper tissues, such as LUCL, which is difficult to assess with physical examination. Management for grade I and II ligamentous sprains is conservative. The acute stage must emphasize management of symptoms (protection, rest, ice and compression and elevation) and, as inflammation subsides, the early stage of rehabilitation must emphasize protection (possibly with taping), mobility work, strengthening of the associated muscles and as soon as possible closed-chain loading activities. Controlled eccentric strengthening of the elbow flexors is to be encouraged to facilitate improved control of any rapid extension movements (Reinold and Wilk, 2003). Electrotherapy, including ultrasound and interferential, may be helpful in the early stages, alongside local and general soft tissue therapy techniques. Chronic ligament injuries and grade III sprains may require reconstruction surgery, which may also include arthroscopic removal of fragments or osteophytes. A range of graft options are available, and most commonly an ipsilateral or contralateral autograft from the tendon of palmaris longus is used. The Achilles, tibialis anterior, plantaris and hamstring tendons may also be considered amenable for autograft or allograft (Aviles *et al.*, 2009). Return to full activity can take 20 weeks or more following reconstruction surgery, and the athlete should only be allowed to return when there is no pain on loading or throwing and where a full rehabilitation programme has been undertaken. Prentice (2004) and others present interval throwing programmes to be initiated at end-stage rehabilitation for throwing athletes, which incorporate specific progressive increments in distance, repetitions, duration and intensity.

Elbow dislocation

Although the elbow has relatively good congruency and stability, dislocations do occur; indeed, the elbow is the second most frequently dislocated major joint in adults (after the glenohumeral joint), and is the most commonly dislocated joint in children. The most common mechanism is a fall onto an outstretched hand, which typically involves a combination of axial compression, supination and valgus stress (Aviles *et al.*, 2009). As the elbow is forced into hyperextension the most likely result is posterior displacement of the radius and ulna with complete disassociation of the articulatory surfaces of the humeroulnar joint (trochlea, trochlear notch and olecranon fossa) (Rettig, 2002; Zernicke *et al.*, 2008). On acute assessment, the olecranon process will be visibly posteriorly malpositioned and the sports therapist should be able to distinguish dislocation from a supracondylar humeral fracture by clarifying that the medial and lateral epicondyles are in normal alignment. Other forceful impact or twisting can also result in dislocation, not necessarily posterior or of the humeroulnar joint. With any dislocation injury, there will also be significant soft tissue damage to the joint capsule, collateral ligaments and possible muscle or peripheral nerve involvement. In some cases there will be associated fracture of the radial head and neck (most common), coronoid process or other bony structure. Immediate management of a dislocation requires first-aid intervention and referral for medical assessment and appropriate closed reduction or possible surgical intervention to reconstruct grade III ligamentous damage.

Following successful reduction and radiographs to confirm such, the elbow is normally splint immobilized and then hinge-braced once swelling has receded. Once cleared for rehabilitation, progressive mobility and strengthening is essential. A common long-term complication of dislocation is reduced functional range of movement, hence protected mobility exercise should be instigated within the first week (Richardson and Iglarsh, 1994). Although there is potential for chronic valgus laxity following complex dislocation, post-rehabilitation recurrent instability is unlikely with simple dislocations (Aviles *et al.*, 2009).

As previously discussed, posterolateral rotatory instability (PLRI) is a pattern of instability associated with post-reduction dislocation. The condition typically presents as a rotational displacement of the ulna from the trochlea alongside radial displacement from the capitulum, and most commonly relates to LUCL insufficiency. The majority of functionally limiting PLRI cases will require operative intervention as conservative management usually fails (Gottlieb and Uzelac, 2006). Alternatives to surgery include activity modification and use of hinged brace, with pronation and extension blocks. Surgery is likely to involve repair or reconstruction of the lateral ligamentous complex (using palmaris longus tendon autograft) (Aviles *et al.*, 2009).

Muscular injuries

Tears of the elbow musculature are common, but the most common type IV rupture affects biceps brachii. Although the biceps long head (originating from the supraglenoid tubercle) is the most common injury site for this muscle, complete rupture of the biceps from its insertion at the radial tuberosity occurs as a result of violent extension (eccentric overload) or overloaded flexion, as may occur in contact and team sports, weight-lifting or sports with potential for falls. The other common sites of injury to this muscle are the musculotendinous junction and the central muscle belly. Biceps rupture injury has a clear mechanism (single acute episode) and presentation. A complete rupture results in the torn tendon retracting towards its origin, with swelling, deep aching and pain in the cubital fossa and possible haematoma (tracked distally with gravity) and weakness and increased pain on movement. The therapist is likely to be able to palpate a recoiled bunching of the biceps muscle belly. Diagnosis is usually clinically obvious, but ultrasound or MRI scan should confirm. Progressive conservative management for a complete biceps insertion tear traditionally has poor functional outcomes, hence surgical repair is usually indicated, especially for young, active athletes (Bruggeman *et al.*, 2003), followed by prolonged rehabilitation. Tears, whether partial or total, can obviously occur in any of the muscles crossing the elbow, yet perhaps strangely, triceps brachii tears are less common. Complete rupture of the triceps tendon is among the rarest of all tendon ruptures in the body but may occur in weight-lifting or result indirectly from a fall onto an outstretched hand ('FOOSH') as the muscle is suddenly eccentrically overloaded. There is, however, a high prevalence of avulsion fractures with this injury. Injury rarely occurs at the musculoskeletal junction, and is more common just proximal to the olecranon (Aviles *et al.*, 2009). Management for type IIIa and IIIb injuries (minor and moderate partial tears), as according to the Munich Consensus Statement on muscle injury classification (Mueller–Wohlfahrt *et al.*, 2013), follows the standard conservative four-stage rehabilitation model. Type IV injuries (previously known as grade III ruptures) generally require surgical repair. Eygendaal and Safran (2006) present the background to flexor–pronator tears, highlighting the potential for such injury particularly in throwing sports and tennis. This injury may be difficult to differentiate from UCL injury, and indeed, both tendon and ligament complexes can be involved. As with all such injuries, the potential for type IV injuries is increased with pre-existing tendon degeneration and pathology, and also in athletes aged under 30 years of age with a history of steroid use.

Management of type IIIa and IIIb muscular injuries and post-operative conditions follow the standard progressive rehabilitation model, but is not complete without inclusion of a shoulder programme and general fitness maintenance (Wilk and Andrews, 2001). The basic criteria for progression through each stage is based on the sports therapist's assessment of the athlete and clarification of their ability to perform each stage correctly and without aggravation or adverse symptom response prior to progression. The main criteria for progression from the early stage, for example, has the athlete presenting with full, pain-free range of movement in the involved elbow, no palpable tenderness, and strength somewhere in the region of 70 per cent of the contralateral limb. Progression from late stage to return to play follows a period of significantly increased rehabilitation activity and no pain, restriction or other adverse response during clinical assessment (Aviles *et al.*, 2009). Different tissues and severities of injury each have their own classic timescale and prognosis for recovery and progression.

Table 7.2 Four-stage rehabilitation model

Stage	Goals, considerations and methods
1 Acute stage	Control inflammation (PRICE/POLICE); protect injury (avoidance of aggravating activity; NWB/PWB) symptom/pain management; minimize effects of immobilization; minimize muscle atrophy; advice
2 Early stage	Promote healing (ultrasound; contrast bathing; soft tissue therapy; thermal therapy); continued symptom/pain management; mobility (active movements; passive physiological and accessory mobilization techniques); proprioception (open to closed chain); early strength (isometric to isotonic; concentric to eccentric; open to closed chain; endurance repetitions; core and peripheral stability); continued protection (taping or support); cryokinetics; flexibility; cardio-vascular training; advice
3 Late stage	Progressive flexibility; strength and conditioning development; power, plyometric and functional exercise; continued mobilization techniques; progressive soft tissue therapy (MFR; MET; STR; NMT); cardiovascular training; advice
4 Return to sport stage	Sport-specific conditioning (emphasizing high-speed; eccentric loading; agility drills; skills and sports movement patterns); prehabilitation techniques; cardiovascular training; advice

Adolescent osteochondroses

There are a number of adolescent osteochondroses, which relate to disorder of the immature articular or non–articular skeletal growth plates. At the elbow, osteochondritis dissicans (OCD), also known as 'little leaguer's elbow', develops as a result of repetitive stress and microtrauma to immature skeletal structure and is characterized by a gradually developing but very localized avascular necrosis and resulting degeneration and fragmentation (loose bodies) of hyaline cartilage and associated subchondral bone. The most common sites where this condition manifests are the knee, ankle and elbow, and it affects males more than females (Jackson *et al.*, 1989). At the elbow, the laterally positioned capitulum or radial head at the radiohumeral joint are damaged by the compressive forces associated with throwing-type movements, hence it is most prevalent in throwing and racquet sports and gymnastics. Forceful throwing-type movements may also cause concurrent valgus stress damage to medial structures. Presenting predominantly in the 13–16-year-old age group, symptoms of the condition include gradual and insidious development of stiffness, local joint pain, swelling, possible medial instability and reduced elbow extension or flexion contracture (Bradley *et al.*, 2010). Articular surfaces can become enlarged and deformed and sufferers may be predisposed to osteoarthritis. Diagnosis is usually confirmed by X-ray, MRI or CT scan, which will show irregular joint surfaces and fragmentation. If identified early and without any fragment displacement, the condition can be self-limiting and is likely to respond well to rest, strict restriction from throwing-type movements for up to three months and graded low-intensity mobility and strengthening exercise. A hinged elbow brace can provide important protection during the protracted conservative recovery period. Surgery is indicated where persistent or worsening symptoms are present. Open surgical reduction and internal fixation of large osteochondral fragments from the capitulum may be performed, possibly with autograft or allograft. Arthroscopic surgery may be offered to remove any smaller detached fragments. As with many of the adolescent sports-related disorders, it is important to structure the exercise training sessions and competition well, allowing for rest days and coaching correct technique (Ashman, 2005; Bradley *et al.*, 2010; MacAuley, 2007; Savoie and Field, 2010).

Panner's disease, another osteochondrosis of the elbow, is also characterized by avascular necrosis and fragmentation, but almost always affects younger male children (i.e. under the age of 11). This condition may result from repetitive trauma, but underlying congenital, hereditary or endocrine causes are also recognized and the onset is acute rather than gradual. Pathologically, the condition develops due to interruption of the direct blood supply to the growing epiphysis and involves complete, rather than partial, fragmentation of the ossification centre of the capitulum. Panner's disease does not usually produce loose bodies, but all other aetiology, signs, symptoms and management are similar to OCD – the conservative approach generally having good outcomes (Rudzki and Paletta, 2004). Panner's disease is the most common cause of lateral elbow pain in children aged under 11 (Franklyn-Miller *et al.*, 2011). Essentially, any child under the age of 11 with a swollen elbow, limitation in extension and a dull, aching pain aggravated by any throwing activity should be suspected as having Panner's disease (Bradley *et al.*, 2010).

Nerve injuries

The three main neural compression problems relating to the elbow region are cubital tunnel syndrome (ulnar nerve), pronator syndrome (anterior interosseous branch of the ulnar nerve) and radial tunnel syndrome (posterior interosseous branch of the radial nerve). Of the three conditions, by far the most common problem is cubital tunnel syndrome (also referred to as ulnar neuritis), where the superficial ulnar nerve coursing under the medial epicondyle is vulnerable to both compression and tensile stress (Anderson *et al.*, 2009; Aviles *et al.*, 2009; Kisner and Colby, 2007). The aetiology and assessment of neural conditions affecting the elbow is presented earlier in this chapter. Management for such problems depends, first, on the severity of symptoms, and, second, on the cause, including any predisposing factors, which need to be addressed if at all possible. Such biomechanical factors as valgus deformity or other irregular bony architecture, ligament laxity, excessive myofacial tension, soft tissue scar tissue or calcification and peripheral neural tensions all need to considered, as do the athlete's movement patterns and equipment. Cubital tunnel syndrome may benefit from night splinting to avoid elbow flexion (Antuna and Barco Laakso, 2010). Care must be taken to avoid excessive tensile stress in the early stage, especially where there are clear neurological deficits (Taylor *et al.*, 2009). Surgical decompression, transposition (relocation) or even nerve fibre repair may be indicated for persistent cases (Antuna and Barco Laakso, 2010). The post-surgical rehabilitation must be based on the consultant's advice, but early protected mobilization is required to minimize adhesions of the neural sheath and to offset other complications such as atrophy, contracture and joint stiffness (Aviles *et al.*, 2009; Buhroo, 2003). Standard management for mild neuropraxia begins with rest from all aggravating activities and as the initial symptoms subside, staged-rehabilitation exercise including local soft tissue therapy, neural mobilization (if indicated) and graded return to functional activities.

Olecranon bursitis

Olecranon bursitis is inflammation of the subcutaneous bursa overlying the olecranon process between the skin and triceps tendon. Smaller, additional bursae have been identified by several authors within the triceps tendon (intratendinous bursa) or between the triceps and joint capsule (subtendinous bursa). Bursitis may be acute, chronic or septic. Injury to the bursa can occur as a result of single trauma (fall onto olecranon process), from continuous friction and pressure from leaning on the elbow – 'student's elbow' or from arthritic or osteophytic irritation. Traumatic bursitis may also cause bleeding into the bursal sac, resulting in a haemabursitis (Regan *et al.*, 2010; Thomas and Field, 2010). Infective (septic) bursitis may originate following local open injury or spread from infection in the hand or forearm, such as paronychia of the nailbed, and may also be accompanied by feelings of malaise or fever (Regan *et al.*, 2010). Acute olecranon bursitis typically presents as a localized swelling, with a distinct, smooth, occasionally reddened and rounded presentation; the elbow is likely to exhibit limited range of flexion. However, there may be inflammation, pain and restriction without the classic observable signs. Management for a mild case of bursitis of traumatic aetiology is likely to be rest, ice and protective padding around the olecranon. As inflammation subsides, warm packs may help to speed absorption of fluid. If the bursitis is more severe or resistant to initial acute management, referral for sterile aspiration is recommended. Repeat aspirations may be necessary. Oral NSAIDs can be useful during the early management phase. Steroid or anaesthetic injection may be considered in resistant cases, but multiple injections are not recommended due to the increased risk of septic bursitis. Recurrent episodes are quite typical and generally these result from much less than the original trauma. Such recurrences lead to chronic bursitis, where significant fibrous thickening of the sac and neovascularization occurs, and if continuously irritating, the bursa may require surgical excision (bursectomy) (Regan *et al.*, 2010; Thomas and Field 2010). Any suspicion of infective bursitis should be referred to a doctor for diagnosis (via needle aspiration and analysis of bursal contents) and antibiotic medication. The bursa, ideally, will be aspirated and undergo saline irrigation. Gout can be an underlying pathology for this condition, and to identify the presence of monosodium urate crystals, the aspirated fluid should be analysed. Complications associated with poorly managed infective bursitis can include osteomyelitis and septic arthritis.

References

Abbot, J. (2001) Mobilization with movement applied to the elbow affects shoulder range of movement in subjects with lateral epicondylalgia. *Manual Therapy.* 6: 170–177

Anderson, M., Parr, G. and Hall, S. (2009) *Foundations of athletic training, prevention, assessment and management*, 4th edition. Lippincott, Williams and Wilkins. Philadelphia, PA

Andrews, J., Wilk, K., Satterwhite, Y. and Tedder, J. (1993) Physical examination of the thrower's elbow. *Journal of Sports Physical Therapy.* 17: 296–304

Antuna, S.A. and Barco Laakso, R. (2010) Elbow injuries. In Margeritini, F. and Rossi, R. (eds) *Orthopaedic sports medicine: Principles and practice.* Springer-Verlag. Milan, Italy

Ashman, E. (2005) Elbow articular lesions and fractures. In O'Connor, F., Sallis, R., Wilder, R. and St. Pierre, P. (eds) *Sports medicine: Just the facts.* McGraw-Hill. New York

Aviles, S., Wilk, K. and Safran, M. (2009) Elbow. In Magee, D., Zachazewski, J. and Quillen, W. (eds) *Pathology and intervention in musculoskeletal rehabilitation.* Saunders, Elsevier. St. Louis, MO

Beam, J. (2002) Rehabilitation including sports-specific functional progression for the competitive athlete. *Journal of Bodywork and Movement Therapies.* 6 (4): 205–219

Biel, A. (2005) *Trail guide to the body: How to locate muscles, bones and more*, 3rd edition. Books of Discovery. Boulder, CO

Bradley, J., Petrie, R. and Tejwani, S. (2010) Elbow injuries in children and adolescents. In Delee, J. Drez, D. and Miller, M. (eds) *Orthopaedic sports medicine principles and practice*, 3rd edition. Saunders, Elsevier. Philadelphia, PA

Bruggeman, N., Steinmann, S., Cooney, W. and Krogsgaard, M. (2003) Elbow, wrist and hand. In Kjaer, M., Krogsgaard, M., Magnusson, P., *et al.* (eds) *Textbook of sports medicine, basic science and clinical aspects of sports injury and physical activity*. Blackwell Science. Malden, MA

Brukner, P. and Khan, K. (2009) *Clinical sports medicine revised*, 3rd edition. McGraw-Hill. NSW, Australia

Buhroo, A. (2003) Observations on rehabilitation of peripheral nerve injuries in Kashmir Valley. *Indian Journal of Physical Medicine and Rehabilitation*. 14: 27–32

Cleland, J., Whitman, J. and Fritz, J. (2004) Effectiveness of manual physical therapy to the cervical spine in the management of lateral epicondylalgia: A retrospective analysis. *Journal of Orthopedic Sports Physical Therapy*. 34: 713–724

Comfort, P. and Abrahamson, E. (2010) *Sports rehabilitation and injury prevention*. Wiley-Blackwell. Chichester, UK

Cook, J.L. and Purdam, C.R. (2009) Is tendon pathology a continuum? A pathology model to explain the clinical presentation of load-induced tendinopathy. *British Journal of Sports Medicine*. 43: 409–416

Coombes, B.K., Bisset, L. and Vicenzino, B. (2009) A new integrative model of lateral epicondylalgia. *British Journal of Sports Medicine*. 43: 252–258

Corrigan, B. and Maitland, G. (2004) *Musculoskeletal and sports injuries*. Butterworth-Heinemann. Edinburgh, UK

Cyriax, J. (1982) *Textbook of orthopaedic medicine Vol 1: Diagnosis of soft tissue lesions*, 8th edition. Balliere Tindall. London, UK

Elliot, B. (2006). Biomechanics and tennis. *British Journal of Sports Medicine*. 40: 392–396

Eygendaal, D. and Safran, M. (2006) Postero-medial elbow problems in the adult athlete. *British Journal of Sports Medicine*. 40: 430–434

Eygendaal, D., Rahussen, F. and Diercks, R. (2007) Biomechanics of the elbow joint in tennis players and relation to pathology. *British Journal of Sports Medicine*. 41: 820–823

Franklyn-Miller, A., Falvey, E., McCrory, P. and Brukner, P. (2011) *Clinical sports anatomy*. McGraw-Hill. NSW, Australia

Frostick, S., Mohammad, M. and Ritchie, D. (1999) Sport injuries of the elbow. *British Journal of Sports Medicine*. 33: 301–311

Glousman, R., Barron, J. and Jobe, F. (1992) An electromyographic analysis of the elbow in normal and injured pitchers with medial collateral ligament insufficiency. *American Journal of Sports Medicine*. 20: 311–317

Gottlieb, J. and Uzelac, P. (2006) *SOAP for orthopedics*. Lippincott, Williams and Wilkins. Philadelphia, PA

Gross, J., Fetto, J. and Rosen, E. (2009) *Musculoskeletal examination*, 3rd edition. Wiley-Blackwell. Oxford, UK

Hamill, J. and Knutzen, K. (2009) *Biomechanical basis for human movement*, 3rd edition. Lippincott, Williams and Wilkins. Philadelphia, PA

Hattam, P. and Smeatham, A. (2010) *Special tests in musculoskeletal examination: An evidence-based guide for clinicians*. Churchill Livingstone, Elsevier. London, UK

Hayes, K.W., Petersen, C. and Falconer, J. (1994) An examination of Cyriax's passive motion tests with patients having osteoarthritis of the knee. *Physical Therapy*. 74: 697–708

Hengeveld, E. and Banks, K. (2005) *Maitland's peripheral manipulation*, 4th edition. Butterworth Heinemann, Elsevier. London, UK

Jackson, D., Silvino, N. and Reinman, P. (1989) Osteochondritis in the female gymnast's elbow. *Arthroscopy*. 5: 129–136

Johnson, D. (section editor) (2008) Pectoral girdle and upper limb. In Standring, S. (ed.) *Gray's anatomy, the anatomical basis of clinical practice*, 40th edition. Churchill Livingstone, Elsevier. London, UK

Jones, M.A., Jensen, G. and Edwards, I. (2008) Clinical reasoning in physiotherapy. In Higgs, J., Jones, M.A, Loftus, S. and Christensen, N. (eds) *Clinical reasoning in the health professions*, 3rd edition. Butterworth Heinemann, Elsevier. Philadelphia, PA

Kaltenborn, F.M. (1999) *Manual mobilisation of the extremity joints: Basic examination and treatment techniques*, 5th edition. Olaf Norlis Bokhandel. Oslo, Norway

Kaminski, T., Powers, M. and Buckley, B. (2000) Differential assessment of elbow injuries. *Athletic Therapy Today*. 5 (3): 6–11

Kisner, C. and Colby, L. (2007) *Therapeutic exercise: Foundations and techniques*, 5th edition. F.A. Davis Company. Philadelphia, PA

Konin, J., Wiksten, D., Isear, J. and Brader, H. (2006) *Special tests for orthopedic examination*, 3rd edition. SLACK Incorporated. Thorofare, NJ

Loudon, J., Swift, M. and Bell, S. (2008) *The clinical orthopedic assessment guide*, 2nd edition. Human Kinetics. Champaign, IL

MacAuley, D. (2007) *Oxford handbook of sport and exercise medicine*. Oxford University Press. Oxford, UK

Magee, D. (2008) *Orthopaedic physical assessment*, 5th edition. Saunders. Philadelphia, PA

Medical Research Council (1976) *Aids to the investigation of peripheral nerve injuries*. HMSO. London, UK

Morrey, B. (2010) Biomechanics of the elbow and forearm. In Delee, J. Drez, D. and Miller, M. (eds) *Orthopaedic sports medicine principles and practice*, 3rd edition. Saunders, Elsevier. Philadelphia, PA

Morrey, B. and An, K. (1983) Articular and ligamentous contributions to the static stability of the elbow joint. *American Journal of Sports Medicine* 11: 315–319

Mueller-Wohlfahrt, H.W., Haensel, L., Mithoefer, K., *et al.* (2013) Terminology and classification of muscle injuries in sport: The Munich consensus statement. *British Journal of Sports Medicine*. 47: 342–350

Ochiai, D. and Nirschl, R. (2005) Elbow tendinosis. In O'Connor, F., Sallis, R., Wilder, R. and St. Pierre, P. (eds) *Sports medicine: Just the facts*. McGraw-Hill. New York

Palastanga, N., Field, D. and Soames, R. (2006) *Anatomy and human movement, structure and function*, 5th edition. Churchill Livingstone, Elsevier. London, UK

Palmer, M. and Epler, M. (1998) *Fundamentals of musculoskeletal assessment techniques*, 2nd edition. Lippincott-Raven. Philadelphia, PA

Petty, N. (2011) *Neuromusculoskeletal examination and assessment, a handbook for therapists*, 4th edition. Churchill Livingstone, Elsevier. London, UK

Pluim, B. and Safran, M. (2004) *From breakpoint to advantage*. Racquet Tech Publishing. Vista, CA

Prentice, W. (2004) *Rehabilitation techniques for sports medicine and athletic training*, 4th edition. McGraw-Hill. New York

Prentice, W. (2011) *Principles of athletic training: A competency-based approach*, 14th edition. McGraw-Hill. New York

Rees, J.D., Stride, M. and Scott, A. (2013) Tendons: Time to revisit inflammation. *British Journal of Sports Medicine*. http://dx.doi.org/10.1136/bjsports-2012-091957, accessed May 2013

Regan, W., Grondin, P. and Morrey, B. (2010) Tendinopathies around the elbow. In Delee, J. Drez, D. and Miller, M. (eds) *Orthopaedic sports medicine principles and practice*, 3rd edition. Saunders, Elsevier. Philadelphia, PA

Reinold, M. and Wilk, K. (2003) Elbow. In Kolt, G. and Snyder-Mackler, L. (eds) *Physical therapies in sport and exercise*. Churchill Livingstone, Elsevier. London, UK

Renstrom, P. and Hach, T. (2005) Insertional tendinopathy in sports. In Maffulli, N., Renstrom, P. and Leadbetter, W. (eds) *Tendon injuries: Basic science and clinical medicine*. Springer-Verlag. London, UK

Rettig, A. (2002) Traumatic elbow injuries in the athlete. *Orthopedic Clinics of North America*. 33 (3): 509–522

Richardson, J. and Iglarsh, Z. (1994) *Clinical orthopaedic physical therapy*. Saunders. Philadelphia, PA

Rudzki, J. and Paletta, G. Jr. (2004) Juvenile and adolescent elbow injuries in sports. *Clinics in Sports Medicine*. 23 (4): 581–608

Safran, M. (1985) Elbow injuries in athletes: A review. *Clinical Orthopaedics and Related Research*. 310: 258

Savoie, F. and Field, L. (2010) Osteochondritis dissicans of the elbow. In Delee, J. Drez, D. and Miller, M. (eds) *Orthopaedic sports medicine principles and practice*, 3rd edition. Saunders, Elsevier. Philadelphia, PA

Scott, A., Docking, S., Vicenzino, B., *et al.* (2013) Sports and exercise-related tendinopathies: A review of selected topical issues by participants of the second International Scientific Tendinopathy Symposium (ISTS), Vancouver, 2012. *British Journal of Sports Medicine*. 47: 536–544

Sewell, D., Watkins, P. and Griffin, M. (2013) *Sport and exercise science: An introduction*, 2nd edition. Routledge. Abingdon, UK

Sexton, M. (ed.) (2006) *Clinics in motion: Practical techniques of physiotherapy examination and treatment: Series 1 Vol 6: Elbow, wrist and hand*. Clinics in Motion DVD. Ireland

Shultz, S., Houglum, P. and Perrin, D. (2000) *Assessment of athletic injuries*. Human Kinetics. Champaign, IL

Starkey, C. and Ryan, J. (2003) *Orthopaedic and athletic injury evaluation handbook.* F.A. Davis Company. Philadelphia, PA

Struijis, P., Daman, P., Bakker, E., Blankevort, L., Assendelft, W. and van Dijk, C. (2003) Manipulation of the wrist for management of lateral epicondylitis: A randomized pilot study. *Physical Therapy.* 87: 608–616

Taylor, C., Nee, R. and Zachazewski, J. (2009) Peripheral nerve injuries. In Magee, D., Zachazewski, J. and Quillen, W. (eds) *Pathology and intervention in musculoskeletal rehabilitation.* Saunders, Elsevier. St. Louis, MO

Thomas, R. and Field, L. (2010) Olecranon bursitis. In Delee, J. Drez, D. and Miller, M. (eds) *Orthopaedic sports medicine principles and practice,* 3rd edition. Saunders, Elsevier. Philadelphia, PA

Tortora, G. and Derrickson, B. (2008) *Principles of anatomy and physiology,* 12th edition. John Wiley and Sons. Upper Saddle River, NJ

Udall, J., Fitzpatrick, M., McGarry, M., Leba, T. and Lee, T. (2009) Effects of flexor–pronator muscle loading on valgus stability of the elbow with an intact, stretched, and resected medial ulnar collateral ligament. *Journal of Elbow and Shoulder Surgery.* 18: 773–778

Whiteside, J. and Andrews, J. (1989) Common elbow problems in the recreational athlete. *Journal of Musculoskeletal Medicine.* 6: 17–34

Wilk, K. and Andrews, J. (2001) Rehabilitation of elbow injuries. In Puddu, G., Giombini, A. and Selvanetti, A. (eds) *Rehabilitation of sports injuries.* Springer-Verlag. Berlin, Germany

Zernicke, R., Whiting, W. and Manske, S. (2008) Upper extremity injuries. In Hong, Y. and Bartlett, R. (eds) *Routledge handbook of biomechanics and human movement science.* Routledge. Abingdon, UK

8

THE WRIST AND HAND REGION

Anatomy, assessment and injuries

Jeanette Lewis and Philip Smith

Functional anatomy of the wrist and hand region

The wrist and hand are the most active and intricate parts of the upper limb and in a way this is what contributes to making the human unique. Many mammals have grasping appendages and humans are not the only primates possessing opposable thumbs; however, what makes the human hand unique is the ability of the small and ring fingers to rotate across the palm to meet the thumb in 'opposition' This allows a unique flexibility for the carpometacarpal joints of these fingers and adds unparalleled grip, dexterity and grasping capability to the human hand. Without the intricate, manoeuvrable joints of the wrist and hand, humans would be unable to complete many normal activities of daily living (ADL) such as eating, writing or self-care. Magee (2008) stated that in addition to being an organ used in communication, the hand has a protective role and acts as both a motor and sensory organ, detecting such information as temperature, texture, depth and shape. Napier (1956) identified that the primary role of the hand itself is grasping and manipulation; however, despite its multiplicity of activities, there are two fundamental prehensile actions: the precision grip and the power grip. It is suggested that precision grips are unique to humans, and these fine movements are controlled by the intrinsic hand muscles in conjunction with the more powerful extrinsic hand muscles of the forearm. High levels of precise neuromotor control and grip strength are required in many sports in order to manipulate racquets, balls or other equipment. For example, athletes competing in tennis, darts and basketball require precise grip and high levels of activity of the flexor musculature of the forearms and hand. Injuries to the wrist and hand are extremely common in sport. Acute traumatic fractures to the distal radius or scaphoid can occur during football, inline skating or snowboarding when falling onto an outstretched hand (commonly known as a 'FOOSH' injury). Additionally, this region is extremely susceptible to repetitive strain injuries (RSI) such as tendinopathies due to the repetitive and forceful upper limb movements in sports such as tennis, golf and gymnastics. Mobility of the wrist and hand is enhanced by movements of the shoulder and elbow, and so although this chapter will discuss the region in relative isolation, it is essential to recognize that any wrist or hand dysfunction or injury will frequently affect or involve the whole upper limb to some degree, just as injuries to the rest of the upper limb are likely to affect wrist and hand function.

The wrist and hand have many functions including (non-verbal) communication (hand signs and gestures), sensation (via peripheral mechanoreceptors, thermoreceptors and free nerve

Table 8.1 Bones of the wrist and hand

Name	Description
Radius	Lateral forearm bone
Ulna	Medial forearm bone
Scaphoid	Lateral proximal carpal bone
Lunate	Middle proximal carpal bone
Triquetrum	Medial proximal carpal bone
Pisiform	Superficial medial proximal carpal bone
Trapezium	Lateral distal carpal bone
Trapezoid	Lateral distal carpal bone
Capitate	Middle distal carpal bone
Hamate	Medial distal carpal bone
Metacarpals	1–5
Proximal phalanges	1–5
Middle phalanges	2–4
Distal phalanges	1–5

Table 8.2 Joints of the wrist and hand

Full name	Abbreviation
Proximal radioulnar joint	PRU joint
Distal radioulnar joint	DRU joint
Radiocarpal joint	RC joint
Midcarpal joints	MC joints
Intercarpal joints	IC joints
Carpometacarpal joints	CMC joints
Intermetacarpal joints	IMC joints
Metacarpophalangeal joints	MCP joints
Proximal interphalangeal joints	PIP joints
Interphalangeal joint	IP joint
Distal interphalangeal joints	DIP joints

endings which provide a sense of touch, pressure, position, temperature and nociception) and, of course, movement and manipulation of objects in one's environment. The bones forming the wrist and hand are as follows: radius and ulna; carpals (eight), metacarpals (five) and phalanges (fourteen). There are numerous joints of the region, the main ones being: the distal (inferior) radioulnar (RU) joint; the radiocarpal (RC) joint; the intercarpal (IC) joints; the carpometacarpal (CMC) joints; the intermetacarpal (IMC) joints; the metacarpophalangeal (MCP) joints and the proximal and distal interphalangeal (PIP and DIP) joints.

Movements of the wrist and hand

The fundamental (uniplanar) movements of the RC and RU joints of the wrist include:

- flexion (movement of the palmar aspect of the hand towards the anterior surface of the forearm);

- extension (movement of the dorsal aspect of the hand towards the posterior forearm);
- pronation (with the elbow bent at 90° and held against the body, this is the action of turning the palm to the floor);
- supination (with the elbow bent at 90° and held against the body, this is the action of turning the palm to the ceiling);
- radial deviation (with the wrist in a neutral or anatomical position, between flexion and extension, this is the action of taking the hand away from the body, towards the radial aspect);
- ulnar deviation (with the wrist in a neutral or anatomical position, between flexion and extension, this is the action of taking the hand towards the body, towards the ulnar aspect).

Normal active ranges of movement (RoM) at the wrist are: flexion 0–85°; extension 0–85°; adduction (ulnar deviation) 45°; and abduction (radial deviation) 15° (Johnson *et al.*, 2008). Wrist flexion range of motion is reduced if flexion is performed with the fingers flexed because of the resistance offered by the finger extensor muscles. Similarly, the range of motion of wrist extension is reduced if the movement is performed with the fingers extended. The close-packed (most stable and congruent) position for the wrist, in which maximal support is offered, is a hyperextended position. The close-packed position for the midcarpal joint is radial deviation. Wrist movements can be combined in a multitude of ways to create a host of complex movements such as those combining to produce circumduction (circling of the wrist), or for the forehand and backhand strokes in tennis or badminton. Wrist movements are also combined with finger movements for precise functional use.

Finger carpometacarpal, metacarpophalangeal and interphalangeal joint movements include:

- Flexion of the fingers: occurs at the metacarpophalangeal joints followed by the proximal interphalangeal joints and the distal interphalangeal joints (movement of the fingertips toward the palm or clenching a fist).
- Extension of the fingers: occurs at the metacarpophalangeal joints followed by the proximal interphalangeal joints and the distal interphalangeal joints (movement of the fingertips away from the palm or opening the hand).
- Abduction of the fingers: movement of the metacarpophalangeal joints away from the middle (third) finger.
- Adduction of the fingers: movement of the metacarpophalangeal joints towards the middle (third) finger.

The MCP joints of the four fingers are condyloid joints allowing movements in two planes: flexion–extension and abduction–adduction. The fingers can flex through 70–90° with most flexion in the little finger and least in the index finger. Flexion, which determines grip strength, can be more effective and produce more force when the wrist is held in 20–30° of extension, a position that increases the length of the finger flexors (Wadsworth, 1985). Finger extension is limited with the wrist hyperextended and enhanced with the wrist flexed. Approximately 20° of abduction and adduction is normal at the MCP joints; however, abduction is limited if the fingers are flexed because the collateral ligaments become taut and restrict movement. The CMC joint of the thumb is classified as a synovial saddle joint, and is the articulation between the trapezium and the first metacarpal. The CMC joint of the thumb has an extensive range of movement, allowing 50–80° flexion and extension, 40–80° abduction and adduction and 10–15° rotation (Wadsworth, 1985). In comparison, the hinged MCP joint of the thumb allows motion in only one plane and enables approximately 30–90° of flexion and 15° extension;

however, this joint is reinforced with collateral ligaments. The various movements of the thumb at the CMC joint can be described as follows:

- Flexion: movement across the palm toward the base of the fifth finger.
- Extension: movement away from the palm but in the same plane.
- Abduction: movement away from the palm with the thumb held at 90° to the palm.
- Adduction: movement towards the palm with the thumb held at 90° to the palm.
- Opposition: movement of the thumb to make contact with the tip of the fifth finger.
- Circumduction: a combination movement of extension, abduction, flexion and adduction to create a circling action of the thumb.

Surface anatomy of the wrist and hand

The anatomy of the hand is complex and intricate. A thorough understanding of the surface anatomy of the hand and wrist will allow the therapist to evaluate common injuries and observe any apparent abnormalities within the region. On visual inspection of the wrist and hand, several significant features can be observed on the palmar (anterior) surface. Running from proximal to distal, there are several creases evident, the most important being: the wrist crease, which identifies the approximate position of the radiocarpal joint line; the thenar crease, which outlines the thenar eminence at the base of the thumb; and the distal palmar crease which gives the approximate position of the metacarpophalangeal joints.

The shape of the hand is created by three arches; two transverse at the lines of the carpal bones and metacarpal heads and a longitudinal arch down the centre of the palm, which are supported by the intrinsic muscles of the hand. The strategic location of these arches enhances the volar projection of the thumb and promotes an efficient pinch unit between the thumb and the index and middle fingers (Hoppenfeld, 1999). The dorsal surface of the hand has fewer features, the most significant being the metacarpal heads (knuckles) where the knuckle of the middle finger (third metacarpal) should be the most prominent when the fist is clenched. The general condition and colour of the fingernails is also important as nail abnormalities can be indicators of anything from local fungal infection to systemic illness. Normal nails are pink in colour with a white crescent at the base (the lunula).

Skeletal anatomy of the wrist and hand

The distal radioulnar (DRU) joint is the distal articulation between the two bones of the forearm and is reinforced by the intra-articular triangular fibrocartilage complex (TFCC), the anterior and posterior RU ligaments and the capsular ligament. Although more usually associated with the elbow joint, it is also an important consideration when assessing any wrist dysfunction due to the inherent relationship; the RU joints account for approximately 70° of pronation and 85° of supination (Hoppenfeld, 1999; Moses *et al.*, 2005). The wrist joint proper is the articulation between the forearm bones and the proximal carpal bones of the hand. There are eight carpal bones in the wrist; however, the complete framework of the hand also incorporates five metacarpals and 14 phalanges. These 27 bones function to enable oppositional grip (Daniels *et al.*, 2004). Within the hand, the proximal row of carpal bones includes the scaphoid, lunate, triquetrum and pisiform. The distal row of carpals comprises the trapezoid, trapezium, capitate and hamate.

The wrist and hand have both a fixed (stable) and a mobile segment. The fixed segment consists of the distal row of carpal bones (trapezium, trapezoid, capitate and hamate) and the

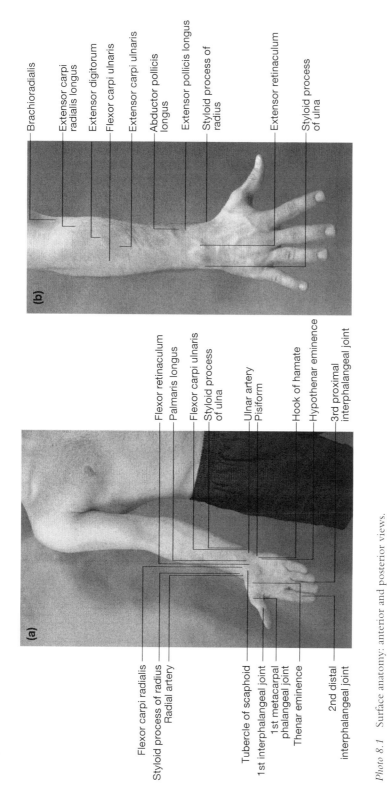

Brachioradialis

Extensor carpi radialis longus

Extensor digitorum

Flexor carpi ulnaris

Extensor carpi ulnaris

Abductor pollicis longus

Extensor pollicis longus

Styloid process of radius

Extensor retinaculum

Styloid process of ulna

(b)

Flexor retinaculum

Palmaris longus

Flexor carpi ulnaris

Styloid process of ulna

Ulnar artery

Pisiform

Hook of hamate

Hypothenar eminence

3rd proximal interphalangeal joint

Flexor carpi radialis

Styloid process of radius

Radial artery

Tubercle of scaphoid

1st interphalangeal joint

1st metacarpal phalangeal joint

Thenar eminence

2nd distal interphalangeal joint

(a)

Photo 8.1   Surface anatomy: anterior and posterior views.

second and third metacarpals; the mobile segment is made up of five phalanges, the first, fourth and fifth metacarpals, as well as the scaphoid, which serves as a link between the distal and proximal rows. All carpal bones contribute directly in wrist function – apart from the pisiform, which is a sesamoid bone embedded within the flexor carpi ulnaris tendon. This skeletal arrangement allows for stability without rigidity, enables the hand to move more discretely and enhances the function of the thumb and fingers when they are used for power or precision grips (Magee, 2008).

Proximal row of carpals

- Scaphoid: the largest proximal bone that forms the radial border of the carpal tunnel. It is somewhat wedge-shaped and slightly larger on the palmar surface, containing a small tubercle, which serves as an attachment point.
- Lunate: a crescent-shaped bone, again slightly larger on the palmar surface than dorsally.
- Triquetrum: a pyramidal-shaped bone with a smooth, distal lateral arc on its palmar surface which articulates with the pisiform.
- Pisiform: a 'pea-shaped' bone which sits superficially on the triquetrum on the palmar surface of the hand.

Distal row of carpals

- Trapezium: an irregularly shaped bone with a palmar tubercle and groove which carries the tendon of flexor carpi radialis.
- Trapezoid: another irregularly shaped bone, rather triangular in outline, and directly distal to the scaphoid.
- Capitate: the largest and most central carpal bone with a roughly triangular distal surface, and a large medial facet which articulates with the hamate.
- Hamate: a wedge-shaped bone with a superficial hook-like process (hook of hamate) on the distal palmar surface. There is also a faint ridge on the dorsal surface (Johnson and Ellis, 2005).

As stated previously, the RC joint is often considered as the wrist joint proper and is classified as a condyloid synovial joint formed between the radius and the TFCC proximally and the scaphoid, lunate and triquetrum bones distally. In the neutral position of the wrist, only the scaphoid and lunate are in contact with the radius. The scaphoid is often considered to be one of the most important carpals, because it supports much of the weight of the arm in many closed-chain activities and transmits much of the force received from the hand to the bones of the forearm and is a key participant in wrist joint actions (Wadsworth, 1985). Furthermore, the scaphoid is seated on the radial side of the wrist and is the only bone that bridges the two carpal rows, creating a mechanical linkage between them (Tan et al., 2009).

The midcarpal joint is formed between the proximal and distal rows of carpal bones and is a synovial plane (gliding) joint supported by the interosseous ligaments between the two rows, as well as the intercarpal ligaments between each pair of carpal bones (Johnson and Ellis, 2005; Moses et al., 2005).

The distal carpal bones articulate with the five metacarpal bones which are long, cylindrical bones expanded into heads distally and bases proximally; these together form the five carpometacarpal joints as follows:

- CMC1: MC1 + trapezium
- CMC: MC2 + trapezium, trapezoid + capitate

- CMC3: MC3 + capitate
- CMC4: MC4 + capitate + hamate
- CMC5: MC5 + hamate.

These are all plane synovial joints with the exception of CMC1, which is a saddle joint articulating proximally with the trapezium, and which allows flexion, extension, abduction and adduction of the thumb. The distal collection of bones in the hand are the 14 phalanges. There are three phalanges in each finger – the proximal, middle and distal, except for the thumb, which has just two phalanges (the proximal and distal). These bones, like the metacarpals, are long and cylindrical, with expansions at both proximal and distal ends of the proximal and middle phalanges. Each distal phalanx terminates as a rounded cone shape. The thumb is also referred to as the 'pollex', just as the great toe is known as the 'hallux' (Johnson and Ellis, 2005; Moses *et al.*, 2005).

Retinaculum

There are also two important retinacula in the wrist; the flexor retinaculum and extensor retinaculum, which are both found at the level of the radiocarpal joint. The extensor retinaculum lies on the dorsal (posterior) aspect and runs from the lateral margin of the radius with the medial border of the ulna to form a thick fibrous band under which the extensor tendons of the forearm run. The flexor retinaculum is a strong, square-shaped fibrous band that crosses the carpal bones transversely to form the roof of the fibro-osseous carpal tunnel. It attaches medially to the hook of the hamate and the pisiform on the ulnar side of the wrist and attaches laterally to the tubercles of the scaphoid and trapezium. The flexor muscles of the fingers and thumb, as well as the median nerve, pass through the carpal tunnel (Johnson and Ellis, 2005; Moses *et al.*, 2005). Both the flexor retinaculum and the palmaris longus muscle are continuous with the palmar aponeurosis, which is a thick sheet of fascia extending throughout the palmar surface of the hand.

Carpal tunnel

The flexor retinaculum is a strong fibrous band that stretches across the front of the carpal bones, enclosing their concavity and forming the carpal tunnel (Waugh and Grant, 2010). The tendons of the flexor muscles of the wrist and fingers, and the median nerve, pass through the carpal tunnel between the tendons of flexor digitorum profundus and flexor digitorum superficialis. Although there is a synovial membrane surrounding the tendons to minimize friction, the tunnel is relatively narrow and so if any of the nine long flexor tendons passing through it become inflamed and swollen, the median nerve can become compressed, which is one of the common causes of carpal tunnel syndrome.

Joint capsule

The wrist is strengthened and lubricated by a synovial membrane, a fibrous capsule and a complex system of ligaments. A loose but strong fibrous capsule lined by synovial membrane completely encloses the joint, attaching to the articular margins (Ateshian *et al.*, 1992). The capsule is sufficiently slack to allow a wide range of movements, while reinforcing ligaments give stability to the joint.

Ligaments of the wrist and hand

The wrist is strengthened anteriorly and posteriorly by the palmar and dorsal radial collateral and ulnar collateral extrinsic and intrinsic ligaments. The extrinsic palmar ligaments provide the majority of the wrist stability; however, the intrinsic ligaments serve as rotational restraints, binding the proximal row into a unit of rotational stability (Dutton, 2012). The wrist is also strengthened laterally by the radial collateral ligament (RCL) and medially by the ulnar collateral ligament (UCL) (Johnson and Ellis, 2005; Moses *et al.*, 2005). The RCL runs from the distal end of the radius to the lateral scaphoid and the UCL from the head of the ulna to the pisiform and triquetrum. The collateral ligaments are active in limiting abduction and adduction at the radiocarpal joint. In adduction, the radial ligament becomes taut while the ulnar ligament relaxes; in abduction the reverse occurs.

Triangular fibrocartilage complex

Further stability is given to the distal radioulnar joint through the triangular fibrocartilage complex (TFCC). The TFCC is formed by the triangular fibrocartilage discus (TFC), the radioulnar ligaments (RUL) and the ulnar collateral ligaments (UCL). The TFC articulates with

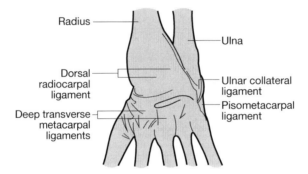

Figure 8.1   Skeletal and ligamentous anatomy dorsal view.

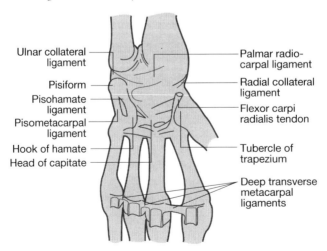

Figure 8.2   Skeletal and ligamentous anatomy palmar view.

the lunate and triquetrum and extends from the ulnar side of the distal radius to attach to the ulnar at the base of the ulnar styloid process (Magee, 2008). The TFCC is important in load transmission across the ulnar aspect of the wrist as it transmits and absorbs compressive forces; however, it can be damaged traumatically by forced extension and pronation and is also vulnerable to repetitive stress and regeneration.

Muscular anatomy of the wrist and hand

The muscular anatomy of the hand and wrist cannot be considered in isolation from the musculature of the forearm since many of the prime movers for wrist and finger actions originate in this area. There are 39 pairs of agonist and antagonistic muscles which work at the wrist and hand (Wadsworth, 1985). However, for the sake of clarity these are usually divided into muscles of the anterior forearm (the flexor group) and those of the posterior forearm (the extensor group), and this convention will be followed below. These muscles can be further divided into superficial and deeper groups.

Muscles of the anterior forearm

The extrinsic muscles provide considerable strength and dexterity to the fingers without adding muscle bulk to the hand. The anterior forearm muscles mainly consist of the wrist flexors and can be arranged into a superficial and deep group.

Superficial muscles of the anterior forearm

Forming the medial border of the cubital fossa at the elbow, pronator teres is the most lateral of the superficial muscles in the flexor compartment of the forearm. It arises from the medial epicondyle of the humerus and terminates on the middle of the lateral surface of the radius.

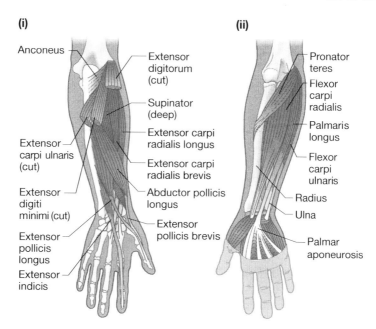

Figure 8.3   Muscular anatomy: posterior (i) and anterior (ii) (source: adapted from Sewell *et al.*, 2013).

Table 8.3 Main muscles of the wrist and hand and their abbreviations

Muscle name	Abbreviation
Extensor carpi radialis	ECR
Extensor carpi ulnaris	ECU
Extensor carpi radialis brevis	ECRB
Extensor carpi radialis longus	ECRL
Extensor pollicis longus	EPL
Extensor pollicis brevis	EPB
Extensor digitorum longus	EDL
Extensor digitorum brevis	EDB
Flexor carpi ulnaris	FCU
Flexor carpi radialis	FCR
Flexor pollicis brevis	FPB
Flexor pollicis longus	FPL
Flexor digitorum profundus	FDP
Flexor digitorum superficialis	FDS
Abductor digiti minimi	ADM
Abductor pollicis longus	APL
Abductor pollicis brevis	APB
Opponens digiti minimi	ODM

Pronator teres pronates the forearm and is supplied by the median nerve (C6–7), while its blood supply is from the anterior ulnar recurrent artery. Flexor carpi radialis also arises from the medial epicondyle of the humerus and inserts onto the base of the second and third metacarpals. Working with palmaris longus and flexor carpi ulnaris, it flexes the wrist and assists in abduction. Also due to its oblique course in the forearm, flexor carpi radialis may aid in pronation (Palastanga *et al.*, 2012). Its nerve supply is from the median nerve (C6–7) and it derives its blood supply from the radial artery. Lying centrally among the superficial flexor muscles of the forearm, palmaris longus again originates from the medial epicondyle of the humerus and inserts into the palmar aponeurosis. Palmaris longus is a weak flexor of the wrist; however, because of its attachment to the palmar aponeurosis, it assists in flexing the MCP joints as it tightens the palmar fascia. Its nerve supply is from the median nerve (C6–7) and it derives its blood supply from the posterior ulnar recurrent artery. The strongest flexor of the group, the flexor carpi ulnaris also originates from the medial epicondyle of the humerus, the olecranon process and the posterior border of ulna (ulnar head). The muscle gains some of its power by encasing the pisiform bone and using it as a pulley to increase mechanical advantage and reduce the overall tension in the tendon before inserting into the base of the fifth metacarpal (Wadsworth, 1985). In conjunction with flexor carpi radialis and palmaris longus, flexor carpi ulnaris flexes the hand at the wrist while assisting in adduction or ulnar deviation. Its nerve supply is from the ulnar nerve (C7–8) and it derives its blood supply from the posterior ulnar recurrent artery. Flexor digitorum superficialis also originates from the medial epicondyle of humerus (humeral head) and the coronoid process (ulnar head) and anterior border of the radius (radial head). It inserts into the base of the middle phalanges of all fingers except for the thumb and it flexes the proximal and middle phalanges while assisting hand flexion. Its nerve supply is from the median nerve (C7–T1) and it receives its vascular supply from both the ulnar and radial arteries.

Deep muscles of the anterior forearm

The flexor digitorum profundus lies deep to the flexor digitorum superficialis on the medial side of the forearm. It arises from the anterior, medial radius and the interosseous membrane, and inserts into the base of the distal phalanges of all fingers (excluding the thumb). The primary function of flexor digitorum profundus is flexion of the distal phalanges of the fingers; however, due to its course it also assists in flexion of the MCP and RC joints. Its nerve supply is from the ulnar nerve (C8–T1), and blood supply is from the anterior interosseous and ulnar arteries. Lying laterally to the flexor digitorum profundus, flexor pollicis longus originates from the anterior surface of the radius and interosseous membrane and inserts into the distal phalanx of the thumb. It is the only flexor of the IP joint of the thumb, and is therefore essential for all gripping activities of the hand. The nerve supply is from the medial part of the median nerve (C8–T1) and blood supply is from the anterior interosseous artery only (Moses *et al.*, 2005). One further muscle in the deep forearm group is the pronator quadratus, arising from the distal anterior ulna and inserting onto the distal anterior radius. This small square-shaped muscle pronates the forearm and is supplied by the median nerve (C8–T1) and anterior interosseous artery (Johnson and Ellis, 2005; Moses *et al.*, 2005).

Muscles of the posterior forearm

The wrist extensors (extensor carpi radialis longus, extensor carpi radialis brevis and extensor carpi ulnaris) originate in the region of the lateral epicondyle and the lateral supracondylar ridge. These muscles are said to have a common extensor tendon (CEO) and become tendinous one-third of the way along the distal forearm. The wrist extensors also offer synergistic contribution to movements at the elbow joint, therefore elbow position is relevant to wrist extensor function and vice versa. The posterior forearm muscles can be discussed in terms of their superficiality and depth.

Superficial muscles of the posterior forearm

Extensor carpi radialis longus lies on the lateral side of the posterior compartment of the forearm and originates from the distal third of the lateral supracondylar ridge of humerus, and inserts into the base of the second metacarpal. Its action is to extend the wrist and abduct the hand and it is supplied by both the radial nerve (C6–7) and the radial artery. More distally, extensor carpi radialis brevis arises from the lateral epicondyle of the humerus via the common extensor tendon (CEO) and inserts into the base of the third metacarpal. Similar to carpi radialis longus, it also extends the wrist and abducts the hand and is supplied by the radial nerve (C6–7) and radial artery. Extensor digitorum also arises from the CEO but then inserts into the phalanges of all of the fingers, excluding the thumb. As its name suggests, it extends the fingers, but also assists in wrist extension. This muscle is supplied by the posterior interosseous nerve (C7–8) and posterior interosseous artery. The CEO is also the origin for the extensor digiti minimi, a small muscle on the medial side of the extensor digitorum which inserts into the base of the fifth proximal phalanx only. It extends the fifth phalanx and is supplied by the posterior interosseous nerve (C7–8) and posterior interosseous artery. One further superficial posterior muscle is extensor carpi ulnaris, which again arises from the lateral epicondyle of the humerus via the CEO, and inserts into the base of the fifth metacarpal. Working with flexor carpi ulnaris and extensor carpi ulnaris, it produces adduction (ulnar deviation) and extension of the wrist. It is supplied by the posterior interosseous nerve (C7–8) and posterior interosseous artery (Johnson and Ellis, 2005).

Deep muscles of the posterior forearm

The only muscle of the deep group to arise from the CEO is the supinator, which inserts onto the proximal third of all surfaces of the radius. As the name suggests, this muscle supinates the forearm and is supplied by the deep radial nerve (C7–T1) and both the radial recurrent and posterior interosseous artery. Abductor pollicis longus originates from the posterior surface of ulna, radius and interosseous membrane and inserts onto the base of the first metacarpal and abducts and extends the thumb. Its nerve and vascular supply is via the posterior interosseous nerve (C7–8) and posterior interosseous artery, respectively. The origin of the extensor pollicis brevis is the posterior surface of the radius and the interosseous membrane and it inserts onto the base of the proximal phalanx of the thumb. Extensor pollicis brevis extends both the CMC and MCP joints of the thumb and is supplied by the posterior interosseous nerve (C7–8) and posterior interosseous artery. Lying deep to extensor digitorum, extensor indicis is the last muscle of the deep group which arises from the posterior surface of the ulna and interosseous membrane, inserting into the dorsal base of the proximal phalanx of the index finger. It extends the proximal phalanx of the index finger and is also supplied by the posterior interosseous nerve (C7–8) and posterior interosseous artery (Johnson and Ellis, 2005; Moses *et al.*, 2005; Palastanga *et al.*, 2012). The interplay between the forearm and intrinsic hand muscles create the complex movements attainable by the wrist, fingers and thumb, while also helping to give the hand its distinctive shape.

Intrinsic muscles of the hand

Working from the thumb to the fifth phalanx, the intrinsic muscles of the hand are arranged as follows: abductor pollicis brevis originates from the flexor retinaculum and the scaphoid and trapezium bones, and inserts into the lateral proximal aspect of the phalanx of the thumb. It is the most lateral and superficial of the three muscles forming the thenar eminence, and its action is to abduct and assist opposition of the thumb. It is supplied by the posterior interosseous artery. Also supplied by the median nerve (C8–T1) and the palmar branch of the radial artery is the flexor pollicis brevis; it originates from the flexor retinaculum and the trapezium, and inserts into the lateral aspect of the proximal phalanx of the thumb. The flexor pollicis brevis is the most medial of the three thenar muscles, and is responsible for flexing the thumb at the MCP and CMC joints. The third and final thenar muscle is the opponens pollicis, which also arises from the flexor retinaculum of the trapezium bone, but in this case inserts into the lateral aspect of the first metacarpal, which it draws forward and medially (in opposition). This muscle is also supplied by both the median nerve (C8–T1) and the palmar branch of the radial artery (Johnson and Ellis, 2005; Moses *et al.*, 2005; Palastanga *et al.*, 2012). The adductor pollicis has a relatively extensive origin from the bases of the second and third metacarpals; the capitate, trapezoid, and the anterior surface of the third metacarpal. It inserts onto the medial side of the proximal phalanx of the thumb, and is a strong muscle that brings the thumb back to the palm from a position of abduction, therefore essential in maintaining the precision grip of the hand (Palastanga *et al.*, 2012). Nerve supply is via the ulnar nerve (C8–T1) and blood supply by the deep palmar arch. Palmaris brevis is a thin, quadrilateral muscle which arises from the palmar aponeurosis. It inserts into, and becomes continuous with, the skin on the ulnar border of the palm. Contraction of this muscle deepens the hollow of the hand. It is supplied by the ulnar nerve (C8–T1) and superficial palmar arch.

The next three intrinsic muscles receive their innervation via the ulnar nerve (C8–T1) and their vascularity via the palmar branch of ulnar artery. Abductor digiti minimi, the most superficial of the hypothenar muscles, originates from both the pisiform bone and the tendon of flexor carpi ulnaris, inserting into the medial side of the base of the proximal phalanx of the fifth phalanx. Abductor digiti minimi pulls the fifth finger away from the fourth finger into a position of abduction. It also helps to flex the MCP joint and is therefore a powerful muscle in grasping a large object with outspread fingers (Palastanga *et al.*, 2012). The proximal phalanx of the fifth phalanx is flexed by flexor digiti minimi brevis, whose origin is the flexor retinaculum of the wrist and the hook of hamate, and the insertion is the proximal phalanx of the fifth phalanx. Finally, the opponens digiti minimi also originates from the flexor retinaculum of the wrist and the hook of hamate, but inserts into the medial border of the fifth metacarpal. This muscle pulls the fifth finger forwards towards the palm and rotates it laterally at the CMC joint.

The muscles of the hand may be remembered using the following mnemonic: 'A OF A OF A' which represents Abductor pollicis brevis, Opponens pollicis, Flexor pollicis brevis, Adductor pollicis (thenar muscles) and Opponens digiti minimi, Flexor digiti minimi and Abductor digiti minimi.

Lumbrical muscles

There are four unique intrinsic lumbrical muscles found in the palm of the hand, and these are arranged in pairs. These muscles are unusual in that they do not attach to bone, instead they attach proximally to the tendons of flexor digitorum profundus and distally to the extensor expansions, therefore creating a greater contractile range. Lumbricals one and two arise from the lateral two tendons of flexor digitorum profundus and insert into the lateral sides of the extensor expansion of digits two and three. Lumbricals three and four originate from the medial three tendons of flexor digitorum profundus, and insert into the lateral sides of the extensor expansion of digits four and five. Lumbricals one and two extend the index and middle fingers at the IP joints, and flex the first and second MCP joints. Their nerve supply is via the median nerve (C8–T1). Similarly, lumbricals three and four extend the ring and fifth phalanx at their IP joints, while allowing flexion at the MCP joints of digits three and four. Lumbricals three and four are innervated by the ulnar nerve (C8–T1). Blood supply to both pairs of lumbrical muscles is from the superficial and deep palmar arches. The lumbrical muscles are essential for coordinating complex, delicate digital movements, especially those which involve both flexion and extension. Collectively they have major functional significance in the dexterity of the hand, which is further enhanced by their rich sensory innervation (Palastanga *et al.*, 2012).

Interossei

Finally, the muscles of the hand are completed by the interossei, which are divided into the dorsal and palmar groups. Both groups are supplied by the ulnar nerve (C8–T1) and the deep palmar arch. Lying superficially in the spaces between the metacarpals on the dorsum of the hand are the four dorsal interossei. These four bipennate muscles arise from the adjacent sides of the five metacarpal bones and insert into the corresponding sides of the proximal phalanges. The first dorsal interosseous is unique in that its insertion is entirely into the base of the proximal phalanx, and therefore it plays a fundamental role in the performance of pinch grips. The dorsal interossei as a group are stronger than the palmar interossei, having twice the muscle mass. Their role is to abduct (palmar) and adduct (dorsal) the MCP joints of the fingers. Situated on the palmar surface of the metacarpal bones are the four smaller palmar interossei. These insert on the opposite sides of fingers to the dorsal interossei and originate from the palmar surfaces of metacarpals two, four and five. It should be noted that the middle finger has no palmar interosseous. These muscles adduct the first (thumb), second (index), fourth (ring) and fifth (little) fingers towards the third (middle) finger (Johnson and Ellis, 2005; Moses *et al.*, 2005;

Palastanga *et al.*, 2012). The interplay between the forearm and intrinsic hand muscles creates the complex movements attainable by the wrist, fingers and thumb, while also helping to give the hand its distinctive shape.

Neural anatomy of the hand

The two main nerves which innervate the hand are the median and ulnar nerves, and these act both as muscular and cutaneous nerves. The median nerve is proximal to the flexor retinaculum and lateral to the tendons of flexor digitorum superficialis, and lies between the tendons of flexor carpi radialis and palmaris longus (Johnson and Ellis, 2005). It then enters the hand through the carpal tunnel, where it splits into palmar digital and recurrent branches. The palmar digital branch innervates the skin over part of the proximal hand, palm and palmar and dorsal surfaces of the medial three and a half digits with the recurrent nerve supplying the muscles above. The ulnar nerve lies superficially to the flexor retinaculum, where it splits into superficial and deep branches. The superficial branch supplies palmaris brevis before dividing into the dorsal and palmar cutaneous branches which supply the lateral border of the hand and lateral one and a half digits. The deep branch supplies the hypothenar muscles, medial lumbricals, dorsal and palmar interossei and adductor pollicis longus. The radial nerve crosses the dorsal surface of the wrist and supplies sensation to the dorsum of the hand not supplied by the median and ulnar nerves (Johnson and Ellis, 2005; Moses *et al.*, 2005).

Circulatory anatomy of the wrist and hand

The hand is well supplied with blood by two main arteries: the radial and ulnar arteries. The radial artery branches at the lateral anterior wrist to form the superficial palmar branch which, on entering the hand, becomes the lateral half of the superficial palmar arch. The other branch runs posteriorly to the dorsum of the hand, where it further divides into the princeps pollicis artery (the principle artery of the thumb). This supplies the thumb and also the radialis indicis artery, which supplies the second finger. It also branches into digital arteries one and two and is the primary contributor to the deep palmar arch, where it terminates. The radial pulse may be felt against the distal border of the radius lateral to flexor carpi radialis, and in the 'anatomical snuffbox' against the scaphoid. The ulnar artery crosses the wrist medially and superficially to the flexor retinaculum, and then divides into a deep palmar branch which contributes to the deep palmar arch. It is the main contributor to the superficial palmar arch, where it meets the radial artery. These arches send out branches which form digital arteries which supply the individual digits.

Venous drainage of the hand follows the digital arteries and then the course of the main forearm arteries. The superficial network is found on the dorsum of the hand which drains into the basilic vein medially, and the cephalic vein laterally, at the wrist. Lymphatic drainage is towards the cubital nodes of the elbow, via lymphatic vessels which generally follow the main venous system (Johnson and Ellis, 2005; Moses *et al.*, 2005).

Grip

Athletes depend on the wrist and hand for adequate strength, grip and range of motion for athletic performance. Furthermore, many athletes are required to hold an instrument or release an object such as a ball, bat, lacrosse stick, javelin or vaulting pole, and this requires precise grip, neuromotor control, strength and endurance. Strength in the hand is most commonly associated with grip strength. A firm grip requires maximum output using the extrinsic muscles; however, delicate actions, such as a pinch grip, use more of the intrinsic muscles to facilitate precise movements. To maintain an object in static equilibrium, sufficient grip forces have to be exerted by the fingertips to counterbalance the object weight (Domalain *et al.*, 2008). Despite the versatility of the hand, there are two main grips that are utilized depending on the activity. These two patterns of movement, which are anatomically and physiologically distinct, provide the basis for all prehensile activities.

A power grip is the maximum gripping force that can be used by the hand, and this requires the fingers to simultaneously flex at the MCP, PIP and DIP finger joints. As the fingers take hold of the object, they are powerfully drawn by the flexor profundus so that they remain in a position which ensures efficient grip. Alternatively, a fine precision grip may only require one or two fingers, and there may be limited flexion at the PIP and DIP joints. The thumb determines whether a precision or power grip position is generated. If the thumb remains in the plane of the hand in an adducted position and the fingers flex around an object, the power position is generated (Jones, 1989; Napier, 1956). The power grip is used extensively within racquet sports, cricket, hockey, rowing and also in athletics for gripping objects such as a javelin or pole. In comparison, a precision (or pinch) grip would typically be required in activities such as darts. Here, the lumbricals and interossei produce and control opposition of the index finger and thumb, which allows the dart to be pinched and subsequently released with defined accuracy.

Therapists must ensure that they specifically address grip strength within their clinical assessment and follow this with adequate rehabilitation exercises to address hand endurance, strength and dexterity in order to minimize the potential risk of functional impairment.

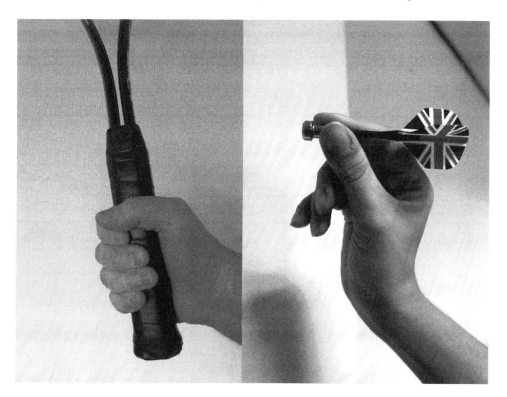

Photo 8.2   Tennis racquet ('power') and dart ('precision') grips.

As the hand does not work in isolation, it is understandable that strength of grip can be enhanced by the position of the wrist and forearm. Waldo (1996) suggested that during gripping activities the muscles of the flexor mechanism in the hand and forearm create grip strength, while the extensors of the forearm stabilize the wrist. During a power grip the wrist is held in extension by the synergistic action of extensor carpi radialis longus and brevis and extensor carpi ulnaris. This wrist position prevents the continued contraction of the long flexors pulling the wrist into flexion and therefore prevents a loss of power in the gripping fingers by 'active insufficiency' of the flexor muscles (Palastanga *et al.*, 2012).

The wrist and hand are capable of many intricate functional movements; however, mobility of this area can be further enhanced by associated movement of other regions in the upper body, including the elbow, shoulder and trunk. A sporting example of this would be the backhand stroke in tennis, which requires simultaneous finger flexion, thumb flexion and adduction, alongside wrist extension radial deviation and supination. These would be combined with elbow flexion, internal rotation and adduction of the shoulder and trunk rotation.

Muscle synergies of the hand

Muscles of the elbow, forearm, wrist and hand coordinate in order to perform common movements ranging from simply opening the hand to throwing an object (Cael, 2010). Synergistic muscular effort between agonist and antagonist muscle groups are required for these movements to occur smoothly and efficiently. Within the arm and forearm, biomechanical constraint can affect independent finger actions. The flexor digitorum profundus has insertions in all four fingers. This multi-tendoned extrinsic muscle, when activated, includes the movements or force production of adjacent fingers when another intended finger moves or produces force (Park *et al.*, 2010).

Practitioner Tip Box 8.1

Muscle synergy of the wrist

Flexion	Flexor carpi radialis
	Palmaris longus
	Flexor carpi ulnaris
	Flexor digitorum superficialis
	Flexor digitorum profundus
Extension	Extensor carpi radialis longus
	Extensor carpi radialis brevis
	Extensor carpi ulnaris
	Extensor digitorum longus
	Extensor digitorum brevis
Radial deviation	Flexor carpi radialis
	Extensor carpi radialis longus
	Abductor pollicis longus
	Extensor pollicis longus
Ulnar deviation	Flexor carpi ulnaris
	Extensor carpi ulnaris

Practitioner Tip Box 8.2

Muscle synergy of the hand

Finger flexion	Flexor digitorum superficialis
	Flexor digitorum profundus
	Flexor digiti minimi brevis
	Lumbricals
	Interossei
Finger extension	Extensor digitorum
	Extensor indicis
	Extensor digiti minimi
Finger adduction	Palmar interossei
Finger abduction	Abductor digiti minimi
	Dorsal interossei
Thumb flexion	Flexor pollicis longus
	Flexor pollicis brevis
	Opponens pollicis
Thumb extension	Abductor pollicis longus
	Extensor pollicis brevis
	Extensor pollicis longus
Thumb adduction	Adductor pollicis
Thumb abduction	Abductor pollicis longus
	Abductor pollicis brevis
Thumb opposition	Opponens digiti minimi
	Opponens pollicis
	Flexor pollicis brevis
	Abductor pollicis brevis

Sports-related movements of the hand

Throwing

Barrett and Burton (2002) describe throwing as *'a unique movement skill, common to a wide range of sports, which allows performers to impact the environment beyond the reach of their body'*. Throwing can be categorized into patterns of arm motion that include overarm, underarm and sidearm. These techniques vary enormously depending on the distance, height and direction of the throw (Palastanga *et al.*, 2012). Throwing requires coordinated movement of all upper limb joints in order to achieve a transfer of momentum from body to ball. The energy for any powerful throw begins in the lower extremity and is transferred through all related kinetic chains to all upper limb joints. Furthermore, for accurate release, the fingers must be under precise neural control in order to absorb the reaction force without injury. During the preparation phase of throwing, segmental rotation occurs from the trunk through to the shoulder girdle. In simplistic terms, the trapezius retracts and depresses the pectoral girdle, while the shoulder joint is abducted by the middle fibres of the deltoid and laterally rotated by the posterior fibres of the deltoid and infraspinatus. Simultaneously, the elbow is extended by the triceps while the wrist is extended by extensors carpi radialis longus, brevis and ulnaris, which all work concentrically (Palastanga *et al.*, 2012).

Catching

In a similar way to throwing, catching also requires substantial coordinated contribution from upper limb joints, primarily the elbow and shoulder. When catching an object thrown at high velocity it is imperative to utilize the other upper limb joints to assist with energy reduction, and this minimizes the stress on any individual muscle within the hand. Chapman (2008) found that by employing several upper limb segments the athlete can achieve a greater range of movement over which force can be applied. Catching also requires synergistic activation of the intrinsic and extrinsic hand and finger muscles in order to control the shape of the entire hand to receive and grip objects. As a consequence of this, the fingers are susceptible to injury mostly through unsuccessful or incorrect catching techniques. Injuries can vary from bruising or lacerations to broken bones, depending upon the direction of force application and its magnitude.

Wrist kinematics

The proximal carpal row act as a mobile segment inserted between the relatively fixed distal radius and ulna and the tightly bound distal carpal row (Tan *et al.*, 2009). During wrist flexion–extension the RC and MC joints synergistically angulate to provide a large motion arc – i.e. in flexion, both RC and MC joints flex, and in extension the opposite occurs. Furthermore, in radial or ulnar deviation, the two carpal rows again angulate synchronously in the coronal plane; however, flexion or extension occurs simultaneously (Tan *et al.*, 2009).

Assessment of the wrist and hand region

Subjective assessment of the wrist and hand

A full clinical assessment of the wrist and hand region begins with a subjective history, but has several unique features. Assessment should be preceded by a brief functional assessment of the entire upper extremity, specifically including the elbow, shoulder and cervical spine. Clearing of these areas can contribute to eliminating any issues such as referred pain from the cervical spine or pain due to the wrist and hand compensating for lack of movement in either of the radioulnar joints or the elbow itself. Evaluation of the acutely injured wrist and hand involves obtaining a detailed patient history that specifically addresses the mechanism of injury, pre- and post-injury state and functional capacity of the hand. Magee (2008) highlights that there are numerous additional questions which should be incorporated within a wrist and hand subjective assessment. These include: What is the patient's age? What is the patient's occupation? Which tasks is the patient able or unable to perform? Which hand is the patient's dominant hand? Such questions allow the therapist to determine a clear direction for the next steps in assessment and for the resulting rehabilitation, and whether there will be any age-related problems (such as osteoarthritic changes). Functional deficits must be investigated.

Objective assessment of the wrist and hand

A thorough physical examination of the wrist and hand is necessary to elicit points of maximal tenderness, assess for strength in the hand and wrist and identify limitations in range of motion, all of which lead to an assessment and determination of the patient's main complaint. The injured hand should also be compared with the opposite hand to determine the patient's normal baseline function. Following initial visual inspection, unless there are any identified contraindications, the patient will be guided to perform all active movements of the wrist and hand (flexion, extension, radial and ulnar deviation, plus circumduction and other combination movements), including forming a clenched fist, followed by passive movements, palpation and any special tests deemed appropriate by the therapist (Hoppenfeld, 1999).

Observation of the wrist and hand

Observation should begin with a thorough inspection of the anterior and posterior forearms, wrists and hands, checking for skin colour, bruising and visible deformities. Chen *et al.* (2009) suggested that the patient's skin should be inspected for any lacerations, abrasions or puncture wounds, as even the smallest puncture wound may be indicative of an open fracture. After assessing for overall appearance, the therapist should closely inspect and compare the bone and soft tissue contours of both upper limbs and note any differences (Magee, 2008). Skin creases should also be noted as muscle wasting on the thenar eminence can indicate peripheral nerve or nerve root injury. Any localized swellings that are seen on the dorsum of the hand should also be recorded and an inspection of the thenar and hypothenar eminences should be conducted to assess musculature. 'Heberden's nodes' are nodular swellings that may be found on the dorsal bases of distal phalanges; and 'Bouchard's nodes' are hardened swellings at the bases of middle phalanges – both are indicative of 'nodal osteoarthritis' of the IP joints, and are more likely to be observed on the older patient (McRae, 2006). The therapist must also observe the condition of the skin of the hand and determine if it is unusually warm or dry. Warmth and/or redness can indicate inflammation or infection, while dryness may indicate nerve damage either at the carpal tunnel or brachial plexus or autonomic disturbance. The fingers should also be observed for any other abnormalities such as 'spoon-shaped' nails, where a concave appearance may be the result of a fungal infection. 'Clubbed nails' are more domed and broader than usual, and may actually indicate underlying heart or respiratory problems (Hoppenfeld, 1999). The most common finger nail infection, paronychia, occurs at the base of the nail and cuticle (McRae, 2006); it may be bacterial (most commonly) or fungal.

Active movements of the wrist and hand

Due to the complexity of the region, it is essential that the therapist develops an efficient, systematic approach to testing both active and passive motion. Passive movement provides information on joint stiffness caused by bony deformity or soft tissue contracture, while active range of motion provides information on general quality, tendon continuity, nerve function and muscle strength (McKenna, 2006), as well as identifying any patient apprehension. In evaluating the range of motion of the wrist and hand, bilateral comparison is most useful in determining the degrees of restriction. When possible, the sports therapist should assess the patient's active flexion and extension of the elbow, supination and pronation of the forearm, flexion and extension of the wrist, and flexion and extension of the fingers (Hoppenfeld, 1999). Each joint or series of joints should be measured in isolation, with the clinician restraining the movements of adjacent joints while assessing the range and quality of each movement. Overpressure should be applied to each movement when there is no significant symptom response. Magee (2008) suggested that if the patient does not have full active RoM and it is difficult to measure the range because of swelling, pain or contracture, the examiner could use a tape measure or ruler to record the distance from the fingertip to one of the palmar creases.

Practitioner Tip Box 8.3

Active movements of the wrist and hand

- Wrist radial deviation 15°
- Wrist ulnar deviation 30–45°
- Wrist flexion 80–90°
- Wrist extension 70–90°
- Finger flexion (MCP) 85–90°
- Finger flexion (PIP) 100–115°
- Finger flexion (DIP) 80–90°
- Finger extension (MCP) 30–45°
- Finger extension (PIP) 0°
- Finger extension (DIP) 20°
- Finger abduction 20–30°
- Finger adduction 0°
- Thumb flexion (CMC) 45–50°
- Thumb flexion (MCP) 50–55°
- Thumb flexion (IP) 85–90°
- Thumb extension (MCP) 0°
- Thumb extension (IP) 0–5°
- Thumb abduction 60–70°
- Thumb adduction 30°

Source: adapted from Magee, 2008.

Passive physiological movements of the wrist and hand

If the patient has illustrated a full range in each active movement, the therapist can apply gentle overpressure to determine the end-feel of the joint in each direction. A springy end-feel is normal and indicates that the ligaments and joint capsules are intact and not restricted by the presence of scar tissue. In contrast, a hard end-feel is usually associated with a limited range of motion in one or more directions and often indicates trauma within the joint, such as a loose body. Finally, an empty end-feel, where the joint moves beyond its normal range without opposition, is indicative of a ruptured ligament or a defect in the joint capsule (Cyriax and Cyriax, 1996). The passive physiological movements should be performed while observing patient response, monitoring range achieved and also watching for the presence of a capsular pattern. At the distal RU joint, a capsular pattern would be categorized as full range, but with pain at the extremes of supination and pronation, and at the MCP and IP joints, the capsular pattern is more limitation in flexion than extension (Magee, 2008). Chen *et al.* (2009) suggest that disproportionate pain with passive movements of the digits is a warning sign of acute nerve compression, fracture or dislocation, therefore a careful approach to clinical assessment is needed to safely eliminate these potential issues.

Practitioner Tip Box 8.4

Normal end-feels of the wrist and hand

- Pronation: tissue stretch
- Supination: tissue stretch
- Radial deviation: bone to bone
- Ulnar deviation: bone to bone
- Wrist flexion: tissue stretch
- Wrist extension: tissue stretch
- Finger flexion: tissue stretch
- Finger extension: tissue stretch
- Finger abduction: tissue stretch
- Thumb flexion: tissue stretch
- Thumb extension: tissue stretch
- Thumb abduction: tissue stretch
- Thumb adduction: tissue approximation
- Opposition: tissue stretch

Source: adapted from Magee, 2008.

Passive accessory movements of the wrist and hand

Passive accessory movements of the wrist and hand should be performed to allow the therapist to identify the quality and range of movement, noting specifically any stiffness, muscle spasm, hypermobility or pain. Passive accessory movements also allow the therapist to grade the range of movement and assist in the decision as to whether to intervene with passive accessory mobilization therapy. The following movements should be tested at the RC, MC and IC joints: anteroposterior (AP) and posteroanterior (PA) glides, medial and lateral transverse glides (MG and LG) and longitudinal cephalad and caudad glides. At the CMC, MCP and IP joints, the following can be assessed: AP, PA, MG, LG, cephalad and caudad glides, as well as medial and lateral rotations (MR and LR) (Hengeveld and Banks, 2005; Ryder, 2006). Following successful completion of all accessory movements of the wrist and hand, the sports therapist should reassess any movements which have been found to reproduce symptoms; this will help to establish the effect of accessory movements on the patient's signs and symptoms.

Resisted movements of the wrist and hand

Muscle tests of the wrist and hand should examine muscle strength, length and isometric muscle testing. The strength of each muscle group should be recorded in a systematic pattern in order to isolate muscles and identify any discrepancies; however, it must be appreciated that there may be compression of certain structures during movement, hence such tests are not always conclusive. Ryder (2006) suggested that a patient may at times be unable to prevent the joint from moving or may hold with excessive muscle activity; either of these circumstances could suggest neuromuscular dysfunction. According to Cyriax and Cyriax (1996), a resisted muscle elicits its maximal contraction while the joint is close to its mid-range position, however, for a more thorough examination of muscle function, the patient should be tested in different positions within the physiological range. Muscle strength will vary between patients; however, the presence of pain or injury to contractive tissue influences the test result. The therapist will ask the patient to perform an isotonic contraction slowly and smoothly, working through the available range of movement and this may be graded according to the Medical Research Council (MRC) scale (1976):

- **Grade 0**: no muscle contraction visible
- **Grade 1**: flicker or trace of contraction
- **Grade 2**: active movement, with gravity eliminated
- **Grade 3**: active movement against gravity
- **Grade 4**: active movement against gravity and resistance
- **Grade 5**: normal strength.

Practitioner Tip Box 8.5

Myotomes of the wrist and hand

Joint movement	Myotome	Muscles
Wrist extension	C6/7	Extensor carpi radialis brevis and longus
	C7	Extensor carpi ulnaris
Wrist flexion	C7	Flexor carpi radialis
	C8	Flexor carpi ulnaris
Wrist supination	C5/6	Biceps
	C6	Supinator
Wrist pronation	C6	Pronator teres
Finger extension	C7	Extensor digitorum
		Extensor indicis
		Extensor digiti minimi
Distal interphalangeal flexion	C8/T1	Flexor digitorum profundus
Proximal interphalangeal flexion	C7/8/T1	Flexor digitorum superficialis
Metacarpophalangeal flexion	C8	Medial lumbricals
	C7	Lateral lumbricals
Finger abduction	C8/T1	Dorsal interossei, abductor digiti minimi
Finger adduction	C8/T1	Palmar interossei
Thumb extension	C7	Extensor pollicis longus and brevis
Thumb flexion	C6/7/8	Flexor pollicis brevis
	T1	Flexor pollicis longus
Thumb abduction	C7	Abductor pollicis longus
	C6/7	Abductor pollicis brevis
Thumb adduction	C8	Adductor pollicis
Opposition of thumb and fifth	C6/7	Opponens pollicis
phalanx	C8	Opponens digiti minimi

Myotome testing

In order to examine the integrity of the peripheral nerves, several tests can be carried out. These include skin sensation tests and muscle strength tests. A loss of muscle strength may indicate either a lesion of the motor nerve supply to the muscle(s) or a lesion of the muscle itself (Ryder, 2006). A working knowledge of the muscular distribution of nerve roots (myotomes) is therefore essential to allow the therapist to assess the severity of the injury.

Dermatome testing

Due to its intricacy, the hand may require more intensive testing; it may therefore be useful for the therapist to return to this area after testing the rest of the upper arm. Examination should take place on both the palmar and the dorsal aspect of the hand, paying special attention to the distribution of the median, ulnar and radial nerves. If an individual nerve or sensory root is affected, all sensory modalities can be reduced. In addition to tests of active, passive, resisted ranges of movement, the therapist should assess the patient's functional movements.

Functional tests of the wrist and hand

Due to the complex operational capacity of the hand, functional evaluation is an important part of any assessment. There is a wide variety of functional tests which can be utilized, some of which focus solely on dexterity, and others which require the integrated use of the upper limb and hand for ADL. Hand functional tests allow the therapist to identify functional limitations, effectiveness of rehabilitation and also suitability for return to sport. For example, the therapist could utilize simple functional coordination exercises, such as turning a door handle or holding a key, which can indicate whether the patient is able to perform a pain-free grip. Simple load-bearing closed kinetic chain and proprioceptive tests can also be employed, such as assessing the patient's ability to perform a four- or three-point kneeling position or a press-up (and its variants), and perhaps utilizing additional challenges such as load-bearing on an unstable surface. These can be progressed to more challenging and sports-related functional tests specific to the athlete and their sport.

Practitioner Tip Box 8.6

Dermatome distribution for the wrist and hand

Radial nerve
- Supplies sensation to the skin on most of the dorsum of the hand

Ulnar nerve
- Palmar aspect of the fifth finger
- Palmar aspect of the medial half of the fourth finger
- Distal half of the dorsal aspect of these fingers

Median nerve
- Palmar aspect of the thumb, second and third fingers
- Lateral half of the fourth finger
- Distal half of the dorsal aspect of these fingers

Grip testing

Functionally, the thumb is the most important digit. In terms of functional impairment, the loss of thumb function affects 40–50 per cent of hand function (Magee, 2008). Grip strength can be assessed using a grip dynamometer, which requires the patient to exert a grip with maximal force; however, the hand should not be fatigued during this test and so the mean value of three trials should be recorded and both hands compared. In addition to this, the examiner may also want to perform a full functional assessment of the patient. This may include testing certain ADL, such as fastening a button or tying a shoelace, which require a combination of movements.

Special tests of the wrist and hand

Special tests of the wrist and hand extend to physiological, neurological and also vascular examinations, to conclude or exclude pathology. Special tests include examinations of soft tissue and joint-related pathology, for the presence of acute inflammation, stress fractures and for underlying medical conditions (Heath, 2010). There are a number of special tests that can be used in respect of the wrist and hand but, as with all special tests, they should only be used to add weight to the therapist's clinical findings, as few are definitive and therefore must not be considered in isolation. The biomechanics and aetiology of the injury must be taken into account before any clinical diagnosis is made (Konin *et al.*, 2006).

Percussion test

The patient sits or stands with the affected finger extended while the therapist firmly taps the tip of the finger. Pain may indicate the presence of a fracture, although this test should not be performed if there is gross deformity of the finger. The 'percussion test' can be modified to simple compression of the finger if a severe fracture is suspected (Konin *et al.*, 2006).

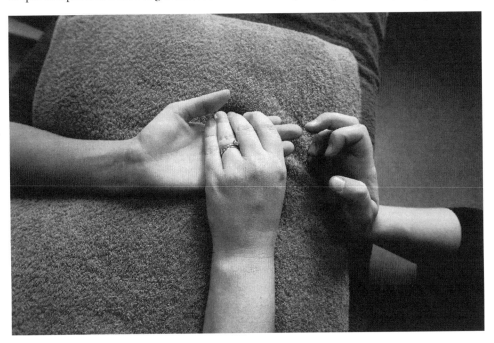

Photo 8.3   Percussion test.

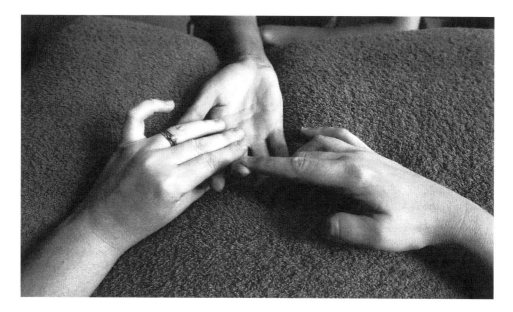

Photo 8.4   Long finger flexion test.

Long finger flexion test

Flexor tests establish the status of the flexor digitorum superficialis and profundus, and determine whether or not they are intact and functioning (Hoppenfeld, 1999). To perform, the therapist holds the patient's fingers in extension – all except for the injured digit. The therapist then isolates first the DIP joint and asks the patient to flex the finger. This process is then repeated at the PIP joint. Failure to flex the DIP joint, but success in flexing the PIP joint, could indicate that the flexor digitorum profundus is compromised, whereas failure to flex either joint indicates a failure of either the flexor digitorum superficialis muscle or both finger flexors. It is useful to check that the joints are capable of full passive range of movement prior to performing this test in order to eliminate soft tissue or joint restrictions (Hoppenfeld, 1999; Konin *et al.*, 2006).

Finkelstein's test

The patient encloses their thumb in a fist. The therapist stabilizes the patient's forearm and holds the patient's fist before gently pushing the patient's wrist into ulnar deviation. To confirm a positive test the patient radially deviates their wrist against resistance. Pain indicates pathology of the abductor pollicis longus and extensor pollicis brevis tendons (De Quervain's disease), which is most commonly a tenosynovitis. The sports therapist must, however, beware of false positive results due to general soft tissue tightness or joint arthropathy (Elliot, 1992; Murtagh, 1989).

Phalen's test

The patient puts the dorsum of both hands together fully so that the wrists are maximally flexed and the therapist applies a mild compressive force to the forearms for one minute. Numbness and tingling in the median nerve distribution indicates carpal tunnel syndrome (CTS), i.e. compression of the median nerve in the tunnel, while more localized pain in the wrist may indicate pathology of the involved joints. The 'reverse Phalen's Test', in wrist extension with the palms this time in opposition, can also be performed in the same manner as an alternative test (Mondelli *et al.*, 2001; Szabo *et al.*, 1999).

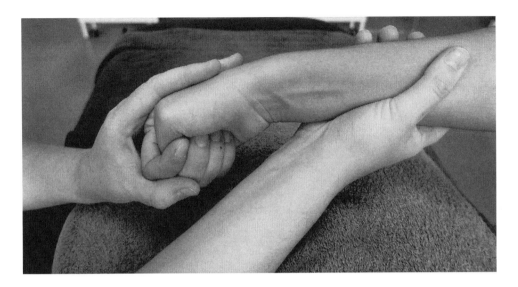

Photo 8.5   Finkelstein's test.

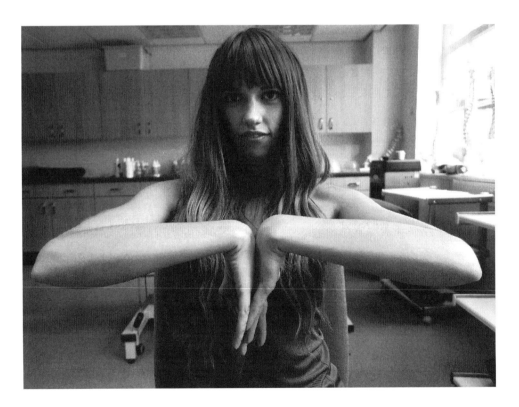

Photo 8.6   Phalen's test.

Tinel's sign

A further indicator for CTS is 'Tinel's sign'. Percussion is performed over the course of the median nerve just proximal to and over the carpal tunnel and at the site of the flexor retinaculum, with the wrist in a relaxed position (20° of extension). A positive test is associated with paraesthesia in the median nerve distribution, or an electric shock-like sensation passing into the hand or forearm (Amirfeyz *et al.*, 2005; Goloborod'ko, 2004).

Various studies have investigated the reliability of Tinel's sign and Phalen's test in the diagnosis of CTS. LaJoie *et al.* (2005) concluded that Tinel's sign is characterized by lower sensitivity in detecting CTS, but false positive results were rare. It is challenging to standardize Tinel's sign as some examiners will use their own fingers to tap the wrist while others use a tendon hammer; the exact site chosen to elicit the percussion may be over the carpal tunnel or proximal to it. In contrast, Phalen's test was found to be the most sensitive procedure for diagnosing CTS, achieving a high inter-rater agreement. Therefore, sports therapists should consider using both procedures within their assessment to gain the most accurate findings.

Allen's test

This test makes it possible to determine whether or not the radial and ulnar arteries are supplying the hand to their full capacities (Hoppenfeld, 1999). The patient is asked to make a fist repeatedly and then hold a clenched fist while the therapist compresses the ulnar and radial arteries at the wrist, using fingers and thumb. As the patient relaxes the hand the pressure from each artery is released in turn and the colour of the hand observed. Any delay (more than a few seconds) in flushing of the ulnar or radial halves of the hand could indicate occlusion of the respective artery. Allen's test should always be performed bilaterally, as a bilateral positive finding is an indication of possible brachial artery involvement (Scavenius *et al.*, 1981; Wendt, 1991).

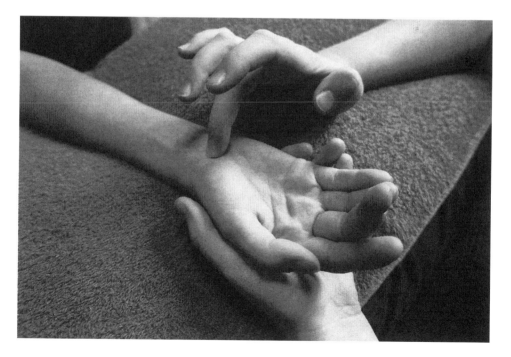

Photo 8.7 Tinel's sign.

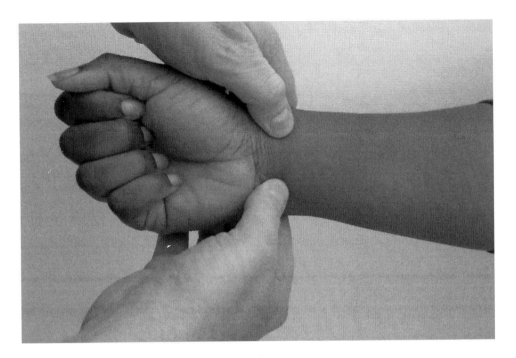

Photo 8.8   Allen's test.

Allen's test is widely used to assess the circulation to the hand; however, its reliability has been questioned and there have been documented cases of hand ischaemia even following a negative Allen's test result (Asif and Sarkar, 2007). Subsequently, it is recommended to employ a modification to the common Allen's test in order to improve reliability. The ulnar artery is compressed using three digits, and then the patient is asked to clench and unclench their hand ten times. The ulnar artery is then released and the time taken for the palm and thenar eminence to become flushed is noted.

Murphy's sign

The therapist notes the position of the third metacarpal (knuckle joint) in the patient's clenched fist. If this is level with the second and fourth metacarpals then a dislocation of the lunate is indicated as this allows the metacarpal to slide proximally (Konin *et al.*, 2006).

Watson's ('scaphoid shift') test

With the patient seated, the therapist stabilizes their forearm at the inferior radioulnar joint. The scaphoid bone is grasped between the finger and thumb of the therapist's other hand and this is mobilized anteriorly and posteriorly while the wrist is moved into ulnar and radial deviation. Excess movement of the scaphoid indicates a carpal ligament tear (Lane, 1993; Wolfe *et al.*, 1997).

Triangular fibrocartilage complex (TFCC) load test

The therapist holds the patient's forearm with one hand and the patient's hand with the other hand. The wrist is then taken into ulnar deviation while moving it into extension and flexion, and pronation and supination. A positive test is indicated by pain, clicking or crepitus in the area of the TFCC (Magee, 2008).

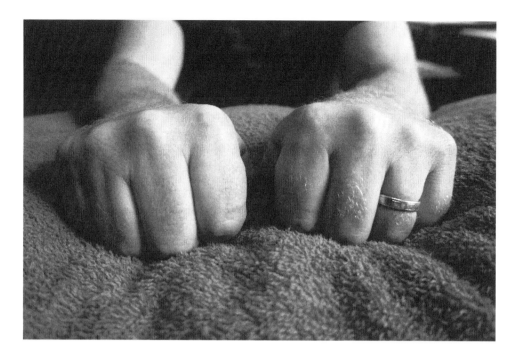

Photo 8.9   Murphy's sign.

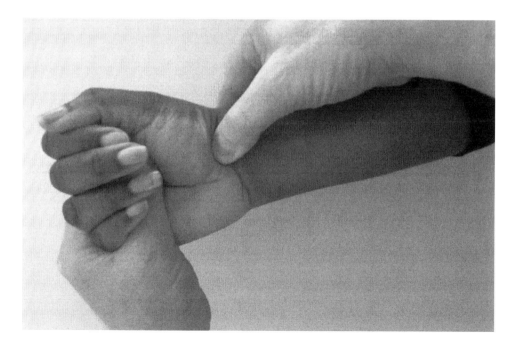

Photo 8.10   Watson's 'scaphoid shift' test.

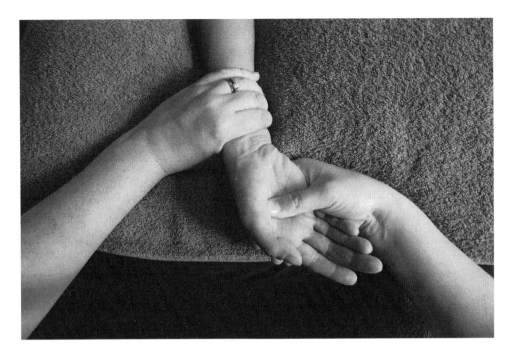

Photo 8.11 TFCC load test.

While provocative wrist tests are routinely used by clinicians to diagnose wrist ligament injuries, there is limited evidence of their accuracy. Prosser *et al.* (2011) compared the reliability of the scaphoid shift test and TFCC load test. The results suggested that both the scaphoid shift test and the TFCC load test appeared to be moderately useful, but diagnostic reliability was very imprecise. Researchers agreed that, while these clinical tests have limited diagnostic use, when utilized alongside MRI they can become statistically significant.

Ligamentous tests

These are usually performed on the digits where each proximal phalanx is stabilized and the intermediate phalanx is forced medially (valgus stress) and laterally (varus stress) in order to gap the joint. This is repeated with stabilization of the intermediate phalanx and pressure on the distal phalanx. Pain and excessive movement (laxity) indicates a sprain at one or both of the collateral ligaments of the IP joint (graded I–III).

Palpation of the wrist and hand

Examination of the wrist and hand must be completed with extreme care due to the complexity and functional importance of the region. The sheer number of joints, bones, muscles and ligaments at the wrist and hand requires the therapist to develop a confident working knowledge of all of these tissues, and how they interact with each other. Palpation will ideally begin with the patient seated and with their forearm, wrist and hand in a relaxed position, with palm facing downwards to enable the dorsal and ulnar aspect of the wrist to be precisely studied (Heath, 2010). Any areas of localized tenderness should be established first, and avoided in the initial part of the examination to help gain the patient's confidence (Waldram, 1999). The basic palpation reference points for the carpal region are the radial and ulnar styloid processes, and

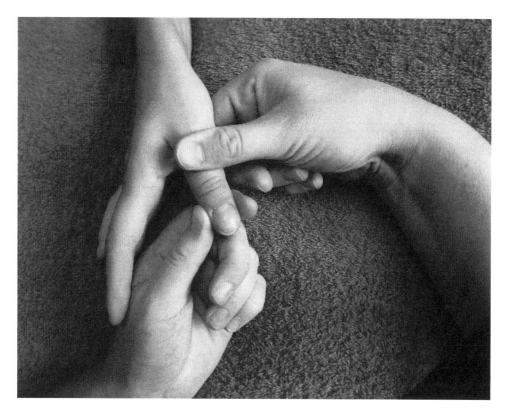

Photo 8.12   IP stress test.

examination should continue distally from here. The radial styloid process is the most lateral bony point when the hand is in the anatomical position (palm facing anteriorly) and is distinguished by a small groove on the lateral edge of the distal wrist crease. The 'anatomical snuffbox' is a small triangular depression located immediately distal and slightly dorsal to the radial styloid process (Hoppenfeld, 1999). The borders of the snuffbox are the tendons of abductor pollicis longus and extensor pollicis brevis (conjoined on its lateral border) and extensor pollicis longus. For palpation of the snuffbox, the patient can extend their thumb laterally away from their fingers, thereby creating a noticeable depression at the base of the thumb. Two important carpal bones can be palpated in the floor of the snuffbox; these are the scaphoid and the trapezium. First, the scaphoid; the largest and most easily fractured proximal carpal bone (Rettig, 2003) can be palpated by moving through passive ulnar deviation of the hand. During this movement the scaphoid pushes against the pad of the palpating finger during ulnar deviation, where it slides out from under the radial styloid process. Severe pain on palpation of this area can be indicative of a scaphoid fracture. Distal to the scaphoid is the trapezium. The first MCP articulation lies immediately proximal to the thenar eminence. The correct identification of the borders of the trapezium can again be achieved through small-range passive extension of the thumb, and here the trapezium remains stationery. On the dorsal aspect of the radius a slight bony prominence (Lister's tubercle) is identifiable. The ulnar side of Lister's tubercle contains EPL, which defines the ulnar border of the anatomical snuffbox. The lunate is palpable in flexion and extension immediately distal to Lister's tubercle, and is commonly damaged by dislocation, fractures and avascular necrosis. In these cases, palpation will usually reveal localized tenderness, and wrist movement will be painful. Distal from Lister's tubercle, the base of the third metacarpal can be palpated. The capitate lies in the distal carpal row between the third metacarpal base and the tubercle of the radius and is the largest of all the carpal bones. The capitate can be located immediately proximal to the base of the third metacarpal (Hoppenfeld, 1999). Proximal to the capitate is the lunate, which can be difficult to locate, however it can be palpated just distal to the radial tubercle. The patient can flex and extend their wrist, moving the bone anteriorly so that the motion at the lunocapitate articulation may be appreciated. The ulnar styloid process is on the medial aspect of the wrist, and is more proximal than the radial styloid process. Using the ulnar styloid as a reference point, the lateral carpals may be palpated. On the distal tip of the ulnar styloid process there is a shallow dorsal groove running longitudinally (Hoppenfeld, 1999). The extensor carpi ulnaris tendon runs through this groove, and can be palpated when the hand is in radial deviation and the muscle is contracted. Distal to the ulnar styloid with the hand held in radial deviation, both the pisiform and triquetral bones can be palpated. The 'pea-like' pisiform can be palpated easily in the hypothenar eminence just distal to the wrist crease on the palmar aspect of the hand (Daniels *et al.*, 2004). The pisiform is located within the flexor carpi ulnaris tendon and on top of the triquetrum, the third most frequently fractured carpal bone. Distal and radial to the pisiform is the hook of hamate, which is located by aligning the therapist's IP joint of the thumb with the pisiform and the tip pointing towards the web space between the patient's index finger and thumb. The hook of hamate then lies under the tip of the thumb, but requires significant pressure as the hook lies beneath the deep fascia of the palm. The hook of hamate has a clinical importance because it forms the lateral border of the tunnel of Guyon, through which run the ulnar nerve and artery to the hand (Hoppenfeld, 1999). The metacarpals can be palpated in order, moving from the index to the little finger. The second and third metacarpals are anchored to the carpus and are consequently immobile, providing the second and third fingers with the stability to perform pinching movements and fine motion (Hoppenfeld, 1999). The first metacarpal, at the base of the thumb, can be found by moving distally from the anatomical snuffbox and feeling for bone continuity; however, the other metacarpals are best palpated at the knuckles while the hand is slightly flexed, causing the heads to become more prominent dorsally. Finally, the 14 phalanges on each hand can be palpated; the proximal and distal interphalangeal joints should be examined for swelling, tenderness and symmetry, and compared to the opposite side (Hoppenfeld, 1999).

Soft tissue palpation

There are six dorsal passageways within the wrist which transport the extensor tendons, and two palmar tunnels which transport the nerves, arteries and flexor tendons to the hand (Hoppenfeld, 1999). The tunnels and structures within them are palpable, and each will be discussed. As explained earlier, the anatomical snuffbox lies dorsal and distal to the radial styloid process. The extensor carpi radialis and brevis tendons can be palpated radially to Lister's tubercle on the dorsal aspect of the radius and this is facilitated if the patient clenches their fist. On the ulnar side of the hand, immediately adjacent to the tubercle, lies the extensor pollicis longus tendon. The extensor digitorum and extensor indicis tendons, lying between the extensor pollicis longus tendon and the inferior radioulnar joint, are best palpable between the carpus and metacarpophalangeal joints with the patient flexing and extending the fingers; or, in the case of extensor indicis; the second finger. The extensor digiti minimi tendon lies directly above the inferior radioulnar joint line, and is elicited by repeated flexion and extension of the fifth finger. Palpation of the flexor tendons can be more challenging in the hand due to the presence of the palmar aponeurosis, which, similarly to the plantar fascia in the foot, provides a covering sheath of fascia to the flexor digitorum tendons. However, regardless of this, several tendons are palpable at the wrist and carpal area. The flexor carpi ulnaris tendon can be palpated at the pisiform bone. It is here that the pulse of the ulnar artery can be found just proximal to the pisiform, by applying gentle pressure against the ulna. Palmaris longus can be palpated in the midline of the anterior aspect of the wrist and is more prominent if the thumb and fifth finger are opposed. The tendon of flexor carpi radialis is situated adjacent to palmaris longus, and is palpated when the patient flexes and radially deviates the hand. One other important area to be palpated is the carpal tunnel, and this is delineated by the pisiform and scaphoid bones proximally and the hook of hamate and trapezium distally. Compression of structures within the carpal tunnel can lead to various symptoms, including atrophy of the thenar eminence due to compression of the median nerve, and this should also be palpated. Normally, it will feel fleshy and mobile to the touch, although therapists should be aware that it may appear more developed on the dominant hand. The hypothenar eminence should also be assessed for atrophy, which can result from ulnar nerve compression (Cyriax and Cyriax, 1996; Hoppenfeld, 1999).

Return to play considerations

As with any injury, the sports therapist must consider several factors before allowing an athlete to return to sport. Specifically at the wrist and hand, such factors may include: the ability to protect the extremity from further injury; the relative stability of fracture or ligament repair; the player's position and sport; and presence of any external social factors (Chen *et al.*, 2009). However, severe injuries, such as unstable scaphoid fractures or distal radius fractures, require the athlete to avoid participation until adequate healing has been demonstrated and the risk of re-injury has reduced. In certain cases, return to play may be possible, providing the injury can be adequately protected. For example, athletes with dislocations of the PIP joint may be able to return to play with 'buddy' taping or splinting within the same game if a stable reduction is achieved; however, this may depend on the player's position, sport and whether there are any other associated injuries. Chen *et al.* (2009) explain how the risks of early return to play are often balanced against pressures related to competition and economic factors, and these can have a significant influence on the sports therapist's decision making.

Injuries of the wrist and hand region

Due to the intricacy of the structures involved, hand and wrist injuries can be complex. Using a systematic examination method, underpinned by confident knowledge of the region's anatomy, can help the sports therapist to avoid missing any underlying pathology. Wherever possible, conservative treatment will be used, but obviously whenever necessary, the patient will be referred to an orthopaedic consultant for medical opinion. Sports-related wrist injuries are relatively common, with the dominant hand being more frequently injured (Hill *et al.*, 1998). Injuries to the wrist and hand may be divided into traumatic and overuse injuries; however, it is important to realize that these distinctions are not clear-cut, and there is an element of trauma in overuse injuries.

Traumatic skeletal injuries to the wrist and hand

Certain clinical conditions will require immediate treatment; these can include the dysvascular hand, acute nerve compression, open fracture or dislocation. The dysvascular hand can be pale or blotchy, and capillary refill may be sluggish. Acute nerve compression is characterized by disproportionate pain relative to examination, pain with passive movement of the digits and paraesthesia or numbness in the thumb, index, middle and ring fingers. An open fracture or dislocation may demonstrate gross deformity, swelling and loss of motion or pain on motion (Chen *et al.*, 2009).

Fractures of the distal radius and ulna

Wrist fractures are relatively common in both athletes and non–athletes; however, the most common mechanism of injury is the result of a fall onto an outstretched hand ('FOOSH'), which is common in sports such as hockey, ice skating and in–line skating (Garnham *et al.*, 2006). As the injury usually occurs at high velocity, there is also a significant risk of concurrent ligamentous injury including damage to the joint capsule; therefore a thorough assessment of ligamentous injury is essential when fractures occur. The most common wrist fracture is termed a Colles' fracture, whereby the radius and/or ulna are displaced posteriorly in a so–called 'dinner fork' deformity. Treatment involves re–alignment of the bones of the forearm and either immobilization in a cast for approximately six weeks or internal fixation with a plate on the anterior (volar) surface of the bones. Following this, treatment aims to incorporate restoration of wrist motion, grip strength and painless loading (Garnham *et al.* 2006; Strømdal *et al.*, 2009).

Fractures of the hand

Onselen *et al.* (2003) recorded fractures of the hand seen in an accident and emergency (A&E) department over one year. The figures considered the population as a whole regardless of gender, age or activity, and showed metacarpals to be the most frequently fractured bones in the hand (although not if the phalanges are considered as a whole). The most frequently injured finger was the fifth phalanx, accounting for approximately 35 per cent of all hand fractures, with the fourth metacarpal being the most commonly fractured metacarpal bone.

Fracture of the scaphoid

The scaphoid is the most commonly injured carpal bone, accounting for 60 per cent of all carpal fractures (Tan *et al.*, 2009), and is often missed on X–ray. The patient typically presents with tenderness in the anatomic snuffbox, tenderness over the scaphoid tubercle and pain on longitudinal compression of the thumb (Chen *et al.*, 2009). Parvizi *et al.* (1998) suggested that these clinical signs are 100 per cent sensitive but lack specificity; therefore therapists should use these three tests in combination to improve specificity while maintaining 100 per cent sensitivity.

If the above symptoms are present, even if X–ray is inconclusive, the wrist should be immobilized, with a follow–up X–ray after 12–14 days to confirm the presence (or absence) of the fracture (Rettig, 2003). Alternatively, the patient can use a rigid thumb spica strapping when not playing or training, and a brace during sports activities. Since the pain from scaphoid fractures can be relatively moderate, players will often ignore symptoms to avoid missing participation, therefore prolonging treatment, and this may occasionally result in malunion or non–union of the bone, requiring a bone graft. In some cases, patients may develop a fibrous (i.e. non–bony) union and this can result in a much higher risk of eventual osteoarthritis of the wrist, significantly affecting wrist and hand biomechanics (Farnell and Dickson, 2010). Avascular necrosis (AVN) is another common complication which is associated with a disruption in blood supply to the distal bony segment of the scaphoid. Wong *et al.* (2005) found that 35 per cent of scaphoid fracture patients presented with an associated carpal ligament or TFCC injury. Various researchers have suggested that many patients with scaphoid fractures will experience some associated intercarpal soft tissue injury (Ho *et al.*, 2000); however, the incidence and severity of these injuries is determined by the energy of trauma. With any fracture, especially for those patients presenting following a traumatic mechanism of injury, there is a high probability of associated soft tissue damage, so this must not be overlooked.

Fracture of the lunate

Acute fractures of the lunate are rare; however, athletes may be seen with Kienböck's disease or AVN of the lunate often due to repetitive trauma typical to activities such as racquet sports or gymnastics (Rettig, 2003). Physical findings of these fractures include tenderness over the lunate or at the radial carpal area, decreased range of movement and decreased grip strength, with the fracture not always evident on X-ray, and only on MRI with difficulty. Treatment is also often challenging, with non-conservative intervention often required in the form of arthrodesis (operative fixation) of the lunate to one or more carpal bones if conservative management (initially with immobilization) is unsuccessful.

Fracture of the hook of hamate

This fracture is relatively rare, accounting for around 2 per cent of carpal fractures (Briones and Mack Aldridge, 2010), with two possible mechanisms suggested for an acute fracture. The first and most common cause is a 'FOOSH'; the second is impact of the hypothenar eminence on the handle of a golf club, baseball bat or similar (Briones and Mack Aldridge, 2010; Garnham *et al.*, 2006). Diagnosis is challenging as often the only clinical finding is pain and tenderness of the hypothenar eminence; however, if pain is presented on resisted fifth finger flexion, a fracture is likely as the hook acts as a pulley for the tendon of flexor digitorum profundus. Treatment normally consists of a period of immobilization, although surgical excision of the hook is also an option if pain persists (Briones and Mack Aldridge, 2010; Rettig, 2003).

Fractures of the metacarpals and phalanges

Metacarpal and phalangeal fractures are often the result of direct trauma, such as a crush injury. In sport, these injuries represent around 24 per cent of all such fractures in all age groups, but 44 per cent in under-18s (Stanton *et al.*, 2007). Treatment, as with other fractures, consists of immobilization or bracing, and non-conservative intervention may be required in cases of extreme displacement or non-union. One consideration here is that there is often significant soft tissue damage within the hand, so early mobilization of fingers may need to be considered in such cases.

Traumatic soft tissue injuries of the wrist and hand

Ulnar collateral ligament sprain ('Skier's thumb')

Injury of the ulnar collateral ligament (UCL) of the first MCP joint is commonly caused by excessive radial deviation of the thumb (Baskies *et al.*, 2007). This injury, although commonly termed 'skier's thumb' (because of the prevalence of fall injuries in skiing which occur while gripping a ski pole), is frequently seen in other sports such as basketball and hockey, where the MCP joint is forced into abduction and hyperextension. Patients typically present with pain and swelling on the palmar aspect of the thumb joint, and will often complain of weakness in pinch grip. The spectrum of UCL injuries can range from a minor grade I sprain, to a grade II partial-thickness tear or full-thickness/complete tear. The following characteristics, as described by Rhee and Cobiella (2007), offer useful classification.

- Grade I: no laxity; pain; minor sprain.
- Grade II: increased laxity with a firm end point; pain; partial thickness tear.
- Grade III: increased laxity with no tensional end-feel; complete tear.

For conservative management, preventative taping can be effective in aiding thumb joint stability, preventing further injury and facilitating early healing. Alternatively, a thumb brace may provide a more durable form of wrist support (Heath, 2010). UCL injuries can be treated with a thumb spica splint, which allows for movement at the IP joint. In addition, grip and thumb strengthening devices can be useful in restoring normal hand and thumb motion.

Referral to an orthopaedic consultant is highly recommended for suspected complete tear of the UCL in order to maximize functional outcomes and offset any long-term disability.

UCL injuries are often associated with other findings, including bony avulsion, volar plate injuries and 'Stener lesions'. Baskies *et al.* (2007) defined Stener lesions as an adductor aponeurosis interposition between the distally avulsed ulnar-collateral ligament and the ligament's insertion into the base of the proximal phalanx of the thumb. Rhee and Cobiella (2007) reported that Stener lesions are observed in many cases of complete rupture of the UCL, with the incidence occurring in 14–87 per cent of cases. In these circumstances, operative intervention is nearly always necessary.

Radial collateral ligament sprain

Injuries to the radial collateral ligament (RCL) are less common than those of the UCL. Diagnosis of RCL rupture is usually confirmed by radial deviation of the proximal phalanx of the thumb; where a deviation of <20° indicates a partial rupture and >20° indicates a complete rupture. Healing usually occurs within 4–6 weeks and immobilization is usually required (Edelstein *et al.*, 2008), followed by progressive clinical therapy and rehabilitation.

Triangular fibrocartilage complex (TFCC) injury

Tears to the TFCC are common in racquet sports such as tennis or badminton, and those that require wrist hyperextension, such as gymnastics, or power gripping activities such as in weight-lifting, golf or rowing. Patients often present with a painful, clicking, weak and unstable wrist. Testing for the TFCC requires the patient to place their wrist in extension and ulnar deviation and then rotate; this movement, as in the forehand volley, relates to overloading of the complex (Heath, 2010). Physical examination of TFCC tears may be associated with tenderness in the ulnar fovea; in addition there may be tenderness along the extensor carpi ulnaris, as its sheath is continuous with the TFCC. The cartilage and ligaments comprising the TFCC are relatively avascular and healing can be complex and protracted. Conservative management may include splinting, non-steroidal anti-inflammatory drugs (where symptoms dictate), progressive mobility and strengthening exercises. Physiological and accessory mobilizations of the DRU and RC joints may be employed, as well as soft tissue therapy and electrotherapy, following the early phase of healing. Intra-articular corticosteroid injections may be considered in chronic presentations. Arthroscopy is the main option if conservative therapy is unsuccessful. It is important to note that a complete tear of the TFCC is almost always associated with injury to associated structures, such as the extensor carpi ulnaris, distal radioulnar joint or lunotriquetral ligament, therefore the therapist should be aware of underlying secondary pathologies.

Extensor tendon rupture ('mallet finger')

Mallet finger refers to disruption of a terminal finger extensor tendon at its insertion on the distal phalanx. Also known as 'drop' or 'baseball' finger, it is mostly caused by forced flexion of the fingertip in sports such as baseball, cricket or basketball (Rettig, 2004). Patients generally complain of pain at the base of the distal phalanx, and may be unable to fully extend their fingertip, however these symptoms may not develop for several days (Bond and Willis, 2010). Avulsion of a small fragment of the distal phalanx is often associated with tendon rupture, and may delay the healing process (Smit *et al.*, 2010). Treatment of this injury depends on the type; however, many authors recommend splinting of the DIP in extension for 6–8 weeks, allowing free PIP motion.

Boutonniere injury

A Boutonniere injury refers to a rupture of the central slip of the extensor mechanism at its insertion into the base of the middle phalanx, either from forced flexion of the middle phalanx or direct trauma (Matzon and Bozentka, 2010; Rettig, 2004). As above, treatment is splinting the finger in slight hyperextension for up to eight weeks before return to sport; however, in sports such as basketball, football and hockey the athlete may continue to play and practise with extension taping as long as the splint is worn at all other times.

Carpal ligamentous injury

Ligamentous injuries are fairly common and often secondary to a 'FOOSH' mechanism (Bond and Willis, 2010). These injuries are often difficult to diagnose correctly. Patients are often misdiagnosed as having a simple sprain and treated conservatively, which in turn can lead to significant morbidity and loss of function, and so correct diagnosis is essential.

Scapholunate injuries

The scapholunate ligament (SLL) complex is the most commonly injured ligament complex in the wrist, often a result of forced and excessive wrist extension with ulnar deviation and intercarpal supination; it can occur with a fall on a pronated hand (Rettig, 2003). Injury to the SLL complex may be partial or complete, depending on the force and position involved. This injury is common in collision and contact sports or in any activity where a fall may occur. With acute injuries, there is usually significant swelling, decreased range of motion, and tenderness, most marked in the scapolunate area and on the dorsal aspect of the wrist. Patients with SLL injuries often clinically present with similar symptoms to someone with a scaphoid fracture, undoubtedly due to the fact that SLL injuries are a common complication of scaphoid and distal radial fractures (Bond and Willis, 2010). Watson's scaphoid shift test should be used for accurate diagnosis, with a positive indication shown by reproduction of pain and a 'pop' sound. Treatment of acute and complete SLL injuries involves arthroscopy of the wrist to confirm the diagnosis and open repair of the scapholunate ligament (Rettig, 2003).

Kienböck's disease

The disease is a traumatic lesion which occurs as a result of a sprain of the wrist and specifically those which involve subsequent tears of the interosseous ligaments and blood vessels. This disturbance of blood supply, in most cases due to repetitive trauma, leads to progressive weakening and potential decay of the affected lunate, which can in some cases lead to total carpal collapse (Garnham *et al.*, 2006). Therapists should be aware that in the early stages of the disease, patients may present with basic symptoms similar to a 'wrist sprain', including swelling, stiffness and pain over the dorsal aspect of the wrist. However, as the disease progresses, patients may report night pain and signs of synovitis, followed by severe wrist stiffness and mechanical symptoms. For accurate diagnosis, an MRI scan may be required to highlight signs of lunate bone marrow oedema. Conservative treatment is only indicated in early-stage Kienböck's disease; however, as it progresses operative management will be essential (Garnham *et al.*, 2006).

Overuse injuries of the wrist and hand

An overuse injury can be described as micro-traumatic damage to a bone, muscle or tendon that has been subjected to repetitive stress without sufficient time to heal (Brenner, 2007).

Overuse injuries may be the most common category of sports injury that therapists may encounter, accounting for 30–50 per cent. These may be classified into four stages:

1. Pain in the affected area after physical activity.
2. Pain during activity without restricting performance.
3. Pain during activity that restricts performance.
4. Chronic, unremitting pain even at rest.

Diagnosis can be difficult, but in many cases specific syndromes can be identified through physical examination (Brenner, 2007; Rettig, 2009).

Carpal tunnel syndrome (CTS)

Compression of the median nerve can occur within the narrow carpal canal, which is formed by the transverse carpal ligament anteriorly, the hook of hamate ulnarly, the trapezium radially and the carpal and volar ligaments dorsally. Nine flexor tendons and the median nerve pass through the carpal tunnel, which is narrowest in its mid portion, and here the median nerve can easily become entrapped between the wrist bones and the transverse carpal ligament (Conrad *et al.*, 1999). Patients may present with complaints ranging from paresthesia throughout the hand to paresthesia only in the long and ring fingers to the more classic distribution in the thumb, index and long fingers, and a portion of the ring finger (Rettig, 2009). In addition, patients may complain of pain on the radial portion of the wrist and in the anatomical snuffbox (Bond and Willis, 2010). These symptoms do not guarantee a fracture, but their absence makes a fracture significantly less likely. The majority of cases occur without obvious cause and are considered to be idiopathic; however, CTS may also be caused by repetitive application of excessive force increasing compression of the median nerve at the wrist and resulting in hand numbness, loss of dexterity, muscle wasting and decreased functional ability at work (Helwig, 2000). Such pathologies interfere with ADL and are recognized as major handicaps (Domalain *et al.*, 2008). Occasionally the younger athlete will present with acute carpal tunnel syndrome due to significant tenosynovitis of the digital flexors secondary to repetitive digital flexion activities. Other aetiology can relate to abnormality of the palmar tunnel, such as an abnormally narrow tunnel or osteoarthritic change; pregnancy; and associated oedema from fluid retention and the presence of adverse neural tension of the median nerve and more proximally from the cervical spine and brachial plexus. Therapists should utilize Phalen's test, the median nerve compression test and Tinel's test (over the carpal tunnel) as well as upper limb neurodynamic tests to determine clear clinical diagnosis. In many cases, symptoms will resolve with rest, functional education and cast immobilization. There is evidence to support the use of steroid injections in resistant cases. In addition, forearm flexibility and strengthening exercises may be used. It is rare that the young athlete will require carpal tunnel release (Fulcher *et al.*, 1998).

Ulnar nerve compression syndrome

A similar condition to CTS is compression of the ulnar nerve as it passes through the pisohamate (Guyon's) tunnel. This can either result from trauma, where the nerve may become compressed as a result of a fracture of the hook of hamate, through chronic pressure typically seen in cyclists who travel long distances while leaning on the handlebars, compressing the ulnar nerve in its canal (hence the term 'cyclist's nerve palsy') (Magee, 2008), or because of adverse neural tension. Treatment for ulnar nerve compression syndrome is similar in principle to that for CTS, where the therapist should consider activity modification and protective splinting alongside manual therapy and rehabilitative exercises. However, if conservative treatment fails or significant weakness is present, surgical intervention may be considered. If the condition is due, in the main, to cycling and handlebar position, this must be addressed.

Wrist flexor/extensor tendinopathies

Tendinopathies have been described in different kinds of sports, with overuse abnormalities caused by repeated movements (Rossi *et al.*, 2005). Achilles tendon disease in runners and epicondylalgia in tennis players are two of the previously most extensively studied conditions (Rettig, 2004). It has been estimated that 50 per cent of all athletes will suffer a wrist injury in their career and 25–50 per cent of these will be an overuse tendinopathy. These syndromes are most frequently seen in racquet sports, rowing, volleyball, handball and gymnastics (Rettig, 2004).

De Quervain's disease

De Quervain's disease (a tenosynovitis or stenosing tendinopathy) is an inflammatory response of tendon synovia of the extensor pollicis brevis (EPB) and abductor pollicis longus (APL) muscles within the first dorsal compartment (Rossi *et al.*, 2005). It is the most common tendinopathy about the wrist in the athlete and is the result of repetitive shear micro-trauma from the gliding of the APL and EPB tendons within their sheath over the radial styloid. For athletes this is often a consequence of grasping in ulnar deviation, for example, holding a tennis or squash racquet, or due to continuous trauma to the radial dorsal region of the wrist, such as in volleyball (Conklin and White, 1960; Rossi *et al.*, 2005). Rossi *et al.* (2005) proposed three clinical indicators for diagnosing De Quervain's disease, which included pain over the first extensor compartment, tenderness to palpation over the first extensor compartment and a positive Finkelstein test. Treatment for this condition could include taping, splinting, local electrotherapeutic modalities, graded local soft tissue and manual therapy alongside a progressive strengthening programme. In some cases an injection of corticosteroid into the tendon sheath may prove beneficial in resistant cases (Garnham *et al.*, 2006).

Intersection syndrome

Intersection syndrome is a bursitis that occurs at the crossing points of the APL and EPB tendons and the radial wrist extensor tendons of extensor carpi radialis longus and brevis. This pathology is often seen in oarsmen, racquet sports, weight training and other activities requiring repetitive wrist extension (Rettig, 2004). Physical examination would reveal tenderness and swelling at the intersection point approximately 6–8 cm proximal to the radial styloid, and frequently crepitus is noted as the wrist is actively extended and flexed. Both intersection syndrome and De Quervain's disease usually resolve with rest and immobilization, although a steroid injection or even surgery may be required in extreme cases (Rettig, 2004; Witt *et al.*, 1991).

Extensor carpi ulnaris tendinopathy

Second to De Quervain's disease, extensor carpi ulnaris tendinopathy is frequently seen in athletes participating in rowing and racquet sports, especially those where the wrist is repeatedly loaded in extension, such as with the two-handed backhand in tennis (Rettig, 2004). Testing for tenderness over the course of the tendon should be performed by supinating the wrist and having the wrist and forearm in supination and asking the patient to extend the wrist (Rettig, 2009). Most ECU tendinopathy conditions can be successfully treated non-operatively with immobilization techniques, equipment modification, conditioning and alteration of athletic techniques (Allende and Le Viet, 2005).

Wrist flexor tenosynovitis

Flexor tendinopathies are rare in athletes; however, flexor carpi ulnaris tendinopathy has been reported in golf and racquet sports such as badminton and squash (Rettig, 2004). This may be the result of compression of the tendon against the pisiform and the golf club or racquet handle (Helal, 1978). Rest, splinting in 25° of volar wrist flexion and corticosteroid injection into the sheath or pisotriquetral joint have resulted in resolution of symptoms in 35–40 per cent of cases (Rettig, 2004).

Trigger finger

This condition may result from direct pressure on the metacarpophalangeal joint flexion crease from repeated racquet use and is occasionally seen in the athlete. It is diagnosed when the joint 'locks' at an angle during extension and then suddenly releases; with or without pain. Initial treatment usually includes icing and injection of corticosteroid into the sheath; this is the preferred treatment in non-diabetics, with cure rates that range from 36 to 91 per cent (Marks and Gunther, 1989).

References

Allende, C. and Le Viet, D. (2005) Extensor carpi ulnaris problems at the wrist: Classification, surgical treatment and results. *Journal of Hand Surgery*. 3: 265–272
Amirfeyz, R., Gozzard, C. and Leslie, I.J. (2005) Hand elevation test for assessment of carpal tunnel syndrome. *Journal of Hand Surgery*. 4: 361–364
Asif, M. and Sarkar, P.K. (2007) Three-digit Allen's test. *Annals of Thoracic Surgery*. 84 (2): 686–687
Ateshian, G.A., Rosenwasser, M.P. and Mow, V.C. (1992) Curvature characteristics and congruence of the thumb carpometacarpal joint: Differences between female and male joints. *Journal of Biomechanics*. 25: 591–607
Barrett, D.D. and Burton, A.W. (2002) Throwing patterns used by collegiate baseball players in actual games. *Research Quarterly for Exercise and Sport*. 73: 19–27
Baskies, M.A., Tuckman, D., Paksima, N. and Posner M.A. (2007) A new technique for reconstruction of the ulnar collateral ligament of the thumb. *American Journal of Sports Medicine*. 35: 1321–1325
Bond, M.C. and Willis, G. (2010) Traumatic injuries of the hand and wrist. *Trauma Reports*. 11: 1–12
Brenner, J.S. (2007) Overuse injuries, overtraining and burnout in child and adolescent athletes. *American Academy of Pediatrics*. 119: 1242
Briones, M.S. and Mack Aldridge III, J. (2010) Hook of the hamate fractures. *Operative Techniques in Sports Medicine*. 18: 134–138
Cael, C. (2010) *Functional anatomy: Musculoskeletal anatomy, kinesiology, and palpation for manual therapists*. Lippincott, Williams and Wilkins. Baltimore, MD
Chapman, E. (2008) *Biomechanical analysis of fundamental human movements*. Human Kinetics. Champaign, IL

Chen, N.C., Jupiter, J.B. and Jebson, P.J.L. (2009) Sports-related wrist injuries in adults. *Sports Health.* 1: 469–477

Conklin, J. and White, W. (1960) Stenosing tenosynovitis and its possible relation to the carpal tunnel syndrome. *Surgical Clinics of North America.* 40: 531–540

Conrad, J., Valis, K. and Stager, J. (1999) Carpal tunnel syndrome: Or is it? *Medicine and Science in Sports and Exercise.* 31: 376

Cyriax, J.H. and Cyriax, P.J. (1996) *Cyriax's illustrated manual of orthopaedic medicine.* Butterworth-Heinemann. London, UK

Daniels, J.M., Zook E.G. and Lynch J.M. (2004) Hand and wrist injuries: Part 1 – Non-emergent evaluation. *American Family Physician.* 15: 1941–1948

Domalain, M., Vigouroux, L., Danion, F., Sevrez, V. and Berton, E. (2008) Effect of object width on precision grip force and finger posture. *Ergonomics.* 51 (9): 1441–1453

Dutton, M. (2012) *Orthopaedics for the physical therapist assistant.* Jones and Bartlett Learning. London, UK

Edelstein, D., Kardashian, G. and Lee, S.K. (2008) Radial collateral ligament injuries of the thumb. *Journal of Hand Surgery.* 33 (5): 760–770

Elliot, B.G. (1992) Finkelstein test: A descriptive error that can produce a false positive. *Journal of Hand Surgery.* 17 (4): 481–482

Farnell, R.D. and Dickson, D.R. (2010) The assessment and management of acute scaphoid fractures and non-union. *Orthopaedics and Trauma.* 24 (5): 381–393

Fulcher, S.M., Kiefhaber, T.R. and Stern, P.J. (1998) Upper extremity tendinitis and overuse syndromes in the athlete. *Clinical Sports Medicine.* 17 (3): 433–448

Garnham, A., Ashe, M. and Gropper, P. (2006) Wrist, hand and finger injuries. In Brukner, P. and Khan, K. (eds) *Clinical sports medicine revised,* 3rd edition. McGraw-Hill. NSW, Australia

Goloborod'ko, S.A. (2004) Provocative test for carpal tunnel syndrome. *Journal of Hand Therapy.* 17: 344–348

Heath, L. (2010) Wrist and hand injuries. In Comfort, P. and Abrahamson, E. (eds) *Sports rehabilitation and injury prevention.* Wiley-Blackwell. Chichester, UK

Helal, B. (1978) Racquet player's pisiform. *Hand.* 10: 87–90

Helwig, A.L. (2000) Treating carpal tunnel syndrome. *Journal of Family Practice.* 49 (1): 79–80

Hengeveld, E. and Banks, K. (2005) *Maitland's peripheral manipulation,* 4th edition. Elsevier, Butterworth-Heinemann. London, UK

Hill, C., Riaz, M., Mozzam, A. and Brennen, M.D. (1998) A regional audit of hand and wrist injuries: A study of 4873 injuries. *Journal of Hand Surgery (European Volume)* 23 (2): 196–200

Ho, P.C., Hung, L.K. and Lung, T.K. (2000) Acute ligamentous injury in scaphoid fracture. *Journal of Bone and Joint Surgery.* 82: 79–86

Hoppenfeld, S. (1999) *Physical examination of the spine and extremities.* Pearson Education. London, UK

Johnson, D. and Ellis, H (2005) Pectoral girdle and upper limb: Wrist and hand. In Standring, S. (ed.) *Gray's anatomy: The anatomical basis of clinical practice,* 39th edition. Churchill Livingstone. London, UK

Johnson, D., Evans, D.M. and Lee, J. (2008) Pectoral girdle and upper limb. In Standring, S. (ed.) *Gray's anatomy: The anatomical basis of clinical practice,* 40th edition. Elsevier, Churchill Livingstone. London, UK

Jones, L.A. (1989) The assessment of hand function: A critical review of techniques. *Journal of Hand Surgery.* 14: 221–228

Konin, J.G., Wiksten, D.L., Isear, J.A. and Brader, H. (2006) *Special tests for orthopedic examination,* 3rd edition. SLACK Incorporated Thorofare, NJ

LaJoie, A.S., McCabe, S.J., Thomas, B. and Edgell, S.E. (2005) Determining the sensitivity and specificity of common diagnostic tests for carpal tunnel syndrome using latent class analysis. *Plastic and Reconstructive Surgery.* 116 (2): 502–507

Lane, L.B. (1993) The scaphoid shift test. *Journal of Hand Surgery.* 18: 366–368

Magee, D.J. (2008) *Orthopedic physical assessment,* 5th edition. Saunders, Elsevier. Canada

Marks, M. and Gunther, S.F. (1989) Efficacy of cortisone injection in treatment of trigger fingers and thumbs. *Journal of Hand Surgery.* 14: 722–727

Matzon, J. and Bozentka, D. (2010) Extensor tendon injuries. *Journal of Hand Surgery.* 35 (5): 854–861

McKenna, D. (2006) Hand assessment. *Emergency Nurse.* 14: 26–36

McRae, R. (2006) *Pocketbook of orthopaedics and fractures,* 2nd edition. Churchill Livingstone, Elsevier. London, UK

Medical Research Council. (1976) *Aids to the investigation of peripheral nerve injuries.* HMSO. London, UK

Mondelli, M., Passero, S. and Gianni, F. (2001) Provocative tests in different stages of carpal tunnel syndrome. *Clinical Neurology and Neurosurgery.* 103 (3): 178–183

Moses, K., Banks, J., Nava. P. and Peterson, D. (2005) *Atlas of clinical gross anatomy.* Mosby, Elsevier. Philadelphia, PA

Murtagh, J. (1989) De Quervain's tenosynovitis and Finklestein test. *Australian Family Physician.* 18 (12): 1552

Napier J.R. (1956) The prehensile movements of the human hand. *Journal of Bone and Joint Surgery.* 38: 902–913

Onselen, E.B., Karim, R.B., Hage, J.J. and Ritt, M.J. (2003) Prevalence and distribution of hand fractures. *Journal of Hand Surgery.* 28: 491–495

Palastanga, N., Field, D. and Soames, R. (2012) *Anatomy and human movement: Structure and function,* 6th edition. Churchill Livingstone, Elsevier. London, UK

Park, J., Kim, Y. and Shim, J.K. (2010) Prehension synergy: Effects of static constraints on multi-finger prehension. *Human Movement Science.* 29: 19–34

Parvizi, J., Wayman, J., Kelly, P. and Moran, C.G. (1998) Combining the clinical signs improves diagnosis of scaphoid fractures: A prospective study with follow up. *Journal of Hand Surgery.* 23: 324–327

Prosser, R., Harvey, L., LaStayo, P., Hargreaves, I., Scougall,P. and Herbert, R.D. (2011) Provocative wrist tests and MRI are of limited diagnostic value for suspected wrist ligament injuries: A cross sectional study. *Journal of Physiotherapy.* 57: 247–253

Rettig, C. (2003) Athletic injuries of the wrist and hand Part I: Traumatic injuries of the wrist. *American Journal of Sports Medicine.* 31: 1038–1048

Rettig, C. (2004) Athletic injuries of the wrist and hand Part II: Overuse injuries of the wrist and traumatic injuries to the hand. *American Journal of Sports Medicine.* 32: 262–273

Rettig, C. (2009) Tests and treatments of overuse syndromes: 20 clinical pearls – sorting through disorders that commonly occur in the upper extremity. *Journal of Musculoskeletal Medicine.* 263

Rhee, S.J. and Cobiella, C. (2007) Gamekeeper's thumb. *Trauma.* 9: 163–170

Rossi, C., Cellocco, P., Margaritondo, E., Bizzarri, F. and Costanzo, G. (2005) De Quervain's disease in volleyball players. *American Journal of Sports Medicine.* 33: 424–427

Ryder, D. (2006) *Examination of the wrist and hand.* In Petty, N. (ed.) *Neuromusculoskeletal examination and assessment: A handbook for therapists,* 3rd edition. Churchill Livingstone, Harcourt. London, UK

Scavenius, M., Fauner, M., Walther-Larsen, S., Buchwald, C. and Neislen, S.L. (1981) A quantitative Allen's test. *Hand.* 13: 318–320

Sewell, D., Watkins, P. and Griffin, M. (2013) *Sport and exercise science: An introduction,* 2nd edition. Routledge. Abingdon, UK

Smit, J., Beets, M., Zeebregts, C., Rood, A. and Welters, C. (2010) Treatment options for mallet finger: A review. *Plastic and Reconstructive Surgery.* 126 (5): 1624–1629

Stanton, J.S., Dias, J.J. and Burke, F.D. (2007) Fractures of the tubular bones of the hand. *Journal of Hand Surgery European Volume.* 32: 626–636

Strømdal Wik, T., Aurstada, A. and Finsenab, V. (2009) Colles' fracture: Dorsal splint or complete cast during the first 10 days? *International Journal of the Care of the Injured.* 40 (4): 400–404

Szabo, R.M., Slater, R.R.J., Farver, T.B., Stanton, D.B. and Sharman, W.K. (1999) The value of diagnostic testing in carpal tunnel syndrome. *Journal of Hand Surgery.* 24: 704–714

Tan, S., Craigen, M.A.C. and Porter, K. (2009) Acute scaphoid fracture: A review. *Trauma.* 11: 221–239

Wadsworth, C.T. (1985) The wrist and hand. *Orthopaedic and Sports Physical Therapy.* 437–475

Waldo, B. (1996) Grip strength testing. *National Strength and Conditioning Association Journal.* 28: 32–35

Waldram, M.A. (1999) Wrist instability. *Trauma.* 1: 133–142

Waugh, A. and Grant, A. (2010) *Anatomy and physiology in health and fitness,* 11th edition. Churchill Livingstone. London, UK

Wendt, J.R. (1991) Digital Allen's test as an adjunct in diagnosis of possible digital nerve lacerations. *Plastic and Reconstructive Surgery.* 88: 379–340

Witt, J., Pess, G. and Gelberman, R.H. (1991) Treatment of De Quervain's tenosynovitis. *Journal of Bone and Joint Surgery (American Volume).* 73: 219–222

Wolfe, S.W., Gupta, A. and Crisco, J.J. (1997) Kinematics of the scaphoid shift test. *Journal of Hand Surgery.* 22: 801–806

Wong, T.C., Yip, T.H. and Wu, W.C. (2005) Carpal ligament injuries with acute scaphoid fractures: A combined wrist injury. *Journal of Hand Surgery (British Volume).* 30: 415

9

THE PELVIS AND HIP REGION

Anatomy, assessment and injuries

Andrew Frampton and Greg Littler

Functional anatomy of the pelvis and hip region

It is important to recognize the complexity of the pelvic girdle and hip (coxal) joint, but even more so their close functional relationship. This region has a multitude of functions, including local weight-bearing and shock absorption, force transmission for locomotion of the lower limb and transference of body weight, in addition to the complementary roles of regional mobility and stability. Each of these are vital to the performance of athletes in sport, and therefore essential for therapists to understand in order to provide effective assessment, treatment and rehabilitation. The anatomy of the hip and pelvic region is required to sustain the excessive stresses of athletic movement (Norkin and Levangie, 2011), and particularly the high shear and tensile forces acting at the sacroiliac and coxal joints (Tyler and Slattery, 2010). When considering anatomy in this region it is essential not to overlook the complex anatomy of the groin, as injuries in this region can often be challenging for the therapist to diagnose and manage (Bizzini, 2011). The hip joint is intrinsically stable except in situations where there is variation in the acetabular depth and femoral head geometry, which results in more reliance on the surrounding soft tissue for stability (Kelly *et al.*, 2003). Despite the relatively high degree of static and dynamic stability provided by its articular architecture and associated fascial, capsular, ligamentous and muscular attachments, the region is still frequently injured in sport.

Skeletal anatomy of the pelvis and hip

The pelvic girdle is composed simply of two innominate bones, the sacrum and coccyx, and two femur bones. Each innominate is composed of an iliac, pubic and ischial bone. The most prominent anterior structure, visible and palpable on the ilium, is the anterior superior iliac spine (ASIS), which provides attachment for the sartorius muscle and inguinal ligament. Slightly inferior and medial to the ASIS is the anterior inferior iliac spine (AIIS), which provides attachment for rectus femoris. The ilium features an anterior surface (the iliac fossa) from where the iliacus muscle originates, and a posterior (gluteal) surface. Posteriorly, the sometimes described 'dimples of Venus' present just medial to each of the posterior superior iliac spines (PSIS), over the left and right sacroiliac joints. The pubic crest, which provides attachment for the rectus abdominis, is located at the anteroinferior aspect of the pelvis, and may be identified

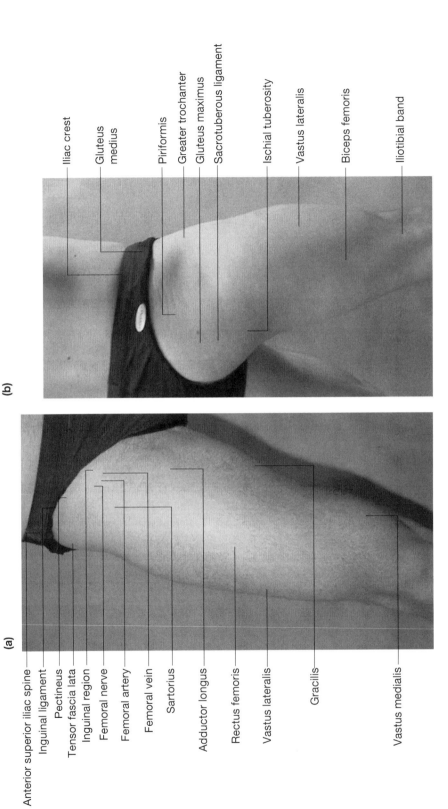

Anterior superior iliac spine
Inguinal ligament
Pectineus
Tensor fascia lata
Inguinal region
Femoral nerve
Femoral artery
Femoral vein
Sartorius
Adductor longus
Rectus femoris
Vastus lateralis
Gracilis
Vastus medialis

Iliac crest
Gluteus medius
Piriformis
Greater trochanter
Gluteus maximus
Sacrotuberous ligament
Ischial tuberosity
Vastus lateralis
Biceps femoris
Iliotibial band

(a)

(b)

Photo 9.1 Surface anatomy: anterior and posterolateral views.

by palpating 15–20cm inferiorly from the umbilicus. The pubic tubercle, where the inguinal ligament and adductor longus have attachment, can be identified medially on the superior aspect of the pubic crest. On the superolateral aspect of the pubic crest is the superior pubic ramus, where pectineus and obturator externus attach. Inferior and lateral to the symphysis pubis is the inferior pubic ramus, where adductor magnus and brevis, and gracilis originate. Located at the most inferior aspect of the posterior pelvis is the ischial tuberosity, which provides attachment for biceps femoris, semimembranosus, semitendinosus, adductor magnus and gemellus inferior.

Practitioner Tip Box 9.1

Skeletal landmarks of the pelvis and hip

Ilium
Anterior superior iliac spine
Anterior inferior iliac spine
Iliac crest
Iliac tubercle
Tuberosity of crest
Posterior superior iliac spine
Posterior inferior iliac spine
Iliac fossa
Gluteal surface
Anterior gluteal line
Posterior gluteal line
Inferior gluteal line
Greater sciatic notch
Superior acetabulum

Pubis
Pubic crest
Superior pubic ramus
Inferior pubic ramus
Pubic tubercle
Anterior inferior acetabulum

Ischium
Ischial spine
Lesser sciatic notch
Ischial ramus
Ischial tuberosity
Obturator foramen
Posterior inferior acetabulum

Sacrum
Base
Apex
S1–5 (fused)
Superior articular process
Sacral promontory
Sacral foramen
Transverse ridges
Lateral masses
Medial sacral crest
Lateral sacral crest
Sacral hiatus
Conus

Coccyx
Cx 1–4 (fused)

Femur
Head
Fovea
Neck
Greater trochanter
Lesser trochanter
Intertrochanteric crest
Intertrochanteric line
Trochanteric fossa
Gluteal tuberosity
Pectineal line

Two palpable landmarks of the proximal femur are the greater trochanter (a bony prominence on the upper lateral aspect), which provides attachment for piriformis, gluteus medius and minimus, obturator internus, gemellus superior and inferior; and the gluteal tuberosity (inferior, and more posteriorly positioned, to the greater trochanter), where gluteus maximus has attachment.

Joints of the pelvis and hip

Although there is a significant articulation between the fifth lumbar vertebra and the sacrum (the 'lumbosacral junction' or L5–S1), and another articulation between the sacrum and coccyx (the 'sacrococcygeal junction'), the three main joints at the pelvis and hip are the left and right coxal (hip) and sacroiliac joints (SIJ), and the anteriorly located symphysis pubis. The coxal joint is a mobile synovial ball-and-socket joint facilitating a variety of multiplanar physiological movements. The joint is an articulation between the acetabulum of the pelvis and head of femur, with approximately 70 per cent of the femoral head in contact with the pelvis (Hamill and Knutzen, 2009). The sacroiliac joints and symphysis pubis are relatively immobile compared to the coxal joints, as these only allow small degrees of translation (linear motion in one direction), rotation (angular motion along an axis) and displacement (angular or linear motion of a rigid body), but still have important roles to play. Medially, superiorly and posteriorly, the sacroiliac joint transmits weight from the spine, while medially, anteriorly and inferiorly, the pubic symphysis functions as a point of central stabilization for both hips (Dougherty and Dougherty, 2008). Transference of force throughout the pelvis is more efficient due to the small movements available at these joints, which reduces the potential for fracture. Articulations, joint types and movements at each of these joints are summarized in Table 9.1.

Acetabular labrum and cartilage of the hip

The acetabular labrum is attached to the bony rim of the acetabulum, and is an incomplete fibrocartilaginous ring which is often triangular in cross-section – although other shapes have been observed in non-pathological hips (Abe *et al.*, 2000; Won *et al.*, 2003). The labrum is

Table 9.1 Joints of the pelvis and hip region

Joint	Type	Articulations	Movements	Comments
Coxal	Synovial ball-and-socket joint	Acetabulum of the pelvis and head of femur	Flexion, extension, abduction, adduction, lateral and medial rotation	Although permitting a large amount of movement, its strong ligaments and musculature make it one of the most stable in the body
Sacroiliac	Synovial irregular plane joint	Postero-medial aspect of ilium and lateral aspect of sacrum	Minimal rotation and translation through all planes of movement	During pregnancy the release of the hormone relaxin allows greater movement at the sacroiliac joint and pubic symphysis to facilitate childbirth
Pubic symphysis	Secondary cartilaginous joint	Medial surfaces of pubic bones	Slight rotation, angulation and displacement	

thinner anteriorly and thicker posteriorly (Kelly *et al.*, 2003), and averages approximately 4.7 mm in width and 5.5 mm in height at its bony attachment (Seldes *et al.*, 2001). Its surface is completed by the transverse acetabular ligament over the acetabular notch; it has been suggested that only the peripheral outer third has a vascular supply (Kelly *et al.*, 2005; Petersen *et al.*, 2003). Evidence suggests that the acetabular labrum has a role in the motion of the hip joint (Suenaga *et al.*, 2002); it deepens the acetabulum (Dy *et al.*, 2008; Narvani *et al.*, 2003; Tan *et al.*, 2001) and increases coxal joint stability (Ferguson *et al.*, 2003; Myers *et al.*, 2011). Some authors have proposed that functions of the labrum are not fully understood (Lewis and Sahrmann, 2006; Smith *et al.*, 2009).

Both the acetabulum and head of femur are covered with articular cartilage, which helps to reduce friction between articulating surfaces. Articular cartilage is avascular, aneural and alymphatic (Poole, 1997), and facilitates smooth articulation and transfer of load across joint surfaces (Eckstein *et al.*, 2006). The cartilage of the acetabulum is thickest at the top of the concavity (Kempson *et al.*, 1971) and is not present inferiorly. The articular cartilage of the head of the femur is thickest in its central sections, and thins at the edges (Hamill and Knutzen, 2009). Atrophy of articular cartilage may occur after long periods of immobilization, and while loading of the joint in sport does not increase its thickness, it may alter the composition (Eckstein *et al.*, 2006).

Joint capsule of the hip

The fibrous joint capsule of the hip is loose but strong, allowing it to be both stable and mobile. The functions of the capsule include: forming a membranous seal to produce and house synovial fluid; maintaining a negative intra-articular pressure; facilitating a vascular supply to the femoral head; passively resisting excess movement; and actively contributing to the process of muscular recruitment and resistance of movement via proprioceptive mechanisms (Ralphs and Benjamin, 1994; Vail and McCollum, 1997). The collagen structure of the hip is similar to that of the shoulder and the elbow (Kaltsas, 1983) and encapsulates the entire femoral head and a significant part of the neck. The hip capsule is composed of both a longitudinal and circular arrangement of fibres, which contribute further to its strength. The superior attachments of the longitudinal fibres are to the acetabular rim and labrum, and margin of the obturator foramen, while inferiorly they attach to the intertrochanteric line, base of the femoral neck and slightly superomedial to the intertrochanteric crest. The circular fibres, known as the zona orbicularis, form a collar around the neck of the femur deep to the inferior aspect of the capsule (Mahadeven, 2008). The capsule is thickest anteriorly and superiorly, while being thinnest posteriorly and inferiorly (Saudek, 1985) because the centre of gravity (CoG) passes behind the joint and there is a tendency for the joint to hyperextend (Ralphs and Benjamin, 1994). The hip joint is reinforced by the iliofemoral, ischiofemoral and pubofemoral ligaments which blend with the capsule.

Ligaments of the pelvis and hip

There are three 'capsular' ligaments which contribute to the stability of the femur in the acetabulum via their attachment to the joint capsule, namely the iliofemoral, ischiofemoral and pubofemoral ligaments, which are generally lax in hip flexion and taut in extension (Kapandji, 2010; Kolt and Snyder-Mackler, 2003; Soderberg, 1986). The iliofemoral ligament is the strongest of the capsular ligaments (Fuss and Bacher, 1991; Martin *et al.*, 2008) and has an inverted 'Y' shape, providing stability anteriorly to the hip joint (contributing to restraint in extension, adduction and lateral rotation). Its apex originates between the AIIS and the acetabular rim, attaching inferolaterally to the intertrochanteric line of the femur. The ischiofemoral ligament provides posterior stability to the hip (restraining extension, adduction and medial rotation) and runs from the acetabulum and posteroinferior ischium to the greater trochanter and posterior aspect of the femoral neck. The pubofemoral ligament is triangular in shape and runs from the superior pubic ramus, obturator crest and acetabular rim to the lower femoral neck (it helps restrain extension, abduction and lateral rotation).

The ligamentum teres and transverse acetabular ligaments have altogether different roles at the hip. Ligamentum teres is a triangular band encompassed by a synovial sleeve, and originates at the acetabular notch from the transverse acetabular ligament, inserting in the fovea of the femoral head. Some authors propose the ligamentum teres has a minor role in restricting adduction (Kolt and Snyder-Mackler, 2003); however, many concur that its function is largely misunderstood (Chen *et al.*, 1996; Kelly *et al.*, 2003; Wenger *et al.*, 2008). The transverse acetabular ligament is a strong, flat structure which continues from the acetabular labrum across the acetabular notch, creating an acetabular foramen. This ligament also has uncertainty over its function; however, most propose it resists anteroposterior widening of the acetabulum during loading of the hip joint (Hak *et al.*, 1998; Konrath *et al.*, 1998; Löhe *et al.*, 1996). There is a lack of cartilage cells in the transverse acetabular ligament's structure, despite its attachments to the cartilaginous labrum.

The inguinal ligament is essentially the thick lower aponeurotic border of the external oblique muscle, and runs from the ASIS to the pubic tubercle (Lytle, 1979). This ligament acts as a retinaculum for structures such as the external iliac artery and vein, femoral nerve and iliopsoas muscle (Moore and Dalley, 2006). Continuous with the deep fascia of the thigh, the inguinal ligament defines the anatomical regions of the thigh and abdominal wall. It also contributes the superior border of femoral triangle, along with adductor longus (medial border), sartorius (lateral border) and pectineus and iliopsoas (floor) (Shadbolt *et al.*, 2001).

Bursae of the pelvis and hip

The bursae of the pelvis and hip function to prevent friction between bony structures and myofascial tissue, as well as between soft tissues themselves. The iliopsoas bursa (sometimes known as the iliopectineal or iliofemoral bursa) is the largest bursa in the body, and lies between the iliopsoas tendon, the superior pubic ramus and the proximal medial aspect of the femur, also functioning to cushion the tendon from the anterior hip joint line (Bianchi *et al.*, 2002). Three bursae contribute to the trochanteric bursa complex; the subgluteus maximus, gluteus medius and subgluteus minimus. The subgluteus maximus bursa lies superolaterally between the gluteus maximus tendon, tensor fasciae latae, gluteus medius tendon and the greater trochanter (Collee *et al.*, 1991). The gluteus medius bursa is anteromedial to the trochanteric bursa and lies between the tendons of the gluteus medius, gluteus minimus and the greater trochanter, while a further small bursa (subgluteus minimus) lies between the gluteus minimus and greater trochanter (Tortolani *et al.*, 2002). The trochanteric bursae also function to absorb the force of blunt trauma to the region (Syed and Shaikh, 2010). The ischiogluteal bursa is located on the inferior aspect of the pelvis at the ischial tuberosity deep to the proximal tendons of the hamstrings, between the ischial tuberosity and gluteus maximus.

The iliopsoas and trochanteric bursae can be irritated during external 'snapping hip syndrome' (Blankenbaker and Tuite, 2006), while a combination of the three trochanteric bursae can be involved in 'greater trochanteric pain syndrome' (GTPS) (Syed and Shaikh, 2010).

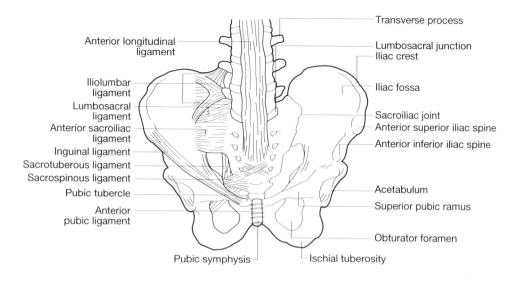

Figure 9.1   Skeletal and ligamentous anatomy: anterior view.

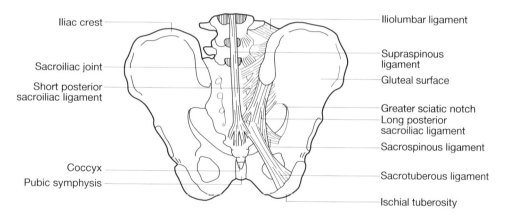

Figure 9.2   Skeletal and ligamentous anatomy: posterior view.

Movements of the pelvis and hip

The hip is a multiaxial, diarthrodial, ball–and–socket joint responsible for flexion, extension, abduction, adduction, lateral rotation, medial rotation and circumduction, plus all combination movements thereof. Accessory movements available at the hip include lateral, anteroposterior (AP) and posteroanterior (PA) glides, as well as longitudinal caudad and cephalad movements. Each of the movements involve articulation of the convex, spherical head of the femur in the concave cavity of the acetabulum, around different axes and angulations.

While there is a certain disparity among authors regarding specific range of motion (RoM) values at the hip, general expectable norms can be ascertained. Flexion and extension occur in the sagittal plane along a frontal axis, with normal active RoM between 110–125° flexion, and 10–30° hyperextension (after going through extension) (Godges *et al.*, 1989; Hoppenfeld, 1976; Mahadeven, 2008). It is important to note the influences of the relative and anatomical positions

531

of the pelvis, spine and knee, as these influence the amount of movement possible. For example, taking hamstrings off stretch in knee flexion reduces the amount of myofascial stretch, restricting full range hip flexion. Abduction and adduction occur in the frontal (coronal) plane, along a sagittal axis, with normal active RoM between 30–50° abduction, and 15–30° adduction, past the anatomical position (Hoppenfeld, 1976; Kapandji, 2010). Medial and lateral rotation occur in the transverse plane, along a vertical axis, with normal active RoM being 30–50° medial rotation, and 30–50° lateral rotation from the anatomical position (Kenyon and Kenyon, 2009; Pressel and Lengsfeld, 1998). Excessive RoM can be indicative of hypermobility syndrome, muscular weakness and atrophy; restricted RoM (hypomobility) may be due to such conditions as arthrosis, local or referred pain, soft tissue pathology (such as muscular damage, tendinopathy or sprain) or mechanical impingement.

The open (loose-packed) position is where the joint is more freely moveable, most unstable and more susceptible to injury (Good, 2000), and for the hip is demonstrated by 30° flexion, 30° abduction and slight lateral rotation (Dutton, 2011). Conversely, the hip is most stable in full extension, medial rotation and abduction (Hertling and Kessler, 1996); this is the close-packed position of the hip, where ligaments are most taut, joint surface congruency is highest and stability maximized (Dutton, 2011). While numerous conditions can lead to limitations in range, flexion is functionally restricted by tension of the posterior joint capsule, gluteus maximus and soft tissue approximation of the thigh and abdomen. Extension is limited by tension in iliopsoas, the anterior joint capsule, and all three capsular ligaments. Abduction is restricted by the pubofemoral ligament, the inferior joint capsule and adductor muscles. Adduction is constrained by soft tissue approximation of the thigh and opposite leg, iliotibial band, superior joint capsule, superior band of the iliofemoral ligament, ischiofemoral ligament and abductor muscles. Medial rotation is limited by tension in the ischiofemoral ligament, posterior joint capsule and lateral rotator muscles; lateral rotation is limited by tension in the iliofemoral and pubofemoral ligaments, the anterior joint capsule and medial rotators.

Muscular anatomy of the pelvis and hip

As a large and stable joint, the hip offers a wide variety of movements in combination with the strength and stability to support the body's weight through stance, gait and all functional and sporting movements. The prime movers for hip flexion are the iliacus, psoas major and rectus femoris muscles. Iliacus originates from the upper two-thirds of the iliac fossa, while psoas major originates from the transverse processes of all lumbar vertebrae and the sides of the vertebral bodies of all lumbar vertebrae, as well as the twelfth thoracic. These muscles merge to create the iliopsoas, and together insert onto the lesser trochanter of the femur. The rectus femoris is the only quadriceps muscle that is biarticular, acting both on the hip and the knee; it originates from the AIIS (and from a groove superior to the rim of the acetabulum), and merges with the other quadriceps muscles (vastus lateralis, medialis and intermedius) at a common tendon (quadriceps tendon) before inserting into the tibial tuberosity via the patella and patellar tendon. Rectus femoris not only contributes to hip flexion and knee extension, but also offers added stability to both joints. The sartorius muscle assists in hip flexion, as well as abduction, lateral rotation and knee extension. Originating from the ASIS and inserting into the anterior medial tibial condyle (as part of the pes anserine tendon), in normal average anatomy this is the longest muscle in the body (Mahadeven, 2008).

The primary hip extensor is the large gluteus maximus muscle, which is also the most superficial of the gluteal group, originating at the posterior gluteal line and the posterior surface of the lower part of the sacrum; its broad attachment incorporates the iliotibial band and gluteal tuberosity. The hamstrings muscle group (excluding short head of bicep femoris) also assist in hip extension, as they are biaxial and act on the hip and also flex the knee. The semimembranosus, semitendinosus and biceps femoris (long head) all originate from the tuberosity of the ischium and insert to the tibia (semimembranosus and semitendinosus) or to the head of fibula (bicep femoris).

Abduction is primarily controlled by gluteus medius and minimus. Gluteus minimus originates from the external surface of the ilium, inserting onto the anterior border of the greater trochanter; gluteus medius also originates from the external surface of the ilium (below medius) and inserts to the lateral aspect of the greater trochanter. The iliotibial band is also on the lateral aspect of the hip, and is a non-contractile fibrous fascia that runs down the lateral aspect of the leg from the anterolateral iliac crest to the lateral condyle of the tibia (at Gerdy's tubercle). This band offers stability to both the hip and knee, and is tensioned by both gluteus maximus and tensor fascia lata.

The primary agonists for adduction are the adductor group, comprising adductor longus, brevis and magnus, assisted by pectineus and gracilis. All of the adductors originate from the pubic rami or pubic symphysis (gracilis), and are distributed onto the femur at the pectineal line of the femur (pectineus), medial to the gluteal tuberosity, middle supracondylar ridge and adductor tubercle (adductor magnus), distal two-thirds of the pectineal line (adductor brevis), middle third of the linea aspera, and the anterior medial tibial condyle (gracilis).

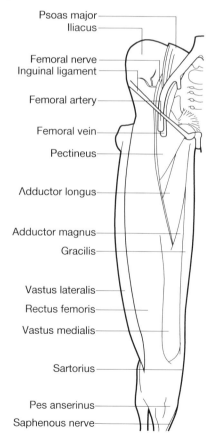

Psoas major
Iliacus
Femoral nerve
Inguinal ligament
Femoral artery
Femoral vein
Pectineus
Adductor longus
Adductor magnus
Gracilis
Vastus lateralis
Rectus femoris
Vastus medialis
Sartorius
Pes anserinus
Saphenous nerve

Figure 9.3 Muscular anatomy anterior view.

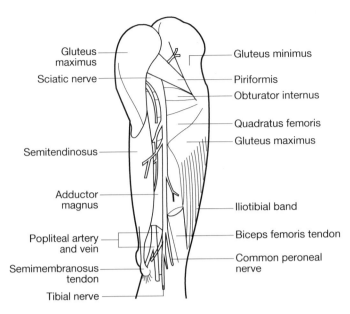

Figure 9.4   Muscular anatomy posterior view.

Table 9.2 Muscular synergy of the hip

Muscle group	Muscles
Hip flexors	Primary: iliopsoas, sartorius, tensor fascia lata, rectus femoris, adductor longus, pectineus Secondary: adductor brevis, gracilis, gluteus minimus
Hip extensors	Primary: gluteus maximus, adductor magnus, biceps femoris, semimembranosus, semitendinosus Secondary: gluteus medius, adductor magnus
Hip abductors	Primary: gluteus medius, gluteus minimus, tensor fascia lata Secondary: piriformis, sartorius, rectus femoris
Hip adductors	Primary: pectineus, adductor longus, gracilis, adductor brevis, adductor magnus Secondary: biceps femoris, gluteus maximus, quadratus femoris, obturator externus
Hip medial rotators	Primary: n/a Secondary: gluteus minimus, gluteus medius, tensor fascia lata, adductor longus, adductor brevis, pectineus, adductor magnus, piriformis
Hip lateral rotators	Primary: gluteus maximus, piriformis, obturator internus, gemellus superior, gemellus inferior, quadratus femoris Secondary: gluteus medius, gluteus minimus, obturator externus, sartorius, biceps femoris

Source: adapted from Neumann, 2010.

There are no obvious absolute prime movers for internal (medial) rotation, although there are several secondary muscles that work in partnership to create this movement, including; gluteus medius and minimus, adductor longus and brevis, as well as tensor fascia lata, semimembranosus and semitendinosus. Piriformis becomes an internal rotator when the hip is flexed above 60°.

External (lateral) rotation of the hip is also performed by differing muscles on the lateral aspect of the hip. The main muscles offering lateral rotation are gluteus maximus and the piriformis. Piriformis originates from the sacrum (anterior pelvic surface) and inserts onto the superior aspect of the greater trochanter. Inferior to piriformis are gemellus inferior and superior, obturator internus and externus, and quadratus femoris. The lateral rotator muscle group also assists in abduction (piriformis, obturator internus and gemellus superior and inferior) and adduction (obturator externus).

Neural anatomy of the pelvis and hip

The peripheral nerve supply to the hip originates from the lumbar plexus and the sacral plexus. The femoral nerve is the largest nerve originating from the lumbar plexus (L2–4); it descends anteriorly through fibres of psoas and emerges on the lateral aspect between psoas and iliacus. The nerve passes through the femoral triangle, innervating the primary hip flexors (iliopsoas and rectus femoris) and secondary hip flexors (pectineus and sartorius). The femoral nerve then splits into its component parts; the anterior compartment containing the anterior cutaneous branches and muscular branches, while the posterior division contains the saphenous nerve and the muscular branches (Mahadeven, 2008). Also from the lumbar plexus (L2–4) the obturator nerve divides and descends anteromedially, innervating the adductors (longus, brevis, magnus, gracilis and pectineus).

The sciatic nerve is the major nerve that runs down the posterior buttock and leg, and stems from the sacral plexus. Originating from L4–S3, it runs laterally and inferiorly between the greater trochanter and the ischial tuberosity. The sciatic nerve then proceeds vertically downwards in the midline of the posterior thigh until it divides into the common peroneal and tibial nerves, just superior to the popliteal fossa (Mahadeven, 2008). The sciatic nerve innervates the majority of the muscles and skin of the posterior thigh (biceps femoris, semimembranosus, semitendinosus and the hamstring part of the adductor magnus), but its divisions continue on to supply the lower leg and foot. The posterior muscles of the hip are innervated by the superior and inferior gluteal nerves of the sacral plexus. The largest gluteal muscle (gluteus maximus) is innervated by the inferior gluteal nerve, while gluteus medius, minimus and tensor fascia lata are innervated by the superior gluteal nerve.

Vascular anatomy of the pelvis and hip

The primary artery responsible for the vascularity of the hip is the femoral artery, which supplies the anterior compartment of the hip. Branching from the external iliac artery, it descends anteriorly into the lateral femoral circumflex artery. In the event of a major cardiac emergency or traumatic sports injury, the femoral artery allows for a strong, reliable pulse to be taken from the mid-inguinal point, halfway between the pubic symphysis and anterior superior iliac spine (Hill and Smith, 1990).

Practitioner Tip Box 9.2

Neural and vascular structures in the femoral triangle

The femoral triangle is significant in that vital vascular and neural structures pass through it. Care should be taken on palpation, when undertaking manual therapy in the region and when looking for major bleeds. Structures passing through the femoral triangle include: the terminal branch of the femoral nerve, the femoral branch of the genitofemoral nerve and the lateral cutaneous nerve, as well as the femoral artery, vein and the femoral canal.

The major blood supply for the femoral head is via the circumflex or retinacular arteries; further blood supply to the femoral head is through the artery housed within ligamentum teres. If blood supply of the femoral head is disrupted (most commonly through intracapsular fractures) avascular necrosis may ensue.

Applied anatomy of the pelvis and hip

Functional relationships

The structures surrounding the pelvis have a strong correlation of function and therefore dysfunction (Brown *et al.*, 2004; Domb *et al.*, 2009; Longjohn and Dorr, 1998; Reiman *et al.*, 2009; Scopp and Moorman, 2001). Movements of the hip have direct relationships with both the SIJ and the lumbar spine, with movements often occurring at all three to assist with primary motion of the hip (Reiman *et al.*, 2009). If the patient has reduced RoM, for whatever reason, in either their hip, lumbar spine or SIJ, this will have an effect on the other two, which need to compensate for the hypomobility.

The relationships between muscle groups must be harmonious due to the large number of muscular attachments to the pelvis, sacrum and proximal femur. When working together they offer the hip dynamic stability as well as active movement. The adductor muscles offer medial stability, with the gluteal group offering lateral stability. Evidence suggests a relationship exists between gluteus medius weakness and adductor muscle tightness and patella femoral pain syndrome (Aminaka and Gribble, 2008; Reiman *et al.*, 2009). Studies have also demonstrated that hip muscle activation controls forces in not only the hip and pelvic region, but also the entire leg (Bobbert and Van Zandwijk, 1999).

Coxa vara and coxa valga

The structure of the proximal femur (in particular, the neck–shaft angle) enhances the stability and congruency of the coxal joint, and contributes towards the mechanics of the whole lower limb. This 'angle of inclination' is a measurement between the neck and shaft of femur in the sagittal plane and is usually between 90–135° (Nordin and Frankel, 2012). If there is an excessive angle of inclination it is termed 'coxa valga'; and a reduced angle is known as 'coxa vara'. Coxa valga will lengthen the limb, and when presenting unilaterally can potentially cause leg length discrepancy, inhibition of abductor muscle efficiency, increased load on the femoral head and decreased stress on the femoral neck (Soderberg, 1986; Spencer, 1978). In coxa vara the opposite effects on the limb will be seen, and it is more commonly seen in athletic females than males (Nyland *et al.*, 2004). Coxa vara can contribute to a genu valgus ('knock-knee') presentation and an increased quadriceps angle (Q-angle); and coxa valga can contribute to a genu varus posture ('bow-legged').

Anteversion and retroversion

Anteversion is the torsional leaning forwards of the femoral neck from the shaft and is measured by the angle made by the femoral neck with the femoral condyles. It has been suggested that the degree of femoral and acetabular rotation is determined by foetal position in the uterus during pregnancy (Hattam and Smeatham, 2010). Between 8–15° of anteversion is considered normal in adults (Magee, 2008); however, an excessive medial torsion beyond this value leads to excessive anteversion where the degree of forward projection from the frontal plane is greater than 15°. Excessive anteversion may cause toeing in at the feet, increased medial femoral and tibial rotation personified by 'squinting' patellae (medially rotated patellae) and subtalar pronation (Riegger-Krugh and Keysor, 1996; Tonnis and Heinecke, 1999). An increased

Q-angle in conjunction with increased anteversion has been strongly linked with overuse knee injuries (Cowan *et al.*, 1996; Eckhoff *et al.*, 1994; Waryasz and McDermott, 2008). The converse is excessive lateral femoral torsion (degree of projection less than 8°: retroversion), which is the leaning backwards of the femoral neck from the shaft. This may also be caused by acetabular retroversion rather than a decreased femoral neck angle (Reynolds *et al.*, 1999), as well as a slipped upper femoral epiphysis, coxa vara, a deep acetabulum or congenital dysplasia (Hattam and Smeatham, 2010). Excessive retroversion would present with the opposite postural dysfunctions to those of anteversion, that is with so-called 'frog-eye' patellae (laterally rotated), instead of squinting, and subtalar supination rather than pronation, for example.

Q-angle and the hip

The quadriceps angle (Q-angle) is a static linear measure taken from one line drawn from the ASIS through the midpoint of the patella, and another from the tibial tuberosity though the midpoint of the patella (Brattstroem, 1964; Greene *et al.*, 2001). Gender differences in this angle have been observed; two reasons suggested for this disparity include the wider pelvic shapes of women (Lyon *et al.*, 1988) and gender height differences (Grelsamer *et al.*, 2005). Other authors have suggested there are minimal differences between sexes (Livingstone and Mandigo, 1999; Skalley *et al.*, 1993). Some researchers have considered that Q-angles greater than 15° may present risk for pathology (Horton and Hall, 1989; Messier *et al.* 1991), although this has not been substantiated in more recent literature. Abnormal Q-angles have been cited as being contributors to lower limb injuries such as stress fractures (Cowan *et al.*, 1996), patellofemoral pain syndrome (PFPS) (Nguyen *et al.*, 2009; Powers, 2003; Tomisch *et al.*, 1996), chondromalacia patella (Aglietti *et al.*, 1983), as well as possible relationships with ankle inversion injuries (Shambaugh *et al.*, 1991). However, the aetiological influence on sports injuries remains controversial as the Q-angle's contribution dynamically is yet to be investigated (Park and Stefanyshyn, 2011). A systematic review into the reliability and validity of Q-angle measurement by Smith *et al.* (2008) found that disagreement exists in methods of clinical measurement, and questioned previously cited relationships to pathology and its significance in clinical assessment.

Male and female differences

Genetic differences in the structure and function of the human anatomy have been well researched and are certainly evident at the pelvis and hip. Researchers have suggested females exhibit larger structural measures such as an anterior pelvic tilt (Medina McKeon and Hertel, 2009), increased femoral anteversion (Medina McKeon *et al.*, 2010; Nguyen and Shultz, 2007) and increased Q-angle (Horton and Hall, 1989; Woodland and Francis, 1992). There are extensive sexual differences in the pelvic shape of men and women, including overall dimensions and more pronounced bony landmarks and generally increased weight mass in men (Mahadeven, 2008). Differences also exist between genders in measures of active RoM (Simoneau *et al.*, 1998) and functional movement (Lephart *et al.*, 2002; Zeller *et al.*, 2003). Muscular strength differences have also been noted, with females having significantly weaker hip abductors and external rotators (Heinert *et al.*, 2008). Other research has shown that males exhibit greater peak isometric and isokinetic strength measures for the hip compared to females (Claiborne *et al.*, 2006; Jacobs and Mattacola, 2005; Wilson *et al.*, 2006). Insufficient hip abduction strength may not be appropriate to resist the external abduction moments at the knee during repetitive athletic movements, predisposing women to knee problems such as ACL injuries (Ireland *et al.*, 2003; Leetun *et al.*, 2004) and patellofemoral pain (Cichanowski *et al.*, 2007).

Sports-related biomechanics at the hip

The hip plays a vital role in gait and represents the junction between passenger (trunk) and locomotor (legs) units of the body (Perry, 1992). The musculature of the hip is fundamental for stability and initiation of movement and limb control in all manner of multiplanar movements, including running, lunging, squatting, turning and jumping. For example, the hip abductors work eccentrically to prevent excessive hip adduction and internal rotation (Lyons *et al.*, 1983); concentrically to produce physiological abduction of the hip; and isometrically to stabilize a standing leg. The pelvis and upper leg move together in most sporting movements – this is known as 'pelvifemoral rhythm', unless the muscles of the trunk are working to restrain pelvic movement. In both open and closed kinetic chain movements there will be pelvic movement to help increase RoM and maintain balance and stability. A football or rugby player initiating open kinetic chain hip extension in order to kick a ball will be aided by anterior tilting of the pelvis to gain maximum back lift in the kicking leg. In the closed kinetic chain weight-bearing leg, there will be at the same time both a mediolateral and a rotational shift in the pelvis towards the standing foot.

Assessment of the pelvis and hip region

The art of effective assessment of a patient is fundamental to forming a clinical impression of the problem at hand and an effective plan to return the athlete to sport. A full subjective history of the patient's complaint, as well as a competent physical examination, will provide the basis for treatment and the setting of rehabilitation goals.

Subjective assessment of the pelvis and hip

During the consultation, questioning of the patient complaining of hip pain must be precise due to the wide variety of injuries and conditions that can present, and as Hengeveld and Banks (2005) profess, extracting the appropriate information requires care and skill to ensure an accurate account of the history is achieved. The subjective assessment must appreciate the potential for referred pain to, or from, the abdominal, lumbar, sacroiliac joint, pelvic, gluteal or knee regions. Due to the relative stability of the pelvis, the mechanism of injury, if known, can be an indicator as to which anatomical structures may be implicated and which functional limitations may present as a result. It is important to identify the specific anatomical region and tissue from which the pain is originating, although this can be particularly difficult with low back, pelvic, hip and groin conditions. A thorough understanding of the functional anatomy and injuries is required if the sports therapist is to synthesize rational clinical impressions of the dysfunction that the patient or athlete presents subjectively.

The onset of pain may indicate specific injuries, depending on whether they are traumatic or insidious. Common traumatic conditions include muscular tears, labral tears, chondral lesions and ligamentous sprains. More insidious conditions include tendinopathy, bursitis, osteitis pubis, hernia, stress fracture, apophysitis and osteoarthritis. It must be noted that some injuries can have a gradual onset but present with acute symptoms, and that chronic syndromes such as fibromyalgia or myalgic encephalomyelitis (ME – chronic fatigue syndrome) can present with severe but diffuse symptoms, including muscle soreness.

The behaviour and response of symptoms is an important indicator of injury; specific aggravating factors affecting this region can include simply walking, ascending or descending stairs and squatting movements, as well as other functional movements such as bending, running or side-stepping. Static postures (such as sitting, standing, stretching, driving, or lying prone,

Table 9.3 Pain at the hip and possible causes

Type of pain	Possible causes
Dull, deep or aching	Osteoarthritis, Paget's disease
Sharp, intense, sudden (on weight bearing)	Fracture
Tingling that radiates	Radiculopathy
Pain in sitting with affected leg crossed	Trochanteric bursitis
Pain in sitting with leg not crossed	Ischiogluteal bursitis
Pain after standing or walking	Hip arthrosis
Pain on weight bearing	Fracture, severe arthrosis
Unremitting or long duration	Paget's disease, cancer, severe arthrosis

Source: adapted from Schon and Zuckerman, 1988.

supine or lying on the side) can also easily aggravate. It is also important to ascertain the patient's perception of easing factors; these may include simple rest or non-weight-bearing postures and asymptomatic ranges of joint movement, as well as unilateral limb dominance (compensation) in activities such as football. Red flags must also be considered in any subjective examination; these may include unremitting night pain, loss of bladder or bowel control or unexplainable recent weight loss (Greenhalgh and Selfe, 2010). Psychosocial issues (yellow flags) must also be considered. Stress, anxiety, depression, fear, avoidance and any other personal concerns can contribute significantly to the patient's inability to effectively adhere to the recommended management plan, and other sources of support (such as via their GP or counsellor) may be required.

Objective assessment of the pelvis and hip

Objective examination usually follows subjective assessment, but only if the therapist is confident that management of the patient's condition is within their scope of practice. For example, if a patient is presenting with red flag symptoms, then assessment should not continue and referral to the patient's GP should be instigated immediately. Petty (2011) suggests that objectivity in physical examination is difficult as the reliability and validity of tests conducted rely heavily on the skill of the therapist, further reinforcing the need for an evidence-based approach to assessment of the hip. Aims of the objective assessment process are to test the clinical impressions from the subjective assessment, reproduce the patient's symptoms (without causing much in the way of aggravation – sports therapists must be aware of the irritability of the condition), assess pain and other symptom response, appreciate the quality and RoM of the hip and related regions, compare bilaterally and exclude structures not implicated.

The collection of objective evidence to confirm or contest the clinical impression is the next step in assessment; it is worth noting the use of the word 'contest' rather than others (such as 'disprove', 'rule out' or 'refute') early on in the examination process. Complete dismissal of potential pathologies before the full objective examination process has been undertaken leaves the therapist at risk of becoming one-dimensional in their approach and potentially missing vital clues in the patient's condition. Atkins *et al.* (2010), in summation of Cyriax's orthopaedic work, propose that negative findings are as important as the positive ones in eliminating those structures seemingly not implicated. In light of this, a flexible, open-minded and non-judgemental approach allows the therapist to explore all avenues of clinical impression; the concept of a 'permeable brick wall' of theoretical and clinical information (Hengeveld and Banks, 2005) could be beneficial. Employing this approach allows the therapist to critically evaluate patients' presentations, but does require a significant depth and breadth of anatomical, functional and pathological knowledge in order to select the impression most indicated.

Superficial palpation of the pelvis and hip

The purpose of examining the tissues around the hip using initial superficial palpation is to assess factors that cannot be observed, build the impression of pathology affecting soft tissue (physiologically and neurologically) and identify potential red flags early in examination. The therapist needs to have an understanding of what is 'normal' for the patient, and should begin with palpation on the unaffected limb and side of the body so they have an outcome measure to compare against. Deeper palpation of tissues should be avoided at this stage of examination so as not to further exacerbate symptoms or interfere with the repair process of damaged tissue. Nociceptors may become more sensitive to the mechanical stimulus from deep palpation, leading to a state of hyperalgesia, potentially giving false positives of pain later in the examination process.

When commencing superficial palpation of structures, the therapist should be feeling for localized sweaty skin (indicative of autonomic disturbance), swelling, effusion or warmth (signs of inflammation), tender or irritable areas of skin, muscular spasm, tightness in superficial fascia and any unusual lumps or other presentations. This palpatory assessment may not be localized specifically to the hip joint, but also surrounding anatomical areas as indicated. The assessment of these areas may commence with the client in prone, supine or side-lying to allow weight-bearing muscles of the lower extremities to be free from unnecessary tension, and permit ease of palpation in a variety of movement ranges. All contralateral abnormalities should be recorded.

Observation and posture of the pelvis and hip

Observational assessment should begin as soon as contact is made with the patient, as vital clues to their condition may be identified without any formal examination taking place. Static posture, functional movements, walking gait, running gait and responses thereof (apprehensions; facial expressions; symptom responses) can all be observed, and each of these allow useful information to be gathered. The patient's facial expressions may exhibit signs of discomfort or additionally underlying illness or fatigue (this may require further subjective assessment). Specific functional movements, such as their ability to sit and stand, as well as undressing (putting shoes on, for example) can all contribute important objective markers to the production of a clinical impression. Hengeveld and Banks (2005) suggest that the body has the ability to adapt, compensate and inform; this fundamental reasoning is why observation of the body's structures, posture and function are integrated into an objective assessment.

Superficial tissues of the body can be examined visually for abnormality, the purpose of which is to provide information on pathology, possible factors that might contribute to pathology, what physical testing needs to be carried out and possible treatment considerations to follow (Petty, 2011). When examining the skin, the therapist should be looking for changes in colour, scars, effusion, swelling, skin creases, bruising, sweating and other signs of abnormality. Changes in colour and texture may indicate circulatory irregularities (for example, a bluish appearance can represent poor circulation; redness suggests inflammation; and a shiny appearance may indicate oedema and fluid retention – which may relate to local joint injury or to impaired vascularity, such as peripheral arterial disease). Local ecchymosis (bruising discolouration), which typically tracks distally due to gravity, may be present with a muscular injury (Bahr and Maehlum, 2004), while effusion strongly indicates a joint injury. Scar tissue is evidence of injury to the skin or previous operative intervention; its appearance can depend on the vascularity and age (red being of recent synthesis, and white older). Abnormal skin creases could be present with underlying defects in the local tissue, or conditions such as acanthosis nigricans (dark, velvety, hyperpigmented skin) or developmental dysplasia of the hip (abnormal hip joint architecture). The pelvis and femur should also be observed for bony deformities that present as a result of injury. Musculature around the hip should be assessed for shape, bulk and tone, with the therapist specifically looking for normality, atrophy and hypertrophy when comparing sides bilaterally. Muscles which are experiencing impaired innervation will ultimately undergo atrophy (Harmon, 2010); this is also common with prolonged immobilization or rest from competitive training; unilateral muscular hypertrophy can be evidence of limb dominance or compensatory movement patterns.

Clinical observation of static posture is rationalized through its simplicity and minimal impact on existing signs and symptoms, particularly with clients presenting with chronic pelvic pain (Montenegro *et al.*, 2009); it provides potential clues to underlying problems, but is far from conclusive. Posture should be assessed three-dimensionally in the anterior, posterior and lateral views, and wherever possible performed in standing. This is to implicate any tissues which may not be functioning appropriately as normal posture in the anatomical position is maintained by balanced, strong and flexible muscles, intact ligaments, freely moving fascia, properly functioning joints and a balanced line of gravity (Gross *et al.*, 2009). Anatomical landmark levels can be assessed bilaterally in the anterior and posterior views, and unilaterally in the lateral view using a plumb-line for reference. Anterior structures (superior to inferior) include the earlobes, clavicles, nipples, antecubital creases, umbilicus, ASIS, greater trochanters, fingertips, base and apex of the patellae, tibial tuberosities, medial and lateral malleoli. Posterior structures to assess include the ears, superior and inferior angles of scapulae, olecranon processes, iliac crest heights, PSIS, greater trochanters, gluteal creases and cleft, fingertips, popliteal creases, medial and lateral malleoli, and calcaneal positioning. An 'ideal posture' has been considered important in sport to make the body more efficient and effective in its functions, delay the onset of fatigue, prevent over-training and decrease the risk of muscular imbalance, joint dysfunction and injury (Kendall *et al.*, 2005). However, experienced practitioners will recognize the clear limitations of static postural assessment. A study by Ferriera *et al.* (2011) suggested that there is no 'true' symmetry in postural alignment and that small asymmetries represent the normative standard for posture in standing and may be a consideration when asymmetry is assessed as not being influentially apparent to a patient's current symptoms. It is, however, fundamental to make an allowance for the considerable effects kinesiology and biomechanics of sport have on the body and the resulting stress and strain likely to be exhibited on musculoskeletal tissues through postural dysfunction (Bartlett, 1999).

Functional observation of the hip at this stage may include gait analysis; other specific functional movement testing would be undertaken after RoM testing has been completed. The RoM needed at the hip during the stance and swing phases of gait are 0–30° flexion and 0–20° extension. If these ranges are not observed then an abnormal gait is considered. The four main causes of abnormal gait are pain, muscular weakness, abnormal RoM and compensation (Gross *et al.*, 2009). The abnormalities can include: antalgic gait (painful, shortened stance phase on injured limb); gluteus maximus gait (where weakness can lead to posterior thoracic movement in

---

Practitioner Tip Box 9.3

True or false limping?

If there is a suspicion of any psychosocial (yellow flag) issues from the patient's history and the legitimacy of objective findings with regards to gait, the sports therapist can consider asking the patient to walk backwards to see if the same limitations are evident.

Table 9.4 Gait disturbances and mechanical faults involving the pelvis and hip

	Gait stage	Pelvic disturbances	Hip disturbances
Stance phase (60 per cent of gait)	Initial contact (heel strike)	Pelvic drop	Excessive flexion – tight iliopsoas Limited flexion – weak hip flexors and gluteus maximus
	Loading response (foot flat)	N/A	Limited extension – tight hip flexors Internal rotation – weak external rotators (femoral anteversion) External rotation (femoral retroversion)
	Mid-stance	Lateral trunk lean – weak gluteus medius Backward trunk lean – weak gluteus maximus Forward trunk lean – weak quadriceps	Excessive lordosis – tight hip flexors Contralateral hip drop – weak gluteus medius Increased knee flexion – decreased hip and back extension
	Terminal swing (heel-off)	Medial heel whip – weak hip external rotators Hip flexion – restriction in hip extension	N/A
Swing phase (40 per cent of gait)	Pre-swing (toe-off)	N/A	Lack of push off – restriction in hip extension
	Swing (acceleration and deceleration)	N/A	Circumduction – weak hip flexors or long leg Hip-hiking – lack of knee flexion or ankle dorsiflexion, weak hip flexors Excessive hip flexion – weak ankle dorsiflexors

Source: adapted from Louden *et al.*, 2008.

stance phase); Trendelenberg gait (weak gluteus medius causing a lateral pelvic shift and angulation away from the affected limb in stance phase); arthrogenic gait (hip restriction can lead to circumduction of the affected limb, and cause exaggerated plantarflexion in contralateral ankle); short leg gait (which produces a lateral shift of the trunk and pelvis towards the affected side in stance phase); and 'stiff hip' gait (where one leg is lifted higher than the other to clear the ground).

Clearing tests for the pelvis and hip

As discussed, the pelvis has multiple functions: supporting the weight of the body, enabling weight transfer between the trunk and lower limb, as well as being the attachment site for a number of muscles. Many of the muscles are biarticular (for example, sartorius, rectus femoris, hamstrings, psoas major and gracilis), which heightens their susceptibility to injury (Latash and Zatsiorsky, 2001). It is important to recognize the relationship between the relationships to joints and tissues above and below the hip, and assess these where appropriate. Clearing of joints above (lumbar spine; SIJ) and below (knee) should be undertaken whenever there is a consideration of problems at the pelvis and hip being generated or influenced by these related regions. Clearing of the lumbar spine can be performed with active flexion, extension, lateral flexion, rotation and quadrant testing, each with overpressure if appropriate; the SIJ can be cleared, to a degree, using the combination movement 'FABER' test, and also via compression and distraction tests. Similarly to the lumbar spine, completion of active physiological movements at the knee (flexion, extension, medial and lateral rotation), with overpressure, will seek to clear the knee of related pathology. Obviously, wherever clearing tests are positive these will need to be investigated further.

Active movement assessment of the hip

Active RoM assessment investigates the patient's willingness to perform movements voluntarily using their contractile tissues (i.e. muscles and tendons) while also gauging some functional appreciation of related nerves, fascia and joints. The main aims of active RoM testing are to (carefully) reproduce the patient's symptoms, looking for quality, control, range, resistance through range, pain, and behaviour of pain through range (Magee, 2008; Petty, 2011); it will provide the therapist with information regarding the patient's flexibility, mobility and strength (Gross *et al.*, 2009). Causes of abnormal active RoM include weakness, spasm, paralysis, shortened or tight tissue, neuromuscular insufficiencies, poor joint–muscle relationships and intra- or extra-articular pathologies.

The therapist should first assess signs and symptoms at rest so that the effect movement has on symptoms can be established and measured appropriately through voluntary movements. When asking the patient to perform active movements of the hip, it is important to explain and demonstrate what is expected, and the uninjured side should be observed first and used as an objective measure of 'normal' if possible. Movements occurring through full range, and in the most efficient pathway (Schmidt and Lee, 1999; Shumway-Cook and Woollacott, 1995), will ensure that all agonistic and synergistic muscles which act on the hip are tested (Magee, 2008). Ensuring that movement only occurs in the desired plane and axis at the joint being assessed can be achieved by fixation or stabilization of others proximally (i.e. with the lumbar spine and sacroiliac joint positioned in neutral).

All physiological movements of the hip should be performed by the patient; these are: flexion, extension, abduction, adduction, medial and lateral rotation. As the hip region is made up of many multi-joint muscles, it is important not to let passive insufficiency influence the RoM the patient is able to perform. For example, in hip flexion, if the knee is in extension, then passive insufficiency of the hamstrings will inhibit range of movement (Clarkson, 2000). In light of this, the therapist should instruct the patient to approximate the attachments of multi-joint muscles to reduce this effect (for example, flexing the knee when performing hip flexion). Overpressure is used at the end of active range or the physiological barrier (Magee, 2008) to test the 'true' range and assess integrity and end-feel at the joint. This is achieved by applying force smoothly and slowly until the end of range is found and an end-feel is picked up by the therapist. Oscillatory movements may also be applied to feel for any resistance within the joint. Active tests of the hip may be modified in terms of start positions (lying on the couch, or in standing, for example), repetitions (for muscular endurance), speed (slow or quick), and the use of combination movements; such approaches more closely mimic functional activity. It is important to observe active movements closely for any compensatory movements such as pelvic tilting and rotation.

In irritable presentations, active movements may also provoke muscular spasm in the gluteal group, quadriceps, hamstrings, adductors, hip flexors or rotators. The sports therapist should consider such questions as: what happens to symptoms through the movement – does it ease, stay the same or get worse? Gentle palpation of the proximal joints may also be used to identify excessive or abnormal movements, suggesting disruption of the kinetic chain.

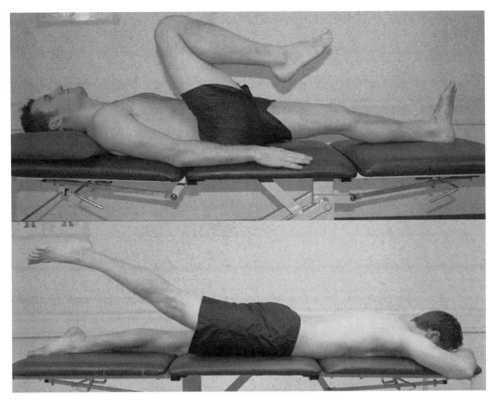

Photo 9.2   Active range of movement assessment: flexion and extension.

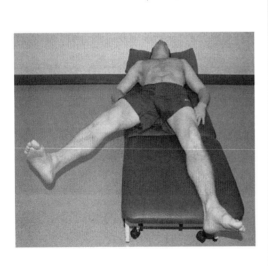
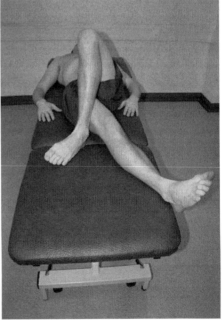

Photo 9.3   Active range of movement assessment: abduction and adduction.

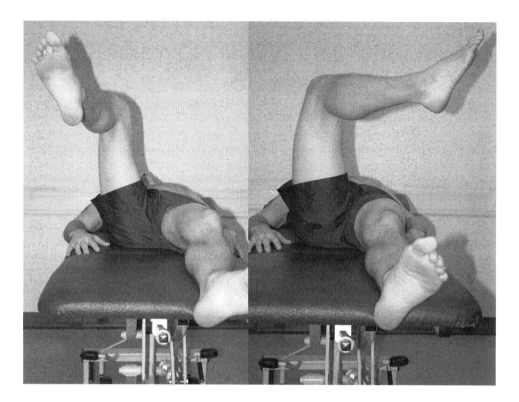

Photo 9.4   Active range of movement assessment: medial and lateral rotation.

Passive physiological movement assessment of the hip

It is important to consider that passive movements not only test non-contractile tissues (ligaments, joint capsules, cartilage, fascia, bursae, nerves), but that they should be used to complement other assessment findings. As a generalization, if contractile tissues are implicated, then active and passive movements are likely to be painful in opposite directions, while non-contractile tissues are likely to be painful in active and passive movements of the same direction (Petty, 2011). For example, muscular damage to rectus femoris at the hip may present with pain in active flexion (shortening) and passive extension (lengthening), while a labral tear at the hip is more likely to present with pain in medial rotation and adduction, both actively and passively. The capsular pattern of the hip must not be overlooked during assessment so that the therapist does not jump to conclusions on restricted RoM; this further justifies the use of bilateral assessment for objectivity. For example, medial rotation is most restricted by the structure of the hip joint, while extension is least limited.

Standard single-plane, passive physiological movements of the hip (flexion, extension, abduction, adduction, medial and lateral rotation) can be undertaken with the patient in prone, supine or side-lying in order to allow the musculature of the hip to be at rest during testing. Hip flexion and extension can be most effectively assessed in side-lying as it allows the tested leg to be taken through the full range (i.e. from full flexion to full extension) rather than just part of the range. The leg can be taken passively through the range in full knee extension; however, passive insufficiency may contribute to decreased range – hence knee flexion is suggested. Care must be taken to stabilize the pelvis and keep the lumbar spine and sacroiliac joint in neutral so as not to permit any compensatory movement. Abduction and adduction can be undertaken with the patient in supine, again taking care to stabilize the pelvis in order to prevent compensatory movement. Medial and lateral rotation is also best performed with the patient supine, with the knee and hip at 90° flexion and the therapist cradling the full lower limb for maximum support. The sports therapist should be assessing the end-feel at the extremes of each physiological movement. As the end ranges are restricted by capsular or ligamentous stretch, normal end-feels at the hip are either a firm and springy soft tissue stretch, or a soft tissue approximation (see Table 9.5).

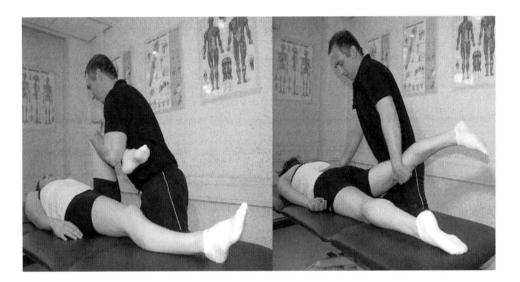

Photo 9.5 Passive range of movement assessment: flexion and extension.

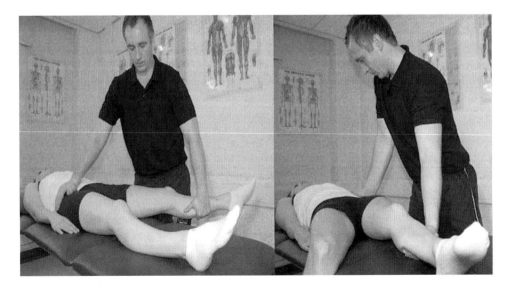

Photo 9.6 Passive range of movement assessment: abduction and adduction.

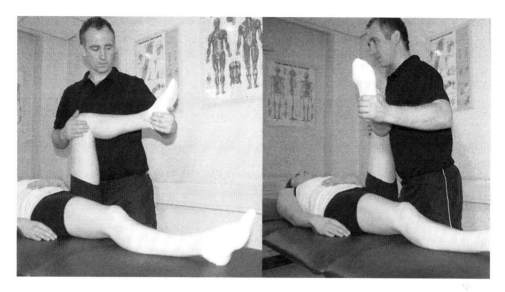

Photo 9.7 Passive range of movement assessment: medial and lateral rotation.

Table 9.5 Normal end feels of the hip

Flexion – soft or springy/elastic
Extension – springy/elastic
Abduction – springy/elastic
Adduction – springy/elastic
Medial rotation – springy/elastic
Lateral rotation – springy/elastic

Passive accessory movement assessment of the hip

Accessory movements are those which cannot be performed actively in isolation, but normally occur in conjunction with physiological movements. When assessing accessory movements, the sports therapist should, as always, be responsive to any visual, verbal and tactile feedback from the patient. Pain, resistance, quality and excessive or diminished ranges of accessory motion should all be considered; the hip may be affected by adhesions, swelling or pathology of its joint capsule, ligaments or articular cartilage. Modifications to the start position in all accessory movements of the hip can be adopted so as to place specific stress on structures around the joint (for example, positions of flexion, extension or rotation, or combinations may be employed). The main accessory movements to assess at the hip are lateral, anteroposterior (AP), posteroanterior (PA), and longitudinal caudad glides. The movements performed are distractions of the femoral head from its resting position in the acetabulum laterally, anteriorly, posteriorly and inferiorly. When undertaking AP and PA glides, the patient can be positioned in side-lying (with hips and knees flexed) and the therapist may use the greater trochanter to move the femur anteriorly and posteriorly. Support (cushion or bolster) should be placed between the knees to keep the hips in neutral. Lateral glides can be undertaken in a neutral, supine position, or in 90° flexion. In neutral, the lateral glide may be performed with one hand on the medial aspect of the thigh – as proximal as possible, and the other laterally – just superior to the lateral femoral epicondyle, applying opposing forces. In flexion, the therapist should clasp their hands around the medial aspect of the thigh as proximally as possible, applying a lateral force while using their shoulder or torso to apply opposition to the distal end of the femur. Longitudinal caudad can also be undertaken in neutral supine, or 90° flexion. In neutral, the sports therapist can grasp the thigh medially and laterally just superior to the femoral epicondyles, carefully pulling on the limb inferiorly. In a more flexed position, the therapist can clasp their hands around the anterior aspect of the thigh as proximally as possible while applying force in the caudad direction. Obviously, where restricted movement, pain or other indicators are present, graded mobilizations of specific accessory movements may be employed as part of a manual therapy strategy.

Active resisted movement assessment of the hip

Assessment of resisted movement provides the sports therapist with an objective measure of the force muscles can produce against resistance, while looking for any pain, weakness, muscular spasm or imbalances left to right. Active resisted movements of the hip primarily seek to implicate contractile tissues, but are also useful in the assessment of neural and osteological pathology. Assessment of muscular strength should be performed bilaterally, and completed in mid-range first; this is to ensure that inert tissues are not on stretch and because muscular forces are likely to be strongest and safest in this position. After testing in mid-range, the inner and outer ranges may be assessed to localize pain to specific tissues and certain parts of those tissues (i.e. proximally or distally). The therapist should resist voluntary contraction of relevant musculature, seeking to prevent any movement from occurring at the joint. The patient can be asked to produce a reaction force relative to therapist pressure and a progressively incremental increase in resistance is requested. Effective handling of the patient is important for mechanical advantage, isolation of muscles and support of the limb, particularly when working with powerful athletes. Outcomes of resisted movement testing can be quantified using a grading scale of 0–5 and compared bilaterally for any discrepancy, although this is most appropriate for use when a neuromuscular pathology is suggested.

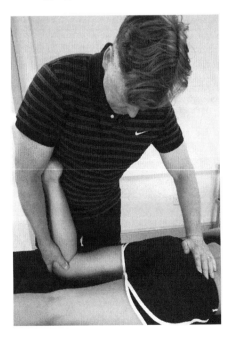

Photo 9.8 Active resisted movement assessment: extension.

Practitioner Tip Box 9.4

Diagnostic accuracy of special tests

Selecting which special tests to utilize with a patient can be challenging as there are so many to choose from. In any presenting situation, certain tests will be more appropriate and useful than others. Different tests have different reliability ratings. Correct patient positioning and handling is crucial, as is interpretation of the test. Sports therapists must recognize the possibility of false negatives and positives, and be recommended to consider sensitivity and specificity ratings of tests, as well as likelihood ratios where available (Cook and Hegedus, 2013; Hattam and Smeatham, 2010). Systematic reviews and meta-analyses of special tests are frequently undertaken and published in the scientific media and therapists must aim to keep up with current evidence.

Special tests of the pelvis and hip

Special tests do not necessarily allow for a clear diagnosis of pathology, and practitioners must recognize the sensitivity and specificity values when selecting special tests. Hattam and Smeatham (2010) explain that *'very few tests can be expected to conclusively rule in or rule out any particular condition, but they should add to the index of suspicion which will inform your clinical reasoning process'*.

FABER test

The FABER test (also known as 'Patrick's test') is named for the movement pattern the hip is required to perform for the test (flexion, abduction and external rotation) and may indicate pathologies such as osteoarthritis, impingement, labral tears and chondral defects. The FABER test is performed with the patient in supine; they are then directed to actively bring their hip

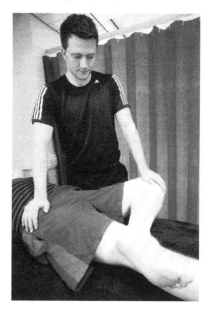

Photo 9.9   FABER test.

into full flexion, and then into full external rotation and slight abduction so that the ankle is resting on the thigh of the non-tested leg. Passive overpressure may be applied on the medial aspect of the knee while stabilizing the pelvis at the ASIS with the opposite hand (Atkins *et al.*, 2010; Hattam and Smeatham, 2010; Petty, 2011). A modified FABER test can be performed passively; Scopp and Moorman (2001) suggest that the stabilizing muscles of the hip will still be activated. Other tests have been proposed for assessing generic hip joint pathology, such as the 'hip scour', 'hip quadrant', 'hip click' and 'resisted straight leg raise' tests; but evidence for the efficacy of these is limited.

FADDIR test

The FADDIR test (flexion, adduction and internal rotation) has been suggested as being effective in the assessment of piriformis syndrome (Fishman *et al.*, 2002), osteoarthritis (DeAngelis and Busconi, 2003), femoroacetabular impingement (FAI) and/or labral tears. Although strong sensitivity data is proposed in literature, most studies on this test were performed retrospectively on patients with known impingement or labral pathology, which questions the specificity of the test. A recent meta-analysis identified that sensitivity ranged from 59 to 100 per cent, while specificity values ranged from 4 to 75 per cent (Reiman *et al.*, 2012). It is suggested that a positive FADDIR test be backed up with further radiological investigation if initial conservative management of symptoms is unsuccessful.

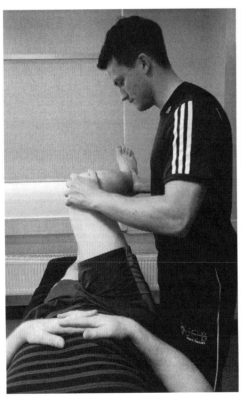 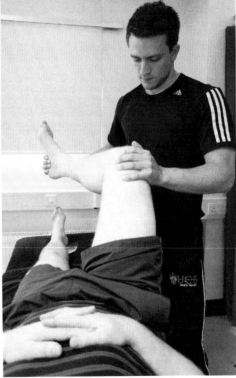

Photo 9.10   FADDIR test.   *Photo 9.11*   McCarthy test.

McCarthy test

The McCarthy test is a test primarily targeting the acetabular labrum. It is performed with the patient supine; their knee is placed in approximately 110° flexion; the therapist then passively takes the tested hip into full flexion (with one hand on the patient's knee and the other supporting their foot); external rotation is then added, followed by slight hip and full knee extension. The test can also be repeated moving the hip into internal rotation if movement into initial hip extension is asymptomatic. If either of these manoeuvres reproduces the patient's symptoms, or a click or pop is heard or felt, labral pathology may be suspected. Combination movements of extension, abduction and external rotation have been advocated for reproducing pain with labral tears by some academics (Fitzgerald, 1995; Klaue *et al.*, 1991); however, these tests have seen little contemporary research, so their diagnostic value is questionable. Labral pathology is often diagnosed clinically via the patient history and physical examination as pain on flexion and rotation of the hip is a common sign (Narvani *et al.*, 2003). Radiological investigations are significantly more diagnostically accurate with labral pathology.

Snapping hip manoeuvre

The snapping hip manoeuvre is similar to the McCarthy test, but performed actively by the patient rather than passively. This test is to distinguish between extracapsular clicking from the iliopsoas tendon (over the femoral head), rather than of intracapsular clicking caused by labral pathology. A positive presentation is when, on descending into extension, a snapping (or clicking) sound is audible, or the patient reports a snapping or popping sensation (Magee, 2008).

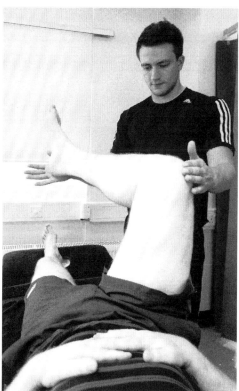

Photo 9.12 Snapping hip manoeuvre.

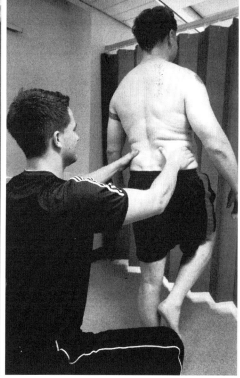

Photo 9.13 Trendelenberg test.

Trendelenberg test

The Trendelenberg test is undertaken in standing, with the therapist asking the patient to stand and flex their hip and knee on the contralateral side. The therapist then observes for any drop of the pelvis on the side of the non-weight-bearing limb. This drop can also be assessed by placing hands on the iliac crests, or by holding the patient's hands while feeling for a shift in bodyweight. The test must be performed bilaterally, and an asymmetric drop indicates weakness in the gluteus medius of the weight-bearing limb (which should be recruiting to stabilize the pelvis). The test may be followed up by observation of a Trendelenberg gait pattern. A study by Bird *et al.* (2001) to assess the sensitivity and specificity of this test for gluteal pathology found favourable outcomes for both; however, research is lacking in its diagnostic capabilities. Passive internal rotation (identifying possible muscular tear) and resisted hip abduction (weakness and/or muscular tear) are other options to assess gluteus medius insufficiency, but have shown only reasonable sensitivity and specificity scores (Bird *et al.*, 2001; Brown *et al.*, 2004; Youdas *et al.*, 2010). The Trendelenberg and resisted hip abduction tests are, however, a strong clinical indicator for weakness of the gluteus medius, which has implications for distal biomechanics and kinematics, particularly at the knee.

Single leg stance test

In a similar positioning to the Trendelenberg test, the patient is asked to stand on one leg by flexing the knee or flexing a straight leg on the contralateral side for 30 seconds. The therapist should ensure there is no trunk deviation during the test. Pain around the posterior greater trochanter suggests a positive test (for what may be termed 'greater trochanteric pain syndrome' – GTPS) as the gluteal muscles contract to stabilize the pelvis. A study by Lequesne *et al.* (2008) found good scores for sensitivity and specificity, although not for a specific pathology (such as tendinopathy, enthesopathy or bursitis), and this has not been backed up by any other notable research. Woodley *et al.* (2008) used MRI and clinical examination to assess lateral hip pain and found that a composite examination including range of movement assessment, muscle strength testing and the Trendelenberg test showed favourable confidence intervals and specificity, but reliability between clinical and radiological findings was poor. GTPS has a number of differential diagnoses, and clinical examination findings using special tests are likely to be non-specific to pathology.

Torque test

The anterior stabilizing ligaments of the hip can be stressed with the torque test (a test for hip instability); this requires the patient to be laid supine, with the symptomatic hip resting over the edge of the treatment couch (Carvalhais *et al.*, 2011; Grimaldi, 2011). The therapist passively extends and medially rotates the hip, followed by the application of a posterolateral glide on the femur for approximately 20 seconds. A positive result is a reproduction of symptoms, or a significant movement in comparison to the unaffected side (Magee, 2008); however, reliability of this test is still open to question. Other tests for hip instability include the 'log roll', 'dial', 'abduction extension external rotation' and 'long axis femoral distraction' tests; however, evidence to support these is lacking, which questions their clinical efficacy, especially because of the potential for muscle guarding, and false negatives and positives, hence they should be used with due consideration.

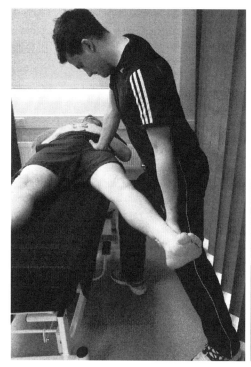 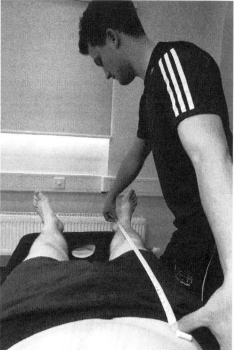

Photo 9.14   Torque test.

Photo 9.15   Leg length discrepancy.

Leg length discrepancy test

It is important for the sports therapist to assess for any leg length discrepancy (LLD) that may result in biomechanical compensations affecting the pelvis and hip, the entire limb, or spinal region. Two simple measures of LLD may be employed initially – apparent and true. Apparent leg length is typically measured with the patient supine-lying, with pelvis squared, from the umbilicus to the medial malleolus. True leg length is commonly measured from either the ASIS or greater trochanter to the medial malleolus. Sports therapists will, however, realize that the ASIS belongs to the pelvis, not the leg; and obviously it is essential to compare left with right. More localized measurements can be taken using key landmarks on the leg to establish specific structural length differences (such as from the greater trochanter to the lateral femoral condyle; or from the lateral tibial condyle to the lateral malleolus). Magee (2008) explains that a LLD of 1–1.5 cm or less is considered normal (however, athletes may require intervention if such a discrepancy exists and if this is a potential cause of pain or dysfunction). Apparent LLD occurs when functionally shortened soft tissues and pelvic imbalances give the impression of leg shortening. This can be assessed by measuring from a central point (such as the umbilicus or xiphoid process) down to the medial malleolus, left and right.

Craig's test

Craig's test is an easy method for assessing femoral anteversion. With the patient lying prone with the knee flexed to 90°, the sports therapist then palpates the greater trochanter with one hand, and with their other hand passively brings the hip into internal rotation. Normal internal rotation in prone can be 8–15°. Any excessive internal rotation indicates femoral anteversion; less than 8° indicates femoral retroversion (Giori and Trousdale 2003; Hattam and Smeatham, 2010).

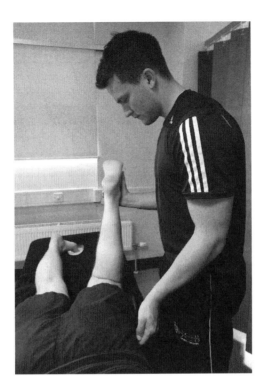

Photo 9.16 Craig's test.

Modified Thomas test

The modified Thomas test can be used to assess for tightness in the rectus femoris and the lateral soft tissues of the hip (tensor fascia lata, iliotibial band and gluteals) (Placzek and Boyce, 2006). First, the patient stands at the edge of the couch, which is high enough to sit in line with the crease of the gluteal muscles. The patient is then laid, with support, into a supine position while holding the knee of their non-tested leg in a position of hip and knee flexion, ensuring there are no gaps between the lumbosacral region and the couch. The tested limb is then allowed to relax into hip extension (Harvey, 1998). The therapist observes the resting angles presenting at the hip and knee; they may also elect to apply slight overpressure to clarify that the patient is relaxed and to confirm end-range position. Accurate assessment requires the use of a goniometer or inclinometer to measure joint angles (Clapis *et al.*, 2008). Normal joint range values will vary between populations (different genders, ages, sports and positions), although generalized norms include approximately: 10° hip flexion; 50° knee flexion; and 15° hip abduction. Variations above and below these values bilaterally may therefore indicate hypo- or hypermobility of joints, or soft tissue shortening.

The original Thomas test is a primary test for a fixed flexion contracture of the hip, assessing the anterior structures including the anterior capsule, hip flexors (iliopsoas and rectus femoris) and labrum. Positioning of the patient should be with the patient in a supine position on the treatment couch. The patient then actively flexes the leg that is not being tested, applying active overpressure with their hands. A normal response is for the leg that is being assessed to remain with slight extension and not raised off the treatment couch. A positive response for fixed flexion contracture is for the tested hip to flex off the plinth. Palpation should then be undertaken to determine if the contracture is caused by soft tissue or a joint restriction (Magee, 2008).

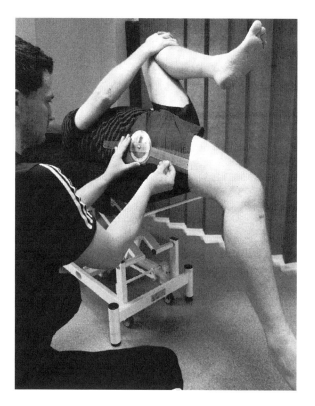

Photo 9.17   Modified Thomas test.

Practitioner Tip Box 9.5

Muscle length tests as screening tools

Muscle (myofascial) length tests may be utilized, not just in the assessment of injured patients, but also to screen for injury risk in non-injured populations. Decreased range of movement due to myofascial shortening may affect joint stability, production of force, cause compensation elsewhere, and alter efficient biomechanics.

Modified Ober's test

The modified Ober's test is adapted from the original test proposed by Ober (1936), which initially aimed to stress the iliotibial band (ITB); however, it is now considered a test for the lateral soft tissues of the hip, including the trochanteric bursae, gluteus medius and tensor fascia lata, as well as the ITB. Although there are variants of the test, the patient is positioned in side-lying with their affected side facing up, and the non-tested leg slightly flexed for stability; the hip is then brought passively into approximately 20° extension, with the knee fully extended. The leg should then be clear from the couch, and lowered into adduction, while stabilizing the squared pelvis. A positive test is reported as reproducing the patient's pain, or an inability to adduct (Gajdosik *et al.*, 2003).

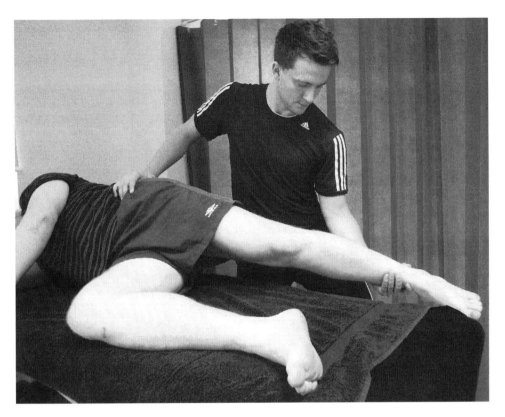

Photo 9.18 Modified Ober's test.

90–90 test

The 90–90 test is used to assess the length of the hamstrings (and associated myofascia) and involves measurement of the knee extension angle (KEA). Davis *et al.* (2008) propose that this test be considered the gold standard for hamstring flexibility measurement. The patient should be in supine-lying with any lumbar lordosis eliminated with a pillow or lumbar roll. The starting position requires the hip to be brought into 90° flexion so the femur is perpendicular with the floor and the knee placed in 90° flexion so the tibia and fibula are parallel with the couch. The sports therapist passively supports the patient into this position as joint position sense may be poor. The patient is then asked to actively extend the knee so a joint angle measurement can be taken (the KEA). As the patient performs the test, an involuntary shaking of the limb may be noted (myoclonus) so the knee should be slightly flexed until the shaking has ceased before measurements are taken. This test can also be performed passively by the therapist and measurements should be taken when a firm point of the springy end-feel is reached. It has been suggested that an active version of the test may provide an 'initial' length of the hamstrings and related soft tissues, while the passive test provides a 'maximal' length (Gajdosik *et al.*, 1993).

Ely's test

Ely's test is commonly utilized to assess the range of hip extension and specifically the length of the rectus femoris muscle. The patient is in prone-lying and the therapist should passively flex the knee of the leg to be assessed so the heel moves towards the gluteals until an end-feel is discovered. Full flexion of the knee to the thigh with no movement in the pelvis is considered

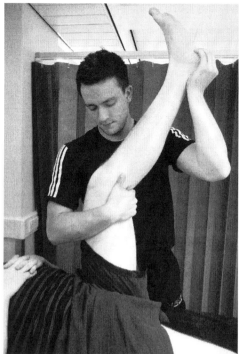
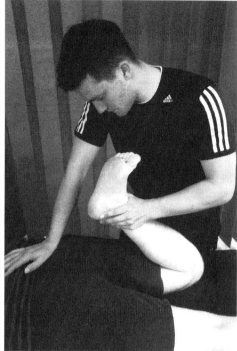

Photo 9.19   90–90 test.

Photo 9.20   Ely's test.

a negative finding, while a test is considered positive if, with flexion of the knee, the pelvis tilts, raising the gluteals from the couch (Braly *et al.*, 2006). Marks *et al.* (2003) suggest the test has good positive prediction value for contracture of the rectus femoris in patients with a stiff knee gait; however, Peeler and Anderson (2008) proposed only moderate intra- and inter-rater reliability values for Ely's test, questioning its clinical efficacy.

Palpation of the pelvis and hip

Skill in palpation is fundamental to the sports therapist's assessment procedure, and requires confident understanding of anatomy and tissue. The therapist must understand what tissues are being palpated and what those tissues should normally feel like. The therapist should assess for abnormalities or differences both locally and contralaterally. Palpatory assessment of the pelvic girdle, hip and groin must be performed with great care and respect for the patient; informed consent is of paramount importance, and when gaining consent the therapist should be clear that they may be placing their hands close to genitalia. Communication is vital to allowing the patient to be aware of the process. This said, sports therapists must respect patient boundaries, especially with regard to males treating females and vice versa.

Towelling techniques can be of great use when palpating the hip to offer a barrier between the therapist and the patient (and specifically covering genitalia); the patient may also be instructed to place their own hands over sensitive areas (palpation may also be performed *through* the patient's hands – accepting that the thickness of the patient's hands will reduce sensitivity). The preceding subjective assessment and rest of the objective assessment informs what palpation is appropriate for the patient. Specifically, any tissue that may be irritable should be palpated last, and in any tissue that is superficially very painful it may not yet be appropriate to palpate the deeper tissues. When palpating the hip, a logical format should be used – from a superior to inferior direction, and palpating anterior, lateral and posterior – so as to reduce the amount of movement the patient has to perform.

Palpatory assessment of the pelvic region is multifaceted. The ASIS may be painful due to a hip pointer, or sartorius dysfunction. Just lateral, the tensor fascia lata and gluteus medius may be palpated. More medially, the area above and below the inguinal ligament must be assessed when inguinal or femoral hernia is suspected. Medial and inferior to the ASIS is the iliopsoas muscle and bursa, and when attempting to palpate the ASIS the rectus femoris may be tender. Palpating the anterior joint line may give indication as to whether there is anterior joint involvement (specifically within the iliofemoral ligament). The pubic symphysis and pubic area generally should be palpated, if possible, in order to assess any adductor dysfunction, osteitis pubis or symphysiolysis. Muscles around the anterior aspect, specifically quadriceps, should be palpated for spasm or tenderness. Tenderness at 'Baer's point', located in the right iliac fossa anterior to the right SIJ, and slightly medial to 'McBurney's point', can indicate disruption of the sacroiliac ligament, or underlying infection (Magee, 2008). Deeper palpation into the posterior aspect of the pelvis may indicate piriformis or sciatic nerve pathology; superficial palpation just inferior to the posterior iliac crest can indicate gluteus medius sensitivity. Tenderness at the ischial tuberosity may indicate hamstring origin tendinopathy, or ischial bursitis. On the medial aspect, the femoral triangle should be palpated for the presence of painful lymph nodes, possibly indicating infection (Petty, 2011). Around the greater tuberosity, tenderness can be due to trochanteric bursitis, gluteus tendinopathy or GTPS. The ITB can be palpated from the lateral aspect, often containing adhesions, and can be tender in runners, especially where there is quadriceps weakness, coxa varus or genu valgus.

Neural assessment of the hip region

A brief summary of important neurological assessment procedures for the hip region is presented here. Further information on this aspect is to be found in Chapter 3.

Straight leg raise test

If a posterior neural aetiology is suspected then the straight leg raise (SLR) test may be used to tension through the sciatic nerve, which originates from nerve roots L2–4. The patient is supine, with the head and neck in neutral. While there are several variant approaches to the SLR, the therapist should raise the patient's leg (with extended knee) to the symptomatic range, keeping the ankle in a neutral position. If symptomatic, it is recommended that the therapist lowers the leg so as to reduce symptoms; the neural structures may then be selectively sensitized and desensitized in order to confirm neural involvement. From this position, the therapist can dorsiflex the ankle (and observe for any symptom response); the patient can also be asked to sensitize the neural pathway by flexing the cervical spine. If neural symptoms (such as dysaesthesia or radiating pain) are prevalent in the posterior leg this may indicate a positive test. This test has seen a lot of interest from practitioners who have generally found good sensitivity scores, but only poor to fair specificity data. The disagreement in findings is likely due to the variability in the procedure undertaken and the potential influences of hamstring tightness in test subjects.

Slump test

Another neural test commonly utilized is the slump test. The patient begins by sitting up straight over the side of the couch, with their arms resting at their side, and the back of their knees in contact with the couch. The patient actively slumps forwards into trunk flexion as far as possible, with the therapist providing slight overpressure. The patient is then asked to extend the knee as far as possible (this can be done passively), followed by active ankle dorsiflexion. Cervical flexion is then added to sensitize neural tissue, and then released into hyperextension to desensitize. If the patient experiences similar symptoms to those they have been experiencing previously, then this suggests a positive test. Variable conclusions to the test's diagnostic value have been proposed in the literature (Rabin *et al.*, 2007; Stankovich *et al.*, 1999), although the scope of studies is limited to only a few. The greater involvement of the spine in implicating the associated nerve roots potentially lends this test to being indicated above the SLR (Majilesi *et al.*, 2008); however, both have their merits and should be used concurrently in clinical practice. There are a number of factors that the sports therapist must appreciate to interpret the test reliably: some discomfort can be quite normal for the patient in the mid-thoracic area or behind the knees; a strong stretching or tingling in the posterior thigh, calf and foot can be normal; restrictions in knee extension or ankle dorsiflexion (left should equal right) are frequently observed; a decrease in discomfort after cervical flexion is released can be normal, as can an increase in RoM after cervical flexion is released.

Dermatome testing of the hip

Dermatomes are defined as areas of skin supplied by specific sensory nerve roots (Magee, 2008; Petty, 2011). When assessing a patient for dermatomal abnormalities through skin sensation responses, the therapist must provide clear instruction regarding what is required of the patient during applications of light, sharp and blunt stimulation. The patient needs to report what they feel, whether right is equal to left and whether they can tell the difference between the sensations. Specifically, when assessing the hip it is important to assess the dermatomes relating to L1–3, as abnormalities can be confused with hip dysfunction.

Myotome testing of the hip

The assessment of the myotomal function is an important element of the sports therapist's assessment of hip dysfunction. Myotomes are defined as a group of muscles supplied (innervated) by a specific nerve root (from a specific spinal segment), and dysfunction of such may be due to local peripheral neural or spinal impingement. Myotomes affecting the hip can be assessed with the patient lying supine, with the tested limb stabilized in a similar manner to that employed when assessing muscular strength. Weakness in force production may be due to muscular weakness (relating to immobilization or local injury), pain inhibition (secondary to injury), or a dysfunction within the neural component (i.e. myotomal). When assessing myotomes of the hip, it is important to assess the quality of the force the patient is producing, as well as how much. Is the patient applying maximal effort with minimal contraction, or is the muscle weak due to acute damage? The 'Oxford Grading Scale' is a method of assessing muscular strength and the neural component of muscular contraction, and should be used when recording patient findings.

Functional tests of the pelvis and hip

While assessing the pelvis and hip through evidence-based, traditional orthopaedic examination techniques is essential, specific functional tests can be used to test patients' combination movement patterns across basic activities of daily living, as well as those required for sports performance. This section merely highlights some of the tests that are available, and is not an exhaustive compilation.

Table 9.6 Myotome assessment

Nerve root	Procedure
L2	Hip flexion with the patient supine. Are they able to actively flex to 90° with a flexed knee? To increase the intensity this could be developed into a straight leg raise. If patient fails the straight leg raise test, and hip pathology is suspected, an X-ray may be appropriate
L3	Knee extension with patient seated. The therapist may apply some overpressure to the lower leg. It is important to not only assess with the knee fully extended, but also in range (+/− 45°), to assess for quality of control
L4	Foot dorsiflexion with patient supine. Resistance can be applied to the dorsum of the foot
S1	Eversion of foot with the patient supine while contracting the gluteals; or knee flexion with the patient prone. Mid-position resistance can be applied with the knee in 90° flexion
S2	Knee flexion in prone. As knee flexion can result from S1/2 dysfunction, the movement is performed as above. It is important to highlight all myotomes for S1/2 and any weakness and dysfunction. S2 can also be assessed via standing on tiptoes, which can also provide functional testing
S3–4	Bladder and bowel dysfunction is often detected in the subjective history rather than on physical assessment. Special questions, and possible red flags, can be highlighted prior to any assessment and appropriate referral to accident and emergency should follow (Greenhalgh and Selfe, 2010)

Squat

There are a number of squat variants (i.e. front, back, wide/sumo, single leg or overhead); the sports therapist may elect to incorporate assessment of ability to perform these with increasing load or repetition. For clinical evaluation, the 'back' and 'single leg' variations are most suitable.

A back squat should begin with the patient standing with feet parallel and a comfortable width apart. In the downward phase the patient should be instructed to keep their back flat, chest up and out and hands either held out in front or holding a bar across their shoulders while keeping their body weight centred through the heels (Chandler and Brown, 2013). As the patient begins to descend, they should be asked to do so under control while the knees flex so they stay over the feet and not in front, which may cause anterior shear. The patient should be asked to descend until the femur is parallel to the floor, or until the trunk begins to round or flex or heels lift from the floor (Baechle and Earle, 2008). In the upward phase, the patient should extend the knees and hips while maintaining a flat back with no forward trunk lean or rounding of the upper back until they reach the standing position (Chandler and Brown, 2013). If the hip is restricted into its capsular pattern the patient will be restricted in both internal rotation and flexion. Common compensatory methods for the hip include low back extension (to decrease hip flexion); hip internal rotation and adduction may point towards a lateral hip weakness of specifically gluteus medius. The squat will also allow for the assessment of the function of the hip and lower limb, but will not offer limitations in spinal (particularly thoracic) and shoulder mobility (which the overhead squat would do).

The single leg squat should begin with the patient holding their arms out in front, or on their hips, standing on one leg. The opposite leg may be placed either straight out in front with hip flexed and knee extended ('pistol' position), or behind with the knee flexed. In the downward phase, the patient should aim to keep their back flat, shoulders and trunk facing forwards and the supporting knee facing forwards in a controlled manner. In the upward phase, the patient should extend the standing knee and hip while maintaining the symmetry of the trunk and upper body. If the hip abductors are weak this may cause the patient's knee to drop into a valgus position on descent. If the hip hikes up on the non-stance side this may be indicative of adductor and/or gluteus medius under-activity in the stance leg, while a hip drop on the non-stance side can indicate under-activity of gluteus medius in the stance leg. If the patient is having difficulty maintaining balance, the reason for inability to control the movement could be due to contractile, non-contractile or neural factors, while a capsular restriction could affect the patient's ability to move into the flexed position. If any specifics are noted, then the contralateral side should be compared for similarities or differences.

Lunge

The lunge can either be performed with the affected side as the front foot or as the stabilizing leg in order to gauge the patient's ability to change and control the motion into flexion and into extension. To begin, the patient should be instructed to stand with feet parallel and arms out in front or on their hips. During the forward phase the patient should take an elongated step forwards with one leg, keeping the trunk and shoulders facing forwards (Chandler and Brown, 2013). The lead foot should point forwards as the knee and hip are flexed under control to approximately 3–5 cm from the floor (Baechle and Earle, 2008), with the knee staying over the foot and not in front to prevent anterior shear. In the backward phase, the patient should forcefully push off the floor with the lead leg, extending the knee and hip and keeping the trunk and shoulders facing forwards until they reach the start position in one smooth movement. When the affected side is brought into flexion the therapist can assess for musculoskeletal dysfunctions. The patient's hip position should be observed to identify whether the patient's centre of mass (CoM) is over the affected hip; if not this may indicate a weak gluteus medius. The inability to get into the flexed position may indicate a joint dysfunction. The patient's knee should be observed to note whether they are able to control hip adduction and internal rotation to prevent knee valgus. If the patient loses balance there may be poor trunk, lumbo-pelvic or ankle instability present; and if they are unable to return to the start position this can indicate a weakness or inhibition to the quadriceps or gluteals.

Reassessment approaches and fitness tests for the hip

Adductor squeeze test

Groin and adductor injury are common in sport (Nicholas and Tyler, 2002). It can be difficult to assess the patient's ability to contract and control their adductor muscle group. A simple method is to use a commercially available sphygmomanometer, or pressure biofeedback unit, which is proven to offer a reliable and valid method of assessing the patient's ability to contract and adduct as a form of biofeedback (Delahunt *et al.*, 2011). When performing this assessment, the targeted tissues are the adductor group (for any pain, strength, weakness and imbalances left to right). Other conditions of the region may, however, also cause symptoms during this test (such as osteitis pubis, inguinal hernia, iliopsoas or rectus femoris injury, or tendinopathy). The test can be performed in three positions, and it is advisable that all three are undertaken in order to assess differences – although literature suggests that 45° hip flexion in supine is the most effective at producing the highest pressure values (Delahunt *et al.*, 2011; Malliaras *et al.*, 2009). The recommended positions are as follows:

1. Patient positioned supine, with sphygmomanometer between knees.

2. Patient supine, with hips flexed to approximately 45° and knees flexed to 90°, with sphygmomanometer between knees.
3. Patient supine, with hips and knees flexed to 90° (legs unsupported), with sphygmomano- meter between knees.

If pre-injury measurements are available then a simple comparison can be made to assess progress and guide return to play. If not, then the therapist can assess the patient's ability to hold the contraction and any differences in values in more progressively difficult positions (Malliaras *et al.*, 2009).

Sport-specific assessment

Sport–specific assessments are fundamental prior to allowing the patient to return to training or competition. For multidirectional sports, it is important that the athlete's ability to pivot and change direction is assessed. The compression and rotation occurring during such movements directly affects the hip – specifically, non-contractile tissues (iliofemoral and ischiofemoral ligaments, and joint capsule), while the musculature controls the movement. A cutting manoeuvre is one of the easiest manoeuvres to assess prior to allowing the patient to progress to full training; the therapist can not only gauge the athlete's pain and their ability to perform the manoeuvre, but also review hip, knee and ankle positions, making sure correct position and control occurs. The therapist can assess bilaterally to make sure that the athlete is able to push off and also land and control the affected hip. Gait patterns should also be assessed prior to

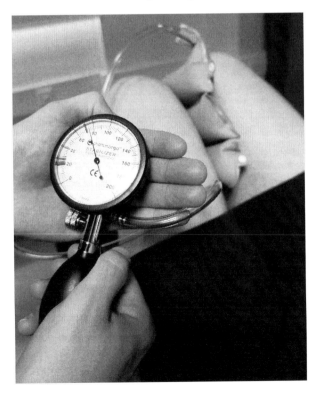

Photo 9.21 Adductor squeeze test.

return to play. Ideally, the athlete should have a full range, normal and pain-free gait pattern, and the therapist may use video recording to analyse regional components (including joint RoM, Q-angles and stride length). For example, knee valgus moments identified during cutting may suggest excessive adduction and internal rotation of the femur which are being caused by weak or underactive gluteal muscles. The sports therapist should assess bilaterally to make sure that the athlete is able to push off, but also land and control their affected hip. Landing and jumping movements are common in many sports, which justifies the inclusion of their assessment before return to play. One method of assessing this is the Landing Error Scoring System, which utilizes a scale of 17 scored items and has shown promising validity and reliability when assessing jumping and landing patterns (Onate *et al.*, 2010).

Injuries of the pelvis and hip region

The pelvis and hip is a complex region of functional anatomy, and as such is at risk of becoming injured through the demands of sport. The following section provides a brief overview of some of the more common conditions affecting the region.

Muscular injuries

Injuries of the musculature of the hip are common; and with the numerous muscles crossing the region, injuries can occur anteriorly, posteriorly, laterally and medially. Mechanisms particularly relate intrinsically to the athlete's conditioning and any previous musculotendinous injuries; and extrinsically to their sport and position. When assessing and reporting muscular injuries of the hip, the classification of acute muscle disorders and injuries presented by Mueller-Wohlfahrt *et al.* (2013) may be employed to allow a contemporaneous definition of the patient's problem to be reported. The first thing to be determined is whether the injury is direct or indirect. Direct injuries to the hip and thigh musculature are common in contact sports such as football, rugby and hockey, and so lacerations and contusions are common presentations. Deep lacerations which penetrate the skin can become infected, so management of bleeding and prompt referral to accident and emergency is recommended. Contusions (as in a 'corked' thigh) are managed acutely with cryotherapy (and possible compression), but must be monitored post-trauma as complications can arise with deep intramuscular haematomas (such as acute compartment syndrome, or myositis ossificans). Smith *et al.* (2006) provide a review of haematoma management. Indirect injuries to hip and thigh musculature are also highly prevalent in sport. The feeling of tightness in muscles, most likely caused by fatigue (a 'type 1A' condition), is very common and may be present as a result of changes in training loads, a change of playing surface or simple over-exertion (Mueller-Wohlfahrt *et al.*, 2013). The delayed onset of muscle soreness (DOMS) (a 'type 1B' condition) is also extremely prevalent in athletes and occurs hours after strenuous exercise, particularly with eccentric or unaccustomed exercise, such as with different movement patterns and increased intensities. DOMS is frequently seen in the gluteal group, hamstrings, quadriceps and adductors. While DOMS may be attenuated to a degree with active recovery methods, cold water immersion (CWI) post-exercise or soft tissue therapy, a preventative approach is considered more applicable with progressively intensive training programmes, including eccentric work.

Indirect muscle injuries can also be the result of neuromuscular disorders, with the cause originating from the spine ('type 2A') or the muscle itself ('type 2B'). Poor neuromuscular control, a structural or functional disorder of the spine and lumbo-pelvic disorders can lead to nerve root compressions in the lumbar plexus, increased muscle tone and neuromuscular misfiring (Mueller-

Wohlfahrt *et al.*, 2013). The sciatic nerve, which may be compressed at its nerve roots, or as it passes through or beneath the piriformis muscle, is the most likely structure linked to these types of muscle injuries around the hip, although increased muscle tone in any muscle may lead to a neuromuscular disorder. Findings of increased tone, symptoms of aching or cramp-like pain, tenderness on palpation and the lack of a clear mechanism of injury should arouse suspicion of a type 2A or 2B muscle injury. Management must focus on treating the symptoms and the cause, therefore spinal mobilizations, soft tissue therapy and neuromuscular training may be employed.

Minor and moderate musculotendinous tears ('type 3A' or '3B' injuries) of the hamstrings, quadriceps, adductors and hip flexors are prevalent in athletes. These occur during both eccentric and concentric actions – specifically kicking, accelerating or decelerating; and these are common in football, rugby and athletics. Most muscle tears are manageable conservatively; so muscular strength, joint RoM, proprioception, neuromuscular control and pelvic stability must be considered in the early stages of rehabilitation, alongside passive modalities. Complete ruptures ('type 4' injuries) of the proximal hamstrings musculotendinous junctions (or avulsions from the ischial tuberosity) usually occur with forced hip flexion (with knee extension). These have been noted in sports including rugby, horse riding and gymnastics; recent research suggests that surgery offers a better prognosis than conservative management for athletes (Birmingham *et al.*, 2011; Pombo and Bradley, 2009; Sarimo *et al.*, 2008).

Bursitis

The hip region has a number of bursae that can become irritated and inflamed by friction from the repetitive movements of overlying soft tissue, or via the direct impact trauma from a fall or a kick, for example. The most common sites at the hip are the iliopsoas bursa separating the iliopsoas tendon and the pubic area of the hip joint; and the trochanteric bursa located between the origin of gluteus medius and minimus and the greater trochanter. However, some believe that pain around the trochanteric bursa is more correctly described as a chronic degeneration of the surrounding soft tissue (specifically tendons of gluteus medius and minimus) (Braun and Jensen, 2007). Patients typically present with localized swelling and pain over the bursa, and tenderness on palpation. Special tests which may reproduce symptoms and possibly indicate hip bursitis can include: modified Ober's, FABER and FADDIR (for all trochanteric bursae); and the prone knee bend, FABER, FADDIR and Thomas test (for the iliopsoas bursa).

Bursitis may be caused by blunt trauma, tight musculotendinous and fascial tissue (particularly TFL and ITB), postural dysfunctions and repetitive irritations. However, an apparent lack of inflammatory cells and oedema in some symptomatic trochanteric bursae presentations does question the involvement of the bursae in lateral hip pain (Shbeeb and Matteson, 1996; Williams and Cohen, 2009). Gluteal tendinopathy, or enthesopathy, is a more likely contributory factor to lateral hip pain than an inflamed trochanteric bursa (Walsh *et al.*, 2011).

Sports therapists can use a variety of management options for bursitis; the focus will typically involve pain reduction and improving function through addressing any dynamic postural and muscular imbalances (Williams and Cohen, 2009). Although evidence is limited for the conservative treatment of hip bursitis, it is generally accepted that cryotherapy can reduce pain (Bleakley *et al.*, 2004; Hamer, 2004). As there are no studies available regarding muscle imbalances and the frequency of bursitis within the hip, studies involving the shoulder joint show a strong correlation with biomechanical changes and bursitis, which may have similar implications with regard to the hip, specifically with gluteus medius weakness and also hip flexor tightness. Some research supports the use of electrotherapy alongside exercise prescription, (specifically the use of pulsed shortwave therapy) (Lustenberger *et al.*, 2011). Where conservative treatment has failed, there is evidence to support the use of injection therapy as an adjunct, specifically if pain is the primary complaint (Hamer, 2004; Williams and Cohen, 2009).

Piriformis syndrome

Piriformis syndrome is a somewhat controversial condition, with some rehabilitation specialists not believing the condition exists (Silver and Leadbetter, 1998). The condition was originally described in 1928 as an irritation of the sciatic nerve by the piriformis muscle, which caused local and referred posterior leg pain. In approximately 16 per cent of people, the sciatic nerve passes through piriformis, and contraction and shortening of the muscle can cause neural pain (Smoll, 2010). The nerve can be damaged, not just irritated, by piriformis as it either passes through the greater sciatic notch or through the muscle itself (Fishman *et al.*, 2002). Further tests which can be carried out to help determine the condition include FADDIR and SLR; pain while palpating or stretching the gluteal muscles or the piriformis may also allow the sports therapist to determine the locality of pain.

Treatment options include soft tissue therapy (Bewyer and Bewyer, 2003), TENS (Ruiz-Arranz *et al.*, 2008) and exercise therapy aimed at incorporating normal movement patterns and strengthening any weakness within the gluteal muscles. There is some evidence to support the use of NSAIDs (Parziale *et al.*, 1996); the sports therapist may feel it appropriate to refer to a GP. Manual treatment is with the patient side-lying, injured side up, knee flexed to 75–85° and resting their foot on the back leg (Fishman and Zybert, 1992). In this position the piriformis is readily palpable and manipulated. In worst-case scenarios decompression surgery can be used; however, limited evidence is available to support this (Foster, 2002). All management should be aimed at the unique presentations of the patient in question, which can include: buttock pain, which commonly refers down the posterior leg; reduced RoM in the hip; inability to sit for long periods; and inability to perform full hip range movements in sport (due to pain and stiffness).

Snapping hip syndrome

Snapping hip, also known as coxa saltans, is a general term used to describe the painful, palpable or audible noise made during movement of the hip joint. It is most common in teenagers and young adults (Lewis, 2010), and may have a higher incidence in sports and activities which involve extreme ranges of hip motion, such as dancing (Winston *et al.*, 2007), and those which require repetitive hip movements, such as football (Ilizaliturri *et al.*, 2006; Wahl *et al.*, 2004) and running (Konczak and Ames, 2005; Provencher *et al.*, 2004). Snapping hip conditions may be split into three classifications based on aetiology – namely intra-articular and extra-articular (internal and external).

Intra-articular snapping hip

Intra-articular cases usually involve associated pathology, such as acetabular labral tears, cartilage defects, loose bodies or fracture fragments (Byrd, 1996; Yamamoto *et al.*, 2004). Signs and symptoms of intra-articular snapping hip include catching, locking, painful clicking or a sharp stabbing sensation (Gruen *et al.*, 2002; Yamamoto *et al.*, 2004). Tests which indicate hip joint pathology are indicated.

Internal extra-articular snapping hip

Internal extra-articular snapping hip is often caused by abnormal movement of the iliopsoas over a bony prominence, typically the femoral neck, lesser trochanter or iliopectineal eminence

(Allen and Cope, 1995; Byrd, 2005; Harper *et al.*, 1987), although research suggests that the iliacus muscle can be more responsible for this than the iliopsoas tendon (Deslands *et al.*, 2008; Winston *et al.*, 2007). The condition may also be linked to iliopsoas bursitis (Wahl *et al.*, 2004), and in rare cases may be due to calcification of the rectus femoris tendon (Pierannunzzi *et al.*, 2010) or ischiofemoral impingement (Ali *et al.*, 2011).

External extra-articular snapping hip

External extra-articular snapping hip is due to abnormal movement of the ITB over the greater trochanter (Pelsser *et al.*, 2001) during lateral rotation and flexion (Battaglia *et al.*, 2011); in rare cases the gluteus maximus may be implicated (Brignall *et al.*, 1993). It is possible that an associated trochanteric bursitis may be present with external extra-articular snapping hip (Kingzett-Taylor *et al.*, 1999), although this association may be low (Choi *et al.*, 2010).

Management of snapping hip syndrome is dependent on its classification and severity, with modalities ranging between therapeutic, medical and operative options. The most utilized treatment conservatively is rest and activity modification, alongside stretching of the associated soft tissues contributing to the condition (including iliopsoas, TFL and associated fascia (Dobbs *et al.*, 2002; Keskula *et al.*, 1999)). Both NSAIDs and soft tissue therapy may be beneficial (Byrd, 2005; Gruen *et al.*, 2002; Konczak and Ames, 2005). Injection of local anaesthetic with corticosteroid into associated bursae to reduce pain has seen positive outcomes when used alongside physical therapy (Flanum *et al.*, 2007; Hoskins *et al.*, 2004; Satku *et al.*, 1990). Operative intervention is often required for intra-articular aetiology. Extra-articular cases may involve endoscopic release, or moderate lengthening of the affected tissue (Hoskins *et al.*, 2004; McCulloch and Bush-Joseph, 2006).

Femoroacetabular impingement

Femoroacetabular impingement (FAI) is the term used to describe abnormal mechanics at the coxal joint which may trap, impinge or erode the acetabular labrum, causing pain and dysfunction. It most typically affects young males and middle-aged females (Byrd and Jones, 2009; Tannast *et al.*, 2007). The highest prevalence of the injury is seen in sports which require repetitive hip flexion, adduction and medial rotation, such as ice hockey, football and rugby (Gerdhardt *et al.*, 2012; Lorentzon *et al.*, 1998; Molloy and Molloy, 2011). This condition can present in three ways: cam-type FAI; pincer-type FAI; or a combined cam–pincer-type FAI, where both cam and pincer situations present together – it is the latter which is most common, seen in over 80 per cent of reported cases (Ganz *et al.*, 2003; Philippon *et al.*, 2009).

Cam-type FAI

Cam-type FAI is present when there is abnormal articulation between the head of the femur and acetabulum in the anterolateral region. This may be due to anatomical abnormalities of the femoral head, neck or junction between the two, or excessive RoM at the coxal joint. As a result, there is impingement of the acetabular labrum and potential separation of the labrum from the acetabular cartilage (Beck *et al.*, 2005).

Pincer-type FAI

Pincer-type FAI is characterized by an abnormality of the acetabulum (socket, cartilage and/or labrum). The acetabular labrum can become compressed against the femoral head or neck anterolaterally, resulting in its degeneration. This may consequently cause posterior subluxation of the femoral head, which in turn can result in posteroinferior acetabular cartilage damage (Parvizi and Ganz, 2005), as well as roughening of the femoral head (Beck *et al.*, 2005).

The aetiology of FAI is still relatively unknown, although a few suggestions have been proposed. These include: abnormal bony prominences on the acetabular rim and femoral head (Wenger *et al.*, 2004); slipped capital femoral epiphysis (Goodman *et al.*, 1997); malunion of femoral neck fractures (Bettin *et al.*, 2003; Eijer *et al.*, 2001); oversized femoral head (Nemtala *et al.*, 2010); flattening of the femoral head due to femoral head necrosis (Kloen *et al.*, 2002); excessive coxal RoM (Parvizi and Ganz, 2005); and acetabulum that is abnormally shaped – deep (coxa profunda), or retroverted (Philippon *et al.*, 2010). Anatomical abnormalities may not be the only aetiology, as the mechanism of injury and influence of repetitive sport-specific movements may also be contributing factors (Kang *et al.*, 2010; Keogh and Batt, 2008). The most common signs and symptoms seen in patients include persistent groin pain (Feeley *et al.*, 2008), pain on movement (particularly flexion and medial rotation) (Ito *et al.*, 2001), and pain during long periods of sitting (Keogh and Bat, 2008). Decreased RoM and decreased performance may also be seen in symptomatic patients (Molsa *et al.*, 1997; Philippon *et al.*, 2007a). A prominent issue with FAI is the difficulty in diagnosis, with the time taken from injury to accurate diagnosis potentially being a long period (Burnett *et al.*, 2006). FAI is strongly linked with other pathologies of the hip joint, including labral tears (Nho *et al.*, 2011), intra-articular acetabular cartilage damage and osteoarthritis (Ganz *et al.*, 2003; Leunig *et al.*, 2005).

Management can be approached both conservatively and operatively, although in a very high percentage of cases surgery is required when symptoms persist. Conservative treatment may involve activity modification, NSAIDs, muscle balance work and core strengthening (Keogh and Batt, 2008; Ng *et al.*, 2010). There are two main approaches to surgery; open and arthroscopic. Open surgery has been most utilized in the past as it allows a full, unobstructed view of the inter-articular structures (Lavigne *et al.*, 2004); however, it is less popular with athletes as it involves dislocation of the hip joint and a lengthy rehabilitation programme (Brunner *et al.*, 2009; Philippon *et al.*, 2007b). Arthroscopic surgery has been shown to be as effective as open techniques with most pathologies involved with FAI (Clohisy *et al.*, 2007; Laude *et al.*, 2009; Lincoln *et al.*, 2009), although accurate classification of the femoral and acetabular morphology is essential when selecting the most effective surgical approach (Bedi *et al.*, 2011). Current surgical procedures include labral repair and debridement, acetabuloplasty, resectioning of the femoral head–neck junction bony prominences and restoration of femoral head sphericity (Kang *et al.*, 2010).

Hip conditions not to be missed...

There is a vast range of pathological conditions which may be implicated at the hip and, although many are rare in the sporting athlete, they should not be discounted from the differential diagnosis of a patient with hip or groin pain. This is particularly the case when treatment and rehabilitation is seen to be ineffective, or the patient's symptoms are getting worse over time. Referral for medical investigation is always an option for consideration where the chronicity of symptoms does not follow an expected pattern.

Osteoarthritis of the hip

Degeneration of articular cartilage can occur at any synovial joint, but due to the significant forces that go through the hip joint during weight bearing (between three to eight times bodyweight according to Hashimoto *et al.*, 2005), the coxal joint is at significant risk. Other contributory factors to osteoarthritis (OA) are obesity, muscular weakness, sports trauma or previous hip joint injury. Typical symptoms of OA include pain on movement, joint stiffness, muscular weakness and easing of symptoms when not weight bearing. Patients suspected of having OA should be referred to their GP for X-ray investigation. Typical radiological findings that suggest OA is present include joint space narrowing, osteophytes (bony spurs), subchondral sclerosis (increased bone formation underneath the articular cartilage) and subchondral cyst formation (Reijman *et al.*, 2004).

Avascular necrosis of the femoral head

Avascular necrosis (AVN, or osteonecrosis) is a condition characterized by a lack of microcirculation in bone, leading to ischaemia (Lieberman *et al.*, 2002). This leads to destruction and death of cells and marrow at the subchondral level of the femoral head, eventually leading to collapse (Malizos *et al.*, 2007). The condition is more common in men (Assouline-Dayan *et al.*, 2002) and can be classified as having traumatic or atraumatic aetiology. Atraumatic causes are typically progressive, and can be linked to alcohol abuse, prolonged steroid use, as well as gastrointestinal, haematological and metabolic diseases. Common traumatic causes, which are actually more common in the athletic population, include displaced intracapsular neck of femur fractures (which affect the retinacular vessels around the head of femur and microvasculature within bone) and hip dislocations (which disturb the blood supply to the fovea of the femoral head within the ligamentum teres) (Lieberman *et al.*, 2002). Patients will often complain of an acute episode of pain which feels deep in the joint or groin, pain on weight bearing and limitations in movement. If suspected, the therapist should refer the athlete for investigation. If confirmed the athlete may require operative decompression of the femoral head, or an arthroplastic procedure, depending on how advanced the condition is on the four-stage 'Ficat Classification', which uses a combination of plain film, MRI and clinical features (Ficat, 1985).

Referred lumbar pathology

As with any other peripheral joint, it is important to assess the joint above (to assist in ruling out referred pathology). Within the hip, it is important to not only rule out SIJ dysfunction (that commonly presents as inner hip pain), but also lumbar referred pain, where the main dermatomal pattern offering referred pain from L1–4 is to the lateral hip. The psoas muscle originates from the lumbar spine, so not only can there be a myotomal effect, but also a biomechanically inefficient muscle. During objective assessment, the therapist must review the lumbar spine in order to highlight any adapted lumbar curvature, such as an increase or decrease in lumbar lordosis, causing the hip to adapt to a change in position that may cause either hypo- or hypermobility of the hip. Various pathologies from the lumbar spine can refer into the hip, specifically within the sporting population discogenic conditions (such as prolapses) need to be assessed and ruled out before a full hip diagnosis can be confirmed. Whether the patient has a history of back injuries or a clear mechanism is the easiest method of highlighting any possible lumbar disc injuries that may have referred to the hip. The most frequent area of referred pain from the lumbar spine is the posterior thigh and buttock (Toth *et al.*, 2005). If the patient presents with posterior thigh and buttock pain when clearing the lumbar spine, it is important to identify whether the patient's pain increases in intensity or centralizes or peripheralizes. Lateral hip pain can be a referral from L5 due to the motor nerve supply to the hip abductors. Furthermore, symptoms may result from the SIJ (S1–3) nerve roots, which often present with an increase in neural tension while assessing neural dynamics via the SLR or slump test (Fagerson, 1998; Walker *et al.*, 2007). Degenerative changes within the lumbar spine (spondylosis) can cause the hips to overcompensate, with increased functional movement to reduce the effort on the lumbar spine (Shum *et al.*, 2005); this affects not only the movement available at the hip, but also general limb coordination. If a patient presents without clear mechanism of injury, or there is suspicion of neural or spinal involvement, these must always be assessed or cleared prior to local assessment of the hip (Hengeveld and Banks, 2005). The management of any hip pain that is originating from the spine (or local neural component) must also not only include local hip treatment, it should prioritize the spinal treatment and dysfunction. A primary goal of the spinal management should be to offer reduction in symptoms during function within the hip region.

Lymphatic metastasis at the groin

The spread of diseases (pathogenic organisms or cancer cells) from one part of the body to another is known as metastasis (Tortora and Derrickson, 2008), and this can occur via the lymphatic system of the lower limb. Lymph nodes play an important role in the human immune response, and the increased activity of lymphocytes (B and T cells) may lead to inguinal lymph nodes becoming inflamed, swollen and tender as a result of injury or infection. As an example, one of the more common lower limb (foot) infections is tinea pedis ('athlete's foot' – a fungal infection) (Crawford, 2009). This usually presents as a mild local unilateral irritation on the skin of the affected foot, often between the toes, with skin breakdown, redness, flaking and itchiness. Occasionally when spreading, this condition can present with other signs and symptoms, such as a painful aching at the groin; with a fairly rapid onset, and no sporting mechanism of injury, the inguinal lymph nodes can become larger and palpably tender. With such spreading of infection (most commonly as a bacterial cellulitis), the popliteal nodes (at the posterior knee) may also become active and inflamed in the popliteal fossa; this may occur prior to any groin pain, and the athlete should be observed for any history of this. It must be noted that serious pathological red flag conditions such as testicular cancer, lymphoma and melanoma may all present pain in this region and must not be dismissed too early in the assessment. Wherever there is the suspicion of infection or other possible serious conditions, referral for medical assessment is essential.

This chapter has provided a foundational overview of the anatomy, relations, functions, sports biomechanics, assessment and management approaches for a selection of common conditions involving the pelvic and hip region. Sports therapists must be advised to seek out further information on all areas discussed, particular by accessing some of the key references cited within the text. Additionally, there are a host of conditions which it has not been possible to include in depth, which sports therapists must also aim to develop their knowledge of – these include: hip-related tendinopathy, inguinal and femoral hernia, osteitis pubis, Legg–Calve–Perthes disease, developmental hip dysplasia, transient hip synovitis, intermittent claudication, total hip replacement (THR) and exercise-associated muscle cramp (EAMC), as well as conditions affecting the SIJ. Some of these conditions are discussed elsewhere in this book.

References

Abe, I., Harada, Y., Oinuma, K., *et al.* (2000) Acetabular labrum: Abnormal findings at MR imaging in asymptomatic hips. *Radiology.* 216: 576–581

Aglietti, P., Insall, J.N. and Cerulli, G. (1983) Patellar pain and incongruence: Measurements of incongruence. *Clinical Orthopaedics and Related Research.* 176: 217–224

Ali, A.M., Whitwell, D. and Ostlere, S.J. (2011) Case report: Imaging and surgical treatment of a snapping hip due to ischiofemoral impingement. *Skeletal Radiology.* 40 (5): 653–656

Allen, W.C. and Cope, R. (1995) Coxa saltans: The snapping hip revisited. *Journal of American Academy of Orthopaedic Surgeons.* 3 (5): 303–308

Aminaka, N. and Gribble, P.A. (2008) Patellar taping, patellofemoral pain syndrome, lower extremity kinematics, and dynamic postural control. *Journal of Athletic Training*. 43 (1): 21

Assouline-Dayan, Y., Chang, C., Greenspan, A., Shoenfeld, Y., Eric, M. and Gershwin, M.C. (2002) Pathogenesis and natural history of osteonecrosis. *Seminars in Arthritis and Rheumatism*. 32: 94–124

Atkins, E., Kerr, J. and Goodlad, E. (2010) *A practical approach to orthopaedic medicine: Assessment, diagnosis and treatment*, 3rd edition. Churchill Livingstone, Elsevier. London, UK

Baechle, T.R. and Earle, R.W. (2008) *Essentials of strength training and conditioning*, 3rd edition. Human Kinetics. Champaign, IL

Bahr, R. and Maehlum, S. (2004) *Clinical guide to sports injuries*. Gazette Bok. Oslo, Norway

Bartlett, R. (1999) *Sports biomechanics: Reducing injury and improving performance*. Taylor and Francis. London, UK

Battaglia, M., Guaraldi, F., Monti, C., Vanel, D. and Vannini, F. (2011) An unusual cause of external snapping hip. *Musculoskeletal Radiology*. 5 (10): 1–6.

Beck, M., Kalhor, M., Leunig, M. and Ganz, R. (2005) Hip morphology influences the pattern of damage to the acetabular cartilage: Femoroacetabular impingement as a cause of early osteoarthritis of the hip. *British Journal of Bone and Joint Surgery*. 87 (7): 1012–1018

Bedi, A., Zaltz, I., De La Torre, K. and Kelly, B.T. (2011) Radiographic comparison of surgical hip dislocation and hip arthroscopy for treatment of cam deformity in femoroacetabular impingement. *American Journal of Sports Medicine*. 39: 20S–28S.

Bettin, D., Pankalla, T., Böhm, H. and Fuchs, S. (2003) Hip pain related to femoral neck stress fracture in a 12-year-old boy performing intensive soccer playing activities: A case report. *International Journal of Sports Medicine*. 24 (8): 593–596

Bewyer, D.C. and Bewyer, K.J. (2003) Rationale for treatment of hip abductor pain syndrome. *Iowa Orthopaedic Journal*. 23: 57

Bianchi, S., Martinoli, C., Keller, A. and Bianchi-Zamorani, M.P. (2002) Giant iliopsoas bursitis: Sonographic findings with magnetic resonance correlations. *Journal of Clinical Ultrasound*. 30 (7): 437–441

Bird, P.A., Oakley, S.P., Shnier, R. and Kirkham, B.W. (2001) Prospective evaluation of magnetic resonance imaging and physical examination findings in patients with greater trochanteric pain syndrome. *Arthritis and Rheumatism*. 44 (9): 2138–2145

Birmingham, P., Muller, M., Wickiewicz, T., Cavanaugh, J., Rodeo, S., and Warren, R. (2011) Functional outcome after repair of proximal hamstring avulsions. *The Journal of Bone and Joint Surgery*. 93 (19): 1819–1826

Bizzini, M. (2011) The groin area: The Bermuda triangle of sports medicine? *British Journal of Sports Medicine*. 45: 1

Blankenbaker, D.G. and Tuite, M.J. (2006) The painful hip: New concepts. *Skeletal Radiology*. 35 (6): 352–370

Bleakley, C., McDonough, S. and MacAuley, D. (2004) The use of ice in the treatment of acute soft-tissue injury: A systematic review of randomized controlled trials. *American Journal of Sports Medicine*. 32 (1): 251–261

Bobbert, M.F. and Van Zandwijk, J.P. (1999) Dynamics of force and muscle stimulation in human vertical jumping. *Medicine and Science in Sports and Exercise*. 31: 303–310

Braly, B.A., Beall, D.P. and Martin, H.D. (2006) Clinical examination of the athletic hip. *Clinics in Sports Medicine*. 25 (2): 199–210

Brattstroem, H. (1964) Shape of the intercondylar groove normally and in recurrent dislocation of patella: A clinical and X-ray-anatomical investigation. *Acta Orthopedica Scandinavica*. 68 (Suppl.): 1–148

Braun, P.P. and Jensen, S.S. (2007) Hip pain: A focus on the sporting population. *Australian Family Physician*. 36 (6):406–413

Brignall, C.G., Brown, R.M. and Stainsby, G.D. (1993) Fibrosis of the gluteus maximus as a cause of snapping hip: A case report. *Journal of Bone and Joint Surgery*. 75 (6): 909–910

Brown, M.D., Gomez-Marin, O., Brookfield, K.F. and Li, P.S. (2004) Differential diagnosis of hip disease versus spine disease. *Clinical Orthopaedics and Related Research*. 419: 280–284

Brunner, A., Horisberger, M. and Herzog, R.F. (2009) Sports and recreation activity of patients with femoroacetabular impingement before and after arthroscopic osteoplasty. *American Journal of Sports Medicine*. 37 (5): 917–922

Burnett, R.S., Della Rocca, G.J., Prather, H., Curry, M., Maloney, W.J. and Clohisy, J.C. (2006) Clinical presentation of patients with tears of the acetabular labrum. *American Journal of Bone and Joint Surgery*. 88: 1448–1457

Byrd, J.W. (1996) Labral lesions: An elusive source of hip pain case reports and literature review. *Arthroscopy.* 12 (5): 603–612

Byrd, J.W. (2005) Snapping hip. *Operative Techniques in Sports Medicine.* 13: 46–54

Byrd, J.T. and Jones, K.S. (2009) Hip arthroscopy in athletes: 10-year follow-up. *American Journal of Sports Medicine.* 37 (11), 2140–2143

Carvalhais, V.O.D.C., Araújo, V.L.D., Souza, T.R., Gonçalves, G.G.P., Ocarino, J.D.M. and Fonseca, S.T. (2011) Validity and reliability of clinical tests for assessing hip passive stiffness. *Manual Therapy.* 16 (3): 240–245

Chandler, T.J. and Brown, L.E. (2013) *Conditioning for strength and human performance,* 2nd edition. Lippinacott, Williams and Wilkins. Philadelphia, PA

Chen, H.H., Li, A.F., Li, K.C., Wu, J.J., Chen, T.S. and Lee, M.C. (1996) Adaptations of ligamentum teres in ischemic necrosis of human femoral head. *Clinical Orthopaedic Related Research.* 328: 268–275

Choi, J.E., Sung, M.S., Lee, K.H., *et al.* (2010) External snapping hip syndrome: Emphasis on the MR imaging. *Journal of the Korean Society of Radiology.* 62: 185–190

Cichanowski, H.R., Schmitt, J.S., Johnson, R.J. and Niemuth, P.E. (2007) Hip strength in collegiate female athletes with patellofemoral pain. *Medicine and Science in Sports and Exercise.* 39 (8): 1227–1232

Claiborne, T.L., Armstrong, C.W., Gandhi, V. and Pincivero, D.M. (2006) Relationship between hip and knee strength and knee valgus during a single leg squat. *Journal of Applied Biomechanics.* 22 (1): 41–50

Clapis, P.A., Davis, S.M. and Davis, R.O. (2008) Reliability of inclinometer and goniometric measurements of hip extension flexibility using the modified Thomas test. *Physiotherapy Theory and Practice.* 24 (2): 135–141

Clarkson, H.M. (2000). *Musculoskeletal assessment: Joint range of motion and manual muscle strength.* Lippinacott, Williams and Wilkins. Baltimore, MD

Clohisy, J.C., Nunley, R.M., Otto, R.J. and Schoenecker, P.L. (2007) The frog-leg lateral radiograph accurately visualized hip cam impingement abnormalities. *Clinical Orthopaedic Related Research.* 462: 115–121

Collee, G., Dijkmans, B.A., Vandenbroucke, J.P. and Cats, A. (1991) Greater trochanteric pain syndrome (trochanteric bursitis) in low back pain. *Scandinavian Journal of Rheumatology.* 20: 262–266

Cook, C.E. and Hegedus, E. (2013) *Orthopaedic physical examination tests,* 2nd edition. Prentice Hall. London, UK

Cowan, D.N., Jones, B.H., Frykman, P.N., Polly, D.W., Jr., Harman, E.A. and Rosenstein, R.M. (1996) Lower limb morphology and risk of overuse injury among male infantry trainees. *Medicine and Science in Sports and Exercise.* 28 (8): 945–952.

Crawford, F. (2009) Athlete's foot. *Clinical Evidence (online)* www.ncbi.nlm.nih.gov/pmc/articles/PMC2907807, accessed June 2013

Davis, D.S., Quinn, R.O., Whiteman, C.T., Williams, J.D. and Young, C.R. (2008) Concurrent validity of four clinical tests used to measure hamstring flexibility. *Journal of Strength and Conditioning Research.* 22 (2): 583–588

DeAngelis, N.A. and Busconi, B.D. (2003) Assessment and differential diagnosis of the painful hip. *Clinical Orthopaedics and Related Research.* 406 (1): 11–18

Delahunt, E., Kennelly, C., McEntee, B.L., Coughlan, G.F. and Green, B.S. (2011) The thigh adductor squeeze test: 45° of hip flexion as the optimal test position for eliciting adductor muscle activity and maximum pressure values. *Manual Therapy.* 16 (5): 476–480

Deslandes, M., Guillin, R., Cardinal, E., Hobden, R. and Bureau, N.J. (2008) The snapping iliopsoas tendon: New mechanisms using dynamic sonography. *American Journal of Roentgenology.* 190 (3): 576–581

Dobbs, M.B., Gordon, J.E., Luhmann, S.J., Szymanski, D.A. and Schoenecker, P.L. (2002) Surgical correction of the snapping iliopsoas tendon in adolescents. *American Journal of Bone and Joint Surgery.* 84 (3): 420–424

Domb, B.G., Brooks, A.G. and Byrd, J.W. (2009) Clinical examination of the hip joint in athletes. *Journal of Sport Rehabilitation.* 18 (1): 3–23

Dougherty, C. and Dougherty, J.J. (2008) Evaluating hip pathology in trochanteric pain syndrome: Pain patterns shared with other conditions often complicate the diagnosis. *The Journal of Musculoskeletal Medicine.* 25 (9): 428

Dutton, M. (2011) *Orthopedics for the physical therapy assistant.* Jones and Bartlett Publishers. Boston, MA

Dy, C.J., Thompson, M.T., Crawford, M.J., Alexander, J.W., McCarthy, J.C. and Noble, P.C. (2008) Tensile strain in the anterior part of the acetabular labrum during provocative manoeuvring of the normal hip. *American Journal of Bone and Joint Surgery*. 90 (7): 1464–1472

Eckhoff, D.G., Montgomery, W.K., Kilcoyne, R.F. and Stamm, E.R. (1994) Femoral morphometry and anterior knee pain. *Clinical Orthopaedics and Related Research*. 302: 64–68

Eckstein, F., Hudelmaier, M. and Putz, R. (2006) The effects of exercise on human articular cartilage. *Journal of Anatomy*. 208: 491–512

Eijer, H., Myers, S.R. and Ganz, R. (2001) Anterior femoroacetabular impingement after femoral neck fractures. *Journal of Orthopaedic Trauma*. 15 (7): 475–481

Fagerson, T.L. (1998). *The hip handbook*. Butterworth-Heinemann Medical. Oxford, UK

Feeley, B.T., Powell, J.W., Muller, M.S., Barnes, R.P., Warren, R.F. and Kelly, B.T. (2008) Hip injuries and labral tears in the National Football League. *American Journal of Sports Medicine*. 36 (11): 2187–2195

Ferguson, S.J., Bryant, J.T., Ganz, R. and Ito, K. (2003) An in-vitro investigation of the acetabular labral seal in hip joint mechanics. *Journal of Biomechanics*. 36 (2): 171–178

Ferriera, E.A., Duarte, M., Maldonado, E.P., Bersanetti, A.A. and Marques, A.P. (2011) Quantitative assessment of postural alignment in young adults based on photographs of anterior, posterior and lateral views. *Journal of Manipulative and Physiological Therapeutics*. 34: 371–380

Ficat, R.P. (1985) Idiopathic bone necrosis of the femoral head: Early diagnosis and treatment. *British Journal of Bone and Joint Surgery*. 67: 3–9

Fishman, L.M. and Zybert, P.A. (1992) Electrophysiological evidence of piriformis syndrome. *Archives of Physical Medicine and Rehabilitation*. 73: 359–364

Fishman, L.M., Dombi, G.W., Michaelsen, C., *et al*. (2002) Piriformis syndrome: Diagnosis, treatment, and outcome. A 10-year study. *Archives of Physical Medicine and Rehabilitation*. 83 (3): 295–301

Fitzgerald, R.H. (1995) Acetabular labrum tears: Diagnosis and treatment. *Clinical Orthopaedics*. 311: 60–68

Flanum, M.E., Keene, J.S., Blankenbaker, D.G. and Desmet, A.A. (2007) Arthroscopic treatment of the painful internal snapping hip: Results of a new endoscopic technique and imaging protocol. *American Journal of Sports Medicine*. 35 (5): 770–779

Foster, M.R. (2002) Piriformis syndrome. *Orthopedics*. 25: 821–825

Fuss, F.K. and Bacher, A. (1991) New aspects of the morphology and function of the human hip joint ligaments. *American Journal of Anatomy*. 192 (1): 1–13

Gajdosik, R.L., Rieck, M.A., Sullivan, D.K. and Wightman, S.E. (1993) Comparison of four clinical tests for assessing hamstring muscle length. *Journal of Orthopaedic and Sports Physical Therapy*. 18 (5): 614

Gajdosik, R.L., Sandler, M.M. and Marr, H.L. (2003) Influence of knee positions and gender on the Ober test for length of the iliotibial band. *Clinical Biomechanics*. 18 (1): 77–79

Ganz, R., Parvizi, J., Beck, M., Leunig, M., Notzli, H. and Siebenrock, K. (2003) Femoroacetabular impingement: A cause for osteoarthritis of the hip. *Clinical Orthopaedics*. 417: 112–120

Gerhardt, M.B., Romero, A.A., Silvers, H.J., Harris, D.J., Watanabe, D. and Mandelbaum, B.R. (2012) The prevalence of radiographic hip abnormalities in elite soccer players. *American Journal of Sports Medicine*. 40 (3): 584–588

Giori, N.J. and Trousdale, R.T. (2003) Acetabular retroversion is associated with osteoarthritis of the hip. *Clinical Orthopaedics and Related Research*. 417: 263–269

Godges, J.J., MacRae, H., Longdon, C., Tinberg, C. and MacRae, P. (1989) The effects of two stretching procedures on hip range of motion and gait economy. *Journal of Orthopaedic and Sports Physical Therapy*. 10 (9): 350–357

Good, C.J. (2000) Passive osteokinematic motion palpation of the peripheral joints. In Broome, R.T. (ed.) *Chiropractic peripheral joint technique*. Butterworth-Heinemann. Oxford, UK

Goodman, D., Feighan, J. and Smith, A. (1997) Sub-clinical slipped capital femoral epiphysis: Relationship to osteoarthritis of the hip. *American Journal of Bone and Joint Surgery*. 79A: 1489–1497

Greene, C.C., Edwards, T.B., Wade, M.R. and Carson, E.W. (2001) Reliability of the quadriceps angle measurement. *American Journal of Knee Surgery*. 14: 97–103

Greenhalgh, S. and Selfe, J. (2010). *Red flags II: A guide to solving serious pathology of the spine*. Elsevier. London, UK

Grelsamer, R.P., Dubey, A. and Weinstein, C.H. (2005) Men and women have similar Q-angles: A clinical and trigonometric evaluation. *British Journal of Bone and Joint Surgery*. 87 (11): 1498–1501

Grimaldi, A. (2011). Assessing lateral stability of the hip and pelvis. *Manual Therapy*. 16 (1): 26–32

Gross, J.M., Fetto, J. and Rosen, E. (2009) *Musculoskeletal examination*, 3rd edition. Wiley-Blackwell. Chichester, UK

Gruen, G.S., Scioscia, T.N. and Lowenstein, J.E. (2002) The surgical treatment of internal snapping hip. *American Journal of Sports Medicine*. 30 (4): 607–613

Hak, D.J., Hamel, A.J., Bay, B.K., Sharkey, N.A. and Olson, S.A. (1998) Consequences of transverse acetabular fracture malreduction on load transmission across the hip joint. *Orthopedic Trauma*. 12: 90–100

Hamer, A.J. (2004) Pain in the hip and knee. In Snaith, M.L. (ed.) *ABC of rheumatology*, 3rd edition. BMJ Books. London, UK

Hamill, J. and Knutzen, K.M. (2009) *Biomechanical basis of human movement*, 3rd edition. Lippinacott, Williams and Wilkins. Philadelphia, PA

Harmon, K.G. (2010) Muscle injuries and PRP: What does the science say? *British Journal of Sports Medicine*. 44 (9): 616–617

Harper, M.C., Schaberg, J.E. and Allen, W.C. (1987) Primary iliopsoas bursography in the diagnosis of disorders of the hip. *Clinical Orthopaedics and Related Research*. 221: 238–241

Harvey, D. (1998) Assessment of the flexibility of elite athletes using the modified Thomas test. *British Journal of Sports Medicine*. 32 (1): 68–70

Hashimoto, N., Ando, M., Yayama, T., *et al.* (2005) Dynamic analysis of the resultant force acting on the hip joint during level walking. *Artificial Organs*. 29 (5): 387–392

Hattam, P. and Smeatham, A. (2010) *Special tests in musculoskeletal examination: An evidence-based guide for clinicians*. Elsevier. London, UK

Heinert, B.L., Kernozek, T.W., Greany, J.F. and Fater, D.C. (2008) Hip abductor weakness and lower extremity kinematics during running. *Journal of Sport Rehabilitation*. 17: 243–256

Hengeveld, E. and Banks, K. (2005) *Maitland's peripheral manipulation*, 4th edition. Butterworth Heinemann, Elsevier. London, UK

Hertling, D. and Kessler, R.M. (1996) *Management of common musculoskeletal disorders: Physical therapy principles and methods*, 3rd edition. J.B. Lippinacott. Philadelphia, PA

Hill, R.D. and Smith, R.B. III. (1990) Examination of the extremities: Pulses, bruits and phlebitis. In Walker, H.K., Hall, W.D. and Hurst, J.W. (eds). *Clinical methods: The history, physical, and laboratory examinations*, 3rd edition. Butterworth. Boston, MA

Hoppenfeld, S. (1976) *Physical examination of the spine and extremities*. Appleton-Century-Crofts. New York

Horton, M.G. and Hall, T.L. (1989) Quadriceps femoris muscle angle: Normative values and relationships with gender and selected skeletal measures. *Physical Therapy*. 69: 897–901

Hoskins, J.S., Burd, T.A. and Allen, W.C. (2004) Surgical correction of internal coxa saltans: A 20-year consecutive study. *American Journal of Sports Medicine*. 32 (4): 998–1001

Ilizaliturri, V.M. Jr, Martinez-Escalante, F.A., Chaidez, P.A. and Camacho-Galindo, J. (2006) Endoscopic iliotibial band release for external snapping hip syndrome. *Arthroscopy*. 22 (5): 505–510

Ireland, M.L., Willson, J.D., Ballantyne, B.T. and Davis, I.M. (2003) Hip strength in females with and without patellofemoral pain. *Journal of Orthopaedic and Sports Physical Therapy*. 33: 671–676

Ito, K., Minka, M.A., Leunig, M., Werlen, S. and Ganz, R. (2001) Femoracetabular impingement and the cam-effect: an MRI-based quantitative anatomical study of the femoral head–neck offset. *British Journal of Bone and Joint Surgery*. 83: 171–176

Jacobs, C. and Mattacola, C. (2005) Sex differences in eccentric hip-abductor strength and knee-joint kinematics when landing from a jump. *Journal of Sport Rehabilitation*. 14 (4): 346–355

Kaltsas, D.S. (1983) Comparative study of the properties of the shoulder joint capsule with those of other joint capsules. *Clinical Orthopaedics*. 173: 20–26

Kang, A.C.L., Gooding, A.J., Coates, M.H., Goh, T.D., Armour, P. and Rietveld, J. (2010) Computed tomography assessment of hip joints in asymptomatic individuals in relation to femoroacetabular impingement. *American Journal of Sports Medicine*. 38: 1160–1165

Kapandji, I.A. (2010) *The physiology of the joints Volume 2*. Churchill Livingstone. Edinburgh, UK

Kelly, B.T., Williams III, R.J. and Philippon, M.J. (2003) Hip arthroscopy: Current indications, treatment options, and management issues. *American Journal of Sports Medicine*. 31: 1020–1037

Kelly, B.T., Shapiro, G.S., Digiovanni, C.W., Buly, R.L., Potter, H.G. and Hannafin, J.A. (2005) Vascularity of the hip labrum: A cadaveric investigation. *Arthroscopy*. 21 (1): 3–11

Kempson, G.E., Spivey, C.J., Swanson, S.A.V. and Freeman, M.A.R. (1971) Patterns of cartilage stiffness on normal and degenerate human femoral heads. *Journal of Biomechanics*. 4 (6): 597–608

Kendall, F.P., McCreary, E.K., Provance, P.G., Rodgers, M.M. and Romani, W.A. (2005) *Muscles testing and function with posture and pain*, 5th edition. Lippinacott, Williams and Wilkins. Baltimore, MD

Kenyon, K. and Kenyon, J. (2009) *The physiotherapist's pocket book: Essential facts at your fingertips*, 2nd edition. Churchill Livingstone. London, UK

Keogh, M.J. and Batt, M.E. (2008) A review of femoroacetabular impingement in athletes. *Sports Medicine*. 38 (10): 863–878

Keskula, D.R., Lott, J. and Duncan, J.B. (1999) Snapping iliopsoas tendon in a recreational athlete: A case report. *Journal of Athletic Training*. 34 (4): 382–385

Kingzett-Taylor, A., Tirman, P.F. Feller, J., *et al.* (1999) Tendinosis and tears of gluteus medius and minimus muscles as a cause of hip pain: MR imaging findings. *American Journal of Roentgenology*. 173 (4): 1123–1126

Klaue, K., Durni, C.W. and Ganz, R. (1991) The acetabular rim syndrome: A clinical presentation of dysplasia of the hip. *British Journal of Bone and Joint Surgery*. 73: 423–429

Kloen, P., Leunig, M. and Ganz, R. (2002) Early lesions of the labrum and acetabular cartilage in osteonecrosis of the femoral head. *British Journal of Bone and Joint Surgery*. 84 (1): 66–69

Kolt, G.S. and Snyder-Mackler, L. (2003) *Physical therapies in sport and exercise*. Churchill Livingstone. Edinburgh, UK

Konczak, C.R. and Ames, R. (2005) Relief of internal snapping hip syndrome in a marathon runner after chiropractic treatment. *Journal of Manipulative Physiological Therapeutics*. 28 (1): e1–e7

Konrath, E.A., Hamel, A.J., Olson, S.A., Bay, B. and Sharkey, N.A. (1998) The role of the acetabular labrum and the transverse acetabular ligament in load transmission in the hip. *Journal of Bone and Joint Surgery*. 80-A (12): 1781–1788

Latash, M.L. and Zatsiorsky, V.M. (eds). (2001). *Classics in movement science*. Human Kinetics, Champaign, IL

Laude, F., Sariali, E. and Nogier, A. (2009) Femoroacetabular impingement treatment using arthroscopy and anterior approach. *Clinical Orthopaedic Related Research*. 467 (3): 747–752

Lavigne, M., Parvizi, J., Beck, M., Siebenrock, K.A., Ganz, R. and Leunig, M. (2004) Anterior femoroacetabular impingement: Part I. Techniques of joint preserving surgery. *Clinical Orthopaedic Related Research*. 418: 61–66.

Leetun, D.T., Ireland, M.L., Willson, J.D., Ballantyne, B.T. and Davis, I.M. (2004) Core stability measures as risk factors for lower extremity injury in athletes. *Medicine and Science in Sports and Exercise*. 36: 926–934

Lephart, S.M., Ferris, C.M., Riemann, B.L, Myers, J.B. and Fu, F.H. (2002) Gender differences in strength and lower extremity kinematics during landing. *Clinical Orthopaedic Related Research*. 401: 162–169

Lequesne, M., Mathieu, P., Vuillemin-Bodaghi, V., Bard, H. and Djian, P. (2008) Gluteal tendinopathy in refractory greater trochanter pain syndrome: Diagnostic value of two clinical tests. *Arthritis Care and Research*. 59 (2): 241–246

Leunig, M., Beck, M. and Dora, C. (2005) Femoroacetabular impingement: Etiology and surgical concept. *Operative Techniques in Orthopaedics*. 15: 247–255

Lewis, C.L. (2010) Extra-articular snapping hip: A literature review. *Sports Health: A Multidisciplinary Approach*. 2 (3): 186–190

Lewis, C.L. and Sahrmann, S.A. (2006) Acetabular labral tears. *Physical Therapy*. 86: 110–121

Lieberman, J.R., Berry, D.J., Mont, M.A., Aaron, R.K., Callaghan, J.J., Rayadhyaksha, A. and Urbaniak, J. R. (2002) Osteonecrosis of the hip: management in the twenty-first century. *American Journal of Bone and Joint Surgery*. 84 (5): 834–853

Lincoln, M., Johnston, K., Muldoon, M. and Santore, R. (2009) Combined arthroscopic and modified open approach for cam femoroacetabular: A preliminary experience. *Arthroscopy*. 25 (4): 392–399

Livingstone, L.A. and Mandigo, J.L. (1999) Bilateral Q-angle asymmetry and anterior knee pain syndrome. *Clinical Biomechanics*. 14 (1): 7–13

Löhe, F., Eckstein, F., Sauer, T. and Putz, R. (1996) Structure, strain and function of the transverse acetabular ligament. *Cells Tissues Organs*. 157 (4): 315–323

Longjohn, D. and Dorr, L. D. (1998) Soft tissue balance of the hip. *The Journal of Arthroplasty*. 13 (1): 97–100

Lorentzon, R., Wedren, J. and Pietila, T. (1998) Incidence, nature and cause of ice hockey injuries: A three-year prospective study of a Swedish elite ice hockey team. *American Journal of Sports Medicine*. 16: 392–396

Lustenberger, D.P., Ng, V.Y., Best, T.M. and Ellis, T.J. (2011) Efficacy of treatment of trochanteric bursitis: A systematic review. *Clinical Journal of Sport Medicine*. 21 (5): 447–453

Louden, J., Swift, M. and Bell, S. (2008) *The clinical orthopaedic assessment guide*, 2nd edition. Human Kinetics, Champaign, IL

Lyon, K.K., Benz, L.N., Johnson, K.K., Ling, A.C. and Bryan, J.M. (1988) Q-Angle: A factor in peak torque occurrence in isokinetic knee extension. *The Journal Orthopedic and Sport Physical Therapy*. 9 (7): 250–253

Lyons, K., Perry, J., Gronley, J., Barnes, L. and Antonelli, D. (1983) Timing and relative intensity of hip extensor and abductor muscle action during level and stair ambulation. An EMG study. *Physical Therapy*. 63: 1597–1605

Lytle, W.J. (1979) Inguinal anatomy. *Journal of Anatomy*. 128 (3): 581.

Magee, D.J. (2008) *Orthopaedic physical assessment*, 5th edition. Saunders, Elsevier, Philadelphia, PA

Mahadeven, V. (2008) Pelvic girdle and lower limb. In Standring, S.L. (ed) *Gray's anatomy: The anatomical basis of clinical anatomy*, 40th edition. Churchill Livingstone. Oxford, UK

Majlesi, J., Togay, H., Ünalan, H. and Toprak, S. (2008) The sensitivity and specificity of the slump and the straight leg raising tests in patients with lumbar disc herniation. *Journal of Clinical Rheumatology*. 14 (2), 87–91

Malizos, K.N., Karantanas, A.H., Varitimidis, S.E., Dailiana, Z.H., Bargiotas, K. and Maris, T. (2007) Osteonecrosis of the femoral head: Etiology, imaging and treatment. *European Journal of Radiology*. 63 (1): 16–28

Malliaras, P., Hogan, A., Nawrocki, A., Crossley, K. and Schache, A. (2009) Hip flexibility and strength measures: Reliability and association with athletic groin pain. *British Journal of Sports Medicine*. 43 (10): 739–744

Marks, M.C., Alexander, J., Sutherland, D.H. and Chambers, H.G. (2003) Clinical utility of the Duncan–Ely test for rectus femoris dysfunction during the swing phase of gait. *Developmental Medicine and Child Neurology*. 45 (11): 763–768

Martin, H.D., Savage, A., Braly, B.A., Palmer, I.J., Beall, D.P. and Kelly, B. (2008) The function of the hip capsular ligaments: A quantitative report. *Arthroscopy*. 24 (2): 188–195

McCulloch, P.C. and Bush-Joseph, C.A. (2006) Massive heterotopic ossification complicating iliopsoas tendon lengthening: A case report. *American Journal of Sports Medicine*. 34 (12): 2022–2025

Medina McKeon, J.M. and Hertel, J. (2009) Sex differences and representative values for 6 lower extremity alignment measures. *Journal of Athletic Training*. 44 (3): 249–255

Medina McKeon, J.M., Denegar, C.R. and Hertel. J. (2010) Sex differences and discriminative value of lower extremity alignments and kinematics during two functional tasks. *Journal of Applied Biomechanics*. 26: 295–304

Messier, S.P., Davis, S.E., Curl, W.W., Lowery, R.B. and Pack, R.J. (1991) Etiologic factors associated with patellofemoral pain in runners. *Medicine and Science in Sports and Exercise*. 23 (9): 1008–1015

Molloy, M.G. and Molloy, C.B. (2011) Contact sport and osteoarthritis. *British Journal of Sports Medicine*. 45 (4): 275–277

Molsa, J., Airaksinen, O., Nasman, O. and Torstila, I. (1997) Ice hockey injuries in Finland: A prospective epidemiologic study. *American Journal of Sports Medicine*. 25: 495–499

Montenegro, M.L.L.S., Mateus-Vasconcelos, E.C.L., Rosa e Silva, J.C., Candido dos Reis, F.J., Nogueira, A.A. and Poli-Neto, O.B. (2009) Postural changes in women with chronic pelvic pain: A case control study. *BMC Musculoskeletal Disorders*. 10: 82

Moore, K.L. and Dalley, A.F. (2006) *Clinically orientated anatomy*, 5th edition. Lippincott, Williams and Wilkins. Philadelphia, PA

Mueller-Wohlfahrt, H.W., Haensel, L., Mithoefer, K., *et al.* (2013) Terminology and classification of muscle injuries in sport: The Munich consensus statement. *British Journal of Sports Medicine*. 47: 342–350

Myers, C.A., Register, B.C., Lertwanich, P., *et al.* (2011) Role of the acetabular labrum and the iliofemoral ligament in hip stability: An in vitro biplane fluoroscopy study. *American Journal of Sports Medicine*. 39: 85S–91S.

Narvani, A.A., Tsiridis, E., Tai, C.C. and Thomas, P. (2003) Acetabular labrum and its tears. *British Journal of Sports Medicine*. 37: 207–211

Nemtala, F., Mardones, R.M. and Tomic, A. (2010) Anterior and posterior femoral head–neck offset ratio in the cam impingement. *Cartilage*. 1: 238–241

Neumann, D.A. (2010) Kinesiology of the hip: A focus on muscular actions. *Journal of Orthopaedic and Sports Physical Therapy*. 40 (2): 82–94

Ng, V.Y., Arora, N., Best, T.M., Pan, X. and Ellis, T.J. (2010) Efficacy of surgery for femoroacetabular impingement: A systematic review. *American Journal of Sports Medicine.* 38 (11): 2337–2345

Nguyen, A.D. and Shultz, S.J. (2007) Sex differences in clinical measures of lower extremity alignment. *Journal of Orthopaedic and Sports Physical Therapy.* 37 (7): 389–398

Nguyen, A.D., Boling, M.C., Levine, B. and Shultz, S.J. (2009) Relationships between lower extremity alignment and the quadriceps angle. *Clinical Journal of Sports Medicine.* 19: 201–206

Nho, S.J., Magennis, E.M., Singh, C.K. and Kelly, B.T. (2011) Outcomes after the arthroscopic treatment of femoroacetabular impingement in a mixed group of high-level athletes. *American Journal of Sports Medicine.* 39 (1): 14S–19S

Nicholas, S.J. and Tyler, T.F. (2002) Adductor muscle strains in sport. *Sports Medicine.* 32 (5): 339–344

Nordin, M. and Frankel, V.H. (2012) *Basic biomechanics of the musculoskeletal system,* 4th edition. Lippinacott, Williams and Wilkins. Philadelphia, PA

Norkin, C.C. and Levangie, P.K. (2011) *Joint structure and function: A comprehensive analysis,* 5th edition. F.A. Davis Company. Philadelphia, PA

Nyland, J., Kuzemchek, S., Parks, M. and Caborn, D.N.M. (2004) Femoral anteversion influences vastus medialis and gluteus medius EMG amplitude: Composite hip abductor EMG amplitude ratios during isometric combined hip abduction-external rotation. *Journal of Electromyography and Kinesiology.* 14 (2): 255–261

Ober, F.R. (1936) The role of the iliotibial band and fascia lata as a factor in the causation of low-back disabilities and sciatica. *American Journal of Bone and Joint Surgery.* 18 (1): 105–110

Onate, J., Cortes, N., Welch, C. and Van Lunen, B. (2010) Expert versus novice interrater reliability and criterion validity of the landing error scoring system. *Journal of Sport Rehabilitation.* 19 (1): 41

Park, S.K. and Stefanyshyn, D.J. (2011) Greater Q-angle may not be a risk factor of patellofemoral pain syndrome. *Clinical Biomechanics.* 26 (4): 392–396

Parvizi, J. and Ganz, R. (2005) Femoroacetabular impingement. *Seminars in Arthroplasty.* 16: 33–37

Parziale, J.R., Hudgins, T.H. and Fishman, L.M. (1996) The piriformis syndrome. *American Journal of Orthopedics.* 25 (12): 819–823

Peeler, J. and Anderson, J.E. (2008) Reliability of the Ely's test for assessing rectus femoris muscle flexibility and joint range of motion. *Journal of Orthopaedic Research.* 26 (6): 793–799

Pelsser, V., Cardinal, E., Hobden, R., Aubin, B. and Lafortune, M. (2001) Extraarticular snapping hip: Sonographic findings. *American Journal of Roentgenology.* 176 (1): 67–73

Perry, J. (1992) *Gait analysis: Normal and pathological gait.* Slack Incorporated. Thorofare, NJ

Petersen, W., Petersen, F. and Tillmann, B. (2003) Structure and vascularization of the acetabular labrum with regard to the pathogenesis and healing of labral lesions. *Archives of Orthopaedic and Trauma Surgery.* 123: 283–288

Petty, N.J. (2011) *Neuromusculoskeletal examination and assessment: A handbook for therapists.* Elsevier. Edinburgh, UK

Philippon, M., Schenker, M., Briggs, K. and Kuppersmith, D. (2007a) Femoroacetabular impingement in 45 professional athletes: Associated pathologies and return to sport following arthroscopic decompression. *Knee Surgery, Sports Traumatology, Arthroscopy.* 15 (7): 908–914

Philippon, M.J., Stubbs, A.J., Schenker, M.L., Maxwell, R.B., Ganz, R. and Leunig, M. (2007b) Arthroscopic management of femoroacetabular impingement: Osteoplasty technique and literature review. *American Journal of Sports Medicine.* 35: 1571–1580

Philippon, M.J., Briggs, K.K., Yen, Y.M. and Kuppersmith, D.A. (2009) Outcomes following hip arthroscopy for femoroacetabular impingement with associated chondrolabral dysfunction: Minimum two-year follow-up. *British Journal of Bone and Joint Surgery.* 91: 16–23

Philippon, M.J., Weiss, D.R., Kuppersmith, D.A., Briggs, K.K. and Hay, C.J. (2010) Arthroscopic labral repair and treatment of femoroacetabular impingement in professional hockey players. *American Journal of Sports Medicine.* 38: 99–104

Pierannunzzi, L., Tramontana, F. and Gallazi, M. (2010) Case report: Calcific tendinitis of the rectus femoris. A rare cause of snapping hip. *Clinical Orthopedics and Related Research.* 468 (10): 2814–2818

Placzek, J.D. and Boyce, D.A. (2006) *Orthopaedic physical therapy secrets.* Mosby, Elsevier. St. Louis, MO

Pombo, M. and Bradley, J.P. (2009) Proximal hamstring avulsion injuries: A technique note on surgical repairs. *Sports Health: A Multidisciplinary Approach.* 1 (3): 261–264

Poole, C.A. (1997) Review: Articular cartilage chondrons. Form, function and failure. *Journal of Anatomy.* 191: 1–13

Powers, C.M. (2003) The influence of altered lower-extremity kinematics on patellofemoral joint dysfunction: A theoretical perspective. *Journal of Orthopaedic and Sports Physical Therapy.* 33: 639–646

Pressel, T. and Lengsfeld, M. (1998) Functions of hip joint muscles. *Medical Engineering and Physics.* 20: 50–56

Provencher, M.T., Hofmeister, E.P. and Muldoon, M.P. (2004) The surgical treatment of external coxa saltans (the snapping hip) by Z-plasty of the iliotibial band. *American Journal of Sports Medicine.* 32 (2): 470–476

Rabin, A., Gerszten, P.C., Karausky, P., Bunker, C.H., Potter, D.M. and Welch, W.C. (2007) The sensitivity of the seated straight-leg raise test compared with the supine straight-leg raise test in patients presenting with magnetic resonance imaging evidence of lumbar nerve root compression. *Archives of Physical Medicine and Rehabilitation.* 88 (7), 840–843

Ralphs, J.R. and Benjamin, M. (1994) The joint capsule: Structure, composition, ageing and disease. *Journal of Anatomy.* 184 (3): 503.

Reijman, M., Hazes, J.M.W., Koes, B.W., Verhagen, A.P. and Bierma-Zeinstra, S.M.A. (2004) Validity, reliability, and applicability of seven definitions of hip osteoarthritis used in epidemiological studies: A systematic appraisal. *Annals of the Rheumatic Diseases.* 63 (3): 226–232

Reiman, M.P., Bolgla, L.A. and Lorenz, D. (2009) Hip function's influence on knee dysfunction: A proximal link to a distal problem. *Journal of Sport Rehabilitation.* 18 (1): 33

Reiman, M.P., Goode, A.P., Hegedus, E.J., Cook, C.E. and Wright, A.A. (2012) Diagnostic accuracy of clinical tests of the hip: A systematic review with meta-analysis. *British Journal of Sports Medicine.* 47 (14): 893–902

Reynolds, D., Lucas, J. and Klaue, K. (1999) Retroversion of the acetabulum. *British Journal of Bone and Joint Surgery.* 81: 281–288

Riegger-Krugh, C. and Keysor, J.J. (1996) Skeletal malalignments of the lower quarter: Correlated and compensatory motions and postures. *Journal of Orthopaedic and Sports Physical Therapy.* 23 (2): 164

Ruiz-Arranz, J.L., Alfonso-Venzalá, I. and Villalón-Ogayar, J. (2008) Piriformis muscle syndrome. Diagnosis and treatment. Presentation of 14 cases. *Revista Española de Cirugía Ortopédica y Traumatología (English Edition).* 52 (6): 359–365

Sarimo, J., Lempainen, L., Mattila, K. and Orava, S. (2008) Complete proximal hamstring avulsions: A series of 41 patients with operative treatment. *American Journal of Sports Medicine.* 36 (6): 1110–1115

Satku, K., Chia, J. and Kumar, V.P. (1990) Snapping hip: An unusual cause. *British Journal of Bone and Joint Surgery.* 72 (1): 150–151

Saudek, C. (1985) The hip. In Gould, J.A. and Davies, G.J. (eds) *Orthopaedic and sports rehabilitation concepts: Orthopaedic and sports physical therapy.* CV Mosby Company. Toronto, Canada

Schmidt, R.A. and Lee, T.D. (1999) *Motor control and learning: A behavioural approach.* Human Kinetics. Champaign, IL

Schon, L. and Zuckerman, J.D. (1988) Hip pain in the elderly: Evaluation and diagnosis. *Geriatrics.* 43 (1): 48

Scopp, J.M. and Moorman, C.T. (2001) The assessment of athletic hip injury. *Clinics in Sports Medicine.* 20 (4): 647–660

Seldes, R.M., Tan, V., Hunt, J., Katz, M., Winiarsky, R. and Fitzgerald Jr, R.H. (2001) Anatomy, histologic features, and vascularity of the adult acetabular labrum. *Clinical Orthopedics.* 382: 232–240

Shadbolt, C.L., Heinze, S.B. and Dietrich, R.B. (2001) Imaging of groin masses: Inguinal anatomy and pathologic conditions revisited. *Radiographics.* 21 (1): S261–S271

Shambaugh, J.P., Klein, A. and Herbert, J.H. (1991) Structural measures as predictors of injury basketball players. *Medicine and Science in Sports and Exercise.* 23: 522–527

Shbeeb, M.I. and Matteson, E.L. (1996) Trochanteric bursitis (greater trochanter pain syndrome). *Mayo Clinic Proceedings.* 71 (6): 565–569

Shum, G.L.K., Crosbie, J. and Lee, R.Y.W. (2005) Symptomatic and asymptomatic movement coordination of the lumbar spine and hip during an everyday activity. *Spine.* 30 (23): 697–702

Shumway-Cook, A. and Woollacott, M.H. (1995) *Motor control: Theory and practical applications* (Vol. 157). Williams and Wilkins. Baltimore, MD

Silver, J.K. and Leadbetter, W.B. (1998) Piriformis syndrome: Assessment of current practice and literature review. *Orthopedics.* 21 (10): 1133–1135

Simoneau, G.G., Hoenig, K.J., Lepley, J.E. and Papanek, P.E. (1998) Influence of hip position and gender on active hip internal and external rotation. *Journal of Orthopaedic and Sports Physical Therapy.* 28: 158–164

Skalley, T.C., Terry, G.C. and Teitge, R.A. (1993) The quantitative measurement of normal passive medial and lateral patellar motion limits. *American Journal of Sports Medicine*. 21 (5): 728–732

Smith, C.D., Masouros, S., Hill, A.M., Amis, A.A. and Bull, A.M.J. (2009) A biomechanical basis for tears of the human acetabular labrum. *British Journal of Sports Medicine*. 43: 574–578

Smith, T.O., Hunt, N.J. and Wood, S.J. (2006) The physiotherapy management of muscle haematomas. *Physical Therapy in Sport*. 7 (4): 201–209

Smith, T.O., Hunt, N.J. and Donell, S.T. (2008) The reliability and validity of the Q-angle: A systematic review. *Knee Surgery, Sports Traumatology, Arthroscopy*. 16 (12): 1068–1079

Smoll, N.R. (2010) Variations of the piriformis and sciatic nerve with clinical consequence: A review. *Clinical Anatomy*. 23 (1): 8–17

Soderberg, G.L. (1986) *Kinesiology: Application to pathological motion*. Williams and Wilkins. Baltimore, MD

Spencer, A. (1978) *Practical podiatric orthopaedic procedures*. Ohio College of Podiatric Medicine. Cleveland, OH

Stankovich, R., Johnell, O., Maly, P. and Wilmer, S. (1999) Use of lumbar extension, slump test, physical and neurological examination in the evaluation of patients with suspected herniated nucleus pulposus: A prospective clinical study. *Manual Therapy*. 4 (1): 25–32

Suenaga, E., Noguchi, Y., Jingushi, S., *et al.* (2002) Relationship between the maximum flexion–internal rotation test and the torn acetabular labrum of a dysplastic hip. *Journal of Orthopaedic Science*. 7: 26–32

Syed, M.I. and Shaikh, A. (2010) *Radiology of non-spinal pain procedures: A guide for the interventionalist*. Springer. New York

Tan, V., Seldes, R.M., Katz, M.A., *et al.* (2001) Contribution of acetabular labrum to articulating surface area and femoral head coverage in adult hip joints: An anatomic study in cadavera. *American Journal of Orthopedics*. 30 (11): 809.

Tannast, M., Siebenrock, K.A. and Anderson, S.E. (2007) Femoroacetabular impingement: radiographic diagnosis: What the radiologist should know. *American Journal of Roentgenology*. 188: 1540–1552

Tomsich, D.A., Nitz, A.J., Thelkeld, A.J. and Shapiro, R. (1996) Patellofemoral alignment: Reliability. *Journal of Orthopedic and Sport Physical Therapy*. 23: 200–208

Tonnis, D. and Heinecke, A. (1999) Acetabular and femoral anteversion: Relationship with osteoarthritis of the hip. *American Journal of Bone and Joint Surgery*. 81: 1747–1770

Tortolani, P.J., Carbone, J.J. and Quartararo, L.G. (2002) Greater trochanteric pain syndrome in patients referred to orthopedic spine specialists. *The Spine Journal*. 2: 251–254

Tortora, G.J. and Derrickson, B.H. (2008) *Principles of anatomy and physiology*, 11th edition. Wiley. Chichester, UK

Toth, C., McNeil, S. and Feasby, T. (2005) Central nervous system injuries in sport and recreation. *Sports Medicine*. 35 (8): 685–715

Tyler, T.F. and Slattery, A.A. (2010) Rehabilitation of the hip following sports injury. *Clinical Sports Medicine*. 29: 107–126

Vail, T.P. and McCollum, D.E. (1997) Fractures of the pelvis, femur and knee. In Sabiston D.C. (ed.) *Textbook of surgery: The biological basis of modern surgical practice*. Saunders. Philadelphia, PA

Wahl, C.J., Warren, R.F., Adler, R.S., Hannafin, J.A. and Hansen, B. (2004) Internal coxa saltans (snapping hip) as a result of overtraining: A report of 3 cases in professional athletes with a review of causes and the role of ultrasound in early diagnosis and management. *American Journal of Sports Medicine*. 32 (5): 1302–1309

Walker, P., Kannangara, S. and Bruce, W.J. (2007) Lateral hip pain: Does imaging predict response to localized injection? *Clinical Orthopaedics and Related Research*. 457: 144–149

Walsh, M.J., Walton, J.R. and Walsh, N.A. (2011) Surgical repair of the gluteal tendons: A report of 72 cases. *Journal of Arthroplasty*. 26(8): 1514–1519

Waryasz, G.R. and McDermott, A.Y. (2008) Patellofemoral pain syndrome (PFPS): A systematic review of anatomy and potential risk factors. *Dynamic Medicine*. 7 (9): 1–14

Wenger, D.E., Kendell, K.R., Miner, M.R. and Trousdale, R.T. (2004) Acetabular labral tears rarely occur in the absence of bony abnormalities. *Clinical Orthopedic Related Research*. 426: 145–150

Wenger, D.R., Mubarak, S.J., Henderson, P.C. and Miyanji, F. (2008) Ligamentum teres maintenance and transfer as a stabilizer in open reduction for pediatric hip dislocation: Surgical technique and early clinical results. *Journal of Children's Orthopaedics*. 2 (3): 177–185

Williams, B.S. and Cohen, S.P. (2009) Greater trochanteric pain syndrome: A review of anatomy, diagnosis and treatment. *Anesthesia and Analgesia*. 108 (5): 1662–1670

Wilson, J.D., Ireland, M.L. and Davis, I. (2006) Core strength and lower extremity alignment during single leg squats. *Medicine and Science in Sports and Exercise.* 38 (5): 945–952

Winston, P., Awan, R., Cassidy, J.D. and Bleakney, R.K. (2007) Clinical examination and ultrasound of self-reported snapping hip syndrome in elite ballet dancers. *American Journal of Sports Medicine.* 35 (1): 118–126

Won, Y.Y., Chung, I.H., Chung, N.S. and Song, K.H. (2003) Morphological study on the acetabular labrum. *Yonsei Medical Journal.* 44: 855–862

Woodland, L. and Francis, R. (1992) Parameters and comparisons of the quadriceps angle of college-aged men and women in the supine and standing positions. *American Journal of Sports Medicine.* 20: 208–211

Woodley, S.J., Nicholson, H.D., Livingstone, V., *et al.* (2008) Lateral hip pain: Findings from magnetic resonance imaging and clinical examination. *Journal of Orthopaedic and Sports Physical Therapy.* 38 (6): 313–328

Yamamoto, Y., Ide, T., Hamada, Y. and Usui, I. (2004) A case of intra-articular snapping hip caused by articular cartilage detachment from the deformed femoral head consequent to Perthes disease. *Arthroscopy.* 20 (6): 650–653

Youdas, J.W., Madson, T.J. and Hollman, J.H. (2010) Usefulness of the Trendelenburg test for identification of patients with hip joint osteoarthritis. *Physiotherapy Theory and Practice.* 26 (3): 184–194

Zeller, B.L., McCrory, J.L., Kibler, W.B. and Uhl, T.L. (2003) Differences in kinematics and electromyographic activity between men and women during the single-legged squat. *American Journal of Sports Medicine.* 31 (3): 449–456

10

THE KNEE REGION

Anatomy, assessment and injuries

Amy Bell and Keith Ward

Functional anatomy of the knee

The knee region has direct relationships proximally with the pelvis, hip and upper leg, and distally with the lower leg, ankle and foot. The load-bearing knee joint complex is essential to such fundamental activities of daily living (ADL) as standing, sitting, walking, negotiating stairs, running and jumping. The knee is crucial to the transmission of force from the hip to the foot and in gross positioning of the feet. As a central component of the lower limb, the knee provides both hinged and rotational open and closed chain leverage for movement. Primarily the knee involves two joints, the tibiofemoral and patellofemoral joints. The tibiofemoral joint (TFJ) is a synovial, modified hinge joint containing a pair of fibrocartilaginous discs (menisci). The TFJ is an articulation between the femur and the tibia, and the medial and lateral condyles of the distal femur articulate with the medial and lateral condyles at the proximal tibia. The TFJ is stabilized by muscles and tendons that cross and strengthen the joint and significant ligamentous structures (intra- and extra-articular); the meniscal cartilages also contribute to its stability. The patellofemoral joint (PFJ) is a gliding synovial joint, and the patella acts as a fulcrum to increase the moment arm of the quadriceps mechanism (Nicoletta and Schepsis, 2005). The patella is pulled by the force of the quadriceps group and glides over the femoral groove (trochlea) during knee motion. The PFJ obtains its stability primarily via: the posterior facet orientation of the patella and the associated congruency occurring in flexed positions; the thin strands of medial and lateral ligaments; the quadriceps muscle group and tendon; the patella tendon; and the medial and lateral retinacula (Mahadevan, 2008). The sesamoid patella bone serves to protect the anterior aspect of the knee while providing a mechanical advantage for the quadriceps muscles to extend the knee; during knee flexion, it maintains the position of the patellar tendon (Blackburn and Craig, 1980). A third joint at the knee is the proximal tibiofibular joint (PTFJ). The PTFJ, fibula, fibular head and associated ligaments contribute to the stability and function of the lower leg and the talocrural joint, but as the fibular head is also a site for attachment of major ligamentous and tendinous structures directly affecting the knee, it must also be recognized as an important component of the knee complex.

The knee is integral to all the forceful and repetitive lower limb movements in exercise, sport and work, and as such is vulnerable to a host of injury problems (direct; indirect; contact; non-contact; overuse; degenerative; pathological; insidious). The knee is often presented as the most commonly injured joint among athletes. This is largely due to the significant rotary torque and compressive stresses, not least ground reaction forces (GRF), which the knee is subjected to particularly in sports such as football, skiing, rugby, basketball and tennis. Injury prevalence to the knee is further enhanced by the acceleration and deceleration forces which are imposed on it by its extensor (quadriceps) and main flexor (hamstrings and gastrocnemius) muscle complexes, particularly during explosive power-based activity, and rapid stop–start and multidirectional work (Franklyn-Miller *et al.*, 2011).

Surface and skeletal anatomy of the knee

Close visual inspection and palpation of the knee region reveals aspects of its skin, bony landmarks, joint lines and capsule, cartilage, ligamentous tissue, muscle and tendinous tissue, fascia, bursae, blood vessels and peripheral nerves.

The contacting surfaces of the three bones which articulate at the knee are covered with hyaline cartilage, and the two main joints share the same synovial capsule (Watkins, 2010).

The femur is the longest, heaviest and strongest bone in the body. The large spherical head (ball) of the femur at its proximal end articulates with the deep acetabular cavity (socket) of the pelvis to form the hip joint. The femur flares at its distal end to create articulatory condyles. The shaft of the femur normally angles medially from the hip (the 'angle of inclination'); at the knee this is described as a genu valgus positioning and is often increased in females due to a wider pelvis. Knee valgus positioning influences the Q (quadriceps) angle. Abnormal tibiofemoral movements tend to cause abnormal patellofemoral movements (Watkins, 2010), and an excessive Q-angle has been identified as a contributing factor in a host of knee injuries such as patellofemoral pain syndrome (PFPS), iliotibial band syndrome (ITBS) and anterior cruciate ligament (ACL) sprain (Emami *et al.*, 2007).

Practitioner Tip Box 10.1

Skeletal landmarks of the knee region

Femur
Shaft
Linea aspera
Medial supracondylar ridge
Lateral supracondylar ridge
Popliteal surface
Patellar surface (trochlear notch)
Adductor tubercle
Medial epicondyle
Lateral epicondyle
Medial condyle
Lateral condyle
Intercondylar fossa

Patella
Anterior surface
Posterior surface
Superior border (base; superior pole)
Medial border

Lateral border
Inferior angle (apex; inferior pole)
Medial facets
Odd facet
Lateral facets

Tibia
Tibial plateau
Intercondylar eminence
Medial condyle
Lateral condyle
Gerdy's tubercle
Tibial tuberosity

Fibula
Head
Neck
Shaft

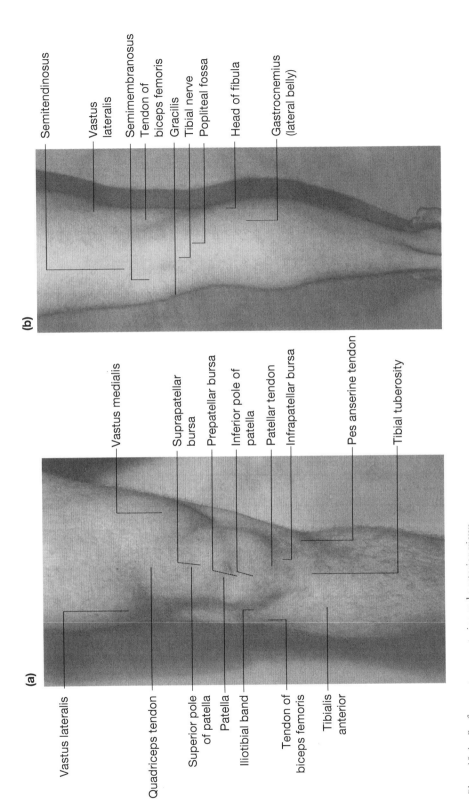

Photo 10.1 Surface anatomy: anterior and posterior views.

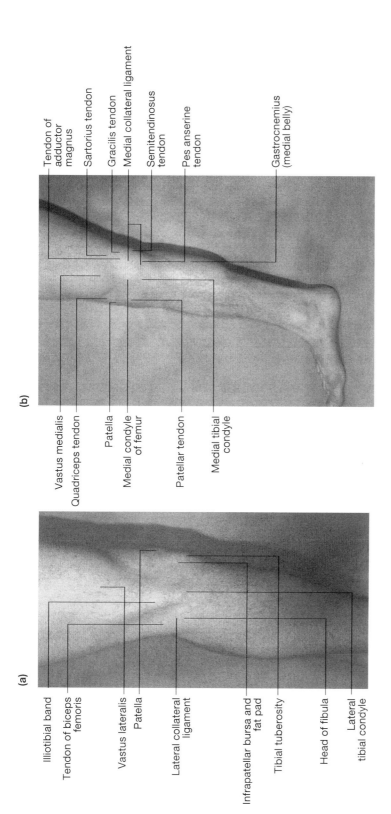

(b)

Tendon of
adductor
magnus

Sartorius tendon

Gracilis tendon

Medial collateral ligament

Semitendinosus
tendon

Pes anserine
tendon

Gastrocnemius
(medial belly)

Vastus medialis

Quadriceps tendon

Patella

Medial condyle
of femur

Patellar tendon

Medial tibial
condyle

(a)

Illiotibial band

Tendon of biceps
femoris

Vastus lateralis

Patella

Lateral collateral
ligament

Infrapatellar bursa and
fat pad

Tibial tuberosity

Head of fibula

Lateral
tibial condyle

Photo 10.2 Surface anatomy: lateral and medial views.

The linea aspera is a vertical ridge with a medial and lateral lip running centrally down the upper posterior aspect of the femur from below the gluteal tuberosity. Distally the linea aspera branches into the medial and lateral supracondylar lines. The medial and lateral femoral epicondyles are distinct, bony prominences situated superior to the femoral condyles. Located on the superior aspect of the medial epicondyle is the adductor tubercle, which is a site of distal attachment for the adductor magnus. The popliteal surface is a slight central depression just superior to the posterior aspect of the femoral condyles. The medial and lateral femoral condyles are the articulatory expansions at the distal end of the femur, and the medial condyle projects more distally than the lateral condyle and has a greater articulatory surface area. The intercondylar fossa, or notch, is a structural depression on the distal and posterior surface between the condyles. The area between the femoral condyles on the anterior surface where the posterior surface of the patella articulates with the femur to form the patellofemoral joint is termed the patellar surface or (femoral) trochlear groove.

The tibia is the larger, medial bone of the lower leg. It is commonly referred to as the shin bone, and is the main weight-bearing long bone of the lower limb. The tibia articulates with the femur superiorly (to form the TFJ), the fibula proximally (to form the PTFJ) and the fibula and talus distally (to form the distal tibiofibular and talocrural joints). Bony landmarks of the tibia at the knee region include the: tibial plateau – a flattened, superior portion of the medial and lateral tibial condyles (the meniscal cartilages are positioned here); intercondylar eminences (small bony projections arising from the central areas on the tibial plateau which provide for situation and attachment of the menisci); medial and lateral tibial condyles – which are the expanded portion of the distal end of the tibia; Gerdy's tubercle – a small projection on the anterolateral aspect of the lateral tibial condyle, and the attachment site for the iliotibial band; and the tibial tuberosity, which is a large bony prominence on the anterior, proximal tibia. This is the insertion site of the quadriceps muscle group via the patellar tendon.

The patella, or kneecap, is a small, roughly triangular bone situated anterior to the femoral patellar surface. The word patella translates literally to mean a 'small plate' (Tortora and Grabowski, 1996). It is essentially a sesamoid bone (the largest in the body) encapsulated within the quadriceps tendon (Mahadevan, 2008). The patella features three borders – medial, lateral and superior. The superior border is also known as the base, and is the superior pole of the patella. The inferior angle is referred to as the apex and is the patella's inferior pole. Its subcutaneous anterior surface is convex, and the hyaline cartilage on the articular surface is the thickest in the body. This indicates the functional stresses that the patella is exposed to. It presents with a number of subtle articular facets; the medial and slightly larger lateral facets are further subdivided into three smaller facets, and the seventh 'odd' facet presents on the posterior medial border (Mahadevan, 2008).

The patellofemoral joint

The PFJ incorporates the femoral trochlea, or patellar surface, which is the groove on which the posterior surface of the patella glides. In full extension, the patella is not tensioned against the trochlea. In mid-range positions of flexion the medial and lateral facets are engaged with the trochlea, and the odd facet approximates at approximately 135° of flexion (Kingston, 2000). Simple walking places 0.3 times body weight (BW) through the patellofemoral joint (Magee, 2008). When ascending stairs this rises to 2.5 times BW; descending stairs it becomes 3.5 times BW; squatting with no resistance can place loads of up to 7 times BW through the joint.

The knee joint receives both static and dynamic stability from surrounding structures. The quadriceps group provides dynamic stability, and the static stability is provided by the congruency and contact architecture of the femoral trochlea and posterior facets of the patella, the medial and lateral patella retinaculum, the small but significant patellofemoral, patellotibial and patellomeniscal ligaments, and the patellar tendon. The medial patellofemoral and patellotibial ligaments actually blend to form part of the medial retinaculum (Nicoletta and Schepsis, 2005), which arises along the midpole of the patella. The medial patellotibial ligament runs from the lower pole and medial patellar facet to insert at the medial aspect of the proximal tibial metaphysis (Miller and Sanders, 2012). The lateral patella retinaculum is formed partly from 'superficial oblique' fascial bands extending from the iliotibial band, and partly from the 'deep transverse' lateral patellofemoral ligament and lateral patellotibial band (Mahadevan, 2008). The lateral aspect of the femoral trochlea is more prominent than the medial aspect. This helps to guide the patella and resist lateral displacement (Kingston, 2000). The medial patellofemoral ligament extends from the superior pole of the patella to the adductor tubercle. Despite being rather thin, it has a mean tensile strength of 208 N, and is another of the primary static restraints to lateral displacement of the patella (Amis *et al.*, 2003; Miller and Sanders, 2012). In combination, these structures and features help to control the movement (tracking) of the patella on the trochlea (Dixit *et al.*, 2007). Dysfunction of the PFJ commonly results from patellar maltracking in the trochlear groove (for local, proximal and/or distal reasons).

The tibiofemoral joint

The TFJ is composed of the femur and the tibia. The articular surfaces of both bones are covered with hyaline cartilage, which acts to decrease friction and maintain congruency of the joint surfaces. The synovial membrane is the largest and most extensive in the body. It begins at the upper border of the patella, passes underneath the patellar tendon, covers the surface of the patella and extends to the intercondylar notch (Mahadevan, 2008). The close-packed and most statically congruent position of the tibiofemoral joint is full, or terminal, extension (Magee, 2008).

The TFJ, a synovial, modified ginglymus, or hinge joint, allows four physiological movements. The two major movements available at the knee joint are flexion (bending) and extension (straightening), which both occur on a sagittal plane about a frontal (or coronal) axis. A degree of medial rotation (tibia rotating inwards) and lateral rotation (tibia rotating outwards) are

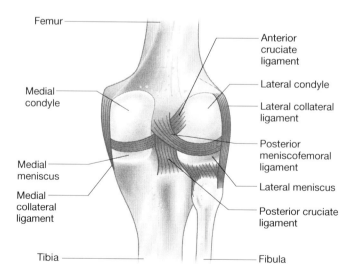

Figure 10.1 Ligamentous anatomy: posterior view (source: adapted from Sewell *et al.*, 2013).

available when the knee is semi-flexed, with lateral rotation being the most extensive. Rotation occurs about the longitudinal axis. During flexion, the articular surfaces of the tibia glide backwards over the femoral condyles in a posterior movement. The cruciate ligaments are relaxed, while the patellar tendon becomes tense as the knee flexes. During extension, the tibia glides forward over the condyles of the femur in an anterior movement; each of the main ligaments are stretched – but not the patellar tendon, which is in a relaxed state in this position. Medial rotation involves rotation of the anterior surface of the tibia toward the mid-sagittal plane (with a flexed knee, turning the foot inwards to rotate the tibia medially). Lateral rotation involves rotation of the anterior surface of the tibia away from the midsagittal plane (with a flexed knee, turning the foot outwards to rotate the tibia laterally). Magee (2008) presents average active ranges of movement (RoM) of the knee complex: flexion 0–135°; extension 0–15°; medial rotation 20–30°; and lateral rotation 30–40°.

The joint capsule and plicae

The knee joint is surrounded by a joint capsule which consists of a synovial and fibrous membrane separated by fatty deposits, both anteriorly and posteriorly. The anterior portion is thin, and it is thicker laterally. It contains the patella, menisci, ligaments and bursae. A number of bursae, fluid-filled sacs, are located around the knee to reduce friction. The outer layer of the joint capsule is richly innervated. Plicae, thickened folds of synovial membrane, are often present deep within the joint capsule. Embryonically, the knee is divided into three separate compartments (by synovium). During the first few months of fetal life, these membranous tissues are resorbed and the knee joint develops a single chamber (Blackburn and Nyland, 2006). There is a possibility, however, that resorption may be incomplete. The remnants of these original synovial membranes are known as plicae. Harty and Joyce (1977) state that plicae are present in just a percentage of the population; they are inconsistent. The most commonly presenting plicae are the suprapatellar plica; infrapatellar plica; medial patellar plica; and, least commonly, the lateral patellar plica. Plicae may present as ridges, cords or sheets, and although they may contribute to increasing the synovial membrane's surface area, and assist the spread of synovial fluid through the joint, they can also be a cause of irritation. A number of synovial plica syndromes exist; plicae can become inflamed or thickened, causing pain and dysfunction, with the medial plica being the most commonly irritated.

Meniscal cartilage

The menisci are a pair of slightly concave, crescent-shaped wedges of fibrocartilage discs which sit on top of the tibial plateau (Chmielewski, *et al.*, 2003; Kingston, 2000). The medial meniscus is situated on top of the medial tibial condyle, and the lateral meniscus on top of the lateral condyle, separated by the intercondylar eminence. The medial meniscus is more 'C-shaped' and the lateral meniscus more circular. Both menisci have an anterior and posterior horn (or tip). They are thinner centrally and thicker peripherally, but as with any structure there are anatomical variations, and the general architecture of menisci can differ between individuals. The anterior horns of the medial and lateral menisci are connected by a transverse ligament (Mahadevan, 2008), which also has attachment to the anterior fibres of the ACL. The coronary (meniscotibial) ligaments attach the perimeter of each menisci to the tibial plateau. Although the menisci are poorly vascularized, each meniscus is supplied by the medial, lateral and middle geniculate arteries, which are branches of the popliteal artery (Brindle *et al.*, 2001). Only 10–30 per cent of the peripheral menisci receive a direct blood supply, and the inner portions are virtually avascular, nourished solely by synovial fluid (Gershuni *et al.*, 1988). Vascularity further declines with age, which, in conjunction with the normal traumatic stress that the knee is exposed to in life, can accelerate degeneration and also increase the risk of injury to the menisci.

The menisci have a number of important functions, including: shock absorption; dissipation of load-bearing and ground reaction stress ('hoop stress'); facilitation of smooth joint movements; and enhancement of joint congruency. The fibrocartilage has relative elastic capacity to distort during loaded movement. They also contribute to fluid diffusion and distribution of synovial lubrication and nutrition to the joint during intermittent loading. Furthermore, the menisci protect the articular cartilage and subchondral bone and contribute to the 'locking' or 'screw-home mechanism' of the knee at terminal extension. The menisci may also provide a small contribution to proprioception (Aagard and Verdonk, 2007; Chmielewski *et al.*, 2003; Mahadevan, 2008). When the peripheral margins are intact, circumferential meniscal stress measurements have shown that 45–70 per cent of the weight-bearing load is transmitted through the menisci (Brindle *et al.*, 2001). During knee movements, the medial meniscus has been shown to demonstrate around 2–5 mm of translation, and the lateral meniscus 9–11 mm (Fu and Baratz, 1994).

Deeper fibres of the semimembranosus muscle have attachment to the medial meniscus, and the associated muscular pull contributes to the posterior meniscal movement during knee flexion. The medial meniscus is more firmly attached to the joint capsule than the lateral one. This is due to a medial thickening of the capsule, generally recognized as the deeper portion of the medial collateral ligament (MCL), which further acts to limit its mobility (Brindle *et al.*, 2001). As a consequence of its relative stability, the medial meniscus is more often injured than the lateral meniscus and is also often injured in conjunction with the MCL and ACL. Simultaneous damage to these three related structures is commonly referred to as the 'unhappy' or 'O'Donaghue' triad (Yu and Garrett, 2007).

The lateral meniscus is more circular in shape than the medial meniscus, and covers a larger proportion of the tibial plateau. Unlike the medial meniscus, its width is often consistent throughout. Its anterior and posterior horns attach to the anterior and posterior aspects of the ACL, respectively. It is attached to the tibia less firmly than the medial meniscus and has no direct attachment to the lateral collateral ligament (LCL), nor does it attach to the capsular ligament posterolaterally, hence it is more mobile than the medial meniscus. The lateral meniscus does, however, have two small ligamentous attachments which are believed to provide secondary support to the posterior cruciate ligament (PCL) and also help control motion of the lateral meniscus (Mahadevan, 2008). The anterior meniscofemoral 'ligament of Humphrey' (aMFL) and the posterior meniscofemoral 'ligament of Wrisberg' (pMFL) both run from the central portion of the posterior horn to the lateral aspect of the medial femoral condyle; the aMFL passes anterior to the PCL; and the pMFL passes posterior to the PCL. The lateral meniscus also has an attachment posteriorly to the deeper fibres of the popliteus muscle, which as an initiator of knee flexion may pull the lateral meniscus posteriorly during such movement.

Main ligaments of the knee

The TFJ is primarily supported by four ligaments, along with the patellar tendon (which is also sometimes referred to as a ligament).

Anterior cruciate ligament

In Latin, cruciate means 'cross'; the anterior and posterior cruciate ligaments cross over each other on the inside of the knee and together work to restrict rotation of the joint. The ACL connects the tibia to the femur. It is an intra-articular but extrasynovial ligament, which is surrounded by its own synovial sheath. The ACL receives its blood supply from a periligamentous plexus which is contained within its synovial sheath. Damage to this plexus is the most common cause of haemarthrosis following ACL injury (Miller and Sanders, 2012). The ACL originates from the anterior aspect of the tibia and passes upwards, backwards and outwards to attach to the medial, posterior aspect of the lateral condyle of the femur (Mahadevan, 2008). A study on the structure of the ACL by Odensten and Gillquist (1985) on 33 normal cadavers revealed the average length of the ligament to be 31 mm (±3). They also measured the angle between the ligament and the long axis of the femur, which on average was 28° (±4) when the knee was flexed to 90°. The ACL consists of two parts: a distinct anteromedial band (AMB) and a posterolateral band (PLB) (Girgis *et al.*, 1975).

The ACL is said to be the second strongest ligament in the knee (after the PCL) and can withstand a maximum load of approximately 2,000 N if the load is applied in the anatomical direction of the ligament (Woo *et al.*, 1991). Its primary function is to prevent anterior displacement (forward movement) of the tibia in relation to the femur. The degree of restriction depends on the degree of knee flexion. Peterson and Renstrom (2005) identified that the ACL can take approximately 75 per cent of the anterior force in full extension, 87 per cent at 30° flexion and 85 per cent at 90° flexion. A study by Fujie and Woo (1995) used the Universal Force Moment Sensor (UFS) testing system to measure the in situ force in the ACL when a 134 N anterior tibial load was applied. The findings showed that the force was greatest at 15° flexion and decreased significantly when approaching 90° flexion. This is clinically relevant and such factors are to be considered during any rehabilitation following ACL injury or reconstruction surgery so as to avoid damage to the healing ligament or graft.

In addition, the ACL has been reported as an important secondary stabilizer against valgus stresses of the knee. The medial meniscus contributes to the resistance of anterior translation of the tibia at all flexion angles and, as mentioned previously, is often injured in combination with the ACL (Brindle *et al.*, 2001). Other structures which resist anterior movement of the tibia are the medial and lateral collateral ligaments, the iliotibial band (ITB) and the joint capsule. Additionally, the ACL has been found to play an important role in proprioception of the knee joint due to the presence of specialized mechanoreceptors, similar to golgi tendon organs (GTO), within the ligament (Shultz *et al.*, 1984). A study by Cerulli *et al.* (1986) confirmed the proprioceptive role of the ACL after discovering Ruffini and Pacinian corpuscles located mainly in the proximal and middle third of the ACL. In a study by Pitman *et al.* (1992), the ACL was stimulated by electrodes which were applied to the femoral end, mid-substance and tibial end of the ligament. Upon stimulation of the ACL, somatosensory evoked potentials (SEP) were recorded at the cerebral cortex, particularly in the mid-substance. These findings support the presence of active proprioceptors within the ACL and may explain why balance is so impaired following injury to the ligament. Proprioceptive training must therefore play an integral role in rehabilitation following injury to the ACL.

The ACL contributes to general stability of the knee and acts as one of the 'four bars' in what is referred to as the 'four-bar linkage mechanism' (Muller, 1983). The other three bars are composed of the PCL, the aspect of the femur between the origin of the ACL and the PCL, and the aspect of the tibia between the insertion of the ACL and the PCL's origin. This is essentially a planar simplification of knee kinematics, but indicates that knee movements are anatomically defined by the lengths of these four bars.

Posterior cruciate ligament

The PCL crosses behind the ACL inside the joint capsule. Like the ACL, it is intra-articular and intracapsular, but extrasynovial (Petersen and Tillmann, 1999), and is housed within its own synovial sheath (Miller and Sanders, 2012). It has a shorter structure than the ACL, but with a wider diameter (approximately 120–150 per cent greater than that of the ACL) (Harner *et al.*, 1995). It originates on the posterior surface of the tibia and passes upwards, forwards and inwards to attach to the lateral side of the medial condyle of the femur. Unlike the ACL, which becomes smaller towards its femoral insertion, the PCL becomes increasingly larger from the tibial to femoral insertions (Harner *et al.*, 1995). At its tibial attachment, it blends with the posterior capsule and periosteum (Saddler *et al.*, 1996). The PCL has two functional components; the anterolateral, which becomes taut in knee flexion, and the posteromedial, which is taut in extension (Irrgang and Fitzgerald, 2000). As mentioned previously, the meniscofemoral ligaments (of Humphrey and Wrisberg) are two additional lateral bundles contributing to the stabilizing role of the PCL. The PCL is the strongest ligament in the knee (marginally stronger than the ACL) and therefore rarely injured; tears to the PCL constitute only 5–10 per cent of major knee ligament injuries (Peterson and Renstrom, 2005). Its primary function is to prevent posterior displacement, or hyperextension, of the tibia in relation to the femur. The PCL is responsible for resisting 93 per cent of the full dynamic extension movement (Piziali *et al.*, 1980). The remaining 5 per cent is stabilized by the collateral ligaments, the popliteus muscle and the posteriolateral aspect of the joint capsule (Hoher *et al.*, 1998). Like the ACL, other functions of the PCL include resisting valgus, varus and rotary stresses (Piziali *et al.*, 1980), as well as offering proprioceptive inputs. The PCL is taut in extension and becomes more lax with increasing degrees of flexion, up to approximately 30°, where it is most relaxed. As flexion continues to increase, the PCL tightens again and is maximally taut at the end of range.

Medial collateral ligament

The medial collateral ligament, or MCL, is a long, broad, strap-like ligament on the inside of the knee and is the most commonly injured of the four major knee ligaments (Fetto and Marshall, 1978). It originates from the anterior aspect of the medial femoral condyle, just below the adductor tubercle, and runs inferiorly to insert onto the anterior medial tibia. The MCL is composed of three portions: the superficial and deep MCL fibres and the posterior oblique ligament (POL), which combine to statically stabilize the medial knee. The deep fibres have attachment to the medial border of the medial meniscus (Warren *et al.*, 1974). The POL is a thickened capsular ligament lying immediately posterior to the deep fibres of the MCL, and becomes slack in flexion. The POL also has an attachment to the medial meniscus at its posterior horn. A tibial collateral bursa may be present and located between the deep and superficial fibres (Miller and Sanders, 2012). The primary function of the MCL is to resist valgus stresses at the knee (Harfe *et al.*, 1998; Miller and Sanders, 2012). The MCL also helps to prevent external rotation of the tibia in relation to the femur. With increasing knee flexion, the degree of laxity of the MCL increases, which allows the joint space to open (referred to as 'medial gapping') (Harfe *et al.*, 1998). When the knee is in an extended position, the MCL is less effective in restraining valgus forces. A study by Grood *et al.* (1981) found that the MCL restrained 57 per cent of the valgus load close to full extension, which increased to 78 per cent of the load in 25° of flexion. This factor is clinically relevant during rehabilitation of the MCL, as the sports therapist should ensure that the ligament is not placed under more stress than can be tolerated during the healing process.

Lateral collateral ligament (and posterolateral corner)

The lateral collateral ligament (LCL) runs on the outside of the knee joint. Unlike the MCL, it is extracapsular and is a shorter, thinner and more cord-like structure than the MCL. It originates from the lateral femoral condyle and runs inferiorly to the head of the fibula on the lateral aspect of the lower limb, where it joins with the biceps femoris muscle to form a conjoined tendon. It is not commonly injured in isolation, but can often be damaged in conjunction with one of the cruciate ligaments. The posteriolateral corner (PLC) complex consists of the LCL, the popliteus muscle and tendon, the lateral head of the gastrocnemius muscle and the arcuate ligament (Miller *et al.*, 1997; Miller and Sanders, 2012). Additionally, Mahadevan (2008) states that the primary stabilizer of the posterolateral knee is the popliteofibular ligament (PFL), which runs underneath the lateral head of the gastrocnemius, from the popliteal tendon to the fibular head and contributes to restrain external rotation forces. A smaller and deeper lateral ligamentous band, the arcuate ligament (AL), runs from the fibular head to the posterolateral femoral condyle (Loudon *et al.*, 2008). Essentially, it runs under the gastrocnemius tendon, over the popliteus tendon, and extends across to the fibula (Mahadevan, 2008). The AL contributes to the arcuate complex (AC), which comprises the AL, LCL, popliteus and lateral head of gastrocnemius – a merging of lateral, posterior stabilizing tissue. Due to its location, it contributes strength to the posterior, lateral aspect of the knee joint. Damage to these tissues is relatively infrequent, but can cause significant functional instability and impairment, and can lead to articular cartilage degeneration (Covey, 2001). The LCL is the primary restraint to varus stress at the knee, and is able to restrain varus stresses more effectively with increasing degrees of flexion. The same study by Grood *et al.* (1981) reported an increase from 55 per cent restraint of the varus force at 5° of knee flexion to 69 per cent restraint at 25° flexion.

Patellar tendon (ligamentum patellae)

The patellar tendon is a continuation of the quadriceps tendon which extends from the patella to the tibial tuberosity and adjacent soft tissue structures and retinaculum (Blackburn and Craig, 1980). It is sometimes referred to as a ligament due to its attachment to its two bones. It is a large (6–8 cm), flat, strong structure integral to the extensor mechanism of the knee joint. The patellar tendon is vulnerable to overuse through repetitive landing and changing direction, which occur in most sporting activities (Cook *et al.*, 2001). Ruptures are rare; when rupture does occur, it is more commonly seen in older populations when significant degeneration is present. An infrapatellar bursa and fat pad separates the synovial membrane of the joint from the posterior aspect of the tendon.

Bursae of the knee

A bursa is a fluid-filled sac, which is usually located close to a joint. Most commonly, a bursa will contribute to reduce friction and hence create smoother, easier movement for tendons over bony prominences and other structures. Bursae may also contribute a modicum of congruency and shock absorption for tissues at a joint. Numerous bursae have been identified around the knee joint. On the anterior aspect of the knee, and superior to the patella, is the large suprapatellar bursa, which is an extension of the joint capsule. Overlying the patella directly is the subcutaneous prepatellar bursa. Inferior to the patella are the subcutaneous superficial infrapatellar bursa and subtendinous deep infrapatellar bursa. At the anteriomedial tibial condyle, the pes anserine bursa lies just under the distal tendon attachment of the sartorius, gracilis and semitendinosus. Laterally overlying the femoral condyle, a bursa may exist under the iliotibial band, and commonly a bursa is present between the LCL and tendon of biceps femoris. Posteriorly, the large popliteal bursa is located between the tendon of popliteus and the lateral femoral condyle, and there are bursae deep to the medial and lateral heads of gastrocnemius. Bursae can easily become irritated and inflamed (bursitis) due to repetitive friction stress, direct trauma or secondary to articular degeneration.

Muscles of the knee

There are a large number of muscles which initiate and control movement at the knee joint (eight flexors; six extensors; five medial rotators; and one lateral rotator). Posteriorly, the hamstring group consists of three muscles located on the posterior thigh and lower leg: biceps femoris, semimembranosus and semitendinosus. Their name actually originates from the eighteenth century, when butchers would hang pig carcasses from their windows by the long tendons at the backs of their knees (as in 'ham-strung') (Biel, 2005). All three muscles are biaxial (two joint muscles) crossing and controlling both the hip and knee. They share a common origin; the ischial tuberosity, on the posterior inferior aspect of the ischium. The biceps femoris has a second origin (short head) from the middle third of the linea aspera and supracondylar ridge. The biceps femoris inserts laterally to the head of the fibula and lateral tibial condyle. The semimembranosus runs to the medial knee and inserts at the posterior medial tibial condyle. The semitendinosus is also directed medially. It is more superficial, and inserts to the anterior, medial tibia at the pes anserinus attachment along with sartorius and gracilis tendons. Pes

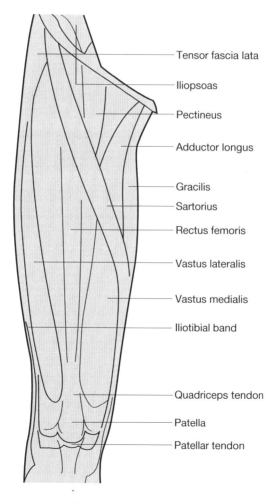

Figure 10.2 Muscular anatomy: anterior view.

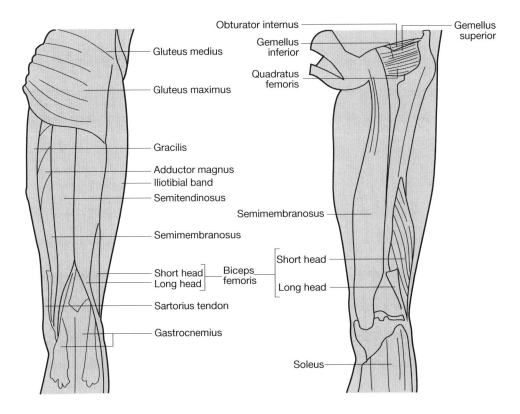

Figure 10.3 Muscular anatomy: posterior view.

anserinus means 'goose foot' in Latin, representing the three tendons which share the same insertion point, also referred to as the 'SGT' point due to the attachment of the above three muscles (Blackburn and Craig, 1980).

As a group, the hamstrings contribute to hip extension and knee flexion. They also rotate the hip and knee joints. The biceps femoris initiates lateral rotation of the TFJ, while the semimembranosus and semitendinosus muscles initiate medial rotation of the tibia. The hamstrings also have a very important role in aiding the ACL in preventing anterior displacement of the tibia (Li *et al.*, 1999). Furthermore, the hamstrings play a vital role in two phases of the gait cycle where they are responsible for producing large forces at the knee and hip. During foot descent the hamstrings must act rapidly to decelerate the thigh. They are also important during foot strike, which is also recognized as the braking phase of the gait cycle.

The gracilis belongs to the hip adductor muscle group and lies on the medial aspect of the thigh, the only adductor which crosses the knee joint. It originates from the ischiopubic ramus and inserts at the anterior, medial tibia at the common pes anserinus tendon. It contributes to medial rotation and flexion at the knee. The long, thin, superficial anterior thigh muscle, sartorius, originates at the anterior superior iliac spine (ASIS) and crosses over the quadriceps group to insert onto the medial tibia at the pes anserinus. Sartorius contributes to medial rotation and flexion at the knee as well as to lateral rotation, abduction and flexion at the hip. The gastrocnemius is a large, superficial biaxial muscle crossing both the knee and ankle. It originates with medial and lateral heads superior to the knee joint at the posterior medial and lateral condyles of the femur and runs distally to insert into the calcaneus via the Achilles tendon. Along with the soleus muscle, it comprises the gastroc-soleus complex, and it acts to flex the knee joint and plantarflex the ankle. It is a weak flexor of the knee, generating peak forces when the knee is in full extension (Li *et al.*, 2002). Popliteus is a short, deep (intracapsular) muscle forming the floor of the popliteal fossa at the posterior knee. It runs medially across the back of the knee from the lateral femoral condyle to the medial tibial condyle. It has attachment to the fibular head via the popliteofibular ligament (which it tensions to help restrain excessive lateral rotation of the tibia) and its tendon divides the lateral meniscus from the LCL (Franklyn-Miller *et al.*, 2011). The popliteus is important as an initiator of knee flexion and in so doing also draws the lateral meniscus posteriorly (Hamill and Knutzen, 2009), hence the popliteus is often referred to as the 'key' that unlocks the knee joint. The popliteus also contributes medial rotation of the tibia on the femur, and inversely during closed chain activity, lateral rotation of the femur on the tibia – which helps to reduce tension on a number of knee ligaments (Mahadevan, 2008). The popliteus also has an integral role when the knee is moving into full extension; the femur medially rotates on the tibia and the medial femoral condyle slots into the medial meniscus to lock the knee joint in place (the 'locking' or 'screw–home mechanism' of the knee).

Plantaris also crosses the posterior knee. It has a short, thin muscle belly, originating at the lateral supracondylar ridge of the femur (just under the lateral head of gastrocnemius), but has the longest tendon in the body, inserting medially at the calcaneus alongside the Achilles. It is absent in 7–20 per cent of the population (Biel, 2005; Spina, 2007) and has been considered to be an almost vestigial accessory muscle – the lower limb equivalent of palmaris longus (Mahadevan, 2008). Although at the knee plantaris may be considered as assisting the gastrocnemius and other knee flexors, both its knee flexor and plantarflexor roles are fairly insignificant (Spina, 2007). Plantaris has been considered to be more important as an organ of proprioception for the plantarflexors of the ankle.

The quadriceps group consist of four large muscles located on the anterior thigh: rectus femoris, vastus lateralis, vastus medialis and vastus intermedius. All four muscles converge at the patella via the quadriceps tendon, and insert via the patella tendon, at the tibial tuberosity. The rectus femoris is a cylindrical, superficial muscle originating at the anterior inferior iliac spine and the superior acetabular rim, and, being biaxial, it is the only muscle of the group to cross both the hip and knee. Rectus femoris is limited as an extensor of the knee when the hip is flexed (Hamill and Knutzen, 2009). The vastus intermedius lies deep to the rectus femoris. It originates at the proximal, anterolateral surface of the femur and is positioned centrally between the vastus lateralis and vastus medialis. The vastus medialis originates as an aponeurosis from the level of the femoral neck (at the intertrochanteric line), the greater trochanter and medial linea aspera. It is often referred to as the vastus medialis oblique (VMO), as the lower fibres, which arise from the adductor magnus, are almost horizontal and attach to the medial border of the patella (Mahadevan, 2008). Although the VMO is recognized as a medial dynamic stabilizer, it has historically been thought to offer significant medial pull on the patella during extension, but Leib and Perry (1971) identified that the quadriceps contract equally throughout this range (Hamill and Knutzen, 2009). The vastus lateralis is the large lateral quadriceps muscle. It also originates from the aponeurosis between the intertrochanteric line, greater trochanter and linea aspera of the femur. It has additional fascial slips from the gluteus maximus and short head of biceps femoris, and superficially it is overlaid by the iliotibial band. Finally, the deep, short and thin articularis genu muscle is located underneath vastus intermedius on the anterior lower third of the femur. Its function is to retract the suprapatellar pouch during knee extension so as to prevent inappropriate folding of the synovium (Mahadevan, 2008).

Practitioner Tip Box 10.2

Muscle synergy of the knee

Flexion	Biceps femoris
	Semimembranosus
	Semitendinosus
	Gastrocnemius
	Popliteus
	Gracilis
	Sartorius
Extension	Rectus femoris
	Vastus lateralis
	Vastus medialis
	Vastus intermedius
	Tensor fascia lata
Medial rotation	Semimembranosus
	Semitendinosus
	Gracilis
	Sartorius
	Popliteus
Lateral rotation	Biceps femoris

Neural anatomy

The knee is served by branches of the obturator, femoral and sciatic nerves. The sciatic nerve (L4–S3) is the largest nerve in the body and is a continuation of the main sacral plexus. The sciatic nerve contains two peripheral nerves loosely bound together; the tibial and common peroneal nerves. In some individuals (around 12 per cent) these nerves are already separate as they exit the pelvis (Moore *et al.*, 2011). The sciatic nerve (including the tibial and common peroneal nerves) innervates the posterior thigh muscles and all lower leg and foot muscles. It also provides sensory supply to much of the skin and joints of the lower leg (Moore *et al.*, 2011). The tibial nerve is the medial terminal branch of the sciatic nerve. It branches from the sciatic nerve at the lower third of the femur and passes through the posterior popliteal fossa to descend inferiorly, before dividing into the medial and lateral plantar nerves below the medial malleolus to innervate the foot. From the popliteal fossa, the tibial nerve branches off to supply gastrocnemius, soleus, popliteus, plantaris, tibialis posterior and flexor digitorum longus. Below the knee, the common peroneal nerve descends laterally to the fibular head, where it runs medially to the biceps femoris tendon. From here it passes to the anterior compartment of the lower leg (superficial to tibialis anterior). It then divides into the superficial and deep peroneal nerves. The superficial peroneal branch runs laterally to supply peroneus longus and brevis, extensor digitorum longus and onwards to the foot. The deep peroneal nerve branches anteriorly to innervate tibialis anterior, extensor digitorum longus, extensor hallucis longus, peroneus tertius and the dorsum of the foot.

The femoral nerve (L2–4) is the largest branch from the lumbar plexus (L1–5). It runs inferiorly from the anterior pelvic region to emerge from under the inguinal ligament in the 'femoral triangle' (which is bordered by the inguinal ligament, adductor longus and sartorius). The femoral nerve runs down the anterior thigh to innervate pectineus, sartorius and the quadriceps group. It has significant cutaneous branches; the saphenous nerve is the largest and longest cutaneous branch of the femoral nerve (Mahadevan, 2008). The obturator nerve (L2–4), also from the lumbar plexus, innervates the adductor muscles of the thigh.

Circulatory anatomy: arteries, veins and lymphatics

The femoral artery is the main artery to serve the lower limb. It arises in the anterior thigh directly from the external iliac artery in the pelvic region, and runs through the 'femoral triangle'. It divides into the deep and superficial femoral arteries just medial to the level of the lesser trochanter. The popliteal artery is a continuation of the superficial femoral artery and arises from the adductor hiatus of adductor magnus. For the knee, there is an intricate system of branching anastomoses supplying the bone and soft tissues of the patellar, femoral and tibial condyles. The genicular, anterior tibial and lateral femoral circumflex arteries are the main direct suppliers of vascularity to the joint (Mahadevan, 2008). The popliteal artery passes posteriorly through the popliteal fossa and divides, just below the popliteus muscle, into the anterior and posterior tibial arteries. The popliteal artery is deep and is particularly important as it supplies the hamstrings, adductor magnus, gastrocnemius and plantaris muscles (Tortora and Derrickson, 2008). The anterior tibial arteries descend through the anterior compartment of the lower leg. They pass through the interosseous membrane which runs between the tibia and fibula. They supply the muscles in the anterior compartment of the leg, the knee joint and the skin covering the anterior leg and foot (Tortora and Derrickson, 2008). The posterior tibial arteries descend through the posterior muscular compartment to the medial malleolus of the tibia. They divide into the medial and lateral plantar arteries, supplying the posterior muscles and structures of the posterior leg and foot.

Although there are superficial and deep, minor and major veins, the main veins that drain venous blood up through and from the knee region towards the common femoral vein (and onward to the external iliac and larger common iliac veins) are the popliteal, long saphenous and short saphenous veins. All the major veins accompany the main arteries of the lower limb. Below the knee are the anterior and posterior tibial veins and the peroneal veins.

Lymphatic vessels, running alongside larger blood vessels from the foot and lower leg, ascend towards the knee. Situated within the fat cells of the popliteal fossa are a small number (6–8) of popliteal lymph nodes, where the lymph is filtered. Larger efferent lymphatics ascend up through the thigh adjacent to femoral blood vessels and course towards the inguinal lymph nodes. Lymph nodes are integral to normal immune functioning. Healthy lymph nodes typically measure 5 mm to 2 cm; they can become more palpable, swollen and painful in the presence of infection.

Clinical assessment of the knee

Any assessment of the knee region must incorporate a recognized, reliable and repeatable protocol. A detailed subjective assessment precedes an appropriate objective assessment. With experience, the sports therapist will prioritize their plan of objective assessment to incorporate the most appropriate techniques for the presenting patient and condition. The resulting assessment must aim to enable the clinician to make a reliably informed decision regarding the presenting injury or condition. Differential diagnoses must be considered, as it is not always possible or appropriate to attempt to reach a confirmative diagnosis, and as such a clinical impression of the involved tissues should be ascertained, importantly including a set of measured examination findings. Cooper (2006) suggests, when presented with a patient complaining of knee pain, that first thoughts could be to consider whether there is a possibility of the patient having one of these common conditions: osteoarthritis, ligamentous injury, meniscal damage or patellofemoral pain syndrome (PFPS). The therapist will also be considering the possibility of musculotendinous injury, bursitis, Osgood Schlatter's syndrome, osteochondritis dissicans, plica syndrome or fat pad impingement. The aim of the complete assessment is to try to identify which structures are affected, the true aetiology of the problem, the symptoms, severity and functional deficits, and the additional individual factors which will influence management and recovery. The therapist must continue to observe and assess the patient during all the treatment or exercise that follows. A thorough assessment of the knee joint can involve the following:

- subjective assessment (the patient history);
- objective assessment;
- general observations;
- specific postural analysis;
- gait assessment;
- clearing of associated regions (lumbar spine, sacroiliac joint, hip, ankle);
- joint movements (active, passive, accessory, and resisted)
- ligament stress tests;
- special tests;
- functional tests;
- palpation.

Subjective assessment of the knee

In the clinical environment, when exploring the patient's main complaint, the focus of the subjective assessment should be on their perception of the cause, pain, weakness and sensory abnormalities. The subjective assessment should clarify the appropriateness of continuing onto the objective assessment – or whether referral would be the appropriate course of action. The 'Ottawa Knee Rules' (OKR) provide clinicians with guidelines for decisions regarding referral for X-ray on suspicion of fracture when the patient presents within seven days of injury (i.e. patient aged 55 years of age or over; isolated tenderness of the patella; tenderness at the head of fibula; inability to flex the knee to 90°; inability to weight-bear for four steps at time of injury or in the clinic) (Stiell *et al.*, 1996). Beyond this, the subjective assessment focuses on the patient's situation and background (name; address; date of birth; telephone and email contact details; GP name and contact details), medical history, current medications and any recent or planned visits to other health care professionals. For the main complaint, an appreciation of the history of the problem must be recorded, whether it is a gradual and insidious onset, with no immediately recognizable cause, or whether it is from one obvious traumatic event. Particularly at the knee, a detailed analysis of the mechanism of injury (MoI) is necessary as the direction and magnitude of the force applied, whether extrinsic or intrinsic, will provide important indicators as to what structures may be damaged. For example, the foot fixed with a twisting impact such as external rotation and valgus may indicate damage to the ACL from a single, traumatic, non-contact event. The novice runner, with an underlying pes planus and genu valgus, and who has begun training for a half marathon, can have a vulnerability to overuse, repetitive stress injuries such as PFPS or ITB syndrome (ITBS) if training has not been carefully progressed or faulty biomechanics addressed.

One of the key aims from history-taking is the working hypothesis of which structures have been damaged or the reason for the patient's symptoms. The therapist should ask about any history of swelling, grinding, locking, catching or giving way of the knee, which can be indicative of osteoarthritis, meniscal injury or ligamentous injury. Certain positions and movements can increase discomfort in the knee joint, hence the therapist must identify what aggravates and what relieves. It is also important to ascertain whether the patient has had any other treatment or surgery on their knee, and whether they have any spinal, hip or ankle issues, as these regions may influence knee function and symptoms (Cooper, 2006).

Objective assessment of the knee

The objective assessment is the practical examination of the patient. Based on orthopaedic principles, using a set of recognized, repeatable and valid test procedures, results are clearly documented on the patient's record form and referred to in any follow-up sessions or communications. The sports therapist should work with a firm rationale for any selected techniques, and it is their responsibility to perform the assessment correctly, eliciting the necessary clinical findings to enable a decision on the suitability of the patient to receive sports therapy intervention. The objective assessment must involve a process of clinical reasoning as the therapist interprets the amalgamated subjective information and the findings from observation, movement, palpation and special tests.

Observation of the knee

Observation begins as soon as the patient is in the view of the therapist – initial impressions can be made on the patient's stance, posture, body type, attitude and approach to movement, gait and general body language. During observation, the patient's skin and superficial tissues are inspected for any abnormal signs. Muscular contours are also observed during observation (general tone; symmetry; atrophy; imbalance between regions). Imbalances of muscle bulk can relate to unilateral hypertrophy of the larger limb or the atrophy on the smaller limb that can occur following prolonged periods of immobilization or interruption to the peripheral nerve supply. Where muscle bulk or joint circumference differences are suspected, a girth measurement can be easily taken by measuring a line from a structural landmark with a tape measure, and comparing left with right. Bony prominences and joint lines should be inspected for signs of deformity, asymmetry, thickening and localized intra-articular swelling or more diffuse joint effusion.

The knee joint should be observed statically, in both standing and seated positions, and if possible, dynamically during walking. The patient should be in shorts and bare feet. The therapist should position themselves appropriately so as to appreciate all required information; this will include getting to eye-level with structures and identifying landmarks with finger and thumb tips. Both knees should be observed and compared anteriorly and posteriorly, and from right and left lateral views. The spinal, pelvic, hip and foot positions must also be assessed. The therapist will observe for any significant bilateral or unilateral postural deviations. Kendall *et al.* (2005) present detailed 'ideal' and commonly deviated postural conditions – however, sports therapists must appreciate that the notion of 'ideal' or 'deviated' postures, and their apparent potential to influence function or identify dysfunction, should be regarded more as a consideration than an absolute.

In the anterior view, the therapist can observe for such presentations as: pelvic shift; lateral pelvic tilt; leg length discrepancy (LLD); anterior or posterior pelvic tilt; hip angle of inclination (coxa vara or valga); femoral anteversion (internal femoral torsion); femoral retroversion (external femoral torsion); genu valgus; genu varus; Q-angle; patellar malalignment; patella baja (inferiorly positioned patella); patella alta (superiorly positioned patella); 'squinting patella' (associated with femoral anteversion); 'frog-eye patella' (associated with femoral retroversion); enlarged tibial tuberosity (indicative of Osgood Schlatter's syndrome); foot angle (associated with both hip angles and tibial torsion); medial longitudinal arch rigidity or insufficiency; 'navicular drop'; hallux valgus; hammer toes. It can be useful to ask the patient to stand with feet together to gain an improved appreciation of any genu valgus (knees touch when feet are apart) and varus (knees are apart when feet touch) (Magee, 2008). Anteriorly, the therapist will be keen to identify surface contours and muscular presentations, including the bulk of the quadriceps group and the possibility particularly of VMO atrophy. The thickness and colour of the patellar tendon can also be observed, as can any localized extra-articular swellings possibly indicative of bursitis (suprapatellar; prepatellar; infrapatellar; pes anserine; ITB), or even a meniscal cyst.

In the posterior view, the therapist will assess hamstring and calf musculature and will again be able to consider pelvic tilting, hip angles and genu valgus or varus. The popliteal creases need to be compared for their levels and angles. At the ankle, valgus heels are commonly associated with pes planus (medial longitudinal arch insufficiency). The Achilles tendon must be observed for any thickening or reddening and for its course down from the calf to the calcaneus, which can be bowed in the presence of valgus heels. Also in the posterior view, the presence of capsular distension may be observed (as in Baker's cyst, which is mostly associated with an arthritic knee).

Laterally, the therapist should observe for excessive or reduced spinal curvatures, the presence of anterior or posterior pelvic tilt (which may be bilateral or unilateral), genu recurvatus (hyperextending knee) or genu flexus (flexed or hypoextending knee). Musculotendinous contours of the lateral thigh (including vastus lateralis, ITB and biceps femoris) and calf (gastrocnemius) may be observed.

If full weight-bearing (FWB) and ambulation (walking) is possible, then the athlete's gait may be assessed. Clinically, the athlete can be asked to simply walk up and down the room, or can be observed on a treadmill. Although it may be considered functional testing, the therapist may elect to include gait assessment prior to other objective tests simply to provide initial clues to irritations and limitations. The therapist should aim to view the athlete from all four sides and be able to identify obvious imbalances or deviations from the norm. The basic gait sequence incorporates stance and swing phases, and the sports therapist will be observing for: basic confidence or apprehension in walking; stride length and width; foot angle; trunk movement and reciprocal arm swing; any linear or angular displacement; and any issues associated with altering cadence and changes in direction. Painful (antalgic) and arthritic and restricted (arthrogenic) compensatory gait patterns can manifest as a reduced stance phase on the affected limb (walking with a limp), or an altered swing phase (circumduction movement). Magee (2008) presents a differential diagnosis of non-antalgic gait limping, including equinus or 'toe-walking' gait (most commonly resulting from tight posterior calf myofascia, congenital clubfoot or cerebral palsy), and Trendelenburg gait (associated with weakened and poorly recruiting hip abductors). At the knee, the therapist should aim to identify limitations in range, especially extension at heel strike and mid-stance, which will be best observed in the lateral view and may result from tight posterior structures (such as hamstrings; gastrocnemius; joint capsule) or mechanical derangement within the joint (such as with a meniscal tear or osteochondral fragmentation). Furthermore, the therapist should aim to identify any patellar maltracking or abnormal tibial motion relative to the femur, which is possibly indicative of instability.

Clearing tests of the knee

When assessing problems affecting the knee, the therapist must establish whether the problem is due to a local injury or if structures above or below the region are involved. Hence, unless it is absolutely clear that the knee injury is a local problem, then the lumbar, pelvic, hip and ankle regions are routinely screened. Generally, active movements, with overpressure (if appropriate) are employed. These are assessed for symptom response and compared contralaterally. If symptomatic, then a more detailed examination will be required.

Lumbar flexion, extension, lateral flexion left and right and rotation left and right can be performed. The therapist may elect to assess active quadrant movements. These are combined movements involving extension, rotation and lateral flexion, left and right, and flexion, rotation and lateral flexion, left and right. Quadrant tests are recognized as being potentially more provocative, particularly to the intervertebral foramen and associated peripheral nerve roots (Petty, 2006). The sacroiliac and pubic symphysis joints can be screened in a number of ways, but a simple compression and distraction technique can offer useful initial impressions of any symptomatic response (Magee, 2008). In a supine or side-lying position, the therapist can use the heels of their hands to compress the lateral aspect of the patient's iliac crests, which can cause an anterior compression at the pubic symphysis and a posterior gapping of the sacroiliac joints. By pressing the heels of their hands against the medial aspect of the patient's iliac crests and anterior superior iliac spines, the therapist can gap the pubic symphysis and compress the sacroiliac joints, again observing for any local or referred symptoms. The hip may be cleared by performing a set of active movements, with overpressure, or by performing a passive combination movement, such as the 'scoop' or hip quadrant test (flexion, medial rotation, adduction and circumduction, with additional longitudinal compression) which may implicate articular hip pathology, such as osteoarthritis or labral impingement (Kenyon and Kenyon, 2009). As highlighted by Loudon *et al.* (2008), Magee (2008) and Petty (2006), mechanical pain relating to a distal joint can sometimes be the cause of pain at a proximal joint, hence the ankle (talocrural) joint can be assessed via active plantar and dorsiflexion with overpressure. The therapist will appreciate that symptoms can occur with assessment of any of the identified regions proximal or distal to the knee and as such they should perform all techniques with great care and recognition of all involved anatomy, especially peripheral nerves and biaxial muscle groups.

The lumbar and sacral plexus supply the leg, and branches of the femoral and sciatic nerve serve tissues of the knee region. Problems affecting the nerve roots or peripheral nerves of the lumbar and sacral plexus (impingements; adverse neural tension; neuropraxia; neurotemesis) commonly lead to referred symptoms such as pain or motor or sensory deficits, which can present at the knee. Increased myofascial tensions and myofascial trigger points of the hip, thigh and calf regions may be the cause of aching around the knee; these can present within the gluteal muscles, deep lateral rotators, TFL, adductors, quadriceps, hamstrings, gastrocnemius, soleus or popliteus.

It is often necessary to explore the nerve supply to the knee region, particularly where there is weakness, atrophy or paraesthesia, or where there are other assessment findings indicative of a neural problem. A myotome is a group of muscles innervated by a particular spinal nerve root. At the knee, L2–4 supply the quadriceps (hip flexion and knee extension), and L5–S2 supply the hamstrings (hip extension and knee flexion). Myotomes are tested with the therapist offering manual resistance against the patient's contraction for a minimum of five seconds (Magee, 2008). A dermatome is the sensory distribution and area of skin relating to a single spinal nerve root. Dermatomes are presented as generalized 'maps' which guide practitioners to the approximate distribution associated with each spinal nerve root. The dermatomes of most relevance to the knee are L2 (the skin overlying the upper anterior thigh), L3 (the lower anterior and medial thigh and knee), L4 (inferior, medial knee and calf), L5 (lateral calf) and S2 (central posterior thigh and calf). Dermatomes relating to the knee are assessed by gauging the patient's response to light or sharp touch. The patient is best positioned in supine-lying with hips and knees flexed, preferably with eyes closed. The therapist slowly traces circumferentially and systematically around the upper leg, knee and calf. The method must compare left with right and allow opportunity for the patient to report any abnormal sensation.

Reflex tests provide further information regarding the functional innervation of the knee region. Deep tendon, or spinal, reflexes assess the integrity of the sensory (muscle spindles and afferent fibres) and motor (efferent) nerve pathways involved in the reflex arc, essentially checking the response of a muscle to being stretched (a stretch reflex). The patient must be relaxed and the muscle placed in a position of slight stretch. The tendon is lightly tapped five or six times. By tapping a number of times, the practitioner may observe an increase or reduction in reflex activity, which can indicate the possibility of upper motor neuron lesion (increased: UMNL) or signs of nerve root involvement, or lower motor neuron lesion (reduced: LMNL). A normal response is an observable or palpable contraction of the tested muscle and slight joint movement. Abnormal reflexes include clonus (very brisk, spasmodic) or exaggerated responses, possibly indicative of UMNL, or diminished or absent responses, which are the more likely presentations in patients attending a sports therapy clinic, indicative of LMNL. Reflexes are not always easy to elicit and can produce false positives. Reflexes are always tested bilaterally and on their own are not conclusive (Magee 2008; Petty, 2006). The patella tap (or knee jerk) reflex relates to nerve roots L3–4 (and the femoral nerve distribution), which can be performed with the patient seated with lower legs hanging off the couch; the patellar tendon is struck with the reflex hammer. The Achilles reflex, relating to the nerve root of S1 (and the sciatic nerve distribution), may also be performed with the patient in the position described above; the therapist should place the foot in a relaxed plantargrade position (neutral 90° angle) prior to tapping the tendon with the reflex hammer. The medial (L5–S1) and lateral (S1–2) hamstring tendons can also be tested, with the patient prone-lying and knee passively flexed (Gross *et al.*, 2009). The therapist's thumb should be placed on the required tendon and they then tap their thumb with the reflex hammer.

Other nerve tests may be required in the presence of suspected nerve root irritation, radicular pain or adverse neural tension; these include the straight leg raise test (SLR – for sciatic nerve distribution and relations), the slump test (for sciatic nerve distribution, dural sheath and spinal cord) and the prone- or side-lying knee bend test (for femoral nerve distribution and relations). Each of the neural dynamic tests may be further modified by way of sensitizing and desensitizing movements to assess for spinal involvement or for assessing individual peripheral nerve branches (Butler, 1991).

Active range of movement of the knee

Active or physiological movement testing is performed to assess the patient's functional ability or apprehension to move affected joints. Active movements should be briefly explained and demonstrated by the therapist and then performed by the patient without assistance from the therapist. They are undertaken initially to assess the patient's willingness to perform the movement, to observe for unwanted or compensatory movements occurring, appropriate movement at associated joints and to clarify where in the range any onset of pain occurs and whether the particular movement alters the intensity or quality of any pain or other symptoms. Active movements should inform the therapist of the possibility of muscle injury, nerve impairment or joint dysfunction, but they are not confirmative. At the knee, full available range flexion, extension, medial and lateral rotation are performed, with overpressure if there is low irritability. Medial and lateral rotation must be performed from a position of knee flexion. If overpressure does not provoke an increase in symptoms, and other findings are normal, then the active movement may be considered normal. Movements of the affected limb should be compared against the contralateral limb and against published norms, but it is important to acknowledge that the patient can have individual factors which need to be considered. Conditions such as hypermobility will show increased movements beyond the normal range, hence, using the contralateral, uninjured knee will provide a more accurate appreciation, with comparison specific to the patient.

Range and quality of movement should be assessed. Range may be measured by way of goniometry, tape measurement or with visual estimation of degrees of movement ('eye-balling'). The patient should be asked to identify where any pain or tightness is felt. Muscle injury, nerve impairment, joint dysfunction (impingement, mechanical derangement, capsule damage, ligamentous damage), pain and swelling may each limit joint range of movement. Therapists should also recognize the possibility of excessive movement (local hypermobility and joint laxity; or a more general 'joint hypermobility syndrome' [JHS]). Initial active movements tend to be performed in a single plane; however, the therapist may decide to ask the patient to repeat movements, perform them at different speeds, observe sustained end-of-range positions or combine particular movements so as to ascertain which specific movements and combinations are most problematic (Loudon *et al.*, 2008; Magee, 2008; Petty, 2006). The findings from active movement assessment must be combined with the results from the passive and resisted tests, along with the rest of the assessment to enable an informed diagnosis.

Practitioner Tip Box 10.3

Active ranges of knee movement

Flexion 0–135°
Extension 0–15°
Medial rotation 20–30°
Lateral rotation 30–40°

Source: adapted from Magee, 2008.

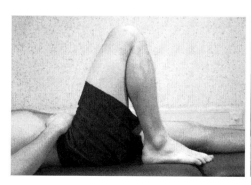

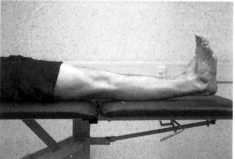

Photo 10.3 Active range of movement assessment: flexion.

Photo 10.4 Active range of movement assessment: extension.

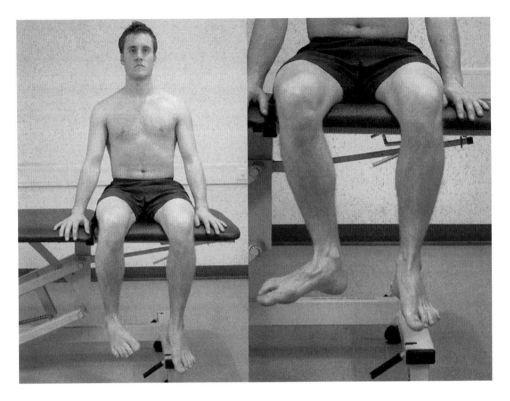

Photo 10.5   Active range of movement assessment: medial and lateral rotation.

Active flexion can be performed in a supine–lying position. The patient should be instructed to slide their heel towards their buttock, as far as they can. The therapist should ask if there is any pain or tightness (possibly around the anterior joint capsule), and if not then they should overpress to appreciate end–feel. Active extension can be performed in the same position (or seated). The patient should be instructed to straighten their knee so it is flat on the couch. The therapist should check for pain then, if appropriate, overpress. Overpressure into end–range extension may involve stabilizing the thigh above the knee and then lifting the posterior aspect of the ankle upwards. Any movement beyond 0° is generally termed hyperextension (or genu recurvatus); similarly, if the knee does not reach full extension it may be termed hypoextension (or genu flexus). In standing, the knee will normally be expected to be in a few degrees of extension beyond zero; any more than this would be classed as hyperextension, which is not an optimal position for the joint. Medial rotation may be performed with the patient either lying supine, with hips and knees flexed to 90°, or seated with lower legs hanging off the couch. The patient is instructed to turn their lower leg and foot inwards and outwards as far as they can, thus rotating the tibia medially and laterally.

Passive range of movement of the knee

Passive physiological movements involve the therapist appropriately positioning the patient so that they can take the joint movement from its start to end position. Passive movements of the knee are usually performed with the patient supine–lying and the therapist must take care to handle the patients limb well (avoiding sudden irritating movements) and to feel and observe the quality and RoM. Simplistically, it is often said that passive movements assess non-contractile (or inert) structures (ligaments; joint capsule; intra-articular tissue). It should be recognized that passive movements may also provoke a symptom response in musculotendinous tissue, especially where there is inflammation, spasm or tendinopathy. Pain can result from any stretching or compression of the injured muscle–tendon unit. The therapist should perform each of the four main movements several times so as to feel the quality and identify where any dysfunction is occurring. Restrictions, tension, laxity, crepitus, and local or referred pain may be present. The therapist should move the joint through its mid-range (feeling the quality) prior to moving towards the point of bind (first appreciation of soft tissue tension) and eventual end-feel. The end-feel, as presented by a range of authors including Cyriax (1982), Magee (2008) and Petty (2006), is how the joint feels to the therapist at the end of its range. At the knee, flexion has been described as having a normal soft tissue approximation end-feel (where the muscles and flesh of the posterior thigh and calf approximate). There are a number of potential constraints or restrictions to flexion, which include: quadriceps tension; pes anserine irritation; anterior capsule tension; anterior or posterior capsular swelling; intra-articular and meniscal damage; quadriceps or patellar tendon injury; patellofemoral joint pain; ITB irritation; bursitis; fat pad impingement and MCL, LCL or other ligamentous injury. Extension has a firm tissue stretch end-feel (where the posterior capsule, posterior muscles, and all main ligaments are placed in tension). Alongside the tissues mentioned, intra-articular damage or meniscal injury can limit range. Medial and lateral rotation also have a normal tissue stretch end-feel, but as these movements are performed when the joint is in its open-packed and least congruent position, there will naturally be less joint restriction. Constraints to rotation movements include: sprains to the collateral ligaments; capsular irritations; musculotendinous injury to hamstrings, popliteus, ITB, pes anserine tendon and gastrocnemius; joint injury; and meniscal damage.

Abnormality in end-feel at the knee may result from a mechanical derangement, such as a meniscal tear, causing a springy end-feel. Arthritic degeneration can cause a harder 'bone to bone' sensation, often with crepitus and muscular spasm, which can cause a tight end-feel. An acutely swollen joint, due to ligament or capsule irritation, will present with a soft but tight end-feel and distinctly reduced range and pain. A more 'empty' end-feel can be associated with joint laxity, reduced muscle tension or atrophy, and also low body fat. The empty end-feel is likely to present as hypermobile, unless pain and a resultant patient apprehension to the movement is a factor (Gross *et al.*, 2009). The PFJ may also reveal itself to be irritated during passive movement testing of the tibiofemoral joint, and the therapist should aim to appreciate such irritation through careful handling and palpation and observation during each of the movements. There are natural or normal constraints to all physiological movements and these directly relate to the state and structure of the joint and associated muscle and other soft tissues.

One further consideration to restricted joint movement is that of the 'capsular pattern', or pattern of limitation, first presented by Cyriax (1982) and expanded by others. This is where injury or inflammation of the joint capsule can result in a capsular contraction leading to a total joint reaction. Hayes *et al.* (1994) described the capsular pattern as '*a joint specific pattern of restriction that indicates involvement of the entire joint capsule*'. Magee (2008) summarizes the capsular patterns associated with the knee as flexion and extension. By comparison, a non-capsular pattern is where there is limitation in a joint which is not characteristic of the capsular pattern, such as when there is mechanical derangement or tendinopathy (Loudon *et al.*, 2008).

As with active movements, passive ranges may be measured by goniometry or other methods, and movements should be compared contralaterally and against published norms. Passive movements must be performed slowly, with correct positioning and confident handling and

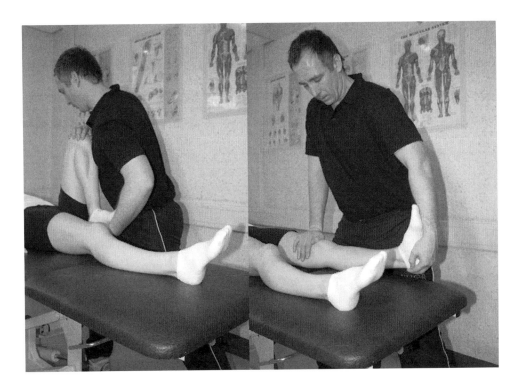

Photo 10.6   Passive range of movement assessment: flexion and extension.

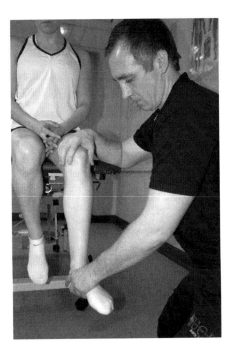

Photo 10.7   Passive range of movement assessment: lateral rotation.

awareness of the potential for symptom response. Magee (2008) suggests that if active movement testing with overpressure has been effectively performed on the knee, then there may be less of a need to undertake passive movements. It may also be considered appropriate to assess combination passive movements of the knee, such as flexion with adduction or rotation. If pain or stiffness is identified, then graded passive physiological mobilization techniques may be considered as part of manual therapy intervention.

Accessory movement assessment of the knee

Accessory movements are the subtle articular joint movements that occur (or should occur) during any gross active or passive physiological movements (Hengeveld and Banks, 2005). Generally classified as being a rolling, spinning or gliding of one articular surface on another, accessory movements allow for normal arthrokinematics. Accessory movements cannot be actively performed in isolation by the individual, but the therapist is able to passively test their range and quality, essentially attempting to clarify normal accessory motion, or identify possible restriction (stiffness or resistance through range), laxity (hypermobility and instability) or pain (or provocation of muscle spasm or any other symptom response). Testing of accessory movements requires precise handling and communication.

A number of accessory movements can be assessed at the knee joint complex. The tibiofemoral accessory movements are generally assessed in a loose-packed position, in the painful position of a free RoM or at the end of a limited RoM (Hengeveld and Banks, 2005). They are normally and initially performed in non-weight-bearing positions, but movements in weight-bearing

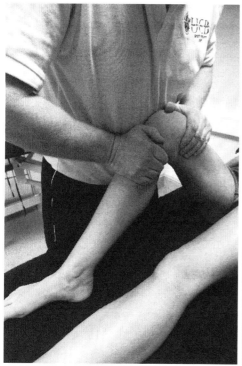
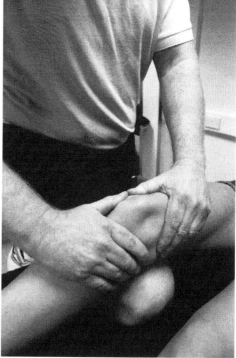

Photo 10.8 Accessory movement assessment: tibiofemoral AP glide.

Photo 10.9 Accessory movement assessment: patellofemoral medial glide.

positions may also be assessed. At the tibiofemoral joint the following may be assessed, initially with the patient supine-lying and the knee flexed to approximately 90°: anteroposterior (AP) glide; posteroanterior (PA) glide; medial glide (MG); and lateral glide (LG). At the patellofemoral joint, the patient's leg is slightly flexed to around 20° (perhaps resting over a bolster or the therapist's flexed thigh): MG; LG; superior, or cephalad, glide; inferior, or caudad, glide; medial tilt (MT); lateral tilt (LT); compression; and distraction. A method for appreciating PFJ mobility has been presented (Halbrecht and Jackson, 1993), which involves dividing the patella longitudinally into four quadrants. A hypomobile medial or lateral glide of the patella will present as movement equalling less than one quadrant. A hypermobile medial or lateral glide will show as more than two quadrants of movement (half a patella width) (Anderson *et al.*, 2009; Magee, 2008). As with physiological movements, where there is pain or restriction, accessory movements (used as mobilization techniques) may be employed to improve the condition.

Resisted movement assessment of the knee

Resistance tests are performed to assess the patient's ability to generate force against the therapist's resistance, identify any pain on contraction or other symptom response, and to gauge the strength or weakness of the working muscles. Isometric resistance tests help to identify the possibility of muscle or tendon injury or nerve impairment and are less likely to incriminate inert joint structures as the involved joint is not moving during the test. The therapist instructs the patient and offers specific resistance to their isometric contractile force, initially in a resting or mid-range position. A progressive incremental resistance is administered, and if the patient can tolerate it they are tested to full strength. For the knee, flexion, extension, medial and lateral rotation are performed. The movement's muscle synergy should also be interpreted. Therapists may choose to localize positioning to assess specific muscles and isotonic resistance may also be used to further evaluate. The therapist should be able to recognize when musculotendinous injury should be suspected by the positive finding of pain on contraction; however, a complete rupture of tissue may not be so painful due to excessive nerve damage. Weakness is a classic feature of muscle injury or nerve impingement or damage. A number of authors (Cyriax, 1979; Magee, 2008; Medical Research Council, 1976) have presented grading systems of muscle strength. For resistance testing, the patient can be instructed to contract their muscles (isometrically) against the therapist's resistance; starting with approximately 30 per cent of maximal strength and gradually increasing the intensity. A patient suffering from a minor muscle injury may find they can actively contract a muscle with no pain, but cannot do so when external resistance is applied. The contralateral limb should be tested first. For resistance testing of the knee, the patient may be prone, supine or seated. It is important that careful positioning takes place, that clear instructions are offered, and that the therapist can handle and resist the patient effectively. Generally, for resistance testing at the knee, so as to begin with optimized length–tension relationships, a mid-range flexion position is adopted, but the therapist may also elect to undertake testing at inner or outer ranges, or with isotonic movement.

Muscle length tests of the knee

Muscle length tests are generally performed as passive movements (although active movements may also be used) to specifically assess for tightness or other symptom response. They are subtly different to standard passive joint movement tests in that they offer important additional information regarding individual myofascial length, tension, imbalance, symptom response and pain provocation. The therapist can also assess antagonist muscle relationships and compare contralateral agonists.

The hamstrings can be assessed as a group by performing passive knee extension from a position of supine-lying hip flexion (to 90°). The therapist should stabilize the patient's anterior thigh (in the 90° flexed position) and gradually extend the knee as far as is comfortable. A generally ideal position will show as the knee comfortably reaching full extension. Loudon *et al.* (2008) describe the passive hamstring SLR test, where the leg, with extended knee, is raised into hip flexion. Less than 80° of hip flexion denotes tightness of the posterior thigh.

The therapist can further gauge tightness in biceps femoris by taking the extended knee into a combination of hip flexion, medial rotation and adduction. Tension in the semimembranosus and semitendinosus complex may be ascertained by combining hip flexion, lateral rotation and abduction. Additionally, the gastrocnemius may also be assessed with the hip in flexion and the knee in extension. The therapist can appreciate the tension in gastrocnemius as they passively dorsiflex the ankle from this position. Gastrocnemius may also be assessed with firm passive dorsiflexion as the patient is in a prone or supine position and their knee extended.

Quadriceps tension may be assessed by flexing the knee in a prone-lying position. The therapist should aim to stabilize the patient's pelvis (with their forearm and hand) as they flex the knee (ideally with the patient's lower leg resting against the therapist's shoulder). This will enable a more localized appreciation of quadriceps tension (if the pelvis is not stabilized it is likely to rotate anteriorly). The therapist must recognize that any swelling of the knee joint, tendinopathy or muscular injury is likely to cause a painful limitation in the range of movement. A similar prone-lying position may be used to gauge appreciation of rectus femoris tension. For this the patient's hip should be placed in a starting position of slight extension (perhaps resting on a bolster or the therapist's thigh). The therapist then carefully and passively extends the patient's thigh, and, importantly, recognizes that knee flexion will be naturally less than that with the hip in neutral.

Of the adductor group, only gracilis crosses the knee, but it may be appropriate to assess the range of both the short and long adductors. Impressions of short adductor tension can be performed with the patient supine-lying, hip and knee flexed to 90°, and their foot resting at the inside of the contralateral knee. The leg is then passively lowered towards the couch and the distance from couch to knee is assessed. Gracilis tension may be assessed, again in supine-lying, with knee extension and abduction. The therapist may offer additional hip flexion and lateral rotation.

General impressions of hip flexor tension can be assessed by the Thomas test (Magee, 2008). Although variants of this test exist (Hattam and Smeatham, 2010), it generally involves the patient lying supine with one leg flexed and the opposite resting in extension. The Thomas test is used to establish resting tensions in psoas, iliacus, rectus femoris, TFL and ITB. The therapist should aim to appreciate that underlying pathology, such as with osteoarthritis, can lead to shortening or contracture of soft tissues. For the standard Thomas test, the patient should be able to maintain normal lumbar lordosis when lying supine. With excessive muscular tension or joint contracture, the affected hip is likely to be observed being held in a position of flexion and possibly increased lumbar lordosis. The therapist will then place a hand under the patient's lumbar spine so as to feel for lumbar movement during the test. The patient is asked to flex their contralateral hip and knee until the lumbar spine flexes and flattens. The patient is then asked to hold their knee with both hands. The therapist observes the resting position of the ipsilateral leg. A negative test shows the leg in a position of extension still flat to the couch. A positive test shows the leg raised to a flexed position. Therapist overpressure may confirm the tension and the patient may show an increased lumbar lordosis. ITB tightness may be indicated if the hip rests in a slightly abducted position; this has been described as a 'J' sign (Magee, 2008). The 'modified Thomas test' has the patient in a similar position, but this time they begin by standing leaning against the edge of the couch and are asked to flex the contralateral leg and hold their knee towards their chest. They are then guided into a supine-lying position (with hip and knee still held in flexion) and the ipsilateral limb's resting position is observed as it hangs off the end of the couch. Therapist overpressure can again be offered to the patient's thigh to ascertain resting tension. From this position, rectus femoris length may be observed by gauging the degree of knee flexion. Excessive tension in TFL and ITB may be gauged again by observing an abducted position. The tibia may also be observed for possible deviation into lateral rotation due to tightness in ITB (Hattam and Smeatham, 2010). Ely's test has also been used to gauge tightness of the rectus femoris (Magee, 2008). The patient is prone-lying and the therapist passively flexes the knee to approximately 90°. Shortening of rectus femoris may be suspected if the hip flexes as the knee is being flexed.

The Ober's and modified Ober's tests are used to assess for tension in the TFL, gluteus medius and ITB (Magee and Sueki, 2011). Both tests have the patient in side-lying (on the contralateral side). The contralateral hip, knee, shoulder and elbow are each flexed to 90° for stability. In the modified Ober's test, the knee is maintained in extension. The therapist stands behind the patient. One hand is used to stabilize and fix the iliac crest and the other hand is used to offer slight extension and abduction as a start position (but maintaining a neutral rotation position); this ensures that the ITB passes over the greater trochanter during the test. The patient is instructed to fully relax the limb and the therapist then lowers it into an adducted position. The test involves observation of the hip adducting onto the couch, or early movement of the pelvis during adduction. Essentially, a positive test is where there is minimal hip adduction (a normal range in the modified test is 10° beyond neutral), where the pelvis moves early in the movement sequence, or where there is a reproduction of the patient's pain (Hattam and Smeatham, 2010). The original Ober's test involves a similar procedure to the modified version, but has the knee in 90° flexion, which emphasizes TFL more than ITB, and a reduced range of normal hip adduction is expected.

Special tests of the knee

Although a host of recognized special tests may be used with varying reliability to assess the integrity and condition of specific tissues of the knee joint, this section aims to present a selection of the most useful (reliable) special tests for assessing structures and conditions. The tests in this section may be single or multi-planar; and they may aim to incriminate a specific structure or simply confirm a (dys)functional condition (such as posterolateral rotatory instability; PLRI). Depending on the test concerned, positive findings may include: pain exacerbation and apprehension; pain reduction; crepitus (grating sensation); clunking (where one or more structural components move inappropriately or suddenly during the test); laxity (excessive joint movement; hypermobility); soft tissue tension; joint stiffness or restriction (reduced movement; hypomobility); weakness or loss of muscle recruitment (due to motor nerve interruption; flaccid paresis); abnormal end-feel (such as 'spongy' – indicative of capsular swelling; or an 'empty' end-feel); or other obvious joint or tissue abnormality. The uninjured limb should always be assessed prior to the affected limb so as to provide a comparison specific to the patient. The therapist must appreciate the potential for false positive or negative test findings. Special tests must be performed correctly (according to best evidence) and with confident handling. They should be repeatable for reassessment and test findings should be reproducible. There are times, particularly in the acute stage of injury, where certain tests and movements are not reliable due to symptoms such as pain or swelling, or not recommended due to the potential for tissue irritation and injury aggravation. The potential for inaccurate diagnostic findings is reduced if the therapist follows the most recent evidence-based recommendations and specific protocols for special tests.

Valgus stress test

This single-plane test is for assessing the integrity of the MCL. The patient is supine and the knee is flexed to approximately 20°. The therapist's medial forearm and waist can be employed to secure the patient's lower leg, and their medial hand can palpate the medial joint line. The therapist's lateral hand is placed over the lateral knee joint and a careful but firm valgus stress is applied as the therapist rotates through their torso. As the test is performed in a loose-packed position, a negative test should present with a degree of normal (slight gapping) end-feel. A positive test is where excessive valgus movement (gapping and laxity) or localized pain is demonstrated. According to Gupta and Funk (2009), medial knee pain alone can be suggestive of MCL injury: a grade I sprain will show pain, tenderness and slight swelling, but with a normal end-feel; a grade II sprain will show with pain, tenderness and local swelling, with an increased gapping prior to end-feel; and a grade III sprain will show as severe pain (at time of injury), significant swelling or haemarthrosis and a loss of definitive end-feel. The test may also be performed with the knee in full extension, which, if demonstrating laxity or pain, can be indicative of injury to the posteromedial corner and posterior oblique ligament, or with loss of end-feel, complete rupture.

Varus stress test

This single-plane test has similar positioning to the valgus stress test and is used to assess for integrity of the LCL (however, the LCL is much less commonly injured than the MCL). The therapist stands inside the patient's slightly abducted leg and the hand positions are reversed. As the varus stress is applied (in 20° knee flexion), a positive test will show with excessive varus

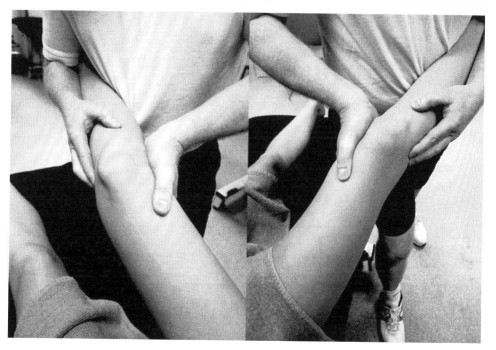

Photo 10.10 Valgus and varus stress tests.

Table 10.1 Grading of MCL and LCL injuries

Grade	Presentation
1	Minimal laxity associated with pain
2	Definite opening, but with a firm end point
3	Gross opening with no firm end point/opening in extension

Source: adapted from Gupta and Funk, 2009.

movement (gapping) or pain on the lateral aspect of the knee. It is normal for the knee to exhibit slightly more movement into varus than valgus. If the test is positive, the therapist should also consider the possibility of injury to the posterolateral corner and arcuate–popliteal complex (Magee and Sueki, 2011).

Anterior drawer test

The anterior drawer is a single-plane test to assess the integrity of the ACL. The patient is supine with knee flexed to approximately 90° (so that the joint is loose-packed and the ACL is

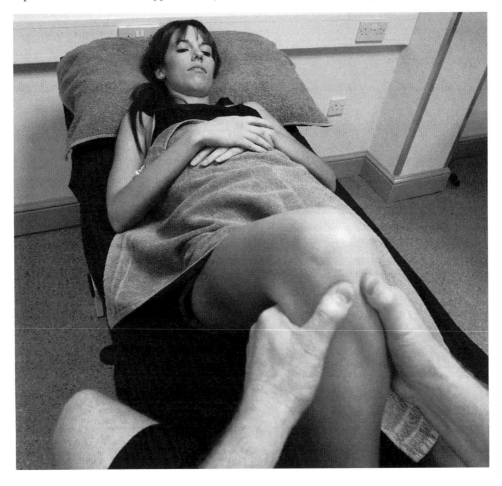

Photo 10.11 Anterior drawer test.

almost parallel with the tibial plateau). The patient's foot must be flat and stabilized by the therapist sitting slightly over and to the side of it. The patient must be encouraged to relax their hip, thigh and calf muscles. The therapist places their thumbs above the tibial tuberosity at the tibiofemoral joint line. Posteriorly, just below the hamstring tendons, the therapist will wrap their hands and fingers around to grasp the tibia. The tibia is then pulled (or drawn) forwards (anteriorly) and the therapist assesses the amount of anterior translation (laxity), end-feel and pain. A positive test is demonstrated when excessive anterior translation (joint laxity) is shown. The severity depends on the grade of ligament tear.

Lachman's test

The single-plane Lachman's test is a reliable test for diagnosing isolated ACL injury (Hattam and Smeatham, 2010). It is similar to the anterior drawer but is performed with less knee flexion (15–30°). A choice of test position may be employed. The patient's upper leg can be slightly abducted and rested flat on the couch. The tibia is then supported off the couch in slight flexion, and as the lateral femur is stabilized with the therapist's proximal hand the tibia is then drawn forward with the therapist's posteromedially positioned distal hand. The alternative position is to have the knee slightly flexed and supported over a bolster or the therapist's thigh. Again, the patient must be encouraged to fully relax as the therapist assesses for anterior laxity, end-feel and pain.

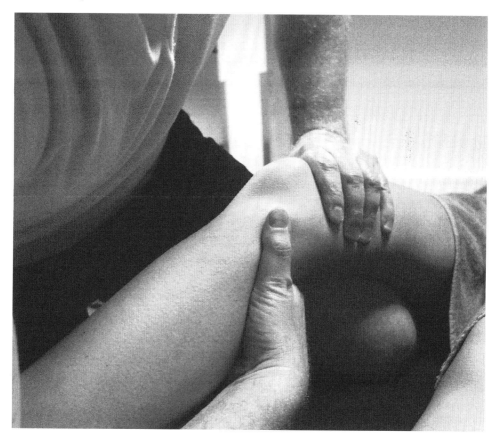

Photo 10.12 Lachman's test.

Table 10.2 Grading of ACL tears in relation to degree of anterior tibial translation

Grade	Anterior translation (mm)
0	0–2 (normal)
1	3–5
2	6–10
3	>10

Source: adapted from Gupta and Funk, 2009.

Anteromedial drawer (Slocum) test

This multi-planar test is a modified anterior drawer test used to establish anteromedial rotatory instability (AMRI). The patient assumes the same start position as for the anterior drawer test, but the lower leg is laterally rotated to 15°, with the foot flat on the couch. It is imperative that the 15° lateral rotation is carefully applied (as any further rotation will place tension on other structures) (Magee and Sueki, 2011). As the therapist draws the tibia anteriorly, they will observe for any increased excursion of the medial aspect of the tibial plateau, as well as for any pain response.

Anterolateral drawer (Slocum) test

This multi-planar test, like the anteromedial drawer test, is a modified anterior drawer test used to establish anterolateral rotary instability (ALRI). The patient assumes the same start position as for the anterior drawer test, but the lower leg is medially rotated to 30°, with the foot flat on the couch. It is imperative that 30° medial rotation is applied (as any further rotation places tension on other structures) (Magee and Sueki, 2011). As the therapist draws the tibia anteriorly, they should observe for increased excursion of the lateral aspect of the tibial plateau, as well as for any pain response.

Pivot shift test

The pivot shift test is a multi-plane test which can reliably assess for both ACL and ALRI. Although a useful test, it can be challenging to produce reliable findings in the acute and painful setting due to the possibility of false negatives if the patient is unable to fully relax (the test is most reliable when the patient is anaesthetized) (Anderson *et al.*, 2000). The patient is supine and supported with their hip flexed to 45° and abducted to 30°. Their knee is flexed to 50° and internally rotated. The therapist supports the patient in the test position by grasping their foot (at the calcaneus) with their distal hand. Their proximal hand is placed over the lateral aspect of the knee joint and the knee is then passively extended (towards end-range) with a valgus and internal rotation stress being carefully applied. The therapist feels for the characteristic 'clunking' (or 'shifting') of the lateral tibial condyle as tension in the ITB causes it to sublux forward on the tibial plateau due to a lax ACL or presence of ALRI. Variations of this test have been presented.

Table 10.3 Comparing anteromedial rotational instability (AMRI) and anterolateral rotational instability (ALRI)

	Typical mechanism of injury	Possibly implicated structures
Anteromedial rotational instability (AMRI)	FWB, fixed foot with external tibiofemoral rotation and possible valgus stress	MCL; medial joint capsule; posterior oblique ligament; ACL
Anterolateral rotational instability (ALRI)	FWB, fixed foot with internal tibiofemoral rotation and possible varus stress	Posterolateral joint capsule; either of the cruciate ligaments; popliteus tendon; LCL; ITB

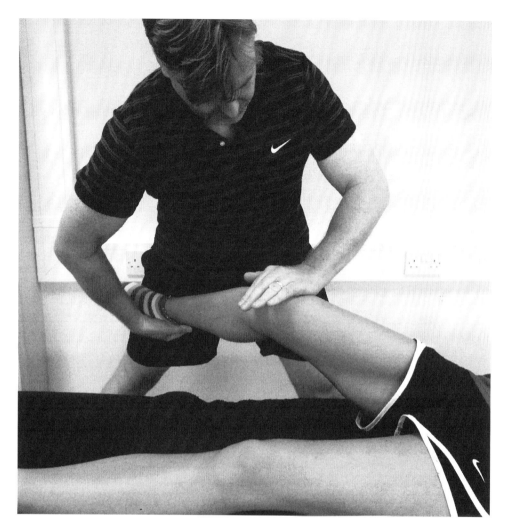

Photo 10.13 Pivot shift test.

Posterior drawer test

This single-plane test has the same positioning as for the anterior drawer test (90° knee flexion; foot on couch; therapist's thumbs, or alternatively their heels of hands, just below the anterior tibiofemoral joint line). The therapist pushes the tibia posteriorly and assesses the end-feel and degree of pain and posterior translation, potentially implicating PCL injury.

Posterior sag test

This single-plane test can be used to indicate the possibility of PCL rupture. The patient is supine-lying, with both hips flexed to approximately 45° and knees flexed to 90°, with feet resting on the couch. Ensuring the patient's feet are in line with each other, the therapist observes for any posterior 'sagging' (tibial translation) at the knee compared to the uninjured side. An alternative test position is again in supine-lying, but with passive flexion at the hip and knee (each to 90°). The knee is observed for any 'sagging' of the tibia at the tibiofemoral joint (Loudon *et al.*, 2008).

Table 10.4 Grading of PCL tears in relation to degree of posterior tibial translation

Grade	Posterior translation (mm)
0	0–2 (normal)
1	0–5
2	5–10
3	>10

Source: adapted from Gupta and Funk, 2009.

Reverse Lachman's test

This single-plane test is performed in a similar manner to the standard Lachman's test, but for this test the patient is prone-lying, their knee passively flexed to approximately 30°; The test is designed to assess integrity of the PCL (as well as possible injury to the posterolateral corner). The therapist initially supports the lower leg in flexion with their caudad hand, and their cephalad hand fixes on the distal femur. The tibia is then passively translated posteriorly with the therapist's caudad hand and assessed for the amount of excursion in comparison to the contralateral knee. The therapist must recognize that this test is less accurate that the posterior drawer and posterior sag tests, and that there is potential for a false-positive result if the ACL is damaged, as the tibia may shift anteriorly with gravity (Magee and Sueki, 2011).

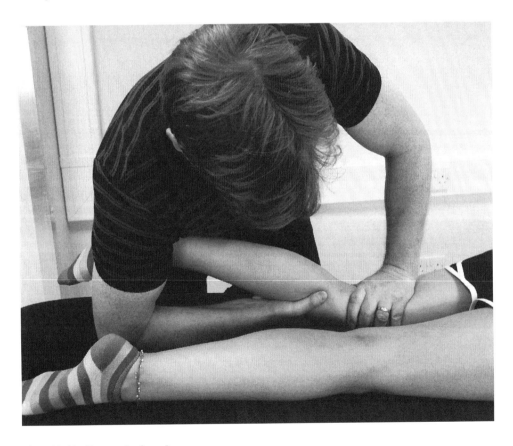

Photo 10.14   Reverse Lachman's test.

Posteromedial drawer test

This test is an adaptation of the posterior drawer test. A multi-planar test of posteromedial rotary instability (PMRI), the start position is the same as for the posterior drawer test, except that the tibia is internally rotated to approximately 30°. As they deliver the posterior drawer manoeuvre, the therapist will observe for increased posterior excursion of the medial tibia.

Posterolateral drawer test

This test is another subtle adaptation of the posterior drawer test. A multi-planar test of posterolateral rotary instability (PLRI), the start position is the same as for the posterior drawer test, except that the tibia is externally rotated to approximately 15°. The therapist observes for any increased posterior excursion of the lateral tibia (Hattam and Smeatham, 2010).

Reverse pivot shift test

This multi-plane test has a similar positioning to the pivot shift test, but is assessing for injury to the posterolateral corner (PLC) and for PLRI. Again, it is most effective when the patient is fully relaxed (or anaesthetized). The patient is supine, with hip flexed to 45°, and the knee flexed to 80°. The therapist supports the patient's limb by placing their distal hand at the ankle and the other hand at the anterior, medial knee. External tibiofemoral rotation is added to the test position, alongside a valgus stress (in this position, the tibia will posteriorly sublux in the presence of PLRI). The knee is carefully extended towards end-range and the therapist observes for reduction ('shifting') of the tibia as ITB tensioning develops at around 20–30° (Hattam and Smeatham, 2010). Several different versions of this test have been presented in the literature.

Dial test

The reliable multi-planar dial (or tibial lateral rotation) test assesses for injury to the PLC and for PLRI. The patient is supine, with their hip slightly abducted so as to allow the knee to be flexed with the lower leg off the couch. The therapist stabilizes the thigh with their cephalad hand and then applies external rotation through the tibia in both 30° and 90° knee flexion. Excessive rotation (beyond 10°) is considered positive (Hattam and Smeatham, 2010).

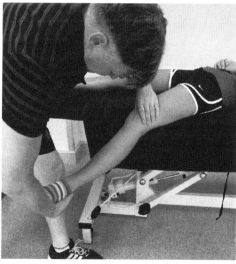 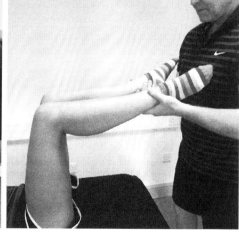

Photo 10.15 Dial test.   *Photo 10.16* Loomer's test.

Gupta and Funk (2009) present an alternative test position, where the patient is prone-lying. The patient's knees are flexed, as before, to approximately 30° and 90°, and in each position the therapist can apply bilateral external rotation by grasping around the ankles. This positioning allows immediate comparison left to right. According to Gupta and Funk (2009), a demonstration of increased external rotation beyond 'normal' is a positive finding: at 30° knee flexion this indicates a PLC injury; at 90° knee flexion this indicates a PLC and PCL injury. Furthermore, Loomer's PLRI test has the patient in a supine position (with hips and knees passively flexed to 90°). The therapist then supports this position bilaterally, and applies the required passive external rotation, assessing for excessive movement (Magee and Sueki, 2011).

External rotation recurvatum test

This multi-planar test assesses for impressions of knee hyperextension, genu varus and rotation of the tibia, which in combination are indicators of PLRI. The patient is supine-lying, and the therapist grasps the big toe of each foot and passively lifts their legs. The patient should remain relaxed, and the therapist compares bilaterally, particularly the positioning of each tibial tuberosity, and the degree of hyperextension, varus and external rotation (Magee and Sueki, 2011).

Table 10.5 Comparing posteromedial rotational instability (PMRI) and posterolateral rotational instability (PLRI)

	Typical mechanism of injury	*Possibly implicated structures*
Posteromedial rotational instability (PMRI)	FWB, foot fixed, external tibiofemoral rotation with valgus stress	PCL; MCL; posterior oblique ligament; posteriomedial joint capsule; semimembranosus tendon
Posterolateral rotational instability (PLRI)	FWB, foot fixed, external tibiofemoral rotation with varus stress	PCL; LCL; arcuate–popliteal complex; biceps femoris tendon; posterolateral joint capsule; ACL

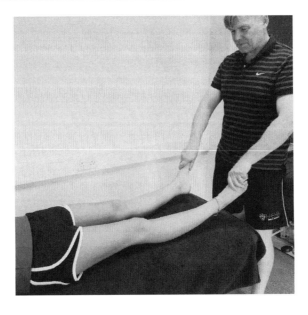

Photo 10.17 External rotation recurvatum test.

McMurray's test

This test of meniscal provocation was first described by McMurray (1942). The patient is supine-lying and the therapist places one hand over the knee joint (with finger and thumb palpating the tibiofemoral joint); the therapist's other hand cups the patient's heel, and their forearm supports the foot. The therapist carefully takes the knee into full flexion, applies external rotation of the tibia and then extends the knee to approximately 90° (Hattam and Smeatham, 2010). The test is then repeated with internal rotation. McMurray (1942) suggested that during external rotation and extension the medial posterior meniscus is stressed, and during internal rotation and extension the lateral posterior meniscus is stressed. The anterior portions of both menisci are less easily evaluated with this test (Magee and Sueki, 2011). The sports therapist should assess for any pain, clicking or patient apprehension during the test. Modifications of the test have been presented, such as combining external rotation with valgus stress (for the medial meniscus) and internal rotation with varus stress (lateral meniscus) while extending the knee (Loudon *et al.*, 2008).

Apley's test (distraction and compression)

This is another test for meniscal provocation. The patient is prone-lying with their knee passively flexed to 90°. With their cephalic knee resting on the patient's posterior distal thigh, the therapist first applies a combination of distraction and rotation (medial and lateral) of the knee by grasping above the ankle and lifting the lower leg upwards. The second part of the test involves delivery of compressive rotary forces through the longitudinal axis of the tibia into the tibiofemoral joint in an attempt to provoke or reproduce symptoms. Pain over the joint line, crepitus and patient apprehension during compression are the positive signs, in addition to a reduction of symptoms during distraction. Any pain exacerbation during distraction can indicate the possibility of ligamentous damage.

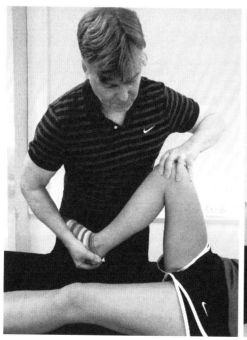

Photo 10.18 McMurray's test.

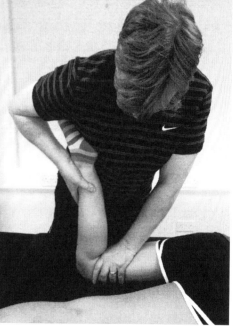

Photo 10.19 Apley's (compression) test.

Thessaly test

This is a multi-planar FWB test for meniscal provocation. Also known as the 'disco test', it is functional in that it replicates aspects of the typical mechanisms for meniscal damage, and has good evidence to support its use (Karachalios *et al.*, 2005). The test involves asking the patient to assume a single-leg weight-bearing stance, with approximately 20° knee flexion (support may be offered). They are then instructed to fully rotate their body over their stance leg (internally and externally). A positive result shows pain, joint locking or patient apprehension which can be indicative of a meniscal lesion. The test may, however, also show as positive where there is other injury or pathology at the knee (such as ligamentous damage or osteoarthritis).

Childress test

This test is also known as the 'duck walk test' and is best reserved for non–acute knee presentations and for identifying the possibility of meniscal damage. The patient is instructed to perform a deep squat and then to walk (as in a 'duck waddle') while in deep knee flexion (and on the balls of their feet). With a posterior meniscal lesion, there is likely to be pain, clicking, inability or apprehension to undertaking the test (Magee, 2008).

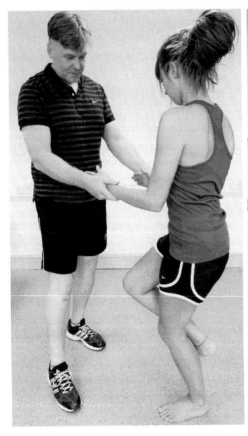
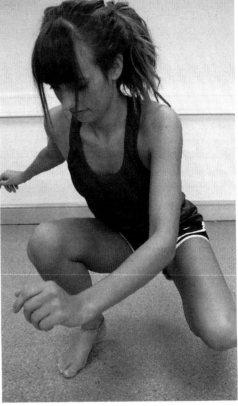

Photo 10.20 Thessaly test. *Photo 10.21* Childress test.

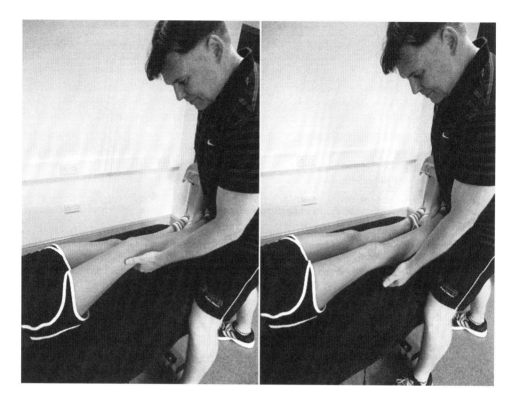

Photo 10.22   Bounce home test.

Bounce home test

This is a simple test for identifying the possibility of mechanical derangement at the knee, and involves having the patient lie supine. The therapist cups the heel of the patient's foot with their caudad hand, and with their cephalad hand placed underneath the knee joint (at the level of the popliteal space), they lift the knee into flexion and then allow it to drop passively into full extension. If full extension is not achieved, or has a 'springy' or 'bouncy' end-feel, then a mechanical derangement (i.e. a possible meniscal lesion) may be suspected (Magee and Sueki, 2011).

Brush test

This test, as described by Magee and Sueki (2011), is used to assess for effusion at the knee. It has also been known as the 'stroke', 'sweep', 'wipe' or 'bulge' test and is performed with the patient supine-lying. The therapist gently 'brushes' synovial fluid upwards from the medial side of the patella, to the proximal edge of the suprapatellar pouch. The therapist should perform two or three upward brushing movements, followed by two or three downward brushing movements, from the suprapatellar pouch to the lateral side of the patella. If a wave of fluid passes to the medial side of the joint and 'bulges' medially and distally, adjacent to the patella, then this is a positive indication of synovial effusion. It may take two or three seconds for the bulge to appear.

Patellar tap test

Also known as the 'ballotable' or 'floating' patella test, the patellar tap test aims to identify swelling of the knee. The patient is supine with knee extended to a comfortable position (slight

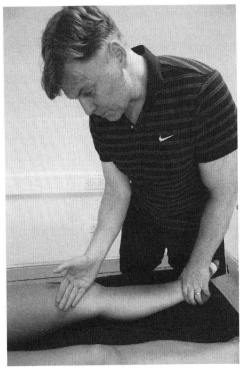

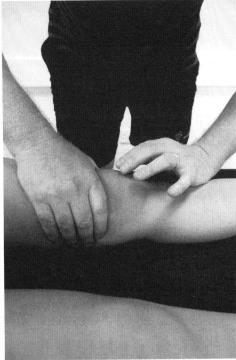

Photo 10.23   Brush test.   *Photo 10.24*   Patellar tap test.

flexion will increase effusion pressure). The therapist applies a light pressure or 'tap' to the patella using thumb or finger tips and observes for any 'floating' of the patella (Shultz *et al.*, 2000). Johnson (2000) describes a two–handed technique, where the therapist gently compresses the suprapatellar pouch with the cephalad hand, followed by the thumb or finger tap onto the patella. Following the downward movement of the patella, a positive result is where the patella is seen to rebound and 'float'.

Patellar apprehension test

This test is used to identify the patient's apprehension to lateral glide, which can be indicative of patellar subluxation or dislocation (Loudon *et al.*, 2008) The patient is supine-lying, with their knee flexed and supported to 30°. Using their thumb tips from the medial aspect of the patella, the therapist then simply delivers a lateral glide to the patella. Patient apprehension with a sensation that the patella will dislocate or a reflexive contraction of the quadriceps are positive signs.

Patellofemoral grind test

This test, also known as the 'Clarke's test', is used to evaluate the integrity of the articular surfaces of the PFJ. The patient is supine-lying, with knees extended but supported on a bolster so as to create articulation of the patella with the femoral trochlea (Nijs *et al.*, 2006). The therapist places one hand just proximal to the superior pole of the patella and applies gentle compression with slight inferior glide. The patient is then asked to contract their quadriceps. The test is positive if it causes pain; however, this test can also cause discomfort in uninjured athletes. The test can be repeated several times, with progressive increases in compressive force

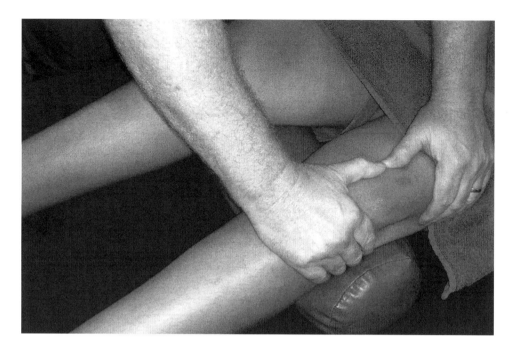

Photo 10.25   Patellar apprehension test.

to the suprapatellar region on each application. The patient can also be asked to perform contractions in different positions of knee flexion (i.e. 30°, 60° and 90°) (Shultz *et al.*, 2000). An alternative patellar grind test has been described by Gupta and Funk (2009). This involves the supine-lying patient being asked to flex and extend their knee while the therapist applies gentle compression over the patella. A positive test is where pain or crepitus are evident, indicating possible chondromalacia patellae (CMP) or patellofemoral pain syndrome (PFPS).

McConnell test

This test, first described by McConnell (1986) and also referred to as the 'critical test' (Loudon *et al.*, 2008), is used to evaluate the integrity of the articular surfaces of the PFJ, and for the identification of CMP (Petty, 2006) or PFPS. The patient is positioned in high sitting (with legs hanging off the side of the couch), and with their tested hip in slight lateral rotation. They are asked to contract their quadriceps isometrically for ten seconds in a range of degrees of flexion (i.e. 0°, 30°, 60°, 90° and 120°). If pain results at any of the ranges, the therapist then applies a medial glide to the patella, which, if it reduces discomfort, can be an indicator of CMP, possible maltracking of the patella and simply pain of patellofemoral origin.

Eccentric step test

Nijs *et al.* (2006) describe the eccentric step test. The patient assumes a single leg stance on a low step (approximately 15 cm high). The patient is instructed to place their hands on their hips, and to step down from the step as slowly and as smoothly as they can. They are, in effect, attempting to flex the stance leg so as to reach the floor in front of the step with the non-stance foot. Anterior pain in the stance knee, or inability to reach the floor with the non-stance foot, are possible indicators for PFPS. Osteoarthritis can be another consideration with a positive test result.

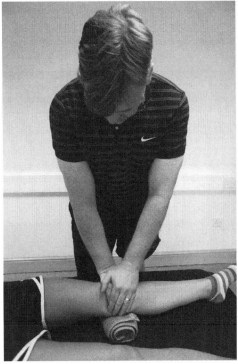 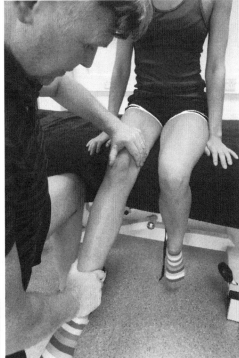

Photo 10.26   Patellofemoral grind (Clarke's) test.   *Photo 10.27*   McConnell (critical) test.

Decline squat test

Warden and Brukner (2003) explain that the 30° decline squat test can be useful for identifying patellar tendinopathy. Such an angled test position places greater load on the patellar tendon than a squat on level ground. Cook and Khan (2002) highlight that the decline squat decreases the contribution of calf muscles and passive ankle structures. Objective measures may be obtained by determining the number of decline squats before the onset of pain, and by asking the athlete to indicate the level of pain on a visual or verbal analogue scale (VAS). Kongsgaard *et al.* (2006) demonstrated that the use of a 25° decline board increased the load and strain of the patellar tendon during unilateral eccentric squats.

Noble's compression test

This test is used to identify iliotibial band syndrome (ITBS), which can develop when the ITB glides repetitively over the underlying bursa on the superior and lateral aspect of the lateral femoral condyle during hip and knee movements. The patient is supine and the therapist supports the knee just proximal to the joint line with their cephalad hand. The therapist must also contact the lateral femoral condyle with the thumb pad of the same hand. With the caudad hand controlling the lower leg, they then passively flex and extend the knee while maintaining contact over the lateral femoral condyle. A positive test is indicated by pain underneath the thumb when the knee is in approximately 30° of flexion (as the band runs over the condyle at this position), indicating irritation or inflammation of local tissues (Starkey and Ryan, 2003).

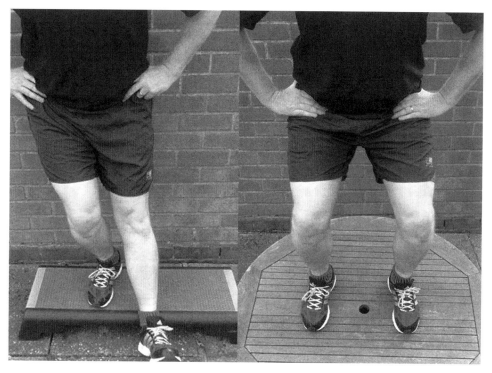

Photo 10.28   Eccentric step and decline squat tests.

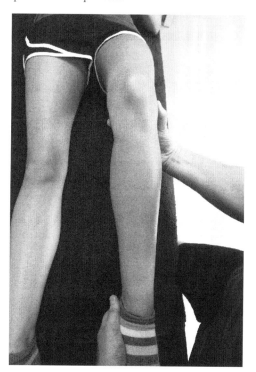

Photo 10.29   Noble's compression test.

Mediopatellar plica test

This test is used to assess for irritation of the mediopatellar plica. The patient is supine with the tested knee supported in 30° flexion. The therapist simply applies a medial glide to the patella and observes for pain as the medial plica (if present) may be 'pinched' between the patella and medial femoral condyle (Magee and Sueki, 2011). Pain may be exacerbated with additional quadriceps contraction.

Stutter test

This is a further test for medial plica syndrome. The patient is high sitting, with the lower leg hanging off the couch. The therapist lightly palpates the patellofemoral joint with the palm of their hand as the patient slowly extends their knee. The therapist assesses for irregular movement ('stuttering') as the knee extends (especially between 40° and 60°), indicating possible catching of the medial plica (if present) on the medial femoral condyle (Starkey and Ryan, 2003).

Q-angle assessment

The Q (quadriceps) angle is formed by two straight and intersecting lines: one running from the ASIS and through the centre of the patella; the other running from the tibial tuberosity and up through the centre of the patella. Shultz *et al.* (2000) describe it as the angle between the quadriceps muscle group and the patellar tendon. An average Q-angle for males is generally recognized as being 10–15° and for females 15–20°. Any significant reduction or increase in the angle can be a contributing factor in knee problems, most commonly PFPS. An increased Q-angle may indicate a tendency to lateral tilt or glide (Rossi *et al.*, 2011). Factors contributing to an increased Q-angle include: coxa vara; genu valgus; increased foot pronation; medial tibial

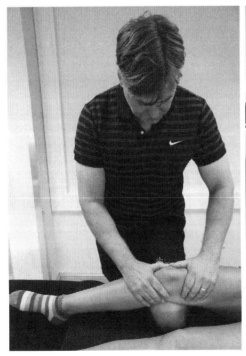

Photo 10.30 Mediopatellar plica test.

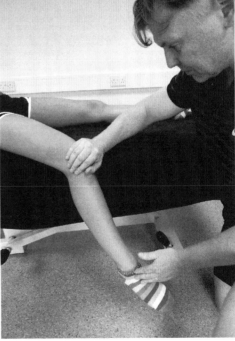

Photo 10.31 Stutter test.

torsion; weakness of vastus medialis oblique (VMO) or gluteus medius; patella alta (superiorly positioned patella); and a laterally positioned tibial tuberosity. To measure the Q-angle, the patient is supine-lying with their knees fully extended. The therapist measures the angle between two lines: the first line from the ASIS to the centre of the patella; the second line from the tibial tuberosity to the centre of the patella. A positive test is where the measured Q-angle falls outside of the accepted 'normal' ranges for males or females. The Q-angle can also be measured in several ways, such as: in different positions of flexion (at 90° knee flexion the normal Q-angle is 0–5°); with quadriceps contraction; and in standing. Each time the sports therapist should ensure that a standardized test is used for each limb (making sure that start position is the same, and that foot angle and position is neutral – as any increase in pronation, supination or tibial torsion can affect the Q-angle). Rossi *et al.* (2011) suggest that the Q-angle be measured at 30° flexion so as to place the patella into the proximal portion of the femoral trochlea (patellar surface).

Leg length discrepancy test

There are number of recognized techniques for measuring for leg length discrepancies (LLD). The therapist may elect to simply have the patient supine-lying, and as straight as possible (by 'squaring the pelvis'), and simply compare visually the relative position of each medial malleolus. The most commonly used general method for comparing leg lengths is by measuring from the ASIS to either the medial or lateral malleolus on the same side, and then comparing on the contralateral side (Magee, 2008). Although this method is often described as being a 'true' leg length assessment, it is not – as the ASIS belongs to the pelvis! The therapist can measure from key landmarks on the leg to establish structural length differences between each leg (such as from the greater trochanter to the lateral femoral condyle; or from the lateral tibial condyle to the lateral malleolus). As Magee (2008) states, an LLD of 1–1.5 cm or less is considered normal (however, athletes may require intervention if such a discrepancy exists and is a cause of pain or

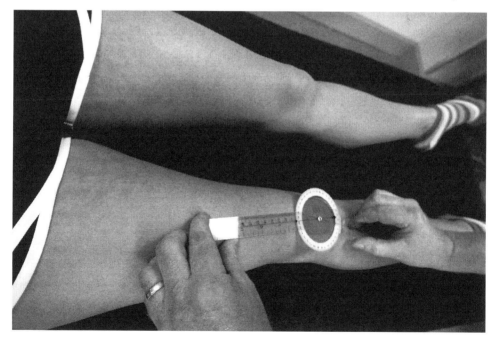

Photo 10.32   Q-angle measurement.

dysfunction). Apparent LLD occurs when functionally shortened soft tissues and pelvic imbalances give the impression of leg shortening. This can be assessed by measuring from a central point (such as the xiphoid process) down to the medial malleolus, left and right (Gupta and Funk, 2009).

Supine to sit test

This test, as described by Wadsworth (1988), is used to identify the possible presence of a unilateral anterior pelvic tilt. The patient is first assessed for LLD (true or apparent) as above. A positive test is indicated when the patient is observed as having one leg appearing longer in supine and shorter in long sitting. This test, like all, must be performed in conjunction with other assessment methods.

Palpation of the knee

Specific and careful palpation is an essential component of clinical knee assessment. It requires good anatomical knowledge and skill in applying appropriate pressure and depth so as to appreciate different tissue structures and abnormalities. Palpation should commence superficially before probing deeper tissues, and should also begin with structures above and below the affected locality of symptoms. Structures that are readily assessed at the knee region include: rectus femoris; vastus medialis; vastus lateralis; vastus intermedius; quadriceps tendon; patella; patellar tendon; tibial tuberosity; bursae (suprapatellar, infrapatellar, prepatellar, pes anserinus; popliteal); femoral condyles; TFJ contours; PFJ contours; biceps femoris; semimembranosus; semitendinosus pes anserine tendon; MCL; LCL; anterior medial meniscus; anterior lateral meniscus; ITB; gastrocnemius; popliteal fossa; popliteus; fibular head; and PTFJ contours.

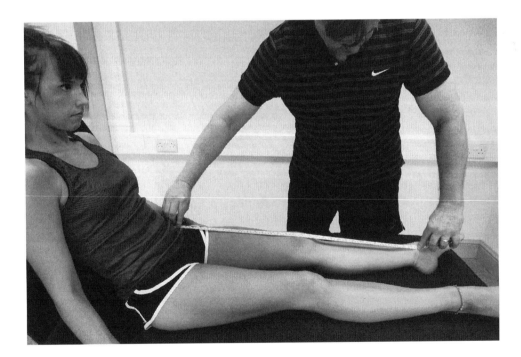

Photo 10.33 Supine to sit test.

Special test	Main structure(s) or condition(s) tested
Valgus stress test	Medial collateral ligament (MCL)
Varus stress test	Lateral collateral ligament (LCL)
Anterior drawer test	Anterior cruciate ligament (ACL)
Lachman's test	ACL
Anteromedial drawer (slocum) test	Anteromedial rotational instability (AMRI)
Anterolateral drawer (slocum) test	Anterolateral rotational instability (ALRI)
Pivot shift test	ACL and ALRI
Posterior drawer test	Posterior cruciate ligament (PCL)
Posterior sag test	PCL
Reverse Lachman's test	PCL and posterior lateral corner (PLC)
Posteromedial drawer test	Posteromedial rotational instability (PMRI)
Posterolateral drawer test	Posterolateral rotational instability (PLRI)
Reverse pivot shift test	PLC and PLRI
Dial test	PLC and PLRI
Loomer's test	PLRI
External rotation recurvatum test	PLRI
McMurray's test	Meniscus
Apley's (distraction/compression) test	Meniscus
Thessaly test	Meniscus
Childress test	Meniscus
Bounce home test	Meniscus
Brush test	Effusion
Patellar tap test	Oedema
Patellar apprehension test	Patellar subluxation
Patellofemoral grind (Clarke's) test	Patellofemoral pain syndrome (PFPS) and chondromalacia patellae (CMP)
McConnell (critical) test	PFPS and CMP
Eccentric step test	PFPS
Decline squat test	Patellar tendinopathy and PFPS
Noble's compression test	Iliotibial band friction syndrome (ITBFS)
Mediopatellar plica test	Medial plica syndrome
Stutter test	Medial plica syndrome
Q-angle assessment	Excessive (or reduced) angle between quadriceps muscles and patellar tendon
Leg length discrepancy (LLD) test	True and apparent LLD
Supine to sit test	Apparent LLD and unilateral anterior pelvic tilt

Functional tests of the knee

The average active supine RoM at the knee is from 0° extension to 135° flexion. Normal daily functioning requires a certain amount of knee flexion and full knee extension, which emphasizes the need for minimizing loss of these movements and regaining functional ranges as soon as possible. For example, reaching for something at a height requires full knee extension, as does walking downstairs, putting on trousers and using the brake pedal while driving. Most daily activities do not require the full 135° of flexion; however, a significant range of flexion is required for everyday activities such as walking up and down stairs, picking up something from the floor, sitting down, going to the toilet and putting on a pair of socks. Functional tests are therefore an important part of the assessment as they can replicate essential movements required for the patient's normal daily functioning. Functional tests enable the therapist to identify the normal approaches to movement, and whether their movement is a contributory factor in their problem. Such tests may be open or closed chain, bilateral or unilateral, and they enable appreciation of trunk, pelvic, hip, ankle and foot movements. Functional tests may enable the practitioner to provoke symptom responses in tissues which were not effectively provoked in other movements and tests. The therapist should observe alignment, range, strength, quality, coordination and steadiness of movement, whether any compensation is present and pain levels. Functional testing also provides the therapist with the opportunity to coach improved technique and assess the patient's ability to undertake improved movement patterns. Simple functional tests for the knee include: standing from a seated position and sitting from standing; bilateral and unilateral squatting (partial or full weight-bearing; partial or full range); lunging; stepping-up and stepping-down; picking up an object from the floor; and reaching a high point on the wall. More challenging functional tests can include: star excursion balance test (SEBT); jogging on the spot; and low-intensity (short-range) jumping and landing (bilateral or unilateral, as in hopping). Such jump tests enable gauging of the athlete's apprehension, ability, pain, stability, proprioception and endurance. During functional testing, the sports therapist must be observant for any abnormal movement patterns occurring at the knee (such as valgus collapse) and the influence of the hip, ankle and foot on knee movements and positioning (such as dynamic pelvic instability, tight adductor muscles or excessive foot pronation). The therapist can request the patient to perform typical movements of their work or sport, such as a football kick (stance and swing positions). Outside of the clinical environment, later-stage functional tests can be undertaken, such as speed and agility testing (Illinois agility test; T-test) and more sports-specific tests (Comfort and Matthews, 2010).

Progressive, functional and sports-specific assessment has become an essential component in the process for improved injury prevention, injury management and sports performance. Barton *et al.* (2012) present an overview of four sequential steps to undertaking lower limb biomechanical assessments: (1) static stance; (2) simple functional movements; (3) dynamic movements; and (4) sports-specific activity. Cook *et al.* (2010) developed the Functional Movement Screen (FMS), a seven-point measurable and graded movement screen, with associated corrective exercise strategies. The screen may be adapted for specific sports.

The seven movements assessed under the standard FMS protocol are:

1. deep squat
2. hurdle step
3. in-line lunge
4. shoulder mobility
5. active straight leg raise
6. trunk stability push-up
7. rotary stability.

Rehabilitation and return to sport

Any rehabilitation plan should reflect the stage of tissue healing – acute, sub-acute or chronic – and the current functional capacity of the individual. In the early stage (acute or inflammatory phase), pain-free mobility and flexibility exercises are key to maintaining joint RoM and tissue extensibility. Passive movements may be useful in assisting mobility, but care must be taken at this stage. The PRICE protocol (protection, rest, ice, compression and elevation) has traditionally been considered vital in order to minimize swelling, assist healing and control pain levels, although its efficacy at improving clinical outcomes in soft tissue injury has been questioned (Collins, 2008; Meeusen and Lievens, 1986). Early strengthening within pain-free ranges should usually be introduced so as to avoid muscle atrophy. This can be performed in a non-weight-bearing position if the client is unable to weight bear at this stage – for example, isometric quadriceps 'setting' in a supine position. Once weight bearing is possible, closed-chain proprioceptive exercises can be gradually introduced to improve balance and spatial awareness. For a knee injury, this could be as simple as unilateral standing on the affected limb (with the knee just 'off-lock' and short of end-range extension). This can be easily progressed as a proprioceptive challenge by turning the head, increasing the length of time, introducing an unstable surface, closing the eyes or adding an external stimulus.

Once the client enters stage two of rehabilitation (sub-acute, repair or proliferation phase), swelling, inflammation and pain levels should be subsiding. The duration of the acute phase largely depends on the severity of the injury, and how effectively it has been managed, as well as patient adherence to the rehabilitation plan. The patient should have achieved a good range of motion, a reasonable degree of strength throughout the full range of the joint and the ability to perform most daily activities. More progressive stretching and strengthening exercises can therefore be introduced at this stage. Strengthening exercises can be progressed in numerous ways; for example, increasing the resistance and repetitions, manipulating the rest period and increasing the complexity of the exercise. Changing the exercises will give the body a new stimulus that it must adapt to, thereby creating overload.

Cardiovascular fitness is an essential part of rehabilitation and should be integrated into the patient's programme where possible. Maintenance of aerobic fitness while managing a knee injury may require creativity. Some gyms have upper-body ergometers; pool-based activities may be an option. It may be that the athlete can undertake use of a cross-trainer or stationary cycle without detriment to their knee injury. Ideally the rehabilitation plan will incorporate a combination of aerobic and anaerobic training, and more emphasis may be placed on one or the other, dependent on the athlete's sporting requirements. Once the patient has regained a reasonable level of flexibility, strength and proprioception, functional activities that form the basis of their sport or daily activity should be gradually reintroduced.

In the later stage (remodelling and maturation phase), the patient should be demonstrating good levels of flexibility, strength and endurance, and joint proprioception. Daily activities should now be relatively comfortable to perform and their condition should not be exacerbated by the rehabilitation exercise. Before return to full activity is advised, the therapist and patient must be confident that movement patterns can be performed at speeds and directions specific to their sport, daily life and work. With graduated, specific training, the patient will relearn motor patterns that they may or may not have mastered prior to injury, and which may need to be improved, depending on the cause. Particularly challenging exercises for the knee include: multidirectional running, hopping and holding, bounding, lateral lunges and any sport-specific movements. Any fitness tests selected depend on the most recent assessments of the patient's condition, the severity of the injury and the sport or work they plan to return to.

Essential markers for return to sport must be assessed prior to the decision being made. First and foremost, the sufficient time constraints to allow tissue healing must have been observed. The client must have achieved good flexibility, strength, endurance and proprioception. They should be pain-free and have full RoM, without compensation or abnormal biomechanics. The patient must have adequate cardiovascular fitness and be regaining sufficient skill levels. The patient must be mentally confident that they are ready to return to sport, as playing with loss of confidence and fear of injury can quite easily result in further damage or reinjury. Progressive sports-specific rehabilitation with SMART (specific; measurable; achievable; realistic; timed) goal-setting, ongoing assessment and full functional fitness testing is a safe platform for return to play. Creighton *et al.* (2010) presented the three-stage 'decision-based model' to guide practitioners towards making the all-important return to play decisions. This model incorporates risk evaluation (clarifying the athlete's health status and their participation risk) in conjunction with a final decision modification component, with consideration to such factors as timing and season, pressures from the athlete and all external stressors (including the coach, family and any conflicts of interest).

Common injuries and conditions of the knee joint

The knee is one of the most commonly injured joints in athletes. This is especially so in sports involving full contact, sudden changes of direction, twisting movements and dynamic landings. The most common acute and traumatic structural injuries of the knee involve tears of the ACL, MCL and the menisci. A rupture of the ACL tends to be the injury of greatest concern for athletes due to the severity of the injury and the lengthy rehabilitation process it requires. Patellar tendinopathy is a common complaint of athletes who have to repeatedly jump and land, such as in basketball. The most common overuse injury of the knee is patellofemoral pain syndrome (PFPS) (Dixit *et al.*, 2007). As a generalized consideration, with regards to gender differences, Atkins *et al.* (2010) explain that young adult males present more commonly with traumatic meniscal lesions associated with rotational injury during sports, while females are more likely to present with general hypermobility, instability and episodes of subluxation and dislocation of the patella.

Ligamentous and joint injuries of the knee

Generally and simply, ligament tears are graded as follows: grade I sprain – a minor partial tear, with mild pain and minimal loss of function; grade II sprain – a moderate sprain, with significant pain and loss of function; grade III tear – a complete rupture with major loss of stability (Gupta and Funk, 2009).

Anterior cruciate ligament injuries

The ACL is one of the most commonly injured ligaments of the knee and accounts largely for prolonged absences from sport caused by knee injury. It is estimated that 70 per cent of all ACL injuries are sports-related (Miyasaka *et al.*, 1991). Significant damage to the ACL will cause abnormal functioning through altering the kinematics of the knee joint (Gillquist, 1990). It also frequently results in degenerative changes in the knee joint. The mechanism of injury generally involves a twisting impact, landing from a jump or decelerating suddenly. Injury to the ACL appears to be most prevalent in a weight-bearing position when a medial or lateral rotatory stress is applied to the tibia with a slightly flexed knee (Feagin and Lambert, 1985). The ACL can be damaged through contact, but is commonly a non-contact, intrinsic injury (Yu and Garrett, 2007). At the time of injury, the player will often report hearing and feeling a loud 'pop' or 'crack'. A rupture of the ACL will cause extreme pain and an immediate cessation of activity. In some instances the player may be able to walk off the pitch, but this does not necessarily mean the ACL is intact. Immediate, severe swelling is an indicator of ACL injury. The patient may describe a feeling of instability and that the knee gives way. It has been reported that approximately 175,000 ACL reconstructive operations take place every year in the United States (Gottlob *et al.*, 1999).

The ACL is frequently damaged alongside the MCL and medial meniscus (injury to all three is known as 'O'Donaghue's Triad'), which is more common in female athletes (Yu and Garrett, 2007). The rate of serious knee injuries sustained by females has increased to twice the level of that in males (Huston and Wojtys, 1996). A combined ACL and MCL injury can result from a laterally applied force to the knee, or a medially applied force to the foot, both of which force the knee into valgus and external rotation, a combination that can lead to an anteromedial rotational instability (AMRI). Conversely, a force to the medial side of the knee can injure the ACL in combination with the LCL and the posterolateral capsule, which presents as an anterolateral rotation instability (ALRI). Combination injuries involving the ACL and PCL are much less common and generally result from an excessive force causing near dislocation of the knee. Significant rotary forces or forced hyperextension or hyperflexion of the knee can cause such injuries to occur.

On objective assessment of the acutely ACL-injured knee, active and passive ranges of movement are likely to be painful and limited. Anterior drawer and Lachman's tests are likely to elicit positive results, especially with grade II and III injuries. The therapist must ensure that the hamstring muscles are relaxed when performing both tests. A 'false negative' may occur if the hamstrings are contracting to stabilize the tibia in place of the damaged ACL, therefore not allowing the tibia to translate forwards, as it would if they were in a relaxed state (Li *et al.*, 1999). This is thought to occur due to the posterior shear force that the hamstrings exert on the tibia (Yu and Garret, 2007). Some studies, however, have reported that the effect is only significant at larger levels of flexion (Beynnon *et al.*, 1995; Li *et al.*, 1999), which emphasizes the importance of using the Lachman's test in addition to the anterior drawer test due to it being performed in a less flexed position. The anteromedial and anterolateral drawer (Slocum) tests are used for identifying AMRI and ALRI, respectively. The pivot shift test may additionally be positive; however, this can be difficult to perform effectively with acute ACL injury as the test relies on the patient being completely relaxed.

Management of ACL Injuries

The majority of partial-tear ACL injuries are managed conservatively. For ACL ruptures, any decision to undertake surgery is based on a number of factors. If the athlete is young and their sport places considerable demands on the knee joint, then surgery may be the preferred option. If they are older and do not wish to return to sport and simply want to function sufficiently to carry out daily activities without pain, then conservative treatment may be the more appropriate management. Patients working in manual or physically demanding occupations may be advised to undertake surgery. Associated abnormalities, damage to other structures and the degree of instability must also be considered. The patient should be provided with information on the benefits and risks of undertaking an ACL reconstruction so as to enable an informed decision based on individual circumstance and future sporting or career aspirations. The patient must be made aware of the importance of adhering to a short pre-operative rehabilitation strategy (reducing swelling; gaining full RoM; and developing strength and proprioception) and a comprehensive and lengthy rehabilitation programme following surgery (Johnson, 2004). If a patient indicates they are unlikely to undertake the necessary rehabilitation, then surgery may not be advisable, as this is integral to a successful outcome. The prevention or reduced potential for osteoarthritis (OA) has been proposed as a possible benefit of operative over conservative management; however, there is limited evidence to suggest this is the case (Lohmander *et al.*, 2007). It has in fact been proposed that there is a higher incidence of OA in ACL reconstructed

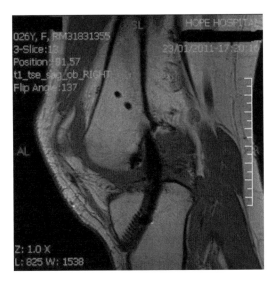

Photo 10.34   MRI image showing ACL reconstruction.

knees compared to those that have not undertaken operative intervention (Gillquist, 1990). Neyret *et al.* (2012) stated that although ACL reconstructions generally have good return to play outcomes, they do not appear to prevent the common evolution to OA (in professional footballers). ACL reconstructions are predominated by 'success stories' in the literature (Frank, 1995; Butryn and Masucci, 2003). However, in many cases, conservative treatment can be just as effective and it should be noted that ACL reconstruction does not guarantee a return to pre-activity levels. It has been suggested that approximately 65–70 per cent of athletes return to their previous level of sport following ACL reconstructions (Irrgang, 2008). Haddad (2012) presents a case for early reconstruction so as to avoid the potential for associated and subsequent problems (such as chondral or meniscal lesions) with delayed surgery.

ACL rehabilitation

Pre-operative rehabilitation should commence from the time of injury, as the reconstruction may not be performed for a number of weeks or months after the injury has occurred. Improved condition of the knee prior to the operation will encourage accelerated healing following surgery, with goals during this period of minimizing swelling, achieving normal RoM and developing quadriceps and hamstring strength (Johnson, 2004). The graft type used for the reconstruction should determine the rehabilitation protocol; however, it is often the same irrespective of graft type (Heijne and Werner, 2007). This is an area requiring ongoing research to confirm key differences in rehabilitation processes for different graft choices.

Some consultants advocate bracing in the early stages following reconstruction to provide additional support during daily activity. A brace should not be relied upon, however, and will offer little support at higher intensities; it is not a substitute for dynamic muscular strength or inherent joint stability. Following surgery, early RoM exercises should be started almost immediately to include active and passive flexion and extension. Johnson (2004) suggests that full extension (0°) and 90° flexion are usual movement goals for stage two rehabilitation, alongside supporting wound healing and strengthening the quadriceps and hamstring muscles. Static strengthening of the quadriceps and SLRs should be introduced at an early stage to prevent muscle inhibition and minimize muscle atrophy. Early active knee extensions following ACL reconstruction are unlikely to increase laxity of the knee joint. The hamstrings must be exercised from an early stage as they are a main agonist to the ACL (Li *et al.*, 1999).

Crutches may be used initially until gait is normal and pain free. Patients should be encouraged to weight bear as soon as possible. ACL injuries can cause large decreases in balance due to the unique proprioceptive properties of the ligament. Therefore, exercises to improve proprioception must be introduced at an early stage and progressed accordingly. Cryotherapy, soft tissue therapy and electrotherapy may all assist with healing in the acute stage following surgery. In the sub-acute phase, cycling may be introduced along with straight line jogging. The accepted length of time before jogging should be commenced after ACL reconstruction is around three months. Hydrotherapy exercises such as pool running can be used to grade a return to jogging on land. Any turning and cutting movements must be avoided at this stage. Eccentric loading should be introduced gradually – stair/step descending and low-intensity jumping on a trampette may be employed.

Later-stage rehabilitation exercises should include more challenging proprioceptive and functional exercises such as hop and holds, multi-directional running, acceleration and deceleration training and sport-specific movements. A combination of both open and closed kinetic chain (OKC and CKC) should be used for optimal results (Fitzgerald, 1997). The amount of anterior shear force must be carefully considered to ensure exercises are safe and effective for the reconstructed ACL. For example, during OKC knee extension, the maximum amount of anterior shear forces occurs at 30° of knee flexion (Lutz *et al.*, 1993). A study by Fleming *et al.* (2003) reported that an increased load of the quadriceps during OKC exercises might further increase the peak ACL strains, while a similar increase of load during a CKC exercise would not. Therefore, to protect the graft, CKC rather than OKC exercises of the quadriceps should play a primary role in rehabilitation following ACL reconstruction (Bynum *et al.*, 1995). Additionally, the inclusion of OKC exercises six weeks post-operatively was found to be superior to CKC exercises alone regarding quadriceps torque. It also allowed a considerably earlier return to sports without complications or compromised joint stability (Mikkelsen *et al.*, 2000).

Evidence suggests that established rehabilitation protocols allow a return to previous sport four to nine months following ACL reconstruction (Hopper *et al.*, 2008). For some patients, however, it may take longer, depending on their circumstances and commitment to rehabilitation, among other factors. It is important to stress that some athletes will never return to the same level of sport following an ACL reconstruction, which must be communicated to patients from the outset. There is research to suggest that some 35 per cent of athletes do not reach their pre-injury level of sport following reconstruction (Irrgang, 2008). The operation can only ever be as good as the rehabilitation; if full RoM is not achieved post-operatively, the outcome may be worse than if no reconstruction was performed (Shellbourne and Gray, 1997). Ultimately, whether a torn ACL is managed conservatively or operatively, a comprehensive, lengthy and specific rehabilitation programme is essential. Fear of re-injury is a concern. Danelon *et al.* (2012) present a case for late (functional) stage on-field rehabilitation (OFR) which is sport-specific. Such strategy emphasizes the development of self-confidence in performing sports movements, in combination with end-stage functional training.

Posterior cruciate ligament and posterolateral corner injuries
The posterolateral corner (PLC) comprises the LCL, arcuate ligament, popliteofibular ligament, fabellofibular ligament and the popliteus tendon. Together, these structures act to restrain lateral rotation and varus angulation of the tibia (Miller *et al.*, 1997). Injury can therefore cause posterolateral rotary instability of the knee, resulting in significant disability for patients. This

injury may occasionally be accompanied by cruciate ligament damage, most commonly the PCL. PCL tears themselves are very infrequent injuries, accounting for only 5–10 per cent of all major knee ligament tears (Covey, 2001). The reason for this may be two-fold; it is a stronger ligament than the ACL, and the knee is much less likely to be subjected to posterior forces in sport than anterior forces. Approximately 30 per cent of PCL tears occur in isolation, while the remaining 70 per cent are combined with other ligamentous damage (Miller *et al.*, 1997).

With regards to mechanism of injury (MoI), the primary cause of posterolateral damage is from a fall or other direct trauma, such as in contact sport or in a road traffic accident (RTA). Specifically, the PCL is recognized as being damaged via a 'dashboard injury' from an RTA, where the tibia is subjected to an excessive posterior force on the anterior aspect of a flexed knee (Baker *et al.*, 1984). Other specific MoI include a direct blow to the anterior tibia such as during a tackle in football, or a fall onto a flexed knee with a plantarflexed foot. A sudden, unexpected hyperextension of the knee can also cause damage to the PCL. Tears of the PCL may cause avulsion fracture at its tibial attachment, more common in adolescents and teenagers due to skeletal immaturity.

The patient will complain of posterior knee pain which is often poorly localized. A PCL injury will generally elicit much less swelling than an ACL tear as it is extrasynovial. An acute injury to the posterolateral corner will cause tenderness over the posterolateral joint line and possibly specific tenderness over the fibular head. This depends upon which structures are damaged, and whether an arcuate (Segond) avulsion fracture is present at the fibular head (Covey, 2001). Pain typically increases with flexion beyond 90°, and a positive posterior drawer test, posterior sag test and reverse Lachman's test may all be present. An avulsion fracture of the tibial insertion of the PCL should be ruled out via X-ray. In some instances, an MRI scan may be needed for diagnosis; however, the reliability of these has been questioned (Rolf and Riyami, 2006). Furthermore, the posteromedial and posterolateral drawer tests may be used to identify posteromedial rotational instability (PMRI) and posterolateral rotational instability (PLRI), respectively. PLRI may also be identified by use of the reverse pivot shift, dial, Loomer's and external rotation recurvatum tests.

PCL injuries can often be managed conservatively with an extensive rehabilitation programme. There is research to suggest that approximately 80 per cent of patients with non-operatively treated isolated PCL tears returned to sport and had successful outcomes (Peterson and Renstrom, 2005). Surgery may be indicated if other structures are damaged in conjunction with the PCL, or if there is significant laxity or rotary instability (Covey, 2001). Greater than 10 mm of posterior translation is considered an indicator for surgery. The most commonly used autografts for PCL reconstructions are from the patellar or hamstring tendons, or an allograft using tissue from a cadaver.

The rehabilitation of a PCL tear should include both OKC and CKC exercises. In the early stages, exercises requiring a large degree of flexion should be avoided so as not to induce posterior translation forces (Schutz and Irrgang, 1994). CKC exercises are indicated in the earlier stages as they reduce the degree of patellofemoral stress and tibial translation via co-contraction of the hamstrings and quadriceps muscles (Lutz *et al.*, 1993). Proprioceptive re-education should commence as soon as possible and can be progressed from NWB to FWB and from static to dynamic exercises.

Medial collateral ligament injuries

The MCL is commonly injured, both in isolation and in combination with other structures, such as the ACL and medial meniscus. Damage to the MCL often occurs through a non-contact valgus stress to a slightly flexed knee. Other MoI include a lateral blow to the knee or lower thigh, which forces the knee into excess valgus, common in contact sports. The MCL is second only to the lateral ankle ligament as the most commonly injured ligament in football (Medina, 2012). Skiing is another activity with high incidences of MCL injury due to excessive external rotary stress mechanisms. The MCL is also commonly injured in breaststroke swimmers as a result of the repetitive combination of rotary and valgus stress. Patients will report pain at the time of injury and tenderness over the medial femoral condyle and medial joint line. Swelling is often minimal – if severe swelling is present then a combination ACL injury may be suspected.

Benjamin (2005) offers descriptions of acute and chronic MCL injury presentations. With an acute injury, the athlete will be likely to describe a mechanism, but it may not be absolutely clear as to the specific mechanism (i.e. it may be missed in the confusion of the episode); the athlete may describe a 'snapping' sound at the time, and report pain all around the knee. They will usually not be able or confident to fully weight bear (i.e. they will 'hobble') and will avoid trying to flex the knee. The knee will usually swell over the following hours, feel warm to touch and continue to ache. The knee will stiffen, both flexion and extension will be difficult and the pain will begin to concentrate around the medial knee. Benjamin (2005) explains that with the chronic MCL injury, the athlete is likely to initially experience 'twinges' when undertaking activities; and gradually the pain begins to settle on the inner aspect of the knee. Swelling may or may not be evident; pain may not be present at the start of activity, may reduce during the activity and then return an hour or so after activity. Gradually the condition tends to worsen, and strenuous activities become difficult.

The valgus stress test will be positive when the MCL is damaged. Increased pain and laxity will indicate a more severe tear. With a complete rupture (grade III), there will be considerable laxity and no discernible end-feel. The patient may report feelings of instability or that the knee 'gives way'.

Zorzi *et al.* (2012) explain that grade I and II injuries (partial tears) are routinely managed conservatively. There is evidence to suggest that patients without surgical intervention may have equally successful outcomes as those who undergo surgery (Zorzi *et al.*, 2012). Where no other structures are damaged, as in an isolated rupture, grade III MCL tears may be managed conservatively with early functional rehabilitation. MCL reconstruction is generally recommended where concomitant or complex injury occurs, such as with ACL rupture or meniscal tear. Later-stage reconstruction is indicated where chronic valgus instability exists (Zorzi, *et al.*, 2012). Normally, post-operatively, the knee will be protectively braced short of end-range extension for a short period (Williams, 2012). A complication to avoid during post-operative rehabilitation is unwanted stiffness in the ligament.

The MCL has excellent healing capacity, and with grade I and II tears, early motion and PWB or FWB should start as soon as possible. Achieving full extension is one of the primary aims, as with any knee ligament injury, as this is essential for normal gait. If the injury was non-contact, measures should be taken to reduce the risk of re-injury by addressing the inherent cause. This may involve improving biomechanics, strengthening the gluteal muscles and stretching the adductors to control valgus stresses at the knee. Athletes may return to sport within 3–8 weeks, depending on the severity of the tear and the quality of their rehabilitation. In elite sport, where swift return to play is an objective, there is low-level evidence to support problematic grade II MCL injuries being injected with PRP (platelet-rich plasma) or sclerosant solutions (Murray *et al.*, 2012).

Lateral collateral ligament injuries

The LCL is less frequently injured than the MCL. This may be because the knee is more likely to be forced into an excessive valgus position than an excessive varus position during sport.

When the LCL is injured, it is frequently caused by a combination of hyperextension and varus force. It is often associated with damage of either of the cruciate ligaments (most commonly the ACL). Ruptures of the LCL are usually sustained with other tissue damage, resulting in a severe knee injury. If PLRI of the knee is present, the LCL may be damaged in conjunction with the PLC, as mentioned in conjunction with the PCL. Clinical tests for assessing the lateral ligamentous structures and for associated instabilities include: the varus stress test; the anterolateral drawer (Slocum) test; the posterolateral drawer test; the reverse pivot shift test; the dial test; Loomer's test; and the external rotation recurvatum test.

Meniscal injuries

Injuries to the medial or lateral menisci are among the most common problems affecting the knee. There are a number of factors which lead to the medial meniscus being more frequently injured than the lateral one: it is more securely attached to the tibial plateau (and therefore less mobile); it has attachment to the deeper fibres of MCL and semimembranosus; the medial condyle of the femur is more pronounced (slightly longer) than the lateral condyle; the knee generally receives greater medial (rather than lateral) load bearing and valgus (rather than varus) stresses; and, in contact sports, there is increased risk of receiving trauma to the outside of the knee, causing tibial external rotation. The classic MoI for meniscal injuries is a load-bearing twisting motion with the knee flexed and foot fixed. Hyperflexion and hyperextension can also cause damage to the menisci, such as landing heavily from a jump with an extended knee. If the foot and lower leg rotate externally in relation to the femur, the medial meniscus will be most susceptible to injury. Conversely, internal rotation of the foot and lower leg relative to the femur will place the lateral meniscus at risk of injury. Football, basketball and netball all have high incidences of meniscal tears due to the high frequency of twisting movements and landings. Meniscal tears can also occur during simple daily movements, particularly in older populations where fibro–cartilage degeneration is present, or in people with a history of knee problems, including previous surgery.

The degree of symptoms will vary greatly with meniscal injuries, depending on the severity and type of tear. With minor tears, there may be little or no pain at the time of injury, but symptoms usually increase gradually within the first 24 hours. An important clinical sign of a meniscal tear is joint line tenderness, which can be palpated most effectively with the knee in a flexed position. Joint effusion may be present, but is often minimal due to the menisci being relatively avascular (Brindle *et al.*, 2001). McMurray's (meniscal provocation) test is reliable (but false positives and negatives are not uncommon); Apley's compression test has shown a lack of sensitivity (Hattam and Smeatham, 2010). The Thessaly test (single-leg weight-bearing, with rotation) is a very useful functional test for meniscal problems (Karachalios *et al.*, 2005). Simple loaded knee flexion may be problematic, and the 'duck walk' (Childress) test may be employed in non-acute presentations. There is likely to be crepitus and palpable tenderness across the joint line. There is likely to be limited movement, especially end-range extension, which may be associated with mechanical blockage or due to pain and swelling. A patient with a meniscal tear may well be apprehensive about the sports therapist moving the knee in the acute phase.

With a more severe tear, such as with a 'bucket-handle' tear, pain can be severe and range of movement will be extremely limited. A primary indication of a bucket handle tear is intermittent locking caused by the torn flap ('handle') becoming lodged between articular surfaces. By manoeuvring and mobilizing the knee into a different position, it may unlock spontaneously, and this is often accompanied by a painful and audible click. In larger bucket handle tears, the torn flap may cause the knee to remain locked, preventing full extension until surgically removed or repaired. A locked knee may be seen as a priority for surgical intervention due to the disabling effect this position has on the knee joint and quadriceps muscles.

Minor tears of the menisci are usually managed conservatively with a comprehensive rehabilitation programme. With severe bucket-handle tears, surgery is required urgently to remove the torn flap and allow normal joint functioning. This is done via arthroscopy with the aim of preserving as much of the damaged meniscus as possible. In the past, the damaged menisci would have been removed (full or partial meniscectomy). More recently, operative interventions tend towards retaining the meniscus if at all possible. Removal has been shown to significantly increase the risk of early onset OA. It has been suggested that the amount of meniscus removed is directly proportional to the degree of degenerative change in the joint. As little as 10 per cent reduction in meniscal contact following a partial meniscectomy resulted in peak joint contact stresses increasing by 65 per cent (Fairbank, 1948; Jones *et al.*, 1978). Furthermore, removal of a whole meniscus has been proposed to increase the stress on the tibial plateau by six to seven times, and nearly double the articular stress on the femur. Meniscal repair (suturing) may be indicated when the tear is peripheral. The potential for successful operative outcomes can depend on the type and location of the tear, the patient's age and sport, as well as the degree of ligamentous stability and type of repair performed (Lelli and Di Turi, 2012). Although repair, as opposed to meniscectomy, is less likely to lead to degenerative changes and may provide a swifter return to play, it is not always possible.

The rehabilitation of meniscal injuries depends on the severity of the tear and whether surgical intervention is performed. An athlete with an isolated meniscal tear may be able to return to sport within four weeks, while a more severe tear may take several months. The key principles following arthroscopy are to control pain and swelling, regain pain-free range of movement, return to FWB via a graduated approach and progressively strengthen the knee muscles, particularly the quadriceps. Atrophy of the quadriceps is a common consequence of meniscal tears. Strengthening should be commenced prior to and immediately following surgery to minimize this. As with any rehabilitation programme, the patient should be closely monitored, and if pain or swelling increases then exercises should be suitably regressed.

Patellofemoral joint injuries

Patellofemoral pain syndrome (PFPS)

Sports therapists will encounter this condition regularly; PFPS has been cited as the most common cause of knee pain in an outpatient setting (Dixit *et al.*, 2007). PFPS is a common problem, particularly among adolescents and young adults, and is characterized by retropatellar or peripatellar pain, particularly when ascending or descending stairs, squatting or prolonged sitting with flexed knees (Heintjes *et al.*, 2003). A combination of factors usually contribute to its development, with the most recognized cause cited as repetitive abnormal loading of the PFJ, which occurs from either proximal, distal or local malalignment affecting the lower extremity and the resultant maltracking of the patella on the femoral trochlea (Herrington, 2000). The PFJ essentially becomes exposed to the imbalanced forces which occur during loaded knee flexion and extension (Dixit *et al.*, 2007). It is often referred to as 'runner's knee' due to its prevalence in this population (however, another 'runner's knee' is that of iliotibial band syndrome – ITBS). It has been proposed that PFPS constitutes 16–25 per cent of injuries to runners (Taunton *et al.*, 2002). Bahr and Maehlum (2004) explain that PFPS may also occur as a result of direct trauma to the PFJ, such as from a fall to the floor. A number of patients who have sustained trauma to the patella have been shown to develop subchondral changes that may contribute to altered stress and pressure through the PFJ.

The patella is a wedge-shaped sesamoid bone which sits in the intercondylar sulcus on the central, distal aspect of the femur (the trochlea). During the first 20° of knee flexion, the position of the patella is largely determined by the interaction of the medial and lateral soft tissue structures (McConnell, 1996). Consequently, any imbalance in these tissues causes the patella to deviate from an optimal position, potentially causing damage to the articular cartilage and other soft tissues around the joint. The most common direction for the patella to track is laterally due to the structures on the lateral side being stronger and more extensive than those on the medial side (McConnell, 1996). A weakness of the vastus medialis oblique (VMO) component may contribute to such a process. The timing and activity of the VMO is critical to PFJ function as it is a key dynamic medial stabilizer of the joint. Ahmed *et al.* (1988) found a 5 mm displacement of the patella laterally when VMO tension was reduced by 50 per cent. The issue of VMO pain inhibition and timing deficits has been discussed by Collado and Fredericson (2010). Even the presence of slight effusion at the knee can lead to reduced muscular firing, and most dramatically at the VMO.

In addition to muscle imbalances, a number of common biomechanical abnormalities can predispose patients to PFPS. These include poor pelvic stability, excessive coxa vara, increased femoral anteversion, patella alta, excessive subtalar pronation (which may be prolonged during mid-stance) and an increased Q-angle; these all increase load through the joint (Dixit *et al.*, 2007). Specifically, the combination of hip adduction, internal rotation, knee abduction, external rotation of the tibia, and excessive subtalar pronation is referred to as the 'valgus collapse' associated with PFPS (Myer *et al.*, 2010; Powers *et al.*, 1997); and essentially it is the characteristic altering of the pressure distribution of the posterior patella on the femur which leads to this condition. Collado and Fredericson (2010) explain how hyperpronation of the foot can be a causative factor in PFPS. With increased pronation during gait, the tibia is forced into prolonged internal rotation during the initial stance phase. This can then prevent the tibia from fully externally rotating during midstance, and also prevent the knee from locking into full extension with its screw-home mechanism. By way of compensation, the femur is likely to internally rotate so as to allow full extension. With increased internal rotation of the femur, increased contact pressure occurs between the posterior patella and the lateral femoral trochlear groove. Overpronation can result for numerous reasons, not least arch insufficiency, but also limited dorsiflexion at the talocrural joint can be a contributory factor. For walking, 10° of dorsiflexion is required; 15–25° is required for running. If dorsiflexion is limited, compensatory overpronation can occur (Collado and Fredericson, 2010). Additionally, an increased Q-angle has been found to negatively influence biomechanics of the PFJ by creating an abnormally high valgus angle, which causes a laterally directed force leading to excessive pressure and, consequently, anterior knee pain (Emami *et al.*, 2007). Some athletes, however, have notable malalignment of their lower limb, but are asymptomatic.

Dixit *et al.* (2007) explained that repetitive stress causing excessive mechanical loading of the PFJ can also create a chemical irritation resulting in inflammation and synovitis. Once inflammation is present, the PFJ can become susceptible to further aggravation by sports and exercise, or even daily activity, depending on severity. Dixit *et al.*, (2007) also differentiate between PFPS and chondromalacia patellae (CMP), which they describe as a condition in which there is softening of the patellar articular cartilage, but which occurs only in a subset of patients who present with anterior knee pain. Furthermore, PFPS may exist in conjunction with other anterior knee conditions such as patellar tendinopathy, plica syndrome or fat pad impingement. It is essential that the sports therapist identifies the key predisposing factors of PFPS in order to address and correct them, as well as managing the initial symptoms.

To assess for PFPS, the therapist will incorporate a full subjective history (including the onset, severity, irritability and nature of the pain). A three-dimensional static and dynamic postural screening must take place, and the patellofemoral grind (Clarke's), the McConnell (critical) and the eccentric step tests may all be employed. Other potential causes of knee pain must also be ruled out. As Cook *et al.* (2012) ascertain, *'the nebulous pathology and lack of sensitive tests to help rule out PFPS when negative, suggests that PFPS may be a diagnosis of exclusion, and may be ruled in after ruling out other contending diagnoses'*.

Management of patellofemoral pain syndrome

As with any condition, an evidence-based approach to rehabilitation must be emphasized. Heintjes *et al.* (2003) conducted a rigorous review to summarize the evidence of effectiveness of exercise therapy in reducing anterior knee pain and improving knee function in patients with PFPS. They concluded that exercise therapy *may* help to reduce the pain of PFPS; that OKC and CKC exercises were equally effective; and that further research to substantiate the efficacy of exercise treatment compared to non-exercising control groups is required. According to Dixit *et al.* (2007), although there have been relatively few long-term studies for the management of PFPS, two studies in which patients were instructed on a programme of home exercises reported successful outcomes in approximately 80 per cent of patients. In another study, 54 per cent of athletes who were instructed on VMO training were pain free, or only had mild ongoing symptoms, after nearly six years. A less favourable outcome may be more likely in patients with a hypermobile patella, bilateral symptoms and in older age groups.

There are various protocols currently prescribed, but treatment of PFPS must ultimately focus on optimizing the position of the patella and improving lower limb mechanics. On the topic of proximal alignment, Herrington (2011) discussed the relationship of the Q-angle to PFPS; decreasing an excessive Q-angle has been shown to be more effective in reducing patellofemoral stress than attempting to increase VMO activity (Elias *et al.*, 2004). Rest may be required in the acute stage to allow any inflammation to subside. Mobilizing tight soft tissues (usually lateral structures such as vastus lateralis, ITB, lateral PFJ ligaments and lateral retinaculum) and improving the activation of the weakened muscles (most commonly VMO training is recommended) should assist in correcting patellar position. Various studies have shown the importance of VMO strength and recruitment in optimal functioning of the PFJ. However, Powers *et al.* (1997) identified no difference between VMO and vastus lateralis (VL) recruitment patterns in symptomatic individuals, which suggests that generalized quadriceps training may be sufficient. A study by Goh *et al.* (1995) reported that VMO atrophy did result in increased loading of the lateral facet of the posterior patella. MRI has been used to demonstrate that a significant number of patients with PFPS had a decreased VMO cross-sectional area (Pattyn *et al.*, 2011). Several studies have discovered negating evidence for the importance of VMO. A study by Conlan *et al.* (1993) reported that the medial patellofemoral and tibial ligaments account for 75 per cent of restraining forces at the joint. There is also significant evidence to suggest that it is difficult to selectively strengthen the VMO individually, and little evidence to say that it is possible (Goh, 2000; Powers *et al.*, 1997). Furthermore, it has been debated as to whether the VMO alone is capable of terminal knee extension (Lieb and Perry, 1971). A study by Elias *et al.* (2004) proposed that decreasing an excessive Q-angle is more effective in reducing stress through the joint than increasing VMO activation. A combination of both open and closed kinetic chain exercises have been advocated as an essential part of the rehabilitation programme to minimize PFJ stress. Exercise modifications may be necessary where the quantity and type of exercise needs to be adjusted according to symptoms and needs.

PFJ taping techniques have also been proposed as effective intervention for decreasing pain, improving alignment and also for promoting earlier activation of VMO and increased quadriceps torque. Taping can create a sustained, low-load stretch to facilitate elongation of shortened tissues (McConnell, 2007). Taping may allow normal tracking of the patella and hence relieve the damaging stresses on the joint surfaces (Herrington, 2000). For example, with a laterally tracking patella, non-stretch tape would be applied from the lateral patellar border and pulled medially just past the medial femoral condyle. However, there is limited evidence to explain how taping achieves its reported effects (Herrington, 2000). With strenuous movement, such as during sport, where it is often used, the tape is likely to loosen in a short time period, thereby reducing its effect. Additionally, Dye *et al.* (1999) concluded that there was little evidence to suggest taping can effectively change alignment of the PFJ in the long term. Whenever taping is applied for such a condition, its usefulness (i.e. its relieving of symptoms) should be immediately apparent – if not, the sports therapist should reconsider the tape application. Taping may be extremely useful, but its effects may only be short-lived and hence should be used in conjunction with a comprehensive rehabilitation programme.

Care must be taken to avoid reoccurrence by ensuring the predisposing factors have been sufficiently addressed. In conclusion, the key areas to focus on for PFPS rehabilitation are overcoming any quadriceps (VMO) inhibition and addressing all main contributing biomechanical abnormalities (such as decreasing an excessive Q-angle), and increasing the functional load tolerance through the joint. This may require specific quadriceps training, gluteus medius work (such as incorporating squat training with resistance bands around the knees), releasing all tight lateral thigh structures and attending to any foot-related issues. Dixit *et al.* (2007) explain that operative intervention for PFPS may be considered for patients who continue to experience symptoms after 6–12 months of thorough rehabilitation, and where other causes of anterior knee pain have been excluded. Local surgical options can range from release of the lateral retinaculum and fascia and articular cartilage procedures to structural realignment of the tibial tuberosity.

Patellar tendinopathy

Patellar tendinopathy is prevalent in athletes who repeatedly jump and land, such as in basketball, volleyball and certain athletic events; it is therefore commonly known as 'jumper's knee'. It is also common in sports involving sudden directional changes. The injury is associated with high demands on the knee extensor mechanism, which obviously occurs in most sports, and is most recognized as an overuse injury. Inflammation is not commonly a factor in its development as the condition is most likely to present to the sports therapist somewhere on the 'three-stage continuum' of tendinopathy as proposed by Cook and Purdam (2009): reactive tendinopathy (an acute episode with homogeneous swelling and pain); tendon dysrepair (a post-acute presentation, with prolonged symptoms and evidence of abnormal repair); or tendon degeneration (tendinosis with collagen disarray and neovascularity). Patellar tendinopathy may coexist with PFPS, as altered biomechanics of the joint increase the mechanical load on the tendon. A host of predisposing factors increase the risk of developing patellar tendon problems (including biomechanical, equipment and terrain factors, as well as the type and frequency of training). The main symptom of patellar tendinopathy is localized anteroinferior knee pain, and specifically, patients will most commonly report pain and tenderness in the tendon just distal to the inferior pole of the patella, which is exacerbated by loading of the tendon, such as when testing with a decline squat. Specific palpation of the tendon lesion may reveal tenderness, although it must be recognized that many athletes will have a tender patellar tendon regardless of any pathological changes. It is recommended that the tendon is palpated in both stretched (patient supine with knee flexed) and relaxed (supine and knee extended) positions, and that the practitioner takes their time to carefully explore the extent and degree of discomfort. There is often thickening of the tendon proximally and in more chronic (degenerative) cases, scarring and adhesions may be palpable. More challenging presentations can exist at the enthesis (attachment site at the tibial tuberosity). Cook *et al.* (2001) explain that the spectrum of presentation may vary from a mildly irritating condition to an acute, irritable and inhibiting pain, subsequently, muscle atrophy of the quadriceps muscles may also be a feature. The degree of pain can often be used as an indicator of severity. Mild pain after strenuous activity would indicate a less severe condition, while pain that is brought on through ADL suggests greater severity. Cook *et al.* (2001) also highlight the predisposing issue of reduced musculotendinous strength such as that caused by a prolonged lay-off from training. Consequently, a situation of structural weakness can leave the tendon vulnerable to an increased risk of symptoms on return to activities.

The Victorian Institute of Sports Assessment scale (VISA scale) is an eight-question subjective tendinopathy questionnaire, taking less than five minutes, which assesses the patient's symptoms and ability to undertake physical activity, and can be useful for monitoring the rehabilitation process (Crossley *et al.*, 2012).

Management requires a multifaceted approach. Cook *et al.* (2001) stress the importance of load modification, specific musculotendinous rehabilitation and interventions to improve the shock-absorbing capacity of the limb. Relative rest and cryotherapy are essential in an acute phase presentation (for one week or so) so as to allow the pain and homogeneous swelling of reactive tendinopathy to settle. Should the condition progress to a situation of tendon dysrepair, the use of cryotherapy may still be employed in the second phase so as to assist with pain. Progressive optimal loading is likely to produce best outcomes, especially in the degenerated tendon. There is good evidence to support controlled progressive, heavy, slow resistance training (Kongsgaard *et al.*, 2009) and eccentric training (Jonsson and Alfredson, 2005). Classic strengthening exercises include: a single-leg squat on a decline board; lunges and lunges with weights (Crossley *et al.*, 2012). Kaeding and Best (2009), Rees *et al.* (2009) and Sharma and Maffulli (2005) have reviewed a range of other interventions including deep tissue friction massage, therapeutic ultrasound and low-intensity laser therapy. Soft tissue therapy may be useful when directed locally to the tendon, with additional techniques applied to address associated soft tissue tightness (such as myofascial release and neuromuscular technique). Patellar taping may also prove useful to offload the patellar tendon (McConnell, 1996). The gastroc-soleus complex is an essential component during the initial jump landing phase, eccentrically absorbing the loads transmitted to the knee (Richards *et al.*, 1996). As calf weakness is often observed in athletes suffering with patellar tendinopathy, calf strengthening to decrease the load on the tendon should be considered early in the rehabilitation plan. In the later stages, eccentric exercises should be included to gradually increase the tendon's tolerance and prepare the athlete for the eccentric loads they will encounter during sport.

Sclerosing injections, nitric oxide (glycerol trinitrate [GTN] patches), extracorporeal shock wave therapy (ESWT) and other pharmacological interventions have been described in the literature, but the evidence for each is still limited. High-volume image-guided injections (HVIGIs) can be a consideration early in the rehabilitation process so as to reduce pain and increase function with a quicker return to play (Chan *et al.*, 2008). If initial conservative treatment fails, then surgery to remove the pathological area may be required. Success rates for patellar tendon surgery vary greatly and depend on which techniques have been performed. Willberg *et al.* (2011) have discussed the option of arthroscopic debridement (ultrasound and doppler-guided tendon 'shaving') of the anterior fat pad from the posterior surface of the patellar tendon (essentially severing the abnormal vascular and neural ingrowth). Coleman *et al.* (2000) explain that there is no guarantee for returning to the same level of sport following more traditional tenotomy procedures; if achieved this can still take 6–12 months.

Muscular injuries

Muscle tears occur when the tension in the fibres exceeds their load tolerance, which causes either partial tearing or complete rupture. Tears of the knee musculature are therefore very common due to the demands placed on the muscles around this joint in both daily and sporting activity. The most commonly affected muscles are those that are biarticular and cross both the hip and knee (hamstrings and rectus femoris) and knee and ankle (gastrocnemius). Tears most commonly occur near to the musculotendinous junction (MTJ). The Munich Consensus Statement on muscle injury classification presents recently recommended terminology (Mueller-Wohlfahrt *et al.*, 2013). Traditionally minor (grade I), moderate (grade II) and severe or complete tears (grade III) have been re-categorized as type 3a, 3b and 4 structural muscle injuries, respectively.

A complete muscular rupture (type 4) results in the torn tissue retracting towards its attachment. Initially, there will be sharp pain and inability to continue. Later, there will be swelling, deep aching and pain and haematoma. Positive symptom responses elicited during active, passive and resistance testing will each contribute towards confirming the diagnosis. On assessment there will be weakness, and pain will increase with movement either due to the fibres having to contract or being stretched. The clinician is likely to be able to palpate a significant lump due to the recoiled bunching of the damaged muscle belly. Diagnosis is usually clinically obvious with a rupture – but if clarification is required, ultrasound or MRI scans should be used to confirm.

Management for type 3a and 3b tears follow a standard conservative four-stage rehabilitation model. Type 4 tears usually require non-weight bearing (NWB) and surgical repair. The basic criteria for progression through each of the four stages is based on the therapist's assessment of the athlete's ability to perform each stage correctly without the presence of adverse symptoms or signs of aggravation or need for regression. For example, the patient must be able to perform within a full and pain-free RoM in the involved knee, should have no palpable tenderness, and strength should be somewhere in the region of 70 per cent of the contra-lateral limb. Cycling and swimming can be recommended in early to late recovery so as to maintain general fitness.

Iliotibial band syndrome (ITBS)

The ITB originates superiorly and superficially from the lateral aspect of the iliac crest and the fascia of the tensor fascia lata (TFL), gluteus medius and maximus muscles, and runs laterally and distally to insert onto the lateral condyle of the tibia at Gerdy's tubercle. Despite its muscular associations, it is a passive structure of the knee. ITBS is most commonly caused by repeated compressive stress between the ITB and the lateral epicondyle of the femur. Such stress does not occur when the knee is extended, as the ITB lies anteriorly to the lateral epicondyle. In flexion, however, the ITB passes over the epicondyle, which can cause irritation (Puniello, 1993). Once the knee is flexed beyond 30°, the ITB becomes posteriorly positioned to the epicondyle. With repeated flexion of less than 30°, such as during running, where the average knee angle is around 21° at foot strike, forces increase and can cause subsequent inflammation of the band or its underlying bursa. It is commonly referred to as 'runner's knee' and is particularly prevalent in downhill and cambered running. Increased subtalar pronation, genu varus, excessive tibial torsion and tightness of the ITB are all associated aetiological factors in this condition (Engebretsen *et al.*, 2003). A lateral pelvic tilt may also predispose the athlete to ITBS through the resulting increased strain on the lateral thigh.

The patient typically describes localized lateral knee pain, which is aggravated by activity, particularly running. There may also be crepitus on movement. In more severe cases, the pain may prevent the patient from exercising. Pain generally subsides with rest. On palpation, tenderness will be present over the lateral epicondyle and lateral joint line. Excess tension may be felt in the ITB, particularly at its distal portion. Ober's test can be used to confirm tightness, and Noble's test for suspecting ITBS. The vastus lateralis muscle should be examined as excessive development can place increased tensile loading on the ITB. Postural and gait analysis should be also conducted. Klimkiewicz (2005) explains that MRI can confirm more chronic cases which have been unresponsive to conservative treatment.

Treatment for ITBS should initially focus on reducing symptoms, typically via cryotherapy, electrotherapy and soft tissue therapy. TFL, hamstring and hip external rotator release, combined with strengthening of hip abductors, is usually successful when combined with activity modification (Klimkiewicz, 2005). Running distance and frequency may need to be reduced in the acute stages to allow symptoms to subside. Any biomechanical abnormalities such as overpronation or a laterally titled pelvis must be addressed. Podiatric orthotics may be required with more severe foot dysfunction. Engebretsen *et al.* (2003) discuss a typical operative procedure to reduce compressive forces between tendon and epicondyle, which involves creation of a 'window' in the tendon in conjunction with a bursectomy.

This chapter has attempted to present the fundamental features and functional anatomical components of the knee region. By understanding and appreciating the tissues, structures and relationships, as well as the requirements for exercise and sports, the sports therapist will be able to make informed clinical assessment and injury management decisions. The chapter has overviewed the process of subjective and objective assessment of the knee and has presented a selection of clinical special tests. Finally, a small collection of common sports-related knee injury problems have been discussed. This chapter does not claim to be comprehensive – indeed, further investigation into any of the topics presented is warranted to further the practitioner's knowledge and understanding of this interesting, yet complex and often troublesome, anatomical region.

References

Aagard, H. and Verdonk, R. (2007) Function of the normal meniscus and consequences of meniscal resection. *Scandinavian Journal of Medicine and Science in Sports.* 9 (3): 134–140

Ahmed, A., Shi, S., Hyder, A. and Chan, K. (1988) The effect of quadriceps tension characteristics on the patellar tracking pattern. *Transactions of the 34th Orthopaedic Research Society conference, Atlanta.* 280–285

Amis, A.A., Firer, P., Mountney, J., Senavongse, W. and Thomas, N.P. (2003) Anatomy and biomechanics of the medial patellofemoral ligament. *Knee.* 10 (3): 215–220

Anderson, A.F., Rennirt, G.W. and Standeffer, W.C. (2000) Clinical analysis of the pivot shift tests: Description of the pivot drawer test. *American Journal of Knee Surgery.* 13 (1): 19–23

Anderson, M., Parr, G. and Hall, S. (2009) *Foundations of athletic training, prevention, assessment and management,* 4th edition. Lippincott, Williams and Wilkins. Philadelphia, PA

Atkins, E., Kerr, J. and Goodlad, E. (2010) *A practical approach to orthopaedic medicine,* 3rd edition. Elsevier. London, UK.

Bahr, R. and Maehlum, S. (2004) *Clinical guide to sports injuries: An illustrated guide to the management of injuries in physical activity.* Human Kinetics. Champaign, IL

Baker, C.L, Norwood, L.A. and Hughston, J.C. (1984) Acute combined posterior cruciate and posterolateral instability of the knee. *American Journal of Sports Medicine.* 12: 204–208

Barton, C., Collins, N. and Crossley, K. (2012) Clinical aspects of biomechanics and sporting injuries. In Brukner, P., Bahr, R., Blair, S., *et al.* (eds) *Brukner and Khan's clinical sports medicine,* 4th edition. McGraw-Hill. NSW, Australia

Benjamin, B. (2005) Collateral damage to knee ligaments. *Sportex Dynamics.* 4: 15–21

Beynnon, B.D., Fleming, B.C., Johnson, R.J., Nichols, C.E., Renstrom, P.A. and Pope, M.H. (1995) Anterior cruciate ligament strain behavior during rehabilitation exercises in vivo. *American Journal of Sports Medicine*. 23: 24–34

Biel, A. (2005) *Trail guide to the body: How to locate muscles, bones and more*, 3rd edition. Books of Discovery. Boulder, CO

Blackburn, T.A. and Craig, E. (1980) Knee anatomy: A brief review. *Physical Therapy*. 60 (12): 1556–1560

Blackburn, T.A. and Nyland, J. (2006) Functional anatomy of the knee. In Placzek, J.D. and Boyce, D.A. (eds) *Orthopaedic physical therapy secrets*, 2nd edition. Elsevier, Mosby. Philadelphia, PA

Brindle, T., Nyland, J. and Johnson, D. (2001) The meniscus: Review of the basic principles with application to surgery and rehabilitation. *Journal of Athletic Training*. 36: 160–169

Butler, D. (1991) *Mobilisation of the nervous system*. Churchill Livingstone. Melbourne, Australia

Butryn, T.M. and Masucci, M.A. (2003) It's not about the book: A cyborg counter-narrative of Lance Armstrong. *Journal of Sport and Social Issues*. 27: 124–144

Bynum, E.B., Barrack, R.L. and Alexander, A.H. (1995) Open versus closed chain kinetic exercises after anterior cruciate ligament reconstruction: A prospective randomized study. *American Journal of Sports Medicine*. 23: 401–406

Cerulli, G., Ceccarini, G., Alberta, P.F. and Caraffa, G. (1986) Neuromorphological studies of the proprioceptivity of the human anterior cruciate ligament. *Journal Sports Traumatology*. 8: 49–52

Chan, O., O'Dowd, D., Padhiar, N., *et al.* (2008) High volume image guided injections in chronic Achilles tendinopathy. *Disability and Rehabilitation*. 30: 1697–1708

Chmielewski, T.L., Mizner, R.L., Padamonsky, W. and Snyder-Mackler, L. (2003) Knee. In Kolt, G. and Snyder-Mackler, L. (eds) *Physical therapies in sport and exercise*. Churchill Livingstone, Elsevier. London, UK

Coleman, B.D., Khan, K.M., Zoltan, S., Bartlett, J., Young, D.A. and Wark, J.D. (2000) Open and arthroscopic patellar tenotomy for chronic patellar tendinopathy: A retrospective outcome study. *American Journal of Sports Medicine*. 28: 183–190

Collado, H. and Fredericson, M. (2010) Patellofemoral pain syndrome. *Clinics in Sports Medicine*. 29: 379–398

Collins, N.C. (2008) Is ice right? Does cryotherapy improve outcome for acute soft tissue injury? *Emergency Medicine Journal*. 25: 65–68

Comfort, P. and Matthews, M. (2010) Assessment and needs analysis. In Comfort, P. and Abrahamson, E. (eds) *Sports rehabilitation and injury prevention*. Wiley-Blackwell. Chichester, UK

Conlan, T., Garth, W.P. and Lemons, J.E. (1993) Evaluation of the medial soft-tissue restraints of the extensor mechanism of the knee. *Journal of Bone and Joint Surgery*. 75: 682–693

Cook, C., Mabry, L., Reiman, M.P. and Hegedus, E.J. (2012) Best tests/clinical findings for screening and diagnosis of patellofemoral pain syndrome: A systematic review. *Physiotherapy*. 98: 93–100

Cook, G., Burton, L., Kiesel, K., Rose, G. and Bryant, M.F. (2010) *Movement: Functional movement systems: Screening, assessment and corrective strategies*. On Target Publications, Apos, CA, USA

Cook, J.L. and Khan, K.M. (2002) What is the most effective treatment for patellar tendinopathy? In MacAuley, D. and Best, T.M. (eds) *Evidence-based sports medicine*. BMJ Books. London, UK

Cook, J.L. and Purdam, C.R. (2009) Is tendon pathology a continuum? A pathology model to explain the clinical presentation of load-induced tendinopathy. *British Journal of Sports Medicine*. 43: 409–416

Cook, J.L., Khan, K.M. and Purdam, C.R. (2001) Conservative treatment of patellar tendinopathy. *Physical Therapy in Sport*. 2: 1–12

Cooper, G. (2006) *Pocket guide to musculoskeletal diagnosis*. Humana Press. Totowa, NJ

Covey, D. (2001). Injuries of the posterolateral corner of the knee. *Journal of Bone and Joint Surgery*. 83: 106–118

Creighton, D., Shrier, I., Shultz, R., Meeuwisse, W. and Matheson, G. (2010) Return to play in sport: A decision-based model. *Clinical Journal of Sport Medicine*. 20 (5): 379–385

Crossley, K., Cook, J., Cowan, S. and McConnell, J. (2012) Anterior knee pain. In Brukner, P., Bahr, R., Blair, S., *et al.* (eds) *Brukner and Khan's clinical sports medicine*, 4th edition. McGraw-Hill. NSW, Australia

Cyriax, J. (1979) *Textbook of orthopaedic medicine Vol 1: Diagnosis of soft tissue lesions*, 7th edition. Baillière Tindall. London, UK

Cyriax, J. (1982) *Textbook of orthopaedic medicine Vol 1: Diagnosis of soft tissue lesions*, 8th edition. Baillière Tindall. London, UK

Danelon, F., Barboglio, A., Pisoni, D. and Rivaroli, S. (2012) Fear of re-injury in football players after ACL reconstruction: Effect of rehabilitation on the field. In Roi, G.S. and Della Villa, S. (eds) *Football medicine strategies for knee injuries: Abstract book*. Calzetti and Mariucci Editori. Italy

Dixit, S., Difiori, J.P., Burton, M. and Mines, B. (2007). Management of patellofemoral pain syndrome. *American Family Physician*. 70 (2): 194–202

Dye, S., Staubli, H., Bierdert, R. and Vaupel, G. (1999) The mosaic of pathophysiology causing patellofemoral pain: Therapeutic implications. *Operative Techniques in Sports Medicine*. 7 (2): 46–54

Elias, J.J., Mattessich, S.M., Kumagai, M., Mizuno, Y., Cosgarea, A.J. and Chao, E.Y. (2004) In-vitro characterization of the relationship between the Q-angle and the lateral component of the quadriceps force. *Proceedings of the Institution of Mechanical Engineers*. 218: 63–67

Emami, M.J., Ghahramani, M.H., Abdinejd, F. and Namazi, H (2007) Q-angle: An invaluable parameter for evaluation of anterior knee pain. *Archives of Iranian Medicine*. 10: 24–26

Engebretsen, L., Muellner, T., Laprade, R., *et al.* (2003) Knee. In Kjær, M., Krogsgaard, M., Magnusson, P., *et al.* (eds) *Textbook of sports medicine: Basic science and clinical aspects of sports injury and physical activity*. Blackwell Science. Malden, MA

Fairbank, T.J. (1948) Knee joint changes after meniscectomy. *Journal of Bone and Joint Surgery*. 30 (4) 664–670

Feagin, J.A. and Lambert, K.L. (1985) Mechanism of injury and pathology of anterior cruciate ligament injuries. *American Journal of Clinical Orthopaedics*. 16: 41–45

Fetto, J.F. and Marshall, J.L. (1978) Medial collateral ligament injuries of the knee: A rationale for treatment. *Clinical Orthopaedics and Related Research*. 132: 206–218

Fitzgerald, G.K. (1997) Open versus closed kinetic chain exercise: Issues in rehabilitation after anterior cruciate ligament reconstructive surgery. *Physical Therapy*. 77 (12): 1747–1754

Fleming, B.C., Ohlen, G., Renstrom, P.A., Peura, G.D., Beynnon, B.D. and Badger, G.J. (2003) The effects of compressive load and knee joint torque on peak anterior cruciate ligament strains. *American Journal of Sports Medicine*. 31: 701–707

Frank, A.W. (1995) *The wounded storyteller: Body, illness and ethics*. University of Chicago Press. Chicago, IL

Franklyn-Miller, A., Falvey, E., McCrory, P. and Brukner, P. (2011) *Clinical sports anatomy*. McGraw-Hill. NSW, Australia

Fu, F.H. and Baratz, M.E. (1994) Meniscal injuries. In: Delee, S. and Drez, D. (eds) *Orthopaedic sports medicine: Principles and practice*, 1st edition. Saunders. Philadelphia, PA

Fujie, H., Livesay, G.A. and Woo, S.L.-Y. (1995) The use of a universal force-moment sensor to determine in-situ forces in ligaments: A new methodology. *Journal of Biomechanics*. 117: 1–7

Gershuni, D.H., Hargens, A.R. and Danzig, L.A. (1988) Regional nutrition and cellularity of the meniscus: Implications for tear and repair. *Sports Medicine*. 5 (5): 322–327

Gillquist, J. (1990) Knee stability: Its effect on articular cartilage. In Ewing, D.D. (ed.) *Articular cartilage and knee joint function: Basic science and arthroscopy*. Raven Press. New York

Girgis, F.G., Marshall, J.L and Monajem, A. (1975) The cruciate ligaments of the knee joint: Anatomical, functional and experimental analysis. *Clinical Orthopaedic and Related Research*. 106: 216–231

Goh, A.C. (2000) Vastus medialis oblique: Are we blind to the evidence? *Physiotherapy Singapore*. 3: 2–3

Goh, C.H., Lee, Y.C. and Bose, K. (1995) A cadaver study of the function of the oblique part of vastus medialis. *Journal of Bone and Joint Surgery*. 77 (2): 225–231

Gottlob, C.A., Baker, C.L., Pellissier, J.M. and Colvin, L. (1999) Cost effectiveness of anterior cruciate ligament reconstruction in young adults. *Clinical Orthopaedics and Related Research*. 367 (10): 272–282

Grood, E.S., Noyes, F.R. and Butler, D.L. (1981) Ligamentous and capsular restraints preventing straight medial and lateral laxity on intact human cadaver knees. *American Journal of Bone and Joint Surgery*. 63: 1257–1269

Gross, J., Fetto, J. and Rosen, E. (2009) *Musculoskeletal examination*, 3rd edition. Wiley-Blackwell. Oxford, UK

Gupta, A. and Funk, L. (2009) *Orthoteers clinical examination book*. Orthoteers, British Orthopaedic Association. Manchester, UK

Haddad, F. (2012) The impact of an acute knee clinic on ACL injury outcomes. In Roi, G.S. and Della Villa, S. (eds) *Football medicine strategies for knee injuries: Abstract book*. Calzetti and Mariucci Editori. Italy

Halbrecht, J.L. and Jackson, D.W. (1993) Acute dislocation of the patella. In Fox, J.M. and Pizzo, W.D. (eds). *The patellofemoral joint*. McGraw-Hill. New York

Hamill, J. and Knutzen, K. (2009) *Biomechanical basis for human movement*, 3rd edition. Lippincott, Williams and Wilkins. Philadelphia, PA

Harfe, D.T., Chuinard, C.R. and Espinoza, L.M. (1998) Elongation patterns of the collateral ligaments of the human knee. *Clinical Biomechanics*. 13: 163–175

Harner, C.D, Xerogeanes, J.W., Livesay, G.A., *et al.* (1995) The human posterior cruciate ligament complex: An interdisciplinary study ligament morphology and biomechanical evaluation. *American Journal of Sports Medicine*. 23 (6): 736–745

Harty, M. and Joyce, J. (1977) Synovial folds in the knee joint. *Orthopaedic Review*. 6: 10 91–92

Hattam, P. and Smeatham, A. (2010) *Special tests in musculoskeletal examination: An evidence-based guide for clinicians*. Churchill Livingstone, Elsevier. London, UK

Hayes, K.W., Petersen, C. and Falconer, J. (1994) An examination of Cyriax's passive motion tests with patients having osteoarthritis of the knee. *Physical Therapy*. 74 (8): 9–19

Heijne, A. and Werner, S. (2007) Early versus late start of open kinetic chain quadriceps exercises after ACL reconstruction with patellar tendon or hamstring grafts: A prospective randomized outcome study. *Knee Surgery, Sports Traumatology, Arthroscopy*. 15: 402–414

Heintjes, E.M., Berger, M., Bierma-Zeinstra, S., Bernsen, R., Verhaar, J. and Koes, B.W. (2003) Exercise therapy for patellofemoral pain syndrome (review). *Cochrane Database of Systematic Reviews*. 4

Hengeveld, E. and Banks, K. (2005) *Maitland's peripheral manipulation*, 4th edition. Elsevier, Butterworth Heinemann. London, UK

Herrington, L. (2000) The effect of patellofemoral joint taping. *Physical and Rehabilitation Medicine*. 12: 271–276

Herrington, L. (2011) Knee valgus angle during landing tasks in female volleyball and basketball players. *Journal of Strength and Conditioning Research*. 25: 262–266

Hoher, J., Harner. C.D., Vogrin, T.M., Baek, G.H., Gregory, J.C. and Woo, S. L-Y. (1998) In situ forces in the posterolateral structures of the knee under posterior tibial loading in the intact and posterior cruciate ligament-deficient knee. *Journal of Orthopaedic Research*. 16 (6): 675–681

Hopper, D.M., Strauss, G.R., Boyle, J.J. and Bell, J. (2008) Functional recovery after anterior cruciate ligament reconstruction: A longitudinal perspective. *Archives of Physical Medicine Rehabilitation*. 89: 1535–1541

Huston, L.J. and Wojtys, E.M (1996) Neuromuscular performance characteristics in elite female athletes. *American Journal of Sports Medicine*. 24: 427–436

Irrgang, J.J. (2008) Current status of measuring clinical outcomes after anterior cruciate ligament reconstruction: Are we good enough? *Operative Techniques in Sports Medicine*. 16: 119–124

Irrgang, J.J. and Fitzgerald, K. (2000) Rehabilitation of the multiple-ligament injured knee. *Clinics in Sports Medicine*. 19 (3): 545–571

Johnson, D. (2004) *ACL made simple*. Springer-Verlag. New York

Johnson, M.W. (2000) Acute knee effusions: A systematic approach to diagnosis. *American Family Physician*. 61 (8): 2391–2400

Jones, R.E., Smith, E.C. and Reisch, J.S. (1978) Effects of medial meniscectomy in patients older than forty years. *American Journal of Bone and Joint Surgery*. 60 (6): 783–786

Jonsson, P. and Alfredson, H. (2005) Superior results with eccentric compared to concentric quadriceps training in patients with jumper's knee: A prospective randomised study. *British Journal of Sports Medicine*. 39: 847–850

Kaeding, C. and Best, T.M. (2009) Tendinosis: Pathophysiology and non-operative treatment. *Sports Health: A Multidisciplinary Approach*. 1: 284

Karachalios, T., Hantes, M., Zibis, A.H., Zachos, V., Karantanas, A.H. and Malizos, K.N. (2005) Diagnostic accuracy of a new clinical test (the Thessaly test) for early detection of meniscal tears. *Journal of Bone and Joint Surgery*. 87 (5): 955–962

Kendall, F., Kendall-McCreary, E., Provance, P.G., Rodgers, M. and Roman, W. (2005) *Muscles: Testing and function; posture and pain*. Lippincott, Williams and Wilkins. Philadelphia, PA

Kenyon, K. and Kenyon, J. (2005) *The physiotherapist's pocketbook: Essential facts at your fingertips*, 2nd edition. Churchill Livingstone, Elsevier. London, UK.

Kingston, B. (2000) *Understanding joints: A practical guide to their structure and function*, 2nd edition. Cengage Learning. London, UK

Klimkiewicz, J.J. (2005) Soft tissue knee injuries (tendon and bursae). In O'Connor, F.G., Sallis, R.E., Wilder, R.P. and St Pierre, P. (eds) *Sports medicine: Just the facts*. McGraw-Hill. New York

Kongsgaard, M., Aagaard, P., Roikjaer, S., *et al.* (2006) Decline eccentric squats increases patellar tendon loading compared to standard eccentric squats. *Clinical Biomechanics.* 21 (7): 748–754

Kongsgaard, M., Kovanen, V., Aagaard, P., *et al.* (2009) Corticosteroid injections, eccentric decline squat training and heavy slow resistance training in patellar tendinopathy. *Scandinavian Journal of Medicine and Science in Sports.* 19: 790–802

Lelli, A. and Di Turi, R.P. (2012) Partial meniscectomy and repair. In Roi, G.S. and Della Villa, S. (eds) *Football medicine strategies for knee injuries: Abstract book.* Calzetti and Mariucci Editori. Italy

Li, G., Rudy, T.W. and Sakane, M. (1999) The importance of quadriceps and hamstring muscle loading on knee kinematics and in-situ forces in the ACL. *Journal of Biomechanics.* 32: 395–400

Li, L., Landin, D., Grodesky, J. and Myers, J. (2002) The function of gastrocnemius as a knee flexor at selected knee and ankle angles. *Journal of Electromyography and Kinesiology.* 12 (5): 385–390

Lieb, F.J. and Perry, J. (1971) Quadriceps function: An electromyographic study under isometric conditions. *Journal of Bone and Joint Surgery.* 53: 749–758

Lohmander, L.S., Englund, P.M., Dahl, L.L. and Roos, E.M. (2007) The long-term consequence of anterior cruciate ligament and meniscus injuries: Osteoarthritis. *The American Journal of Sports Medicine.* 35 (10): 1756–1769

Loudon, J., Swift, M. and Bell, S. (2008) *The clinical orthopedic assessment guide,* 2nd edition. Human Kinetics. Champaign, IL

Lutz, G.E., Palmitier, R.A., An, K.N. and Chao, E.Y. (1993) Comparison of tibiofemoral joint forces during open-kinetic-chain and closed-kinetic-chain exercises. *Journal of Bone and Joint Surgery.* 75: 732–739

Magee, D. (2008) *Orthopaedic physical assessment,* 5th edition. Saunders. Philadelphia, PA

Magee, D. and Sueki, D. (2011) *Orthopaedic physical assessment atlas and video.* Elsevier Saunders. Philadelphia, PA

Mahadevan, V. (2008) Pelvic girdle and lower limb: Knee. In Standring, S. (ed.) *Gray's anatomy: The anatomical basis of clinical practice,* 40th edition. Elsevier, Churchill Livingstone. Edinburgh, UK

McConnell, J. (1986) The management of chondromalacia patellae: A long term solution. *Australian Journal of Physiotherapy.* 32 (4): 215–223

McConnell, J. (1996) Management of patellofemoral problems. *Manual Therapy.* 1: 60–66

McConnell J. (2007) Rehabilitation and non-operative treatment of patellar instability. *Sports Medicine and Arthroscopy Review.* 15 (2): 95–104

McMurray, T.P. (1942) The semilunar cartilages. *British Journal of Surgery.* 29: 407–414

Medical Research Council (1976) *Aids to the investigation of peripheral nerve injuries.* HMSO. London, UK

Medina, D. (2012) MCL injuries in football. In Roi, G.S. and Della Villa, S. (eds) *Football medicine strategies for knee injuries: Abstract book.* Calzetti and Mariucci Editori. Italy

Meeusen, R. and Lievens, P. (1986) The use of cryotherapy in sports injuries. *Sports Medicine.* 3 (6) 398–414

Mikkelsen C., Werner S. and Eriksson, E. (2000) Closed kinetic chain alone compared to combined open and closed kinetic chain exercises for quadriceps strengthening after anterior cruciate ligament reconstruction with respect to return to sports: A prospective matched follow-up study. *Knee Surgery Sports Trauma Arthroscopy.* 8: 337–342

Miller, M. and Sanders, T. (2012) Patellar instability. In Miller, M. and Sanders, T. (eds) *Presentation, imaging and treatment of common musculoskeletal conditions: MRI–arthroscopy correlation.* Saunders, Elsevier. Philadelphia, PA

Miller, T.T., Gladden, P., Staron, R.B., Henry, J.H. and Feldman, F. (1997) Posterolateral stabilizers of the knee: Anatomy and injuries assessed with MR imaging. *American Journal of Roentgenology.* 169: 1641–1647

Miyasaka, K.C., Daniel, D.M. and Stone, M.L. (1991) The incidence of knee ligament injuries in the general population. *American Journal of Knee Surgery.* 4: 3–8

Moore, A.M., MacEwan, M., Santosa, K.B., *et al.* (2011). Acellular nerve allografts in peripheral nerve regeneration: A comparative study. *Muscle and Nerve.* 44 (2): 221–234

Mueller-Wohlfahrt, H.W., Haensel, L., Mithoefer, K., *et al.* (2013) Terminology and classification of muscle injuries in sport: The Munich consensus statement. *British Journal of Sports Medicine.* 47: 342–350

Muller, W. (1983) *The knee: Form, function, and ligament reconstruction.* Springer. New York

Murray, D., Jain, N. and Kemp, S. (2012) Knee injuries in elite professional footballers: The findings of one English premier league team. In Roi, G.S. and Della Villa, S. (eds) *Football medicine strategies for knee injuries: Abstract book.* Calzetti and Mariucci Editori. Italy

Myer, G.D., Ford, K.R., Barber Foss, K.D., *et al.* (2010). The incidence and potential pathomechanics of patellofemoral pain in female athletes. *Clinical Biomechanics.* 25 (7): 700–707

Neyret, P., Duthon, V.B. and Servien, E. (2012) ACL surgery in football players. In Roi, G.S. and Della Villa, S. (eds) *Football medicine strategies for knee injuries: Abstract book.* Calzetti and Mariucci Editori. Italy

Nicoletta, R.J. and Schepsis, A.A. (2005) The patellofemoral joint. In O'Connor, F.G., Sallis, R.E., Wilder, R.P. and St Pierre, P. (eds) *Sports medicine: Just the facts.* McGraw-Hill. New York

Nijs, J., Van Geel, C., Van der Auwera, C. and Van de Velde, B. (2006) Diagnostic value of five clinical tests in patellofemoral pain syndrome. *Manual Therapy.* 11: 69–77

Odensten, M. and Gillquist, J. (1985) Functional anatomy of the anterior cruciate ligament and a rationale for reconstruction. *Journal of Bone and Joint Surgery (American Volume).* 67 (2): 257–262

Pattyn, E., Verdonk, P., Steyaert, A., *et al.* (2011) Vastus medialis obliquus atrophy: Does it exist in patellofemoral pain syndrome? *American Journal of Sports Medicine.* 39 (7):1450–1456

Petersen, W. and Tillmann, B. (1999) Structure and vascularization of the cruciate ligaments of the human knee joint. *Anatomy and Embryology.* 200 (3): 325–334

Peterson, L. and Renstrom, P. (2005) *Sports injuries: Their prevention and treatment*, 3rd edition. Taylor and Francis. London, UK.

Petty, N. (2006) *Neuromusculoskeletal examination and assessment: A handbook for therapists*, 3rd edition. Churchill Livingstone. London, UK

Pitman II, M., Nainzadeh, N., Menche, D., *et al.* (1992) The intraoperative evaluation of the neurosensory function of the anterior cruciate ligament in humans using somatosensory evoked potentials. *Arthroscopy.* 8: 442–447

Piziali, R.L., Seering, W.P. and Nagel, D.A. (1980) The function of the primary ligaments of the knee in anterior–posterior and medial–lateral motions. *Journal of Biomechanics.* 13: 777–784

Powers C., Landel, R., Sosnick, T., *et al.* (1997) The effects of patellar taping on stride characteristics and joint motion in subjects with patellofemoral pain. *Journal of Orthopaedic and Sports Physical Therapy.* 26 (6): 286–291

Puniello, M.S. (1993) Iliotibial band tightness and medial patellar glide in patients with patellofemoral dysfunction. *Journal of Orthopaedic Sports Physical Therapy.* 17 (3): 144–148

Rees, J.D., Maffulli, N. and Cook, J. (2009) Management of tendinopathy. *American Journal of Sports Medicine.* 37: 1855–1867

Richards, D.P., Ajemian, S.V., Wiley, J.P. and Zernicke, R.F. (1996) Knee joint dynamics predict patellar tendinitis in elite volleyball players. *American Journal of Sports Medicine.* 24 (5): 676–683

Rolf, C.G. and Riyami, M. (2006) Can we really trust MRI in diagnosing knee injuries in athletes? *Imaging Decisions MRI.* 10 (1): 2–7

Rossi, R., Dettoni, F., Bruzzone, M., Cottino, U., D'Elicio, D.G. and Bonasia, D.E. (2011) Clinical examination of the knee: Know your tools for diagnosis of knee injuries. *Sports Medicine, Arthroscopy, Rehabilitation, Therapy and Technology.* 3: 25

Saddler, S.C., Noyes, F.R. and Grood, E.S. (1996) Posterior cruciate ligament anatomy and length–tension behavior of the PCL surface fibres. *American Journal of Knee Surgery.* 9: 194–199

Schutz, E.A. and Irrgang, J.J. (1994) Rehabilitation following posterior cruciate ligament injury or reconstruction. *Sports Medicine and Arthroscopy Review.* 2: 165–173

Sewell, D., Watkins, P. and Griffin, M. (2013) *Sport and exercise science: An introduction*, 2nd edition. Routledge. Abingdon, UK

Sharma, P. and Maffulli, N. (2005) Current concepts review: Tendon injury and tendinopathy, healing and repair. *Journal of Bone and Joint Surgery.* 87-A (1): 187–196

Shellbourne, K.D. and Gray, T. (1997) Anterior cruciate ligament reconstruction with autogenous patellar tendon graft followed by accelerated rehabilitation. *American Journal of Sports Medicine.* 25: 786–795

Shultz, A.R., Miller, C.D., Kerr, C.S. and Micheli, L. (1984) Mechanoreceptors in human cruciate ligaments. *Journal of Bone and Joint Surgery.* 66A: 1072–1076

Shultz, S., Houglum, P.A. and Perrin, D.H. (2000) *Assessment of athletic injuries.* Human Kinetics. Champaign, IL

Spina, A.A. (2007) The plantaris muscle: Anatomy, injury, imaging, and treatment. *Journal of the Canadian Chiropractic Association.* 51 (3): 158–165

Starkey, C. and Ryan, J. (2003) *Orthopedic and athletic injury evaluation handbook.* F.A. Davis Company. Philadelphia, PA

Stiell, I.G., Greenberg, G.H., Wells, G.A., *et al.* (1996) Prospective validation of a decision rule for the use of radiography in acute knee injuries. *Journal of the American Medical Association.* 275: 611–615

Taunton, J.E., Ryan, M.B., Clement, D.B., McKenzie, D.D., Lloyd-Smith, D.R. and Zumbo, B.D. (2002) A retrospective case-control analysis of 2002 running injuries. *British Journal of Sports Medicine.* 36: 95–101

Tortora, G. and Derrickson, B. (2008) *Principles of anatomy and physiology*, 12th edition. John Wiley and Sons. Princeton, NJ

Tortora, G.J. and Grabowski, S.R. (1996) *Principles of anatomy and physiology*, 8th edition. Harper Collins. New York

Wadsworth, C.T. (1988) *Manual examination and treatment of the spine and extremities.* Williams and Wilkins. Baltimore, MD

Warden, S.J. and Brukner, P. (2003) Patellar tendinopathy. *Clinics in Sports Medicine.* 22: 743–759

Warren, L.A., Marshall, J.L. and Girgis, F. (1974) The prime static stabilizer of the medial side of the knee. *American Journal of Bone and Joint Surgery.* 56: 665–674

Watkins, J. (2010) *Structure and function of the musculoskeletal system*, 2nd edition. Human Kinetics. Champaign, IL

Willberg, L., Sunding, K., Forssblad, M., Fahlström, M. and Alfredson, H. (2011) Sclerosing polidocanol injections or arthroscopic shaving to treat patellar tendinopathy: A randomised controlled study. *British Journal of Sports Medicine.* 45: 411–415

Williams, A. (2012) Surgical treatment of NCL injuries. In Roi, G.S. and Della Villa, S. (eds) *Football medicine strategies for knee injuries: Abstract book.* Calzetti and Mariucci Editori. Italy

Woo, S.L.-Y., Hollis, J.M., Adams, D.J., Lyon, R.M. and Takai, S. (1991) Tensile properties of the human femur–anterior cruciate ligament tibia complex: The effects of specimen age and orientation. *American Journal of Sports Medicine.* 19 (3): 217–225

Yu, G. and Garrett, W.E. (2007). Mechanisms of non-contact ACL injuries. *British Journal of Sports Medicine.* 41: 147–151

Zorzi, C., Condello, V., Madonna, V., Cortese, F. and Piovan, G. (2012) Who needs MCL surgery? In Roi, G.S. and Della Villa, S. (eds) *Football medicine strategies for knee injuries: Abstract book.* Calzetti and Mariucci Editori. Italy

11

THE ANKLE AND FOOT REGION

Anatomy, assessment and injuries

Keith Ward, Troy Douglin, Hannah Boardman and Adam Hawkey

Functional anatomy of the ankle and foot region

The ankle and foot play a major role in stable bipedal posture, locomotion and balance of the human body. These structures have a direct functional relationship with the hip and knee (Ferber *et al.*, 2009). While the supporting structures within the ankle and foot display some similarity to those of the wrist and hand, the differences between these two anatomical units reflects the differences in their functional demands (Oatis, 2009). The anatomy of the ankle and foot is largely dictated by the need to bear the total body mass during activities such as standing, walking, stair-climbing and running. The ankle and foot are composed (in average populations) of a complex structure of 28 bones, 55 articulations (including 30 synovial joints), more than 100 ligaments, and over 30 muscles (Dutton, 2008). All of these structures ideally interact harmoniously, with the overriding aim being the achievement of smooth and stable motion of the lower limb.

Gross *et al.* (2009) explain how generally the ankle lies lateral to the body's centre of gravity (CoG) and therefore is exposed particularly to both varus and compressive loading. The ankle and foot system contributes significantly to the function of the entire lower limb through being the body's primary contact with the ground. Under normal conditions, it does this extremely efficiently, performing in a number of complex roles, such as: acting as a loose adaptor to uneven surfaces during contact (Hunter and Fortune, 2000); acting as a natural shock absorber (Soutas-Little *et al.*, 1987); providing a stable platform or base of support (BoS); and providing a mechanism to both dissipate ground reaction forces (GRF) during heel strike in the initial stance phase of gait, and to generate propulsion by producing a rigid lever for pushing off during terminal stance (Norkin and Levangie, 2001).

One important facet of the ankle and foot complex is its ability to remain stable even while absorbing large dynamic and multidirectional forces during load-bearing. Activities such as running, walking and stair-climbing may transmit forces up to 14 times an individual's bodyweight through the foot and ankle. The requirement to be stable under extreme force is offset by a need to offer a wide range of movement (RoM); and this flexibility is used to facilitate mobility in a diverse spectrum of environments from running on uneven terrains to swimming in water. However, due to the complexity of the system, injury or other pathology affecting the support structures around the ankle and foot can cause the region to become unstable (Hamilton and Ziemer, 1981). Understanding how the ankle and foot are structured, and how they function normally, is crucial to the sports therapist as this forms a basis for detection and treatment of problems.

Surface and skeletal anatomy of the ankle and foot region

Close visual inspection or palpation of the ankle and foot region reveals aspects of its skin, superficial and deep bony landmarks, ligamentous tissue, musculotendinous tissue, fascia, blood vessels and nerves. The ankle and foot complex consists of 28 bones (when including the tibia and fibula). The tibia and fibula have a large influence on the RoM at the ankle and foot. The distal tibia flares medially and extends distally to form the medial malleolus. This bony landmark serves as the medial constraint and the superior articular surface of the ankle mortise. In contrast, the distal fibula flares laterally to form the lateral malleolus, which serves as a lateral constraint to the ankle mortise. It is important to note that the lateral malleolus extends more distally than the medial malleolus, making it significant in ankle stabilization.

The remaining 26 bones include the tarsals, metatarsals and phalanges. The tarsals consist of the talus, calcaneus, navicular, cuboid and three cuneiforms (medial, intermediate and lateral). The talus sits superiorly to the rest of the tarsal bones and features in transmitting the entire body mass to the arches within the foot during normal human gait. This bone is made up of four main parts – the body, neck, head and dome (trochlea); it has an unusual retrograde arterial blood supply. The head of the talus is wider anteriorly than posteriorly, making it wedge-shaped. The articulating surface of the talus can be palpated distal to the anterior tibia while plantarflexing and dorsiflexing the ankle. The neck and subsequent head of the talus can be located distally to this. The head of the talus can also be palpated on the medial side, proximal to the navicular tubercle, especially when the foot is everted.

The calcaneus, the largest of the tarsal bones, sits inferiorly to the talus and is a key base component of the medial and lateral longitudinal arches of the foot. Together, the talus and calcaneus compose the skeletal components of the hindfoot. The sustentaculum tali of the calcaneus, a small ridge-like structure, can be found distal to the space between the medial malleolus and the calcaneal body (the sustentaculum tali helps to 'sustain the talus' on its medial aspect). On the lateral side of the calcaneus, the peroneal tubercle can be palpated distal to the lateral malleolus. On the anterolateral aspect of the ankle is the sinus tarsi; this is a distinct and palpable structural cavity which is the anterolateral aspect of the subtalar joint, and is where, at the talus, the anterior talofibular ligament (ATFL) attaches distally.

On the posterosuperior prominence of the calcaneus is the retrocalcaneal bursa, deep to the Achilles tendon. The anterior wall of the bursa is invested with fibrocartilage, while the posterior wall is more tendinous. The function of the bursa is to reduce friction between the Achilles tendon and calcaneus. The plantar surface of the calcaneus at the heel is partially covered by the subcalcaneal fat pad. This is composed of dense strands of elastic fibrous tissues which help to orientate bound adipose tissue. The subcalcaneal fat pad has an average thickness of 18 mm (Mahadevan, 2008a), and functions as a shock absorber (compression and shear) to help dissipate forces directed to the plantar surface of the foot during standing, walking, running and landing. It is believed that the fat pad absorbs 17–46 per cent of energy during walking (Gefen *et al.*, 2001). Atrophy of the fat pad can be a constant source of rearfoot pain, and causes of this can include: genetic factors; age-related degeneration; significant weight loss; arch abnormalities; walking barefoot excessively; or wearing thin-soled shoes.

Structurally, the midfoot is made up of the navicular, cuboid and the three cuneiforms. These five bones join the hindfoot to the forefoot and contribute to the shock-absorbing

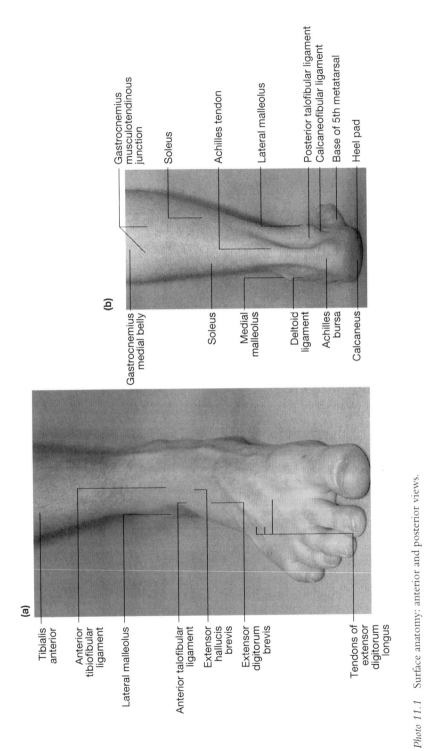

(a)

Tibialis
anterior

Anterior
tibiofibular
ligament

Lateral malleolus

Anterior talofibular
ligament

Extensor
hallucis
brevis

Extensor
digitorum
brevis

Tendons of
extensor
digitorum
longus

(b)

Gastrocnemius
musculotendinous
junction

Soleus

Achilles tendon

Lateral malleolus

Posterior talofibular ligament
Calcaneofibular ligament
Base of 5th metatarsal
Heel pad

Gastrocnemius
medial belly

Soleus

Medial
malleolus

Deltoid
ligament

Achilles
bursa

Calcaneus

Photo 11.1   Surface anatomy: anterior and posterior views.

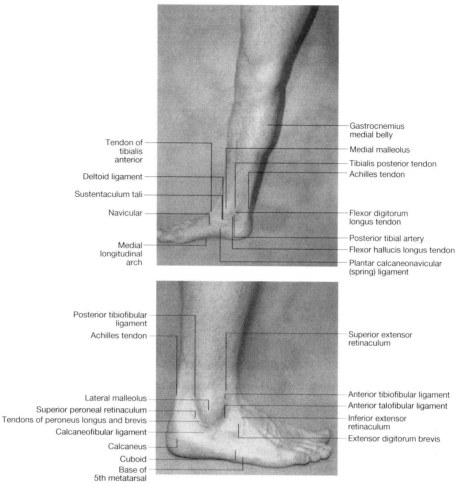

Gastrocnemius
medial belly

Medial malleolus

Tibialis posterior tendon

Achilles tendon

Tendon of
tibialis
anterior

Deltoid ligament

Sustentaculum tali

Navicular

Flexor digitorum
longus tendon

Posterior tibial artery

Flexor hallucis longus tendon

Medial
longitudinal
arch

Plantar calcaneonavicular
(spring) ligament

Posterior tibiofibular
ligament

Achilles tendon

Superior extensor
retinaculum

Lateral malleolus

Superior peroneal retinaculum

Tendons of peroneus longus and brevis

Calcaneofibular ligament

Calcaneus

Cuboid

Base of
5th metatarsal

Anterior tibiofibular ligament

Anterior talofibular ligament

Inferior extensor
retinaculum

Extensor digitorum brevis

Photo 11.2   Surface anatomy: medial and lateral views.

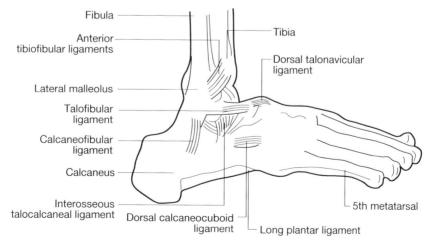

Fibula

Anterior
tibiofibular ligaments

Lateral malleolus

Talofibular
ligament

Calcaneofibular
ligament

Calcaneus

Interosseous
talocalcaneal ligament

Tibia

Dorsal talonavicular
ligament

5th metatarsal

Dorsal calcaneocuboid
ligament

Long plantar ligament

Figure 11.1   Skeletal and ligamentous anatomy: lateral view.

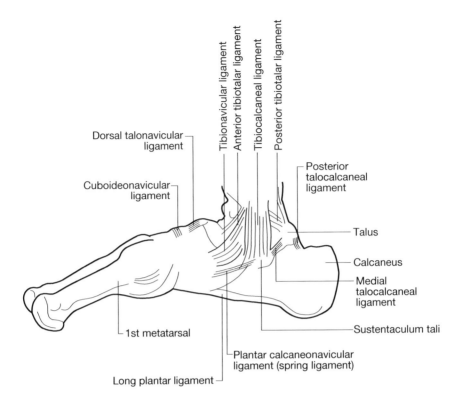

Figure 11.2 Skeletal and ligamentous anatomy: medial view.

qualities of the foot during load-bearing. The navicular is situated on the medial aspect of the foot located between the head of the talus and the posterior aspect of the three cuneiform bones; laterally it articulates with the cuboid. The most notable bony landmark of the navicular is its tuberosity – prominent on its medial aspect, and an insertion point for tibialis posterior. The plantar calcaneonavicular (spring) ligament provides support to the talus, and the medial longitudinal arch, and runs from the sustentaculum tali to the navicular. Lateral to the medial cuneiform are the intermediate and lateral cuneiforms, respectively. The cuboid is situated lateral to these three bones on the lateral aspect of the foot. Located at the distal end of the plantar surface of the cuboid is a groove for peroneus longus. Proximal to this is the cuboid tuberosity, which possesses a facet that often articulates with a sesamoid bone housed within the tendon of peroneus longus.

There are five metatarsals, two sesamoid bones and 14 phalanges, which complete the forefoot. The five metatarsals correspond to the five individual toes (including the great toe – the hallux). Each metatarsal is composed of a base, shaft and head region. The plantar surface of the forefoot (and the 'balls' of the foot) are also partially covered by a complex structure composed of fascial layers and adipose tissue (metatarsal fat pad). This framework is also used to dissipate force directed towards the plantar surface of the foot in order to reduce injury risk. Situated at the lateral aspect of the base of the fifth metatarsal is a tuberosity (or styloid process). This is an insertion site for peroneus brevis and tertius. At the plantar surface of the head of the first metatarsal are two sesamoid bones; they help to distribute force during locomotion, and facilitate flexion of the hallux by increasing the tendon moment arm (similar to the role of the patella at the knee). Each individual toe has three phalanges (proximal, middle and distal), with the exception of the great toe (hallux) which has only a proximal and a distal phalanx.

On the dorsal aspect of the foot the transverse arch is apparent, as are the five 'rays' (functional load-bearing units running from the tarsal to the phalanges). There are three medial rays (from the medial cuneiform to the first metatarsal; from the middle cuneiform to the second metatarsal; and from the lateral cuneiform to the third metatarsal); and two lateral rays (running from the cuboid through the fourth and fifth metatarsals). Finally, superficially on the plantar surface of the foot, running from the heel (mainly from the medial tubercle of the calcaneous) via its medial, central (largest) and lateral components and distal digital slips to the heads of the metatarsals and bases of the phalanges, is the thick, fibrous plantar fascia (aponeurosis).

Of the muscles and tendons of the ankle and foot, a number present superficially. Anteriorly, running from the lateral tibia to the medial cuneiform and first metatarsal is the tibialis anterior; its prominent tendon crosses the talocrural joint. Laterally adjacent to tibialis anterior on the lower leg is extensor digitorum longus; its distal tendons are apparent overlying the dorsal surface of the second to fifth distal phalanges. The tendon of flexor hallucis longus runs to the base of the first distal phalanx. Medially, winding their way inferiorly under the medial malleolus are the tendons of tibialis posterior, flexor digitorum longus and flexor hallucis longus, the latter two of which run to the plantar surface of the second to fifth distal phalanges and the first digital phalange respectively. On the lateral aspect of the ankle and foot running from the fibula are the peroneal tendons. Peroneus longus winds under the lateral malleolus to pass via the cuboid and underside of the foot to insert at the medial cuneiform and first metatarsal. Peroneus brevis also runs under the malleolus

---

Practitioner Tip Box 11.1

Skeletal landmarks of the ankle and foot region

Distal tibia
Medial malleolus

Distal fibula
Lateral malleolus

Talus
Head
Neck
Trochlea (Talar dome)
Medial tubercle
Lateral tubercle
Sinus tarsi

Calcaneus
Tuberosity of calcaneus
Peroneal trochlea
Sustentaculum tali

Navicular
Navicular tuberosity

Cuboid
Cuboid tuberosity

Cuneiforms
Lateral cuneiform
Middle cuneiform
Medial cuneiform

Metatarsals
Base
Shaft
Head
Tuberosity at base of fifth metatarsal

Phalanges
Base
Shaft
Head

Practitioner Tip Box 11.2

Average ranges of movement at the ankle

- Dorsiflexion 20°
- Plantarflexion 50°
- Inversion 30°
- Eversion 20°

Source: adapted from Clarkson, 2013; Loudon *et al.*, 2008; Magee, 2008; Palmer and Epler, 1998.

---

to attach at the base of the fifth metatarsal; tertius, however, runs over the lateral malleolus to insert more dorsally on the base of the fifth metatarsal. Posteriorly, gastrocnemius and soleus feed into the Achilles tendon and attach to the posterior surface of the calcaneus.

Joints and movements of the ankle and foot region

The motions of the ankle and foot are classified as single and multiplanar (Dutton, 2008). The major movements of the ankle (talocrural joint) are uniplanar, occurring in the sagittal plane, and are dorsiflexion (raising the foot upwards) and plantarflexion (pointing the foot downwards). The frontal plane movements of inversion (turning the heel and sole inwards) and eversion (turning the heel and sole outwards) occur primarily at the subtalar joint, with some contribution from the transverse tarsal joints. Many of the functional movements of the foot are complex, primarily due to the variety of large and small joints, irregularly shaped articular surfaces and the manner in which movements of many joints are required to occur around multiple axes. Pronation and supination may be described as rotational movements of the foot below and distal to the talus. Supination is a triplanar movement and a combination of inversion (via the subtalar joint) with plantarflexion (via the talocrural joint) and adduction (of the midtarsal joint). Pronation is also triplanar and combines eversion, dorsiflexion and abduction (Muscolino, 2006; Pansky and Gest, 2012). The metatarsophalangeal joints allow for some flexion, extension, abduction and adduction. The interphalangeal joints allow flexion and extension of the toes.

The ankle comprises a complex arrangement of joints which facilitate its RoM – the four primary joints are the distal (inferior) tibiofibular, talocrural, subtalar and (transverse) midtarsal. The distal tibiofibular joint is an articulation where the concave surface of the distal tibia sits in the convex surface of the distal fibula. The joint is classed as an amphiarthrodial, or fibrous syndesmotic, joint. An interosseous membrane between the tibia and fibula allows the fibula to contribute to load–bearing during stance and locomotion. It is important to recognize the accommodating accessory movements occurring at the distal and proximal tibiofibular joints during dorsiflexion and plantarflexion (Palastanga *et al.*, 2008). Despite transmission of approximately 10 per cent of body mass through the fibula during locomotion, the average movement at the distal tibiofibular joint is approximately 2.4 mm inferiorly, with approximately 1 mm of widening typically occurring; without this movement superiorly, the ankle itself may lose its normal range and can become stiff (Rupp, 2008). However, the significant restriction of movement at the end of range also helps to stabilize the joint during load bearing.

The talocrural (ankle) joint is classified as a ginglymus (hinge) joint, and is the articulation between the talar dome, tibial plafond (distal tibia), medial malleolus and lateral malleolus. While the architecture of the talocrural joint facilitates torque to be transmitted from the internal and external rotation movements of the lower leg to the foot during closed–chain activity (Hertel, 2002), the primary motions of the talocrural joint occur in the sagittal plane, namely plantarflexion and dorsiflexion. Plantarflexion involves an accessory gliding action of the talus anteriorly, and is the movement of the ankle and foot away from the tibia. Dorsiflexion involves an accessory gliding action posteriorly, with the dorsum of the foot approximating with the anterior aspect of the tibia. During dorsiflexion the wedge-shaped talar head is compressed between the medial and lateral malleoli and reaches the end RoM in a close-packed highly congruent position. Plantarflexion, therefore, is the joint's loose-packed (and most unstable) position.

Active plantarflexion may range anywhere between 20° and 58°, but an average range (assessed from a plantargrade, neutral 90° start position) is approximately 50° (Magee, 2008; Palmer and Epler, 1998). Average active dorsiflexion is reported to range from 12° to 30° (AAOS, 1969; Boone and Azen, 1979; Luttgens and Hamilton, 1997; Roass and Andersson, 1982). Greater ranges of dorsiflexion, up to 40°, have been achieved – especially while performing heavy weight-bearing activity such as squats (Brown and Yavarsky, 1987). The amount of dorsiflexion RoM required for normal efficient gait is approximately 10°. However, variations will present, and healthy older individuals typically exhibit reduced dorsiflexion compared to their younger counterparts, who are likely to display greater RoM during gait (Hamill and Knutzen, 2009).

The talocrural joint is stabilized by the joint capsule, bony congruency and a number of ligaments. The medial collateral (deltoid) ligament complex provides strong restraint medially. This structure includes tibiocalcaneal, tibiotalar and tibionavicular components and primarily prevents excessive eversion of the hindfoot and movement of the talus. The lateral collateral ligament complex includes the following ligaments: the anterior talofibular (ATFL), the calcaneofibular (CFL) and the posterior talofibular (PTFL). These primarily prevent excessive inversion of the hindfoot and movement of the talus.

The subtalar joint also converts torque between the lower leg and foot (Hertel, 2002), and is an arthrodial (gliding) joint which forms an articulation between the talus and calcaneus at posterior, medial and anterior joint surfaces. The subtalar joint is inclined by approximately 42° from the horizontal plane, and deviates towards the medial side by approximately 23° (Sarrafian, 1993). The posterior surface, sometimes termed the posterior subtalar joint, has its own synovial capsule. The medial and anterior surfaces, sometimes termed the talocalcaneonavicular joint, share a synovial capsule together. The separate articulations are divided by the tarsal tunnel. The configuration of the three articulating surfaces allows for inversion and eversion, but also a small degree of plantarflexion and dorsiflexion. While it is possible for either eversion and inversion, or dorsiflexion and plantarflexion, movements to be achieved on their own while the joint is in neutral alignment, joint orientations away from neutral result in movements occurring concurrently. This has led to the joint being described as functioning about a universal axis.

Average subtalar joint movement ranges between 20° and 37° for inversion, and between 10° and 28° for eversion (AAOS, 1969; Boone and Azen, 1979; Roass and Andersson, 1982). While gait on even ground requires approximately 5° inversion and eversion, it is likely that locomotion on uneven ground utilizes a greater proportion of the available RoM. The subtalar joint maintains its stability through a number of intrinsic and extrinsic ligaments. The primary intrinsic structures responsible for stability are the interosseous talocalcaneal (subtalar) and cervical ligaments; Viladot *et al.* (1984) described these as the '*cruciate ligaments of the subtalar joint*'. The extrinsic structures responsible for stability include the CFL, the lateral and posterior talocalcaneal and tibiocalcaneal ligaments. Together, these intrinsic and extrinsic structures prevent excessive hindfoot inversion and eversion.

The transverse midtarsal ('Chopart's') joint, which is classed as an arthrodial joint, is an 'S-shaped' articulation between the talus and navicular bones medially, and the calcaneus and cuboid bones laterally. The talonavicular articulation can be classed as a small ball-and-socket joint, with the neck of the talus providing the axis. The calcaneocuboid joint is a saddle-shaped configuration with the calcaneal body forming the axis. These orientations allow the joint surfaces to glide over each other harmoniously. When the lateral border of the foot is raised during eversion, the navicular moves inferiorly to the talus, allowing for greater pronation of the forefoot. Similarly, when the medial surface of the foot is raised, the cuboid can move inferiorly relative to the calcaneus, allowing for increased forefoot supination. The joint separates the hindfoot from the midfoot, which subsequently allows both the hindfoot and forefoot to act as stabilizers during weight-bearing, irrespective of each other. On uneven terrain, this allows the hindfoot to be stable and remain in contact with the ground with little influence from a potentially unstable forefoot and vice versa. The midtarsal joint is stabilized by several ligaments; the role of these is to prevent excessive separation of the hindfoot from the midfoot and to restrict aberrant movement of the joint. The ligaments involved in this feature include the plantar calcaneonavicular, calcaneonavicularcuboid and calcaneocuboid; as well as the dorsal talonavicular and calcaneocuboid ligaments.

The tarsometatarsal joints (also known as 'Lisfranc's joint') include articulations between the cuboid and the three cuneiforms with the five metatarsal bases. The second and third metatarsals share a joint capsule, as do the fourth and fifth metatarsals. The movements which occur at these joints are primarily flexion, extension, inversion and eversion. Very little movement occurs at these joints, with the first and second metatarsals demonstrating less movement compared with the fourth and fifth metatarsals. One of the main purposes of this small movement range at the tarsometatarsal joints is to assist the midtarsal joints with maintaining foot contact with the ground. Joint stability is maintained through dorsal, plantar and interosseous ligaments.

There are four intermetatarsal and five metatarsophalangeal joints. The intermetatarsal joints permit a small degree of flexion, extension, abduction and adduction, alongside accessory gliding. The metatarsophalangeal joints, between the heads of the metatarsals and the bases of the proximal phalanges, are condyloid; these permit flexion, extension, abduction and adduction of the toes. Generally, there is a significantly greater degree of extension compared to flexion at these joints; and active abduction is also usually performed in conjunction with extension. Extension at the first metatarsophalangeal joint is crucial to facilitate the 'Windlass mechanism' via the plantar fascia for ideal propulsion during heel lift in terminal stance of gait. The interphalangeal (ginglymus, or hinge) joints, between the heads and bases of adjacent phalanges, allow flexion and extension (Pansky and Gest, 2012).

Arches of the foot

The foot is composed of three important arches – the transverse arch and the medial and lateral longitudinal arches, each of which contribute greatly to foot functioning during loading. The three arches allow the foot to act as a tripod-like structure, which allows the foot to remain extremely stable on almost any terrain, no matter how uneven. The transverse arch runs across the midfoot, while the medial and lateral arches run longitudinally, creating an elastic shock-absorbing system (Hamill and Knutzen, 2009). The arches are maintained mainly by the foot's skeletal architecture (i.e. the shape and articulatory relations of each of the tarsals and metatarsals) and associated tensioning of the intrinsic foot ligaments and plantar fascia; and partly by the dynamic activity of the foot's musculature. In static stance, several researchers have identified that extrinsic foot muscles are relatively inactive, and that arch integrity is maintained primarily by the skeletal architecture and plantar fascia (Basmajian and Stecko, 1963; Huang *et al.*, 1993). Indeed, even the intrinsic musculature may only be recruited under heavy loading.

The transverse arch is formed by the effective wedging of the tarsals (principally the second and third cuneiforms) and the bases of the second to fourth metatarsals. The lateral longitudinal arch is formed by the calcaneus, cuboid, and lateral metatarsals. It is relatively flat compared to the medial longitudinal arch, and is limited in its mobility. It has been suggested that due to the lateral arch being lower it may make contact with the ground and contribute to load-bearing during gait, consequently playing a role in supporting the foot (Hamill and Knutzen, 2009). Structurally, the medial longitudinal arch is formed from the calcaneus, talus, navicular, cuneiforms and medial metatarsals. Proximally, the plantar calcaneonavicular (spring) ligament offers important medial support to the elevated talus. The more mobile medial longitudinal arch has greater flexibility than its lateral equivalent and makes a significant contribution to shock absorption on ground contact. It is believed that these structures support the arch dynamically, such that they deform (flatten) during load bearing, and allow for supporting many times an individual's body weight without damage (Kim and Voloshin, 1995; Soderberg, 1986). Aside from individual articular ligaments, the long plantar ligament (from the calcaneous to the bases of second and third metatarsals) and the short plantar ligament (from the calcaneous to the cuboid) offer particularly important hind and midfoot support.

The dynamic stability of all three arches is maintained, in part, by the unique plantar aponeurosis (fascia) which prevents foot collapse by virtue of its anatomical orientation and pure tensile stiffness. The plantar aponeurosis originates from the medial tubercle at the base of the calcaneus, and although there are medial and lateral components, the central component extends distally via its digital slips to the bases of all the metatarsals to the proximal phalanges. Stretch tension from the plantar fascia prevents excessive spreading of the calcaneus and the metatarsals, and maintains the medial longitudinal arch (Fuller, 2000; Sarrafian, 1987; Viel and Esnault, 1989). The well-recognized 'Windlass mechanism' intrinsically associated with the plantar fascia gives stability to the arches during ambulation (Hicks, 1954). The main Windlass mechanism begins as extension of the hallux at the first metatarsophalangeal joint occurs during the propulsive phase of gait. Extension of this joint during propulsion winds the plantar fascia around the head of the metatarsal and, because of its resistance against tensile stress, functionally shortens the distance between the calcaneus and metatarsals to elevate the medial longitudinal arch. This results in a more rigid foot which is better for propulsion (Fuller, 2000; Kwong *et al.*, 1988; Lombardi *et al.*, 2002; Sammarco and Hockenbury, 2001; Sarrafian, 1987; Whiting and Zernicke, 1998). Activation of tibialis posterior during this phase of gait provides additional support medially as it helps to lift the arch (Basmajian and Stecko, 1963). Similarly, it has been proposed that at heel strike, where the foot and toes are actively dorsiflexed, contraction of the tibialis anterior, extensor digitorum longus and extensor hallucis brevis may serve to help initiate the Windlass mechanism and increase medial arch height to increase potential to absorb GRF (Caravaggi *et al.*, 2001).

Depending on the presentation of the longitudinal arches, individuals can be grouped into different categories. These categories, which can be considered predisposing risk factors for certain injuries, are based on the height of the medial longitudinal arch and are referred to as 'normal' (average), pes planus ('flat foot'), or pes cavus ('high arch') (Neeley, 1998). These latter presentations can also be described as being flexible or rigid, respectively. With pes cavus, the midfoot does not make contact with the ground during standing or gait and will typically exhibit limited eversion or inversion. The pes planus foot is more characteristically hypermobile, often exhibiting overpronation; this can lead to a weakening of the medial side of the ankle, foot splaying, and an increased risk of plantar fasciopathy (Gill, 1997; Hamill and Knutzen,

2009). Both pes cavus and planus presentations demonstrate reduced shock absorbing capacity and have been shown to be a risk factor for recurrent lower limb stress fractures in athletes (Korpalainen *et al.*, 2001).

Retinaculum of the ankle and foot region

There are several retinacula of the foot and ankle. These are thickened bands of fascia which serve to help position, support and prevent translation of anatomic structures, such as tendons, blood vessels and nerves. At the distal lower leg and ankle there are extensor, flexor and peroneal retinacula. The extensor retinaculum is subdivided into superior and inferior portions. The superior extensor retinaculum portion, sometimes named the transverse crural ligament, is situated on the distal anterolateral surface of the tibia. It attaches to the tibia medially, whereas laterally it attaches to the fibula. The inferior extensor retinaculum is a 'Y-shaped' band which prevents translation and the bow-stringing of several key ankle and foot extensor muscles. The stem of this Y-shaped structure attaches laterally, in front of the depression for the interosseous talocalcaneal ligament, on the upper surface of the calcaneus (Mahadevan, 2008a). The proximal band of the inferior extensor retinaculum attaches to the tibia, whereas the distal band extends medioinferiorly, and blends with the plantar fascia. The peroneus tertius, extensor digitorum longus, extensor hallucis longus and tibialis anterior all run under the extensor retinacula. The deep peroneal nerve and anterior tibial vessels also run beneath the extensor retinaculum.

On the lateral side of the ankle lie the superior and inferior peroneal (fibula) retinacula. These two structures are extremely important as they bind the sheath of peroneus longus and brevis in place during their course around the lateral calcaneus. The superior peroneal retinaculum originates at the lateral malleolus and attaches distally at the calcaneus; damage to this retinaculum can cause instability (and subluxation) of the peroneal tendons (Mahadevan, 2008a). The attachment of the inferior peroneal retinaculum at one end blends with the inferior extensor retinaculum; at the other end, it attaches inferolaterally at the calcaneus.

The flexor retinaculum of the ankle and foot prevents translation of the tibialis posterior, flexor digitorum longus and flexor hallucis longus as they pass inferiorly to the medial malleolus towards the plantar surface of the foot. The posterior tibial artery and nerve also run beneath the flexor retinaculum (in the 'tarsal tunnel') as they too pass towards the plantar surface of the foot. The flexor retinaculum originates from the medial malleolus and attaches inferiorly at the medial calcaneus.

Muscular anatomy of the ankle and foot region

Gross movements of the ankle are provided by four muscle groups which can be classified simply as: plantarflexors, dorsiflexors, evertors and invertors. The plantarflexors include the gastrocnemius, flexor digitorum longus, peroneus longus, plantaris, soleus and tibialis posterior. The gastrocnemius muscle is separated into medial and lateral bellies. The two heads of gastrocnemius originate on the posterior aspect of the medial and lateral epicondyles of the femur, respectively. The medial and lateral heads of gastrocnemius merge at the musculotendinous junction (MTJ) and continue via the Achilles tendon to insert at the posterior surface of calcaneous. The gastrocnemius shares this insertion with the soleus muscle, which lies deep to both the medial and lateral heads.

The soleus originates on the upper third of the posterior shaft of the fibula, the posterior surface of the head of the fibula and the popliteal line and middle third of the medial border of the tibia. It merges deep to the gastrocnemius to insert into the calcaneus via the Achilles

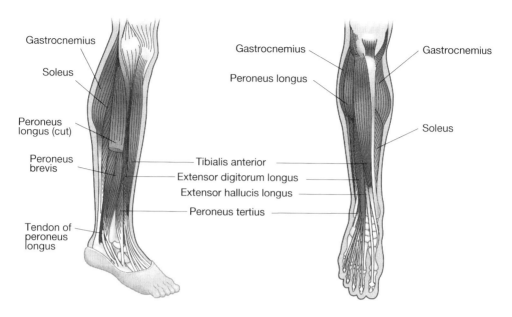

Figure 11.3 Muscular anatomy: anterolateral and anterior (source: adapted from Sewell *et al.*, 2013).

tendon. Since both the gastrocnemius and soleus (muscles capable of extremely large contraction forces) merge into the Achilles, the tendon itself is required to be extremely resistant to load. It has been shown to withstand loads of over 5,000 N prior to rupture. Together, gastrocnemius and soleus, combined with plantaris, are sometimes referred to as the triceps surae, meaning three-headed muscle (Marieb and Hoehn, 2009). Plantaris is the short, thin muscle attached laterally just above the knee between the gastrocnemius and soleus muscles. The proximal attachment is on the posterior surface of the lateral epicondyle of the femur, while its distal attachment is at the posterior surface of the calcaneus. The muscle belly of the plantaris is approximately one-third of the length of the gastrocnemius, with its tendon making up the majority of the length. It has been hypothesized that the plantaris could be vestigial; however, the large number of sensory organs within the muscle indicate a proprioceptive function providing a kinaesthetic sense of limb position and muscle contraction (Menton, 2000).

In addition to assisting ankle plantarflexion, flexor digitorum longus also facilitates interphalangeal flexion of the second to fifth toes. It is especially important for lower limb fine motor control, such as when standing on tiptoes or uneven surfaces, and manipulating objects on the ground with the plantar surface of the foot. Its origin is located on the middle third and posterior aspect of the tibia. The proximal tendon of flexor digitorum longus enters a synovial sheath prior to passing posteriorly and inferiorly to the medial malleolus. The sheath reduces friction and allows the tendon to move more freely. Both the tendon and the sheath run beneath the flexor retinaculum before the tendon exits the sheath on the plantar surface of the foot. The tendon then diverges to attach to the distal phalanx of each of the four lesser toes. The final posterior lower leg muscle is flexor hallucis longus; its origin is at the lower two-thirds, posterior aspect of the fibula, and its insertion is at the base of the distal phalanx of the first toe. In addition to being responsible for interphalangeal flexion, it also contributes to plantarflexion.

The peroneus (fibularis) longus is primarily an everter of the foot; it also contributes to plantarflexion. It is an important stabilizer of the ankle during standing and ambulation. Delayed activation of this muscle is associated with functional ankle instability (Donahue *et al.*, 2013). It originates from the lateral proximal surface of the tibia and the upper two-thirds of the lateral aspect of the fibula. The distal tendon of peroneus longus begins slightly superiorly to the lateral malleolus, surrounded by a tendinous sheath. It runs behind the lateral malleolus beneath the superior fibular retinaculum, and exits the sheath anteroinferiorly to pass by the peroneal trochlea. The insertions of peroneus longus are at the inferior aspect of the foot, medial cuneiform and the first metatarsal. Peroneus brevis, like longus, contributes to eversion and plantarflexion. Its origin is the lower two-thirds of the lateral aspect of the fibula, and its insertion is at the inferolateral aspect of the base of the fifth metatarsal. The peroneus tertius muscle in humans, although sometimes absent, is believed to be important for bipedal walking and running. The lack of peroneus tertius in other primates, and the variance in insertion point in humans, are believed to highlight this evolutionary adaptation required necessary for bipedal locomotion (Jana and Roy, 2011; Jungers *et al.*, 1993). Because of its path distally from the fibula to the fifth metatarsal over (rather than below) the lateral malleolus, peroneus tertius contributes to eversion and dorsiflexion. During walking and running gait, peroneus tertius contracts along with extensor digitorum longus during the swing phase to level the foot and help the toes clear the ground (Jungers *et al.*, 1993). Its origin is located on the lower third of the anterolateral surface of the fibula, and most frequently inserts to the superior aspect of foot, at the base of the fifth metatarsal.

Tibialis posterior is the primary dynamic stabilizer of the medial longitudinal arch of the foot and is important in maintaining optimal foot posture (Basmajian and Stecko, 1963). It performs this function by combining plantarflexion with inversion, which serves to lift the medial longitudinal arch (Kohls-Gatzoulis *et al.*, 2004). It originates at the middle third of the posterolateral surface of the tibia and the middle third of the posteromedial surface of the fibula, while its insertions are located at the plantar surface of the foot – the lower inner surfaces of the navicular, the three cuneiforms and the second and third metatarsals. Similarly to flexor digitorum longus, the tibialis posterior tendon enters a synovial sheath prior to passing the medial malleolus, and runs beneath the flexor retinaculum. It exits its sheath on the plantar surface of the foot.

The talocrural dorsiflexors are composed of tibialis anterior, peroneus tertius, extensor digitorum longus and extensor hallucis longus. Tibialis anterior is responsible for dorsiflexion and inversion, and has origins on the lateral condyle of tibia and the upper two-thirds of the anterolateral aspect of the tibia. Its tendon enters a synovial sheath at the distal tibia, just distal to its musculotendinous junction. This sheath spans across the talocrural joint running beneath both the superior and inferior extensor retinaculum. The distal tendon exits its sheath as it passes the talus, and inserts to the medial cuneiform and first metatarsal.

Adjacent to tibialis anterior, extensor digitorum longus has origins on the lateral condyle of the tibia and the upper three-quarters of the anterior aspect of the fibula and interosseous membrane; it continues distally across the talocrural joint and along the superior aspect of the foot. The insertions of extensor digitorum longus are at the middle and distal phalanges of the four lesser toes. It is linked to three types of movement; extension of the four lesser toes, dorsiflexion and eversion.

Extensor hallucis longus is responsible for both dorsiflexion and extension of the great toe; it will also contribute to eversion. Its origin is on the middle aspect of the anterior fibula; its insertions are at the superior aspect of the foot, and base of the distal phalanx of the great toe. As with tibialis anterior, both extensor digitorum longus and extensor hallucis longus run beneath the superior and inferior extensor retinaculum; these two muscles enter their synovial sheaths more distally along the tibia and exit on the dorsum of the midfoot.

The smaller, intrinsic musculature of the foot contribute to general foot function and arch stability, as well as specific toe flexion, extension, abduction and adduction. These include: extensor digitorum brevis, extensor hallucis brevis, flexor digitorum brevis, flexor hallucis brevis, abductor hallucis, adductor hallucis, abductor digiti minimi, flexor digiti minimi, quadratus plantae, the dorsal and plantar interossei and the first to fifth lumbricals (Mahadevan, 2008a).

Neural anatomy of the ankle and foot region

There are six primary peripheral nerves associated with motor and sensory functions of the lower leg, ankle and foot; these all extend from the sciatic nerve. They are: the tibial nerve (L4–S1); the common peroneal nerve (L4–S1); the superficial peroneal nerve (L4–S1); the deep peroneal nerve (L4–S1); the lateral plantar nerve (S2–3); and the medial plantar nerve (L5–S3). Mahadevan (2008b) provides important detailed overview of the cutaneous distributions of the main peripheral nerves and their segments of origin.

Approximately 4–7 cm above the posterior knee (the bifurcation is variable), the sciatic nerve divides into large tibial and common peroneal branches (Mahadevan, 2008b). The tibial nerve passes between the heel and medial malleolus in the tarsal tunnel; its branches innervate gastrocnemius, soleus, plantaris, tibialis posterior, flexor digitorum longus, and flexor hallucis longus. The tibial nerve divides under the flexor retinaculum into the medial and lateral plantar nerves. The medial plantar nerve innervates flexor digitorum brevis, flexor hallucis brevis, abductor hallucis and the first lumbrical. The lateral plantar nerve serves abductor digiti minimi, flexor digiti minimi, adductor hallucis, the interossei, and the second to fourth lumbrical muscles (Hamill and Knutzen, 2009; Marieb and Hoehn, 2009; Oatis, 2009).

Laterally on the lower leg, just inferior to the fibular head, the common peroneal nerve divides into the superficial and deep peroneal nerves. The superficial branch innervates the peroneus longus and brevis, and continues to serve some of the smaller intrinsic foot muscles; the deep branch innervates tibialis anterior, extensor digitorum longus, extensor hallucis longus, peroneus tertius and some intrinsic muscles.

Circulatory anatomy

The foot is served by a complex network of arteries, veins and lymphatic vessels which work to maintain blood perfusion and allow drainage. The posterior tibial artery passes under the medial malleolus in the tarsal tunnel, where it sits between the tendons of flexor digitorum longus and flexor hallucis longus; its pulse can be palpated here. The dorsalis pedis artery of the foot is a continuation of the anterior tibial artery (itself derived initially from the femoral artery, and then the popliteal artery) and arises at the anterior aspect of the ankle joint midway between the malleoli (Mahadevan, 2008b). This vessel extends along the tibial side of the dorsum of the foot and terminates at the posterior aspect of the first intermetarsal space. Here, it divides into two branches, the first dorsal metatarsal artery and the deep plantar artery. The dorsalis pedis artery is also clinically important in assessing peripheral circulation; its pulse can be palpated just lateral to the tendon of extensor hallucis longus at the distal part of the navicular. The medial and lateral plantar arteries are continuations of the posterior tibial artery; these divisions start beneath the origin of adductor hallucis and pass forward medially and laterally, respectively (Mahadevan, 2008b). The medial plantar artery extends forwards beneath the abductor hallucis and then, further along, passes between both the abductor hallucis and the flexor digitorum brevis. The artery divides into three digital arteries at the base of the first metatarsal, which then continue to form the common digital arteries. The lateral plantar artery, much larger than the medial artery, runs anteriorly and laterally, first deep to the abductor hallucis and then deep to the flexor digitorum brevis muscle. At the base of the fifth metatarsal it then turns medially to the interval between the bases of the first and second metatarsal bones and completes the dorsal arch by joining the deep plantar branch of the dorsalis pedis artery.

Venous drainage from the foot and ankle occurs via superficial and deep veins; the superficial veins are subcutaneous, while the deeper veins are subfascial (Mahadevan, 2008b). The main superficial veins (distal to proximal) are the dorsal venous arch (draining blood from the fore- and midfoot), and the short (lateral) and long (medial) saphenous veins; these drain into the larger, deeper femoral vein.

The lymphatics draining from the foot and ankle can also be divided into superficial and deep vessels. The superficial vessels mainly originate subcutaneously from the skin of the toes and the sole of the foot and heel; these can be divided further into medial and lateral systems which eventually drain into the superficial inguinal lymph nodes (at the groin) and the popliteal lymph nodes (at the knee), respectively. The deeper vessels can be further subdivided into dorsalis pedis and anterior tibialis lymphatics, plantar and posterior tibialis lymphatics and peroneal lymphatics. All three of these channels terminate at the popliteal lymph nodes (Kelikian and Sarrafian, 2011).

Assessment of the ankle and foot region

A systematic approach to clinical assessment ensures the investigation is thorough, while minimizing the possibility of missing any important information. The effectiveness of assessment is dependent upon the sports therapist having a solid theoretical underpinning and also being well-practised. A thorough discussion of fundamental principles and generic components of the clinical assessment process is presented in Chapter 2; this includes an overview of gait assessment.

When first assessing any patient/athlete complaining of ankle or foot pain, and obviously depending upon the background and subjective history, early considerations might include whether there is a possibility that they have one of the more common conditions, such as: calf muscle tear; lateral ankle ligament sprain; peroneal tendon subluxation; mid-portion Achilles tendinopathy; plantar fasciopathy; neural entrapment; or a metatarsal stress fracture. The sports therapist will also be able to consider the possibility of other musculotendinous or ligamentous injuries, as well as whether a less common condition, serious underlying pathology or possible psychosocial issue is present. The aim of the completed assessment is to identify which structures are affected, the aetiology of the problem, the current symptoms and severity, the functional deficits, and the additional individual factors which can influence management and recovery.

The SOAP model (i.e. subjective; objective; assessment; plan) provides a valuable standardized approach for assessment. The subjective aspect is where information is carefully obtained from the patient/athlete, with any appropriate additional information gathered from previous medical notes or athlete screening (Magee, 2008; Petty, 2011). The subjective history provides a narrative to the patient's chief complaint. It must aim to include: information regarding the mechanism with which the injury occurred (mechanism of injury – MoI); the severity, irritability and nature (SIN) of the injury; main aggravating and easing factors; and relevant features of the patient's previous medical history. In completing the subjective assessment, the sports therapist should have formulated a differential diagnosis and clinical impression (hypothesis) of the nature of the complaint. The objective assessment then aims to confirm (or refute) this, and characteristically includes the undertaking of reliable, valid, measurable and repeatable physical examination techniques applicable to the presenting complaint. This will incorporate the assessment and recording of active, passive and resisted ranges of movement, palpation, and the patient response to specific special tests; the sequence and specifics of these will be clinically reasoned with reference to the individual's subjective history. The results from the subjective and objective assessment are used to inform the overall assessment and analysis of findings, which then provides information for diagnosis and a guide to formulate a set of goals (short and long term) and a resulting plan of action (for specific therapeutic intervention and rehabilitation).

While establishing an accurate patient diagnosis is important, sometimes this is challenging (such as when the athlete presents with an acutely inflamed condition), hence the ability to identify key patient symptoms, limitations and problems are an equally valuable feature of an effective patient assessment. However, an accurate diagnosis is important, for several reasons; first, it allows the practitioner to consider a working prognosis for their patient; second, it allows the practitioner to prescribe accurate and effective treatment; and third, it allows the practitioner to create an accurate and effective rehabilitation plan. On occasions where an exact diagnosis cannot be made, specific pathologies can still usually be ruled out and abnormalities identified. Both establishing and addressing the patient-centred concerns and goals have been shown to be important features of patient satisfaction with treatment overall.

Subjective assessment of the ankle and foot

The standard approach for assessing a patient begins with a detailed subjective assessment. This is an extremely important section of an assessment as it forms the basis for the other features of patient assessment. By the end of the subjective assessment the practitioner should have an idea of the following: the patient's functional abilities; the MoI; their symptoms; levels of irritation and ease; potential contraindications or precautions; their general expectations; and list of hypotheses that are most likely.

Establishing the SIN factors is an important feature of subjective assessment. This information can be used to generate a baseline against which to measure improvement, and plays an important part in planning the objective assessment. For example, it is better to wait until the end of the objective assessment to attempt movements which result in relatively high amounts of pain and take a long time to return to normal levels. When completing the subjective assessment for the ankle or foot area, particular attention should be paid to establishing a precise MoI. Injuries associated with an acute onset may be more traumatic in nature, whereas injuries with a more insidious onset are more likely due to repetitive trauma. The position that the ankle was in when the injury occurred or is most symptomatic is also of importance. Forced movements at end of range in the frontal plane often result in injury to the contralateral side. For example, inversion injuries are more likely to relate to lateral structures suffering damage, and eversion injuries are more likely to relate to the medial structures being implicated. Foot position may also indicate which type of structures are implicated; if an injury occurs when the foot is in dorsiflexion, it is more likely to relate to bone, whereas injuries that occur in plantarflexion are more likely to cause ligamentous injury. Where an external rotation force is indicated, particularly in combination with dorsiflexion, it is possible that a syndesmotic injury is implicated. The amount of force is also a key factor in determining which structures are affected, with soft tissue injuries often being associated with low forces and bony injuries being associated with higher forces, such as with high impacts and high accelerations (Birrer *et al.*, 1999). The patient should be asked questions regarding the intensity of the force, the general conditions in which they found themselves, the terrain, their footwear and the condition of their ankle or foot both before and immediately after the incident.

Practitioner Tip Box 11.3

Common ankle and foot injury mechanisms to consider

Bone injury?	Ligament injury?
Foot was dorsiflexed	Foot was plantarflexed or inverted
High velocities were involved (>20 mph)	Low velocities were involved (<20 mph)
Fall from a height	

Practitioner Tip Box 11.4

Common sports-related ankle and foot injuries

Sport	Injury
American football	Achilles tendinopathy; plantar fasciopathy; ATFL sprain
Basketball	Achilles tendinopathy, plantar fasciopathy; ATFL sprain
Gymnastics	ATFL sprain; stress fractures
Long/triple jump	Achilles tendinopathy/rupture; navicular stress fractures
Tennis	Calf muscle tear; ATFL sprain; plantar fasciopathy
Running	Achilles tendinopathy; plantar fasciopathy; tibial stress fracture; fifth metatarsal stress fracture; tarsal tunnel syndrome
Football	Achilles tendinopathy; plantar fasciopathy; ATFL sprain; tenosynovitis; osteochondritis; extensor retinacula tear; turf toe

---

The potential for re-injury at the ankle is particularly high. It is therefore important to question the patient/athlete on any previous injuries affecting the area; previous ligamentous injuries, fractures, tendinopathies and repetitive muscle tears are significant. Due to possible weakening of the joint attributed to certain health conditions, these should also be noted and discussed; particularly conditions such as osteoporosis, arthritis, diabetes, hyperthyroidism, as well as the use of any steroid or seizure medications.

During the subjective assessment questions should be directed towards the patient/athlete in regards to their everyday and recreational activities which may contribute to the injury. Epidemiological studies have shown many sports to have common injuries specific to the activity demands (Birrer *et al.*, 1999). Hence, once the sport or activity has been identified, considerations need to be made with regards to the sport's demands globally and locally to the ankle and foot, while also considering the intensity of training, direction of forces and the associated intrinsic and extrinsic risk factors. These considerations need to be made not only with regards to the requirements of any particular sport, but also to the specifics of the athlete's position within that sport.

It is important for the sports therapist to ascertain the behaviour of symptoms, and to investigate which factors aggravate them in comparison to which factors ease them. Common aggravating factors for ankle and foot injuries include simply weight bearing or walking, but also prolonged standing, pivoting, inclines, heel raises, running or jumping (Loudon *et al.*, 2008). Other significant questions include the length of time that it takes for the symptoms to be produced and, once irritated, how long it takes for the symptoms to ease. These questions will aid the practitioner in confirmation of symptom relationship while also providing information regarding how irritable the condition is and therefore what order to perform movements in the physical examination. The therapist could also use this opportunity to discuss with the patient the overall nature of the pain, such as ascertaining whether symptoms refer to other regions, and whether any neurological symptoms such as anaesthesia or paraesthesia are present.

In general, the subjective assessment of the injury is an important process in diagnosing and treating injuries. Information in the subjective assessment helps to generate hypotheses regarding what the injury may be and incriminates structures by behaviour. This part of the assessment also aids in giving direction to the objective assessment. Importantly, the subjective assessment also identifies the patient/athlete's current functional ability alongside their expectations, and therefore gives indications of areas to consider when looking at the aims of the treatment plan. In a majority of situations the subjective assessment will provide a relilable working hypothesis, or at least allow certain pathologies to be ruled out.

Objective assessment of the foot and ankle

The objective assessment is a physical examination. It is essential at this point that a thorough subjective assessment has already been undertaken; there should already be in the therapist's mind key conditions that relate to their patient, and the subjective assessment should have a direction for the physical examination. The methods and test procedures used should be measurable, valid and repeatable. It is of utmost importance that all tests carried out are documented, and that the results and implications of these are understood. This allows for information to be used when undertaking follow-up reassessment and continuation of treatments, and also for any forms of communication which may be required.

The physical examination should be logical and systematic; however, this approach is flexible and is dependent upon the therapist's experience, the patient's presenting symptoms and their irritability. The level of function of the patient or their irritability are major factors influencing how the assessment is performed, and may affect the order in which tests are carried out, or whether specific tests are included or excluded. Responsibility for the thoroughness and accuracy in assessment lies with the sports therapist; therefore a firmly justified rationale for their approach is required (Magee, 2008; Petty, 2011; Shultz et al., 2000).

The physical examination should start with the uninvolved limb, which will provide a baseline or set of norms for the practitioner for that specific patient. While assessing the involved limb, the physical examination should progress from pain-free areas to the specific area affected. This will increase the amount and accuracy of information that the clinician gains from the examination (Birrer et al., 1999). Similarly, the assessment should progress from the movements which aggravate injury the least through to those that aggravate the most. If the practitioner

Practitioner Tip Box 11.5

Clinically reasoning the objective assessment

If, during subjective assessment, the patient highlights particular movements that cause irritation, the sports therapist should assess these movements last in the objective assessment. Care must be taken to avoid exacerbation of symptoms and possible clouding of findings.

causes too much irritation early on in the assessment it may blur the results and give an untrue representation of the condition, leading to confusion for the practitioner or misdiagnosis.

Observation of the ankle and foot

Observation begins as soon as the practitioner sees the patient; this is of particular importance when assessing the ankle and foot problems relating to their gait. An antalgic gait or limp, characterized by apprehension and reduced weight bearing on the affected foot, can give an indication as to the severity of the injury. Similarly, gait abnormalities such as reduced plantarflexion at toe-off, or hip circumduction (arthralgic compensation), may be indicative of functional impairments which could be contributing to the patient's pathology. The clinician should also pay attention to details such as quality of movement, where the movement is occurring and the facial expressions of the patient. It is also beneficial to note the patient's stance, posture, body type, approach to movement and general body language. The patient is observed throughout the assessment process, with particular attention being paid to their facial expressions in response to the tests. The sports therapist must ensure that the patient is suitably dressed, exposing their toes, feet, ankles, shins, knees and thighs, and that they are able to access landmarks around the pelvis. If the patient is able to stand, the therapist should remember to not only focus their observations on the ankle and foot, but also up the lower kinetic chain to the ankle, knee, hip and pelvis. Both hip and knee presentations, whether with internal rotation, external rotation, genu valgus or varus, have a direct link with ankle and foot function. It is important to note whether the forefoot or rearfoot are overpronated with pes planus ('flat foot'), typically with a 'navicular drop' or valgus heel presentation, or supinated with pes cavus (high-arched, rigid foot); also whether there is any hallux valgus or hammer toe. The therapist should note any abnormalities of the skin, acknowledging any abrasions, lacerations, discolouration (bruising or reddening), oedema, callouses, corns, scarring or other conditions. It is also significant to note whether the patient can load bear fully, bilaterally, unilaterally, statically and/or dynamically.

Clearing tests for the ankle and foot

When assessing the ankle and foot it is obviously essential to establish whether the problem is due to injury or dysfunction at the ankle or foot, or if it originates further up the kinetic chain (i.e. the knee, hip or lumbosacral regions). Usually, following observations, these related regions should be cleared before local assessment. Clearing may simply involve standard active range of movement (ARoM) plus overpressure if asymptomatic. If during the subjective assessment it has been highlighted that neural tissue may possibly be implicated in the condition presented, then the lumbar spine may be initially cleared via ARoM plus overpressure, or use of quadrant

---

Practitioner Tip Box 11.6

Footwear inspection

Footwear should be inspected for any areas of localized wear – which may be indicative of underlying biomechanical issues. Additionally, the sports therapist should ascertain if the patient/ athlete's training shoes are appropriate for the intended function.

(combination) movements as these are considered more provocative. Further regional assessment may be required if symptoms are reproduced; similarly, further assessment of the peripheral nervous system may be required. Functional movements, such as the squat, can also help in clearing associated regions (Petty, 2011).

Active movement assessment of the ankle and foot

When completing physical examination of this region it is valuable to consider the position of the knee joint, particularly with regard to the attachment sites of the gastrocnemius. The position of the knee will have an effect on the RoM of the ankle. Also, while the foot is statically and kinetically reliant on the ankle – which in turn is reliant on the tibia – the tibia, fibula and femur should also be considered during the assessment. When the therapist assesses the active movements of the ankle and foot it is important that they observe for the quality, range and symptom reproduction. Any compensatory movements, jerks or shakes should be noted during each movement. If, once the patient has reached their end of range, no pain is reported, then overpressure should be applied; this enables appreciation of the end-feel of the joint and for any symptom production in that position.

The therapist can measure the full available ARoM via use of a goniometer. This provides an objective measure and allows for assessment of improvement during the session or in follow-up sessions (Petty, 2011). The main movements to assess are plantarflexion, dorsiflexion, inversion and eversion; however, for conditions involving the mid- and forefoot, movements involving the joints of this region will need to be assessed. The order in which movements are completed is dependent primarily on the findings from the subjective assessment.

Practitioner Tip Box 11.7

Rearfoot versus forefoot goniometry

Cailliet (1997) indicates that the RoM of the ankle joint should be assessed by measuring movement of the calcaneus – and that observing movement at the forefoot may result in false readings.

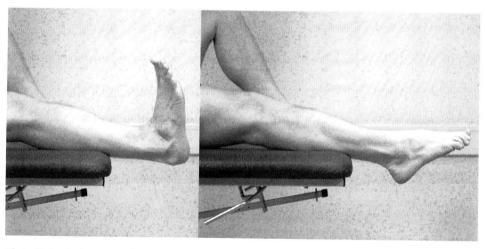

Photo 11.3   Active range of movement assessment: dorsiflexion and plantarflexion.

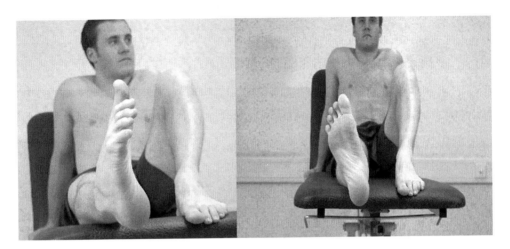

Photo 11.4   Active range of movement assessment: inversion and eversion.

Passive range of movement assessment of the ankle and foot

Passive physiological movements are completed by the practitioner. In order for the passive assessment to be accurate, the patient is required to fully relax and the practitioner is required to confidently move the selected joint. The passive section of the objective assessment tests the integrity of the joint and other associated non-contractile structures. At end of range, the practitioner should note that contractile structures can become stretched and hence may become more symptomatic. The patient is best positioned on the couch for this aspect of the assessment.

For dorsiflexion of the talocrural joint, the therapist may cup the heel of the foot with one hand, and use their forearm along the sole of the patient's foot to apply pressure and force the joint into dorsiflexion. Plantarflexion can be achieved with the same positioning, with the added application of the other hand over the top of the forefoot. In order to assess the inversion and eversion in the subtalar joint the lower leg should be held in one hand while the practitioner's other hand holds the calcaneus in a dorsiflexed position. This will fix the talus in the mortise of the tibia/fibula, preventing any medial and lateral rotation and allowing for more precise movement of the subtalar joint (Cailliet, 1997). To test the metatarsal joints, the therapist should hold the calcaneus with one hand while their other hand grasps the forefoot above the metatarsal joint. The therapist then pronates, supinates, adducts and abducts the patient's forefoot.

Testing of the movements between the individual metatarsals and cuneiforms or cuboid requires each to be tested individually. This is completed by the practitioner fixing with one hand above the tarsometatarsal (TMT) joint while grasping with their free hand the individual metatarsals. The base of the second metatarsal only allows plantarflexion and dorsiflexion, the third to fifth metatarsals plantar- and dorsiflexion while also allowing a counteracting rotation to the first metatarsal (Cailliet, 1997).

The assessment of the toes can be carried out by the therapist fixing the forefoot just above the metatarsalphalangeal (MTP) joint of the selected toe, and using their other hand to fix the proximal phalanx between their index finger and thumb. The therapist is then able to move the joint through flexion, extension, abduction and adduction. At the interphalangeal (IP) joints the therapist can fix the proximal phalanx with one hand's index finger and thumb grasping the middle phalanx, and with their other hand's finger and thumb they can then apply flexion and extension to the joint. This technique can then be applied to the distal IP joint. It is important

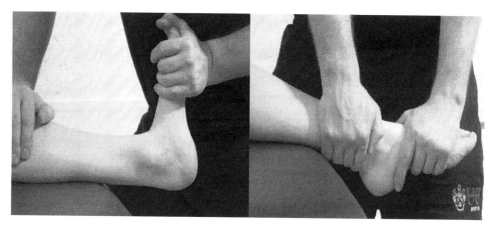

Photo 11.5 Passive range of movement assessment: dorsiflexion and plantarflexion.

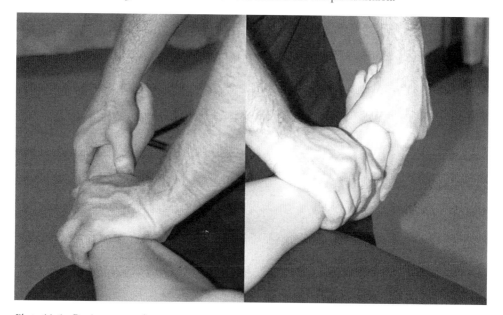

Photo 11.6 Passive range of movement assessment: inversion and eversion.

to note that the subjective assessment will dictate in which order to carry out the movements, especially if the patient's condition is highly irritable.

Accessory movement assessment of the ankle and foot

The accessory movements of the ankle and foot occur within joints during normal gross physiological movements, but cannot be performed actively in isolation. Therapists are able to test the range and quality of accessory movements, essentially attempting to identify the presence of normal motion, restriction (stiffness or resistance through range), pain or provocation of muscle spasm or any other symptom response. As a general rule, the sports therapist will usually fix (stabilize) the proximal segment, and then assess the mobility of the distal segment. At the inferior tibiofibular (syndesmosis) joint, the main accessory movements to test are anteroposterior

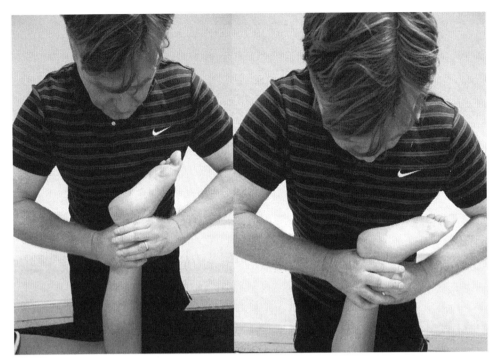

Photo 11.7 Accessory movement assessment: anteroposterior and posteroanterior glides of the talus.

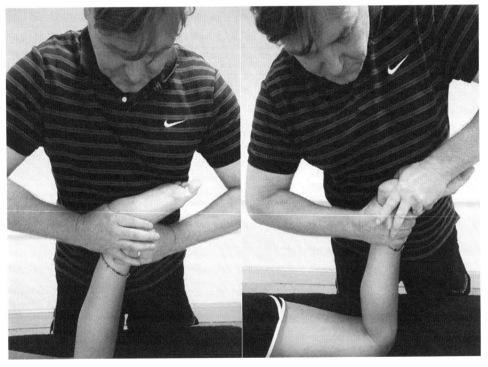

Photo 11.8 Accessory movement assessment: posteroanterior and anteroposterior glides of the calcaneus.

and posteroanterior glides of the fibula (via passive movement of the lateral malleolus). At the talocrural joint, distraction of the talus, anteroposterior, and posteroanterior glides of the talus may be tested. At the subtalar joint, the main accessory movements to test are: distraction (caudad glide) of the calcaneus; anteroposterior and posteroanterior glides of the calcaneus; and medial and lateral glides of the calcaneus. At the tarsometatarsal joints, the main accessory movements are anteroposterior and posteroanterior glides of the bases of the metatarsals. At the metatarsophalangeal joints, the main accessory movements are anteroposterior and posteroanterior glides of the bases of the phalanges. At the interphalangeal joints the main accessory movements are anteroposterior and posteroanterior glides of the bases of the phalanges. Passive, accessory rotations (medial and lateral) may also be assessed at the tarsometatarsal, metatarsophalangeal and interphalangeal joints.

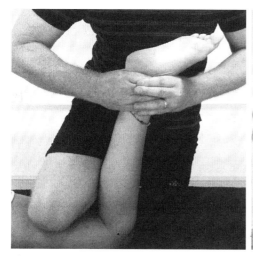

Photo 11.9 Accessory movement assessment: distraction of the calcaneus.

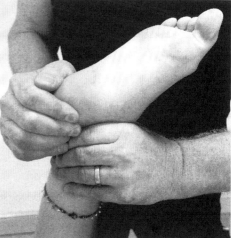

Photo 11.10 Accessory movement assessment: medial glide of the calcaneus.

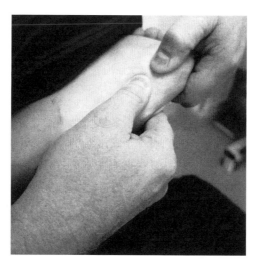

Photo 11.11 Accessory movement assessment: anteroposterior or posteroanterior glide of a metatarsal head.

Resisted movement assessment of the foot and ankle

Resisted testing of the ankle and foot should ideally be carried out in the same order that the active and passive movement tests were carried out so as to avoid over-irritation of the patient's condition. This section of the assessment allows the therapist to test the contractile structures in the area, and provides opportunity to identify any pain on contraction (possibly indicating injury to the musculotendinous unit) or any decrease in expected strength. Resisted dorsiflexion, plantarflexion inversion and eversion of the ankle, and flexion, extension, abduction and adduction of the toes are the main movements which can be tested. The joint will normally be placed in a mid-range position of the movement being tested; and an isometric test is usually performed before any isotonic testing. Confident handling and clear instructions are required, and the therapist should aim to gradually increment the resistance so as to avoid unnecessary stress to the affected tissues. Due to the expected strength of the gastrocnemius, it is sometimes more appropriate to test the resisted strength in a functional manner; this can be achieved by asking the patient/athlete to stand on their tip toes, and can be performed both bilaterally and unilaterally, depending on their functional ability. The sports therapist should grade the patient's strength according to the Oxford Grading Scale (OGS) or Modified Medical Research Council Scale, both of which score the strength output on a scale of 0–5 (0/5 if no contraction is produced; and 5/5 if normal, full strength is observed).

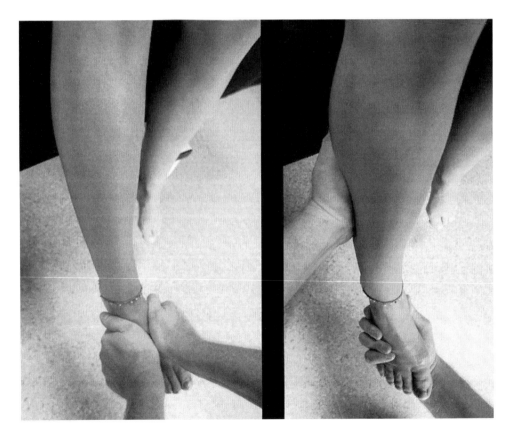

Photo 11.12 Resisted range of movement assessment: dorsiflexion and plantarflexion.

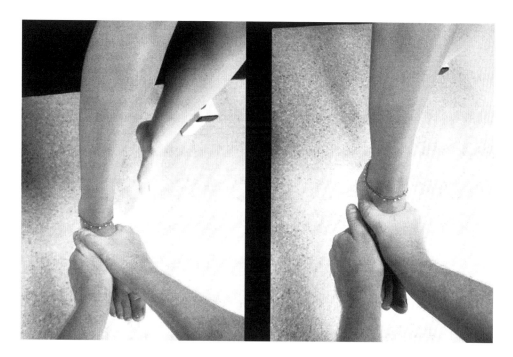

Photo 11.13   Resisted range of movement assessment: inversion and eversion.

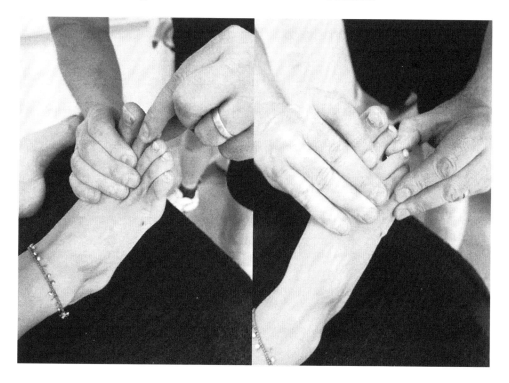

Photo 11.14   Resisted range of movement assessment: interphalangeal flexion and extension; and abduction and adduction.

Muscle length tests of the foot and ankle

Assessment of muscle/myofascial length is an important feature of the objective assessment; abnormally lengthened myofascia may indicate muscle imbalance and inhibition or functional weakness, whereas shortened myofascia indicates functional tightness and potential over-activity (Kendall *et al.*, 2005). Such findings can help the therapist decide whether weakened muscles need to be re-trained, or shortened muscles lengthened, in order to bring about a positive change. While assessing the functional length of ankle plantarflexors, it is important to appreciate differentiation between the biarticular and uniarticular muscles. Gastrocnemius is biarticular (affecting both the ankle and knee), hence its function (and length) is influenced by both ankle and knee positioning. Therefore, to differentiate, passive dorsiflexion of the ankle can be assessed with the knee in extension (for gastrocnemius) and flexion (for soleus). The discrepancy between these two methods demonstrates the degree to which biarticular muscles affect dorsiflexion; and this then influences the therapist's decision as to whether muscles need to be lengthened with the knee flexed or extended.

Special tests of the ankle and foot region

When selecting special tests it is important to remember that they are not a diagnostic tool as such – they are merely part of the process. Tests should be utilized to confirm or rule out what at this point the sports therapist already suspects; therefore there should be good clinical reasoning for any of the tests selected. It is also important to consider when compiling the special tests for selection that the therapist remembers that it is the quality rather than the quantity of tests selected. A larger quantity of tests can become counterproductive as they may reveal conflicting results, and can lead to confusion (Hattam and Smeatham, 2010). As with many motor skills, practise is essential to improve handling and increase accuracy. It is also important to remember that while many special tests have good evidence to support their use, they should be carefully selected for each particular patient presentation.

Ligament stress tests of the foot and ankle

Anterior talofibular ligament stress test

The anterior talofibular ligament (ATFL) stress test is utilized to detect a sprain. In the test described by Hattam and Smeatham (2010), the patient is positioned in long sitting and the therapist cups around the patient's calcaneus with one hand, and with their other hand grasps over the dorsal aspect of the foot (the medial border of their hand needs to fix closely over the talus to localize stress to the ATFL). In an initial position of slight calcaneal plantarflexion, the dorsal hand applies further plantarflexion and inversion to specifically stress the ligament. A positive test would be indicated by the presence of pain over the lateral aspect of the ankle and/or joint laxity.

Practitioner Tip Box 11.8

Stress testing the ATFL is more accurate when the acute swelling phase has passed.

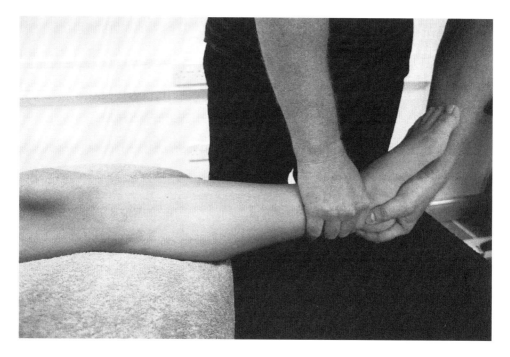

Photo 11.15 Anterior talofibular ligament stress test.

Calcaneofibular ligament stress test

This test is very similar to the talar tilt test, but with more emphasis on establishing end-feel in the presence of minor ligamentous injury (Hattam and Smeatham, 2010). The patient is positioned as per the ATFL stress test, and the therapist again cups the calcaneus with one hand, and with their other hand they grasp around the dorsal ankle – this time with fingers fixing (neutral, 90°) over the talar dome and thumb under the sole. An inversion force is then applied from a plantargrade position to stress the ligament. A positive test is represented by pain over the lateral aspect of the ankle and/or joint laxity. The CFL is most tensioned in a position of dorsiflexion and inversion, and in this position, there is less tensioning of the ATFL.

Calcaneocubiod ligament stress test

The calcaneocuboid ligament (CCL) stress test is designed to detect a sprain of this complex. The CCL can be injured via adduction, inversion-type forces, and it is important to distinguish this from the more common inversion sprains. In the test described by Hattam and Smeatham (2010) the patient is again positioned in long sitting, and the therapist cups the calcaneus with one hand. With the other hand, the therapist grasps around the dorsal aspect of the foot, with the medial border (of the hand) just distal to the calcaneocuboid joint line. The calcaneus is stabilized in a neutral, plantargrade position (to negate tensioning of the ATFL and CFL) as the forefoot is moved into adduction and inversion. A positive test is detected through localized pain at the calcaneocuboid joint and lateral forefoot at end-range and/or joint laxity.

Practitioner Tip Box 11.9

Calcaneocuboid ligament stress test

In the CCL stress test, the calcaneus must be maintained in either a neutral, or slightly everted, position so as to avoid incrimination of the ATFL or CFL.

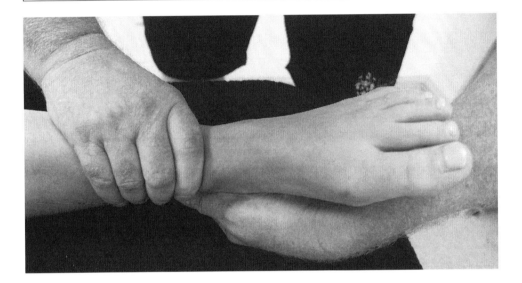

Photo 11.16   Calcaneofibular ligament stress test.

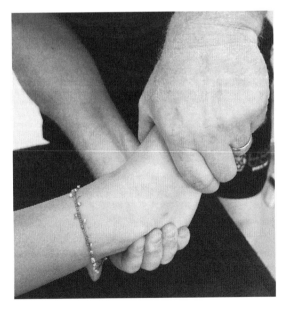

Photo 11.17   Calcaneocuboid ligament stress test.

Deltoid ligament stress test

The deltoid (or medial collateral ligament) stress test is devised to stress the deltoid ligament to detect sprain; it is most applicable to the assessment of superficial tissue damage – which may follow from a dorsiflexed, eversion-type force. The patient is positioned in either long sitting or supine-lying. The therapist cups the calcaneus with one hand, as their other hand then grasps around the dorsal foot with the medial border (of the hand) fixing over the navicular. With the ankle in a neutral, plantargrade position, the therapist imparts a valgus force to the calcaneus with their (calcaneal) hand, which is then reinforced with an eversion stress via their other (navicular) hand. A positive test is represented by local medial ankle pain (most likely at end-range) and/or excessive joint play (Hattam and Smeatham, 2010).

Practitioner Tip Box 11.10

The deltoid ligament is a strong and thickened fibrous sheet – the syndesmosis above or the medial malleolus can both be more vulnerable to injury than the ligament itself to sprain during forceful eversion stresses.

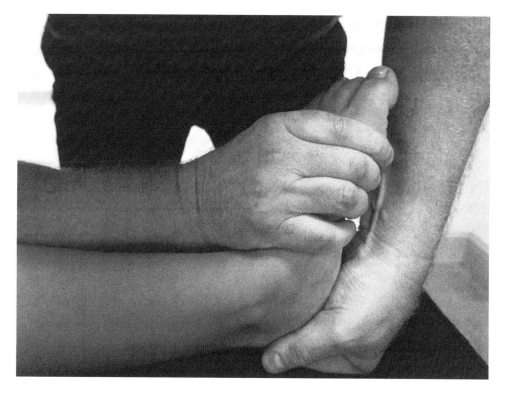

Photo 11.18   Deltoid ligament stress test.

Kleiger's test

Kleiger's (external rotation stress) test assesses injury to the inferior tibiofibular syndesmosis. In order to complete this test the patient is supine or seated on the couch with the knee of the affected leg flexed to 90°, the therapist grasps the patient's heel with one hand, and with the lower leg stabilized and the ankle placed in a neutral (plantargrade) position, a passive external rotation stress is applied to the foot. The test is deemed positive if pain is produced over the inferior tibiofibular joint (Cook and Hegedus, 2013; Hattam and Smeatham, 2010; Prentice, 2009).

Practitioner Tip Box 11.11

Approximately 10 per cent of all ankle sprains are syndesmotic ('high ankle sprain') injuries.

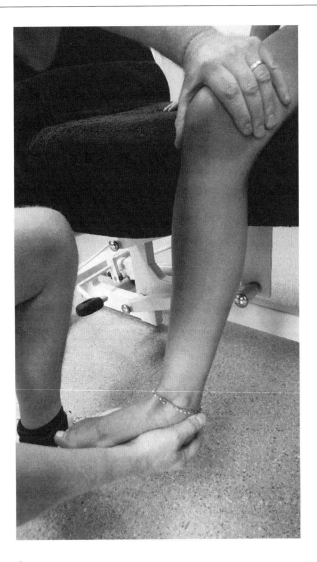

Photo 11.19   Kleiger's test.

Anterior drawer test

The anterior drawer test aims primarily to test the integrity of the ATFL and the degree of anterior talus displacement relative to the tibia (Cook and Hegedus, 2013); it may also implicate the CFL or inferior tibiofibular syndesmosis. There are a number of versions. In the test described by Hertel *et al.* (1999) and Magee (2008), the patient is supine, the therapist grasps under the heel of the foot, and with the ankle in plantarflexion (20°) an anterior glide of both the calcaneus and talus is performed. An inversion bias during the test increases the stress on the ATFL and CFL. Hattam and Smeatham (2010) describe a version where the patient is supine, with their knee flexed to 90° and their foot resting on the couch. While stabilizing the midfoot dorsally, the therapist then applies a downward and posterior movement to the distal, anterior tibia (in this version the tibia is moved backwards rather than the ankle being moved forwards). In both tests, the therapist observes for excessive displacement (on the lateral side of the joint), possible clunking and painful or absent end-feel, and also for a characteristic 'dimple' sign as the lateral malleolus is shifted posteriorly and the joint's negative pressure draws the superficial soft tissues inwards.

Talar tilt test

The talar tilt test is designed to test the integrity of the collateral ligaments (primarily CFL, and to a lesser degree the ATFL, laterally and deltoid ligament complex medially). In this test the patient is supine-lying, and the therapist fixes their distal lower leg at the malleoli with their proximal hand, and with their distal hand grasps the patient's heel (in a neutral, plantargrade position) and applies either inversion or eversion with due consideration to the end-feel and pain response. A difference in range of movement between the involved ankle and the normal joint (>5–10 per cent) is indicative of a sprain of the respective collateral ligaments (Birrer *et al.*, 1999; Cook and Hegedus, 2013; Hattam and Smeatham, 2010; Prentice, 2009).

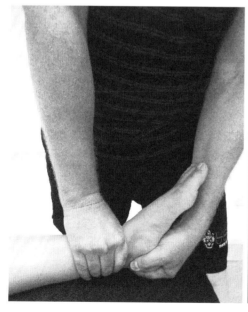
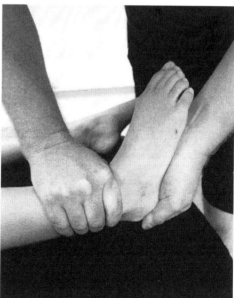

Photo 11.20 Anterior drawer test.　　*Photo 11.21* Talar tilt test.

Ottawa ankle rules

While a large proportion of ankle injury patients seen in A&E departments undergo ankle or foot radiographs, only a small percentage of these (15 per cent) demonstrate bony abnormalities (Stiell *et al.*, 1992a; 1992b). The Ottawa Ankle Rules (OAR) are evidence-based guidelines which can be used to highlight ankle patients who are unlikely to require radiography since they have negligible risk of fracture (Stiell *et al.*, 1992a; 1992b); and, conversely, can be important in guiding referral for such. The rules stipulate that an ankle X-ray series is only required if there is any pain in the malleolar zone and any one of the following: bony tenderness along the distal 6 cm of the posterior edge or tip of the medial malleolus; bony tenderness along the distal 6 cm of the posterior edge or tip of the lateral malleolus; or the patient demonstrates an inability to weight bear both immediately, or in the clinic, for four normal steps. The rules also suggest that a foot X-ray series is required only where there is any pain in the midfoot zone and any one of the following are present; bony tenderness at the base of the fifth metatarsal; bony tenderness at the navicular bone; and again, where the patient demonstrates an inability to weight bear immediately after injury, or in the clinic, for four normal steps (Stiell, 1996).

The OAR have been observed to be an accurate objective assessment tool for excluding fractures in healthy adults and children above the age of six. Pooled analysis of studies has shown the rules to have a sensitivity of almost 100 per cent, with modest specificity (Bachmann *et al.*, 2003). However, the accuracy of the test for some patient sub-groups, such as young children, pregnant women and patients with diminished sensation or comprehension, has not been established.

Weight-bearing lunge test

There have been a number of weight-bearing lunge tests described; also known as the 'knee to wall test', this test of weight-bearing ankle dorsiflexion has been shown to be reliable and valid (Bennell *et al.*, 1998; Cejudo *et al.*, 2014; Konor *et al.*, 2012), and it provides a more functional assessment of ankle movement. While there are variants, the standard version has the patient standing barefoot in a lunge-type position, facing and lightly supported against a wall (Konor *et al.*, 2012). The patient is directed to place their test foot onto a tape measure which is perpendicular to the wall, and then is asked to lunge forward while keeping their heel in contact with the floor so that their knee touches the wall. Their foot is then moved further away from the wall until the knee can only make slight contact with the wall. This test places the ankle into maximal (loaded) dorsiflexion, and allows for the distance from the hallux to the wall to be measured (in centimetres). The sports therapist may also utilize an inclinometer (positioned at the level of the tibial tuberosity) or a goniometer (positioned on the outside of the ankle with the stationary arm on the floor and the moving arm in line with the fibula) to record the dorsiflexion RoM in degrees. This test may be better performed with the ankle and foot in a subtalar neutral position as an overpronating foot may allow a greater angle of dorsiflexion. For this, manual guidance may be provided or a wedge may be placed under the medial longitudinal arch; also, the patient should be instructed to move their knee in an anterior direction towards the wall in line with their second toe.

Windlass test

There are two main versions of this test. In the non-weight-bearing version, the patient is seated with legs hanging off the couch; the therapist passively dorsiflexes the first metatarsophalangeal joint with the ankle stabilized in a plantargrade position. In the more provocative and specific weight-bearing (standing) version, the same procedure is performed

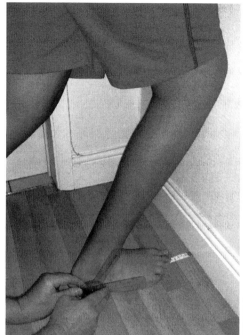
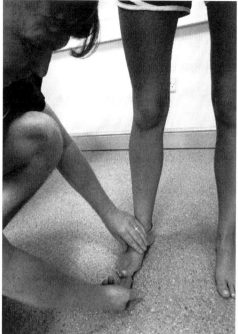

Photo 11.22   Weight-bearing lunge test.

Photo 11.23   Windlass test.

(De Garceau *et al.*, 2003; Mulligan, 2012). Bolgla and Malone (2004) explain how dorsiflexion (during the propulsive phase of gait) shortens and winds the plantar fascia around the head of the first metatarsal, which in turn shortens the distance between the calcaneus and metatarsals, and therefore elevates the medial longitudinal arch – which is the essential principle of the windlass mechanism. The windlass test can be used to identify any restriction (or pain) with first metatarsophalangeal extension (dorsiflexion), or reproduction of the patient's pain at the origin and proximal section of the plantar fascia (which is indicative of plantar fasciitis).

Peroneal subluxation test

The peroneal subluxation test assesses for any subluxation or dislocation of the peroneus longus and brevis tendons as they wind under the lateral malleolus. For this test, the patient is long seated on the couch, and the therapist palpates over the tendons as the patient actively dorsiflexes and everts their foot. In the event of a positive test the therapist will simply feel the tendons subluxing out of position. Localized pain can also be indicative (Hattam and Smeatham, 2010).

Metatarsal squeeze test

The metatarsal squeeze test is designed to detect a possible Morton's neuroma (and is therefore sometimes referred to as 'Morton's test'. To complete this test, the patient is positioned in sitting or supine. The therapist then grasps around the patient's midfoot (medial and lateral borders) with one hand and gently squeezes towards the middle of the foot. While squeezing the foot, the therapist may also palpate the sensitive area with their free hand. A sharp pain is indicative of a positive test (Cook and Hegedus, 2013; Hattam and Smeatham, 2010). It is important to differentiate the possibility of interdigital neuroma from metatarsalgia (which may be better identified via careful palpation).

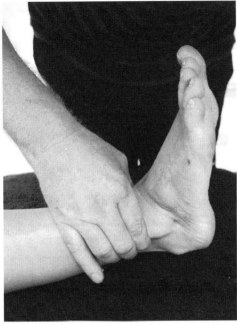

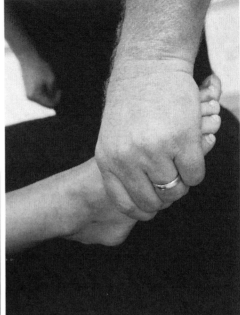

Photo 11.24 Peroneal subluxation test.   *Photo 11.25* Metatarsal squeeze test.

Thompson squeeze test

The Thompson (or 'squeeze') test aims to detect an Achilles tendon rupture. For this test the patient lies prone, ideally with their feet overhanging the end of a couch. The therapist then places both hands on the widest part of the calf with their fingers on one side and thumbs on the other and squeezes the calf musculature. The test is classed as positive if there is a lack of plantarflexion and would be suggestive of a complete rupture (Birrer *et al.*, 1999; Hattam and Smeatham, 2010; Prentice, 2009). In reality, this test is most useful as part of an immediate injury assessment, as in most clinical circumstances a completely ruptured Achilles tendon would normally have been previously identified – either pitch-side, or in an A&E department.

Homan's sign

The Homan's sign is a test which is designed to indicate the possibility that a patient has a deep vein thrombosis (DVT), which is most commonly seen in the lower limb (calf) region. It is important that this test is used in conjunction with an efficient subjective history, which should employ probing questions to explore background which may suspect a DVT (such as: previous history of DVT; recent prolonged immobility; pregnancy; taking oral contraception or hormone replacement therapy; chronic heart disease; obesity; family history of DVT; or an underlying thrombophilia) (Tidy and Kenny, 2012). Homan's test is carried out with the patient in a supine position, with their knee extended. The therapist passively dorsiflexes the patient's foot, and pain in the calf is the positive sign. Other clues to suspect DVT may include calf oedema, with possible redness and warmth. The differential diagnosis includes a calf muscle tear or skin infection (such as cellulitis), but if there is any doubt and Homan's test is positive, along with any suspicious subjective findings, the patient must be referred for medical assessment immediately (Prentice, 2009).

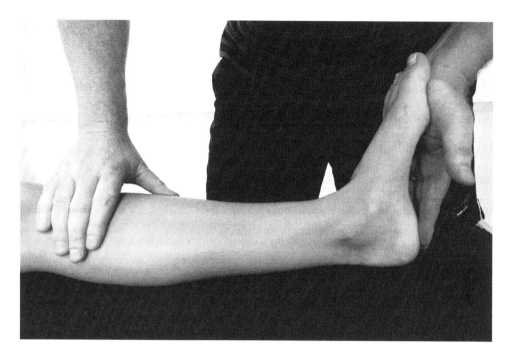

Photo 11.26 Homan's sign.

Palpation of the ankle and foot

Palpation of the ankle and foot should be approached with care in positioning and in type and depth of contact so as to avoid unnecessary stress to affected tissues; the sports therapist should proceed in a logical way so as to identify any abnormalities in tissue integrity or pain response. It is important to recognize that problems involving the ankle or foot may also involve structures more proximally or distally up and down the kinetic chain. Anatomical landmarks for palpation can include major bony landmarks, joint lines, ligaments (attachment sites and mid-substance), muscle bellies and their often multiple tendinous attachments, plus other specific tissue structures such as the plantar fascia, fat pads, bursae, blood vessels, nerves and skin. Certainly, palpatory assessment is very different to simply identifying anatomical structures; and the sports therapist must work with an understanding of what may be considered normal in the tissues (and in the tissue response to palpation) and what may be considered abnormal (such as the degree of tenderness, referral of pain, presence of heat or swelling, thickening, fibrosis, tension, laxity or malpositioning). The unaffected limb will usually be assessed first to allow for appreciation of normal (assuming no abnormalities). The sports therapist may elect to palpate the ankle and foot region while the patient is seated, supine, prone, crook-lying (supine with hips and knees flexed, with feet flat on the couch), side-lying or in weight-bearing positions. Bolsters may be useful when in lying positions. Palpation should begin superficially prior to any deeper probing; and it is essential to maintain dialogue with the patient during assessment. Regions and structures above and below the symptomatic area must be considered.

Palpatory skills are also used to establish the circulation of the foot; this may be required in the presence of any peripheral arterial condition, suspected compartment syndrome or acute traumatic ankle injury. This can be carried out through assessing the patient's pulse(s). Pulses can be taken at the posterior tibial artery (posterior to the medial malleolus) and the dorsalis pedis artery (between extensor hallucis longus and extensor digitorum longus at the distal most prominent aspect of the navicular bone). The sports therapist should also be mindful of the presence of any abnormalities within the venous system, such as varicosities in the long saphenous vein (the main superficial vein in the leg), particularly in overweight, pregnant or elderly populations. Varicose veins, which result due to a failure of small non-return valves in the veins, present as localized bulging in the affected vein, with a twisted appearance; they may be blue or purplish in colour (Knott and Kenny, 2013).

Table 11.1 Structures to palpate in the ankle and foot region

Skeletal structures	Soft tissue structures
• Medial malleolus	• Anterior muscle compartment (tibialis anterior; extensor digitorum longus; extensor hallucis longus; and peroneus tertius; and associated fascia)
• Lateral malleolus	
• Inferior tibiofibular joint line	
• Talocrural joint line	
• Talus (head; neck; trochlea/dome; medial tubercle; lateral tubercle)	• Distal tendons of above muscles
	• Deep posterior muscle compartment (tibialis posterior; flexor digitorum longus; and flexor hallucis longus; and associated fascia)
• Subtalar joint line	
• Sinus tarsi	
• Calcaneus (tuberosity of calcaneus; peroneal trochlea; sustentaculum tali)	• Distal tendons of above muscles
	• Superficial posterior muscle compartment (gastrocnemius; and soleus) and associated fascia
• Midtarsal joint line	
• Intertarsal joint lines	• Achilles tendon
• Navicular (tuberosity)	• Lateral muscle compartment (peroneus longus and brevis; and associated fascia)
• Cuboid (tuberosity; peroneal groove)	
• Medial, middle and lateral cuneiforms	• Distal tendons of above muscles
• Tarsometatarsal joint lines	• Anterior tibiofibular ligament
• Metatarsals 1–5 (base; shaft; head; tuberosity of fifth metatarsal)	• Posterior tibiofibular ligament
	• Anterior talofibular ligament
• Metatarsophalangeal joint lines 1–5	• Posterior talofibular ligament
• Phalanges (base; shaft; head)	• Calcaneofibular ligament
• Interphalangeal joint lines	• Deltoid ligament complex
	• Plantar calcaneonavicular (spring) ligament
	• Calcaneocuboid ligament
	• Plantar fascia
	• Calcaneal fat pad
	• Metatarsal fat pad
	• Retrocalcaneal bursa
	• Tibial artery and pulse
	• Dorsalis pedis artery and pulse
	• Short and long saphenous veins

Practitioner Tip Box 11.12

An ankle anatomy mnemonic

Tom, Dick AN' Harry (To remember structures passing under the medial malleolus)
- **T**ibialis posterior
- Flexor **D**igitorum longus
- Tibial **A**rtery
- Tibial **N**erve
- Flexor **H**allucis longus

Practitioner Tip Box 11.13

Dermatomes of the ankle and foot

- L4 relates to the medial anterior and posterior ankle and foot
- L5 relates to the midline anterior ankle and foot and midline foot plantar surface
- S1 relates to the lateral anterior ankle and foot, posterior heel and lateral foot plantar surface

Practitioner Tip Box 11.14

Myotomes of the ankle and foot

- Dorsiflexion (L4–5)
- Inversion (L4–5)
- Eversion (L5–S1)
- Plantarflexion (L5–S2)

Practitioner Tip Box 11.15

Reflexes of the ankle and foot

- Achilles (S1)
- Lateral plantar surface (Babinski's sign – for possible upper motor neurone lesion)

Practitioner Tip Box 11.16

Muscle synergy of the ankle and foot region

Plantarflexion	Gastrocnemius
	Soleus
	Tibialis posterior
	Flexor digitorum longus
	Flexor hallucis longus
	Peroneus longus
	Peroneus brevis
	Plantaris
Dorsiflexion	Tibialis anterior
	Extensor digitorum longus
	Extensor hallucis longus
	Peroneus tertius
Inversion	Tibialis anterior
	Tibialis posterior
	Flexor digitorum longus
	Flexor hallucis longus
Eversion	Peroneus longus
	Peroneus brevis
	Peroneus tertius
	Extensor digitorum longus

Functional tests of the foot and ankle

Any ankle or foot assessment requires an assessment of the functional capability of the joint. Bipedal stance may indicate if patients favour the uninvolved over the injured side. Tasks such as single leg balance and the ability to single leg squat with the patient's eyes open or closed may help to establish impairments in foot posture, stability, motor control, proprioception or functional strength. In addition, the patient may be asked to walk normally, on their toes, their heels, or their medial or lateral borders; they may also be assessed hopping on each foot, jumping, running in a straight line or with changes in direction, and stair climbing (Birrer *et al.*, 1999; Prentice, 2009). These tests will assess the patient's ability in utilizing full range of movement and dynamic balance skills.

Injuries of the ankle and foot region

Within the following section a selection of some of the more common ankle and foot conditions are discussed in terms of their basic aetiology, characteristic presenting features and management strategies and considerations.

Ankle sprains

Inversion and eversion sprains

The ankle region accounts for upwards of 45 per cent of all sports injuries (Ferran and Maffulli, 2006; Kaminski *et al.*, 2013). Approximately 75 per cent of all ankle injuries which occur during sport are sprains, with the majority of these affecting the lateral ligaments (inversion sprains) (Fong *et al.*, 2007). These ligaments, predominantly including the ATFL and CFL, are often damaged following forced inversion of the foot while changing direction during walking or running. Ankle sprains can lead to long-term disability, with over 50 per cent of individuals requiring more than one year to fully recover (van Middelkoop *et al.*, 2012). Predisposing factors to ankle sprain include impaired balance, reduced proprioception, strength, coordination and previous ankle sprain injury (Willems *et al.*, 2005; van Middelkoop *et al.*, 2012). Patients are often able to recall precisely when the injury occurred and frequently describe inversion as the MoI. Pain on the lateral side of the ankle is often present. Furthermore, sudden changes in direction, cutting manoeuvres and landing on uneven ground are classic mechanisms. An eversion mechanism and pain on the medial side can implicate the deltoid ligament. Precise palpation and handling during ATFL, CFL, CCL and eversion stress tests will greatly improve the accuracy of diagnosis; however, Kerkhoffs *et al.* (2013) highlight that delayed physical diagnostic examination (four to five days after the event) will provide a more reliable diagnostic result once swelling has subsided. Kerkhoffs *et al.* (2013) describe a sensitivity of 96 per cent and a specificity of 84 per cent for delayed physical examination. The sports therapist must recognize the differential diagnoses and also the possibility of comorbidity. Fractures are commonly associated with forceful MoI at the ankle, and the OAR must be utilized.

Residual problems following ankle sprain include pain, reduced RoM, chronic ankle instability (CAI) and ligamentous laxity, proprioception deficits and reduced strength (Kaminski *et al.*, 2013). Indeed, McKeon and Mattacola (2008) identify that 30 per cent progress to CAI. CAI, as described by McCaig (2012) is a combination of mechanical factors (pathological laxity, arthrokinetic restriction and degenerative changes) and functional deficits (impaired proprioception and neuromuscular control), possibly with the addition of psychosocial factors (such as 'perceived instability'). Ankle sprains are most frequently managed in the immediate stage by protecting the area from further damage, rest, ice, compression and elevation (PRICE). With grade I and II sprains this is followed by the introduction of movement (optimized loading) and progressive functional rehabilitation once initial symptoms have subsided (Cooke *et al.*, 2003). During early rehabilitation, lace-up or semi-rigid braces (rather than elastic support) have been recommended, as has the use of athletic taping (Kerkhoffs *et al.*, 2013). Long-term treatment is aimed at returning functional impairments to normal. RoM activities, balance training and strengthening have all been shown to be effective in treating ankle sprains (Punam and Chhaya, 2013; Kaminski *et al.*, 2013). Such components must be progressed to incorporate multidirectional single leg squatting, jumping and landing. During the rehabilitation process, clinical modalities including ultrasound, joint mobilizations and soft tissue therapy may be utilized, but Kerkhoffs *et al.* (2013) in their systematic review found little evidence for such. Return to play criteria should take into account athlete perception of function, alongside functional performance testing (such as with single leg hop tests and the star excursion balance test [SEBT]), and the injured limb's performance should equal at least 80 per cent of the non-injured limb (Kaminski *et al.*, 2013).

High ankle (syndesmotic) sprains

The high ankle sprain involves disruption of the distal (inferior) tibiofibular joint (syndesmosis) (Read, 2008). The mechanism is traumatic and classically involves a load-bearing, forcefully dorsiflexed and rotated ankle. Sports involving frequent cutting and turning manoeuvres, or stiff boots (such as in hockey and skiing), have higher incidences of this injury (Mulligan, 2012). The injury may involve the anterior inferior tibiofibular ligament (AITFL) and the interosseous membrane; in severe cases the medial malleolus can also be fractured, as in a 'Pott's' or 'Maisonneuve' fracture (Karlsson, 2006). Rupp (2008) explains that a syndesmotic injury will alter normal talocrural joint mechanics and can lead to chronic ankle pain, instability and arthrosis. Unlike inversion sprains, the high ankle sprain does not usually produce significant swelling. A confident subjective history, combined with careful observations, movement testing, local palpation and use of 'Kleiger's' (external rotation) test can indicate the condition. A 'squeeze test' of the lower leg may also be provocative. Fractures of the malleolus frequently require open reduction fixation procedures; while syndesmosis injuries without fracture but with chronic instability (i.e. with radiographic evidence of mortise widening indicative of diastasis) may require arthroscopic debridement and reconstruction (Park, 2014). The rehabilitation period tends to be longer than for inversion sprains. A secure, compressive ankle brace may be required in the early stages, and end-range dorsiflexion, external rotation and eversion should be avoided until a progressive dynamic stability regime has been successfully undertaken. Usual interventions such as ultrasound, joint mobilizations and soft tissue therapy may all be considered for supporting rehabilitation.

Muscular injuries

Muscle tears are among the most frequent injuries which affect sportspeople. In the lower limb, gastrocnemius injuries can account for up to 12 per cent of all muscular problems in sporting populations (Volpi *et al.*, 2004), and the most frequently affected section is the musculotendinous junction (MTJ). The MoI of calf tears often involves forceful activation of the gastrocnemius muscle, commonly when the contraction type changes from eccentric to concentric (Orchard *et al.*, 2002). Patients often complain of acute onset of pain and discomfort in the calf region following a sports task. Immediate treatment should include PRICE. Following the immediate injury, patients will often report stiffness, increased pain on activity and impaired function during load-bearing activities such as walking or stair climbing. On examination, resisted muscle contraction is often painful and reduced strength may be present. Diagnostic ultrasound or MRI may be required to confirm muscle injury and its extent. Long-term rehabilitation of these injuries involves the return of normal RoM and muscle function. Early management modalities may include interferential muscle stimulation, soft tissue therapy (cautious deep transverse friction techniques) and stretching (not during the first week) to increase RoM until it equals that of the uninjured side (Muller-Wohlfahrt *et al.*, 2013). Outcome measures such as use of ankle goniometry and observation of a weight-bearing lunge can help to establish when normal RoM has been achieved (Bennell *et al.*, 1998; Konor *et al.*, 2012).

Avoiding unwanted muscle atrophy is an important feature of muscle injury rehabilitation. Allowing patients to use muscles functionally within pain-free limits can reduce some of the negatives associated with long-term immobilization. With time, as muscle function returns, a strengthening programme should commence. Early goals include improving muscular endurance with reduced load. This can be progressed to increasing strength and power. Complexity of contraction may also be progressed from isometric to concentric or eccentric.

Functional tasks such as walking or running may be introduced and then progressed by increasing speed, duration or incline. The transition from therapeutic exercise to more pure training therapy, with an emphasis on sport-specific, closed-chain loads must be made (Muller-Wohlfahrt *et al.*, 2013). Demanding functional tasks such as sprinting, running with changes of direction or plyometric activities should be incorporated near the end of the athlete's rehabilitation once RoM and functional strength have returned to near previous levels. While integrating these types of activities into the rehabilitation programme, it is important to note the velocity, volume, size and types of contraction the athlete will be performing during training and performance to ensure the programme is realistic and valid.

Achilles tendinopathy

Achilles tendinopathy is a frequent occurrence in athletes and recreational sportspeople. Achilles tendon pain has traditionally been described as a tendonitis, though this is often deemed semantically inaccurate due to the reduced role of inflammation in this pathology. While tendinosis can affect any of the tendons of the ankle and foot, Achilles tendinopathy appears to be the most common. Within the general population, the lifetime cumulative incidence is approximately 5.9 per cent, but this can be as high as 50 per cent among elite endurance athletes (Kujala *et al.*, 2005). The aetiology of tendinopathy is complex and multifactorial (factors include: decreased vascularity in older-aged athletes; stress-shielded vulnerability in underused tendons; biomechanical irregularities; and anatomical musculoskeletal abnormalities such as the 'Haglund's deformity' bone spur which can occur on the superior aspect of the posterior calcaneus) (Den Hartog, 2009). Achilles tendinopathy is associated with both overpronating and pes cavus foot presentations, and forefoot varus has also been found to be a factor in the development of both paratendonitis and insertional complaints – the cavus foot is less efficient in shock absorption and can place increased stress on the lateral aspect of the Achilles tendon (Den Hartog, 2009). Inappropriate training frequency or progressions can lead to overuse, and the resulting overload and inefficient recovery can lead to a failure in the process of collagen synthesis. The precise aetiology, pathogenesis and risk factors are yet to be described entirely (Alfredson and Cook, 2007; Cook and Purdam, 2009; Rees *et al.*, 2013; Scott *et al.*, 2013; Sharma and Maffulli, 2005). The three-stage continuum model as proposed by Cook and Purdam (2009) provides a pragmatic explanation of reactive tendinopathy (acute episodic tendon response, which if managed carefully has good potential for swift resolution), tendon disrepair and degenerative tendinopathy. A chronic, degenerative Achilles tendinopathy presents with established collagen cleavages, abundant abnormal neovascularity, fat infiltration and neural ingrowth, which results in a thickened, restricted, weakened, painful and vulnerable (to rupture) tendon. Typically, the athlete will be able to pinpoint the tenderness within the tendon complex, which can be located anywhere between 2 and 7 cm above the insertion. Crepitus may also be present, and other classic symptoms include morning stiffness and local pain and stiffness after an increase in activity. Symptoms sometimes ease with the application of heat or with mild activity, although while there may be a reduction in symptoms they are likely to return once activity is stopped (Alfredson and Cook, 2007). Diagnostic ultrasound can help to confirm diagnosis. The Victorian Institute of Sports Assessment Achilles scale (VISA-A scale) is a subjective questionnaire assessing the patient's symptoms and physical function. It has been shown to be a reliable index of subjectively grading the severity and changes in recovery of specific tendinopathies in relation to life activities (Robinson *et al.*, 2001).

Activity modification (i.e. avoiding or reducing running activities; and also avoiding incline and decline running until rehabilitation has been progressed) and possible protection via taping techniques (either conventional athletic support or kinesiology taping) – alongside the addressing of underlying causative factors – may efficiently help to resolve reactive tendinopathy. Chronic degenerative tendinosis, however, with pathological alteration in structure, can be more resistant to remedial action; and additionally the individual is vulnerable to tendon rupture with any sufficiently intensive singular overload. Numerous modalities have been used to treat mid-portion Achilles tendinopathies. Eccentric loading appears to be one of the most effective, low-risk and low-cost treatments for tendinopathies (Magnussen *et al.*, 2009). Ranson (2013) suggests the mechanism of effect following eccentric loading may be due to a combination of factors, including: the destruction of aberrant vessels; the normalization of the tendon matrix; an increase in collagen turnover; an improved length–tension relationship of involved muscles; stronger muscles; and the resulting development of a denser Achilles tendon. One of the most frequently used protocols was described by Alfredson *et al.* (1998). This 12-week programme utilizes eccentric loading of the tendon both with the knee extended and flexed, to maximize the activation of the soleus muscle. Three sets of 15 repetitions have been recommended for both exercises. This method has been observed to have a good long-term prognosis with successful outcome in 65–88 per cent of cases (Gärdin *et al.*, 2010; Ohberg *et al.*, 2004). While some mild pain may remain, 40 per cent of cases have been observed to be completely pain free five years post-injury. In cases where tendons do not respond to eccentric loading, other modalities such as shockwave therapy, prolotherapy and surgical interventions have been shown to be beneficial (Alfredson *et al.*, 2013; Alfredson and Ohlberg, 2005; Rasmussen *et al.*, 2008; Yelland *et al.*, 2011). Although robust evidence is still lacking (Joseph *et al.*, 2012), anecdotal evidence is plentiful, and sports therapists may also utilize joint mobilizations and soft tissue therapy to address movement restrictions involving the lower limb and also localized deep transverse frictions (DTF) or instrument assisted soft tissue mobilization (IASTM) targeted at the focal degeneration. Patients with insertional Achilles tendinopathies present with pain at the calcaneal tuberosity. This diagnosis can also be confirmed using diagnostic ultrasound. It is believed that this injury has poorer prognosis compared with mid-substance tendinopathies (Alfredson and Cook, 2007). Conservative management of insertional tendinopathy is also favoured; similarly to mid-substance tendinopathies, this includes modalities such as eccentric loading and shockwave therapy, although more research into this area is needed (Kearney and Costa, 2010; Rowe *et al.*, 2012).

Achilles tendon rupture

While diagnosing Achilles tendon pain, it is important to differentiate between tendinopathy, insertional tendinopathy and Achilles tendon rupture. The possibility of Achilles tendon rupture can be confirmed using the Thompson squeeze test. Achilles ruptures often occur during forced, extreme contraction of the calf muscles (such as occur when landing from a jump or fall), and ruptures tend to occur most commonly at the tendon's narrowest point (i.e. approximately 3–5 cm above its insertion) (Carnes and Vizniak, 2012). During the rupture event, the athlete will experience a sudden, sharp, audible snapping (and commonly it is reported that they feel as though they were hit or kicked from behind). Achilles tendon rupture has an annual incidence of 18 per 100,000, being most common among men 30–50 years of age (Alfredson and Cook, 2007; Leppilahti *et al.*, 1996). The injured athlete may be still able to walk with compromised movements. Risk factors for these injuries include corticosteroid use, limb ischaemia and local vascular compromise, anabolic steroids, chronic pain, previous Achilles rupture and rheumatoid arthritis (Kakkar *et al.*, 2011). Histological findings from ruptured Achilles tendons have shown marked degenerative changes and collagen disruption (Maffulli, 1999). This may indicate that acute Achilles ruptures occur as a consequence of more long-term damage. Achilles ruptures may be managed either operatively or conservatively. While there can be a greater number of soft tissue complications associated with operative management (Willits *et al.*, 2010), Park (2014) suggests that surgical repair results in a much lower recurrence rate. In conservative management, the athlete will normally be cast immobilized for two weeks (in full plantarflexion) followed by an average of eight weeks non-weight-bearing. Alfredson *et al.* (2012) recommend early mobility and isometric strengthening as the cast or brace allows (i.e. toe movements and low-grade plantarflexion isometrics). With both operative and conservative management, an accelerated functional rehabilitation programme should be completed, not only to strengthen and align the developing scar tissue, but also to address the resulting atrophy of the calf musculature. This usually comprises around six more weeks of early protected weight bearing in an ankle brace or adjustable walking boot device which can maintain a degree of dorsiflexion throughout the gait cycle. This will then be followed by a further eight-week exercise programme designed to increase weight bearing independently and normalize residual strength and RoM deficits (Carnes and Vizniak, 2012; Mulligan, 2012). A heel raise may be employed during this phase. High-impact activities should be avoided during the rehabilitation process.

Plantar fasciopathy

Plantar fasciopathy (previously referred to as plantar fasciitis) is a common cause of heel pain and is estimated to account for up to 15 per cent of all foot injuries (Buchbinder, 2004). Histological findings have shown the pathology to include degeneration and fragmentation of the plantar fascia (Lemont *et al.*, 2003). Risk factors for plantar fasciopathy include reduced ankle dorsiflexion, obesity, middle-age and work related weight bearing (Riddle and Schappert, 2004). Patients typically present with pain of insidious onset located on the heel on the plantar surface of the foot. The plantar fascia consists of three main bands, and the medial band is the thickest and most commonly implicated. Some episodes may coincide with increases in load-bearing activity such as standing, walking or running. Other contributory factors include biomechanical overpronation, pes planus and cavus, improper footwear, training on hard surfaces, weak dorsiflexor muscles and short plantarflexor muscles. Mulligan (2012) explains how an overpronating, planus foot maintains perpetual tension on the fascia, while a cavus foot is inherently tight and causes repeated bowstring-loading during each step. Acute trauma is considered a less common cause (Carnes and Vizniak, 2012). With chronic irritation, inferior calcaneal traction spurs may develop, but their presence is not necessarily an indication of severity. Fuller (2000) explains that the spur develops in a direction horizontal to the ground as that is the direction of tensile stress from the fascia on the calcaneus. Hallux rigidus (or 'limitus') – restricted first metatarsophalangeal joint extension – can be a feature. This may be due to underlying pathological osteoarthritis, or can be a functional limitation secondary to a tight fascia (Fuller, 2000).

Patients will often complain of increased pain with (initial) standing and walking, and pain which is worse after a period of rest (such as first thing in the morning). Some athletes will begin to compensate for the condition by oversupinating to avoid loading the painful site. Alongside, lower limb observations (for biomechanical deviations), active, passive and resisted tests, the 'windlass test' may be used in assessment. Commonly, pain will be elicited during active heel raises and heel walking. Palpation of the inferior heel (at the medial calcaneal tuberosity and a few centimetres distally) frequently elicits intense focal tenderness. The differential diagnosis for plantar fasciopathy includes calcaneal stress fracture, long or short plantar ligament sprain, intrinsic foot muscle tear, neurogenic pain and inflammatory arthritis. Achilles tendinopathy and calcaneal bursitis should also be considered.

Management should be initially aimed at reducing pain, minimizing stress on the fascia and addressing all underlying aetiological factors (Mulligan, 2012). Interventions used to treat plantar fasciopathy may include cryotherapy (for pain relief), mobilizing and stretching exercises (including self-massage techniques), orthotic shoe inserts (including heel cups, silicon heel pads and 'doughnut-type' heel pads), night-splints (such as the 'Strassbourg sock') and steroid injections (Cole and Gazewood, 2005). Stretching exercises have been shown to result in successful outcomes in 65 per cent of cases (Rompe *et al.*, 2010); however, repeated steroid injections should be avoided as these can lead to weakening of the fascia (predisposing to rupture) alongside skin and fat pad atrophy (Park, 2014). Ultrasound, joint mobilizations (to the talocrural and first metatarsophalangeal joints), soft tissue therapy (including myofascial release and deep transverse frictions) and plantar fascia taping support have all been used in traditional sports therapy settings and may all be clinically reasoned for inclusion. A rigid 'low-Dye' taping method has been shown to be helpful (Landorf *et al.*, 2005). Progressive strengthening of all intrinsic foot and main ankle muscles must be recommended. Rathleff *et al.* (2014) found that a high-load strength training programme compared to a more traditional plantar fascia stretching programme improved outcomes. For this study they used heavy and slow (three seconds concentric up, two second isometric hold and three seconds eccentric down) single-leg calf-raises with a towel positioned to maximally dorsiflex the toes. A 12-repetition maximum (RM) for three sets was used for the initial period, progressing to 8-RM by week four or five, with increased sets (five were recommended). The proposed mechanisms for the positive outcomes resulting from this protocol include increased collagen synthesis, increased load tolerability of the plantar fascia, increased intrinsic foot and ankle dorsiflexor muscle strength and improved ankle dorsiflexion RoM (Rathleff *et al.*, 2014). Cases which do not respond to conservative methods may benefit from surgical intervention (Stoita and Walsh, 2010). An open or arthroscopic plantar fascia release may be undertaken (most commonly the proximal, medial segment is the target); however, prognosis is uncertain and even with successful surgery, return to training can take weeks (Park, 2014).

Stress fractures of the lower leg and foot

Stress (micro or 'fatigue') fractures are partial or complete breaks in bone. In athletes, their cause is frequently attributed to overuse (and excessive compressive or torsional loading), with insufficient recovery and therefore failure of the required remodelling process. These injuries occur when repetitive mechanical loads, often in the form of GRFs, cause micro-damage and deformation to bones. Over time, the summation of these forces and subsequent damage (in the absence of adequate rest to allow for remodelling and adaptation) results in partial or complete fractures, which may be vulnerable to displacement. Similarly to other overuse pathologies, stress fractures are frequently associated with inappropriate alterations in training, such as changes in duration, speed, distance, surface, footwear or exercise frequency or intensity. Intrinsic risk factors can include reduced bone mineral density, poor nutritional intake, leg length discrepancies and deconditioning, alongside biomechanical factors. Biomechanical factors, such as pes planus and cavus, are associated with increased risk for stress fractures of the foot.

Areas of the foot and ankle which have relatively high incidences of stress fractures include the metatarsals (most common) and the navicular, although the talus and calcaneus are also vulnerable; proximally the tibial shaft is also a common site for stress fractures. Jose *et al.* (2011) describe a higher incidence of proximal posteromedial cortex tibial stress fractures in recreational and competitive runners; ballet dancers and jumping athletes (such as basketball players) more commonly experience stress fractures in the anterior cortex. Jose *et al.* (2011) also clarify the clinical challenge to distinguish a tibial stress fracture from a medial tibial stress syndrome (MTSS) presentation. Regarding metatarsal stress fractures, Mulligan (2012) describes a classic process of overpronation and hypermobility of the first ray, which can lead to increased stress to the three central metatarsals. Some individuals have abnormal lengths of their metatarsal bones and when involved in repetitive loading activities can be predisposed to stress fractures. The most common site is at the neck of the second metatarsal (Agosta and Holzer, 2012). A metatarsal fracture is also commonly referred to as a 'march fracture'. Navicular stress fractures more commonly result from excessive compressive stress between the talus proximally and the cuneiforms distally, especially where ankle and foot biomechanics are less than ideal (such as with reduced talocrural dorsiflexion and resulting compensatory mobility through the midfoot). Like the majority of stress fractures, a distinct and often palpable focal centre of pain is evident; in navicular stress fractures this has been termed the 'N spot' (Agosta and Holzer, 2012). After the navicular, the second most common site for tarsal stress fracture is at the calcaneus (Agosta and Holzer, 2012). This is more likely to result from (among other factors) heavy heel strike during running or landing.

Assessment of potential stress fractures must include a full appreciation of the patient/athlete's history, which is likely to include an increase in repetitive loading, and is unlikely to include recent history of macrotrauma. The patient/athlete is likely to describe a gradual, insidious onset of pain. Objectively, posture and movement assessments can be helpful in providing clues, but careful palpation is extremely important because stress fractures often present with localized tenderness at the fracture site. Indirect digital percussion of the affected bone may prove painful as the vibration travels to the fracture site. A careful 'squeeze test' of the affected bone is another technique which may also elicit a localized pain response. Additionally, active or passive movements may invoke pain at the site. Stress fractures are not normally visible in their early stage on X-ray, hence the suspicion of diagnosis is usually made clinically. Bone scans and MRI may be used for confirmation (Beck, 2012). It is obviously also important to appreciate the differential diagnosis – hence the sports therapist must be familiar with local anatomy and other regional pathologies. The majority of stress fractures respond to rest from aggravating activity (i.e. to a threshold below symptoms), followed by a period of reduced loading which can enable sufficient remodelling; a graded increase in activity is often sufficient – in conjunction with full consideration of aetiological factors (including: training; equipment; biomechanics; and nutrition). Where pain on weight bearing is a continuing feature (or where athlete adherence to activity modification is a concern) a short leg cast can be helpful; later, taping or foam cut-outs can be used to reduce local stress (Mulligan, 2012). Beck (2012) advises avoiding the following when acutely injured: any excessive stretching of adjacent muscles; performing local muscle strengthening exercises; engaging in pain-producing activities; and training on unusually soft or uneven surfaces when injured. In cases where malunion of fractures persist, surgical fixation may be required.

Medial tibial stress syndrome

MTSS is another common cause of exercise-induced lower leg pain and discomfort. Historically it has been termed 'shin-splints' and periostitis. In some physically active populations, the incidence has been observed to be as high as 35 per cent (Yates and White, 2004). Patients often present with focal tenderness along the mid- to distal portions of the tibial crest's posteriomedial border. The pain can be either continuous or intermittent; it typically intensifies with initial exercise, and may subside during exercise in the early stages, but is often made worse with weight-bearing activity (Kortebein *et al.*, 2000; Rathleff *et al.*, 2011). Neurological symptoms are rare, and pain does not usually continue during walking (Harradine, 2013). Excessive tensile and compressive forces from loading (vertical loading rate [VLR] and associated GRFs), tensile and compressive loading from myofascial forces and shear stress from torsional bone forces are considered the key factors in the development of MTSS (Harradine, 2013)

Results from bone scans may appear abnormal in the last phase of injury, demonstrating involvement of the bone and periosteum, with high-resolution CT scans also showing the tibial cortex to be osteopenic as a sign of remodelling (Gaeta *et al.*, 2006; Moen *et al.*, 2010). While stress reaction of the tibia is currently recognized as the key presenting issue, the condition is multifactorial, also locally involving tendon and periosteal dysfunction (particularly with relation to tibialis posterior, tibialis anterior and soleus attachment) (Galbraith and Lavallee, 2009). The onset often accompanies a change in physical activity. This may be an increase in speed, distance or a change in terrain. Other factors may include footwear or the style of running, such as downhill fell running. Care must be taken to differentiate between this pathology and tibial stress fractures or chronic exertional compartment syndrome (CESC). Established tibial stress fractures may be confirmed via X-ray, or more effectively with bone scanning or MRI; compartment syndromes can be diagnosed by measuring intra-compartmental pressure invasively. MTSS is usually managed conservatively, with an emphasis on behaviour modification to prevent overuse and to introduce a more gradual change in activity. The objective must be to strengthen the tibial cortex, increase tibial remodelling and encourage resorption of micro-damage (Harradine, 2013). In overpronators, the employment of motion control training shoes or medially posted orthotics can be helpful. Weight loss in overweight runners can be recommended. Graded running programmes, which slowly increase distance (importantly reducing fatigue factors), speed and intensity, have been shown to be effective. Fatigue is associated with a reduced tolerance for impact. Other training errors must also be addressed. Taping applications to help control foot motion may be useful; however, the addition of stretching, strengthening and the wearing of ankle braces may not be of benefit to all patients (Moen *et al.*, 2010; 2012). In recalcitrant cases, posterior fasciotomy is the commonly performed operative procedure (Galbraith and Lavallee, 2009).

Tarsal tunnel syndrome

Tarsal tunnel syndrome (TTS) is not as well-recognized as carpal tunnel syndrome (CTS) of the wrist. However, it is where the posterior tibial nerve becomes irritated posteroinferiorly to the medial malleolus in the fibro-osseous tunnel created superficially by the flexor retinaculum and deeply by the medial wall of the talus and calcaneus (Birrer *et al.*, 1999; Mulligan, 2012). The condition is most often seen in sports which are associated with repetitive loading (such as running, racquet sports and basketball). Additional risk factors include poorly fitted shoes, overpronation and training errors. The condition can also result from an eversion sprain, direct impact trauma, osteophytic bone projection, fibrous tumour or other fibrosis, or adverse neural tension. Initial presentations may include local pain, burning (or intermittent shooting) radiating pain into the plantar aspect of the foot, as well as paraesthesia. These symptoms tend to occur during weight bearing and in positions of dorsiflexion combined with eversion. The athlete will typically report aggravation with activity and easing with rest. Diagnosis may be suspected with a positive Tinel's sign, or prolonged local digital compression (for 60 seconds). Nerve conduction studies or MRI may be required for confirmation (Joyce, 2010). Management of TTS usually incorporates relative rest from aggravating activities and attendance to any underlying overpronation (via shoe modification, orthotics or taping). Cryotherapy, ultrasound, soft tissue therapy and neurodynamic therapy may be incorporated into treatment with clinical reasoning for assisting the reduction of any oedema, fibrosis or mechanical irritation. Surgical release of the tunnel may be indicated in persistent cases.

Peroneal subluxation

While assessing patients with lateral ankle pain, it is important to identify or exclude the presence of peroneal injury or dysfunction. Peroneus longus and brevis originate on the lateral aspect of the lower leg on the fibula. As they wind their way in a subtle groove (the retromalleolar sulcus) under and around the lateral malleolus they pass under the lateral retinaculum. Peroneal subluxation and dislocation are associated in sports which require changes in direction, particularly where the peroneal muscles are required to perform sudden and forceful contraction from a dorsiflexed and inverted position, and where the ankle is subjected to large varus and valgus GRFs (Scholten *et al.*, 2012). During such mechanisms, the lateral retinaculum can tear, which results in peroneal tendon instability. Patients often present with posterolateral ankle pain, ankle instability, weakness during eversion with dorsiflexion and may complain of clicking or snapping along the lateral aspect of the ankle. A positive peroneal subluxation test will confirm the possibility of pathology. Conservative methods of treatment may include taping or cast immobilization, but if the injury does not respond to these methods, surgical intervention may be of benefit (Tan *et al.*, 2003; Vega *et al.*, 2013). Surgery may aim to reconstruct the retinaculum, deepen the groove or re-route the tendons under the CFL (Mulligan, 2012).

Anterior synovial impingement

If the athlete is reporting persistent anterolateral ankle pain which follows recurrent ankle sprains it could be indicative of synovial impingement. Synovial impingement can result from a chronically swollen, hypertrophied synovial membrane that gets pinched in the ankle mortise during dorsiflexion movements (Birrer *et al.*, 1999). The patient will report pain during activity, which is characteristically worsened by sudden stops and starts. During objective assessment, tenderness will be located on the anterior aspect of the mortise, and the athlete will report discomfort during passive dorsiflexion. Cook and Hegedus (2013) detail a set of clinical prediction rules for anterior impingement (anterolateral ankle joint tenderness; anterolateral ankle joint swelling; pain with forced dorsiflexion; pain with single-leg squat; pain with activities; and possibly an absence of instability). MRI is not considered sufficiently sensitive, therefore arthroscopy is the preferred investigation and is recommended for chronic post-ankle sprain pain (Molloy *et al.*, 2003). While conservative approaches, including joint mobilization and soft tissue therapy, may prove effective, arthroscopic debridement of the impinging soft-tissue (synovectomy) alongside possible bony decompression in chronic presentations is considered effective (Molloy *et al.*, 2003). The sports therapist must be mindful of the differential diagnosis, which includes anterior tibiofibular or talofibular sprain, sinus tarsi syndrome, osteochondral lesions of the talar dome and anterior tendinopathy (i.e. extensor digitorum longus).

Sinus tarsi syndrome

Sinus tarsi syndrome (STS) relates to anterolateral ankle pain, which most commonly can be secondary to overuse and overpronation of the subtalar joint, or due to an acute anterolateral inversion/plantarflexion trauma (Karlsson, 2006). The sinus tarsi is an observable and palpable structural cavity which is the demarcated anterolateral aspect of the subtalar joint. Whilst there are extrinsic ligaments contributing to stability of the subtalar joint (i.e. the CFL laterally and the deltoid ligament medially), there are also a set of intrinsic ligaments (the talocalcaneal, interosseous and cervical). Laxity or rupture of the intrinsic subtalar ligaments can lead to increased movement of the subtalar joint that in turn results in instability (overpronation and/ or supination) and possibly impingement of the subtalar synovium; additionally, the connective tissues of the joint contribute to proprioception of the ankle, which can then be compromised following injury (Helgeson, 2009). In chronic presentations, inflammation can be prolonged and fibrosis can develop to perpetuate symptoms. The condition classically presents with a pre-history as mentioned; the patient/athlete will be able to localize their pain to the sinus tarsi, and the pain can be provoked with palpation. Movement tests are likely to reproduce local symptoms, subtalar accessory movements may be lax or painful; together with ankle instability, these signs indicate STS. Helgeson (2009) highlights how balance and proprioceptive training, muscle strengthening, bracing, taping and foot orthoses have been recommended for managing STS, but that robust and specific evidence is lacking. When conservative management has failed, arthroscopic exploration, synovectomy, arthrotomy, reconstruction of the interosseous or cervical ligaments or even arthrodesis may be indicated.

Os trigonum

Rathur and colleagues (2009) describe the classic features and causes of posterior impingement syndrome, which is characterized by posterior ankle pain when exposed to forceful plantarflexion movements. Soft tissue, bony projections (such as the os trigonum), unfused ossicles (or osseous fragments) entrapped posteriorly between the tibial plafond and the calcaneus can lead to the symptoms. According to Birrer *et al.* (1999), around 5–14 per cent of the population has a small accessory bony development which is located posterior to the posterior tubercle of the talus. The os trigonum, when present, is a prominent posterolateral projection of the talus (it may be fused or separated); it is the most common reason for posterior impingement syndrome. With this condition, the accessory bone may be present congenitally, or there may have been a history of an ankle injury (particularly those involving forced dorsiflexion) in the weeks to months prior to the patient consultation. Birrer *et al.* (1999) suggest that there is persistent posterior and posterolateral pain, with persistent swelling and ankle instability being classic features. During objective examination, a 25° decrease in plantarflexion may be noted, accompanied by pain on palpation between the Achilles and the tibia. Pain will be increased through forced plantarflexion of the ankle or resisted plantarflexion of the great toe, hence it is a common dance-related condition (in ballet the 'en-point' position can be an exacerbating factor). It is obviously important to differentiate the condition from other causes of posterior ankle pain, such as talar fracture, Achilles tendinopathy or other (more medial) tendinopathies (i.e. involving flexor digitorum longus or tibialis posterior). Conservative management may involve initial relative rest from aggravating activities and anti-inflammatory medication, followed by manual therapy and possibly local steroid injection. In non-responsive cases, referral for orthopaedic consultation is recommended. Park (2014) describes an arthroscopic excision procedure with good prognosis for full return to sport within six to eight weeks post-operatively.

Morton's neuroma

Morton's neuroma is a peripheral nerve pathology within the intermetatarsal regions of the foot. Affecting one of the interdigital plantar nerves, a benign neuroma (localized enlargement), presents most commonly in the third or fourth intermetatarsal web space. While the exact cause is not always certain – it may relate to abnormal biomechanics or osteoarthritic changes leading to compressive and shearing forces – ultrasonic imaging is likely to show a hypoechoic (dark) mass of neuroma. The common presentation is the patient with a hypermobile foot, particularly during midstance and propulsion. Patients typically present with local pain alongside radiating anaesthesia, paraesthesia or burning pain from the midfoot to the toes. Patients will often note an unwillingness to want to walk or in extreme cases just to place their foot on the ground. The possibility of neuroma involvement can be confirmed using the 'metatarsal squeeze test'. Conservative management can include reducing activities which exacerbate pain and footwear modification to address overpronation or off-load painful areas (such as use of a metatarsal pad placed proximal to the metatarsal heads) (Hassouna and Singh, 2005; Mulligan, 2012). If symptoms do not respond to conservative treatment, operative management may be required (such as decompression or excision of the neuroma).

This chapter has presented the main anatomical structures and functional relationships regarding the lower leg, ankle and foot regions. Clinical assessment approaches have been discussed, and a set of special and functional tests presented. While there are a multitude of reasons for ankle and foot (and related lower leg) pain and dysfunction, a selection of the more common injury conditions have been presented. The sports therapist is recommended to undertake further investigation into advanced clinical assessment and clinical reasoning strategies so as to be able to deliver specific progressive exercise rehabilitation and, where appropriate, manual therapy, electrotherapy and taping techniques. It is essential to keep abreast of the latest research findings so as to support the effective functional recovery of injured athletes.

References

AAOS (American Academy of Orthopaedic Surgeons) (1969) *In joint motion: Method of measuring and recording.* E. and S. Livingston. Edinburgh and London, UK

Agosta, J. and Holzer, K. (2012) Foot pain. In Brukner, P., Bahr, R., Blair, S., *et al.* (eds) *Brukner and Khan's clinical sports medicine*, 4th edition. McGraw-Hill. NSW, Australia.

Alfredson, H. and Cook, J. (2007) A treatment algorithm for managing Achilles tendinopathy: New treatment option. *British Journal of Sports Medicine.* 41: 211–216

Alfredson, H. and Ohlberg, L. (2005) Neovascularization in chronic patellar tendinosis: Promising results after sclerosing neovessels outside tendon challenges need for surgery. *Knee Surgery, Sports Traumatology and Arthroscopy.* 13 (2): 74–80

Alfredson, H., Pietilä, T., Jonsson, P. and Lorentzon, R. (1998) Heavy-load eccentric calf muscle training for the treatment of chronic Achilles tendinosis. *American Journal of Sports Medicine.* 26 (3): 360–366

Alfredson, H., Cook, J., Silbernagel, K. and Karlsson, J. (2012) Pain in the Achilles region. In Brukner, P., Bahr, R., Blair, S., *et al.* (eds) *Brukner and Khan's clinical sports medicine*, 4th edition. McGraw-Hill. NSW, Australia.

Alfredson, H., Andersson, G., Backman, L., Bagge, J., Danielson, P. and Forsgren, S. (2013) US doppler-guided surgical treatment based on immunohistochemical findings in mid-portion Achilles tendinopathy shows good clinical results and fast return to activity. *British Journal of Sports Medicine.* 47 (9): e2

Bachmann, L.M., Kolb, E., Koller, M.T., Steurer, J. and ter Riet, G. (2003) Accuracy of Ottawa ankle rules to exclude fractures of the ankle and mid-foot: A systematic review. *British Medical Journal.* 326: 417

Basmajian, J.V. and Stecko, G. (1963) The role of muscles in arch support of the foot: An electromyographic study. *Journal of Bone and Joint Surgery.* 45: 1184–1190

Beck, B.R. (2012) *ACSM current comment: Stress fractures.* www.acsm.org/docs/current-comments/stressfractures.pdf, accessed May 2014

Bennell, K., Talbot, R., Wajswelner, H., Techovanich, W., Kelly, D. and Hall, A.J. (1998) Intra-rater and inter-rater reliability of a weight-bearing lunge measure of ankle dorsiflexion. *Australian Journal of Physiotherapy.* 44: 175–180

Birrer, R., Fani-Salek, M., Totten, V., Herman, L. and Politi, V. (1999) Managing ankle injuries in the emergency department. *Journal of Emergency Medicine*. 17 (4): 651–660

Bolgla, L.A. and Malone, T.R. (2004) Plantar fasciitis and the windlass mechanism: A biomechanical link to clinical practice. *Journal of Athletic Training*. 39 (1): 77–82

Boone, D.C. and Azen, S.P. (1979) Normal range of motion of joints in male subjects. *Journal of Bone and Joint Surgery*. 61: 756–759

Brown, L.P. and Yavarsky, P. (1987) Locomotor biomechanics and pathomechanics: A review. *Journal of Orthopedic and Sports Physical Therapy*. 9: 3–10

Buchbinder, R. (2004) Plantar fasciitis. *New England Journal of Medicine*. 350 (21): 2159–2166

Cailliet, R. (1997) *Foot and ankle pain*, 3rd edition. FA Davies Company. Philadelphia, PA

Caravaggi, P., Pataky, T., Günther, M., Savage, R. and Crompton, R. (2001) Dynamics of longitudinal arch support in relation to walking speed: Contribution of the plantar aponeurosis. *Journal of Anatomy*. 217 (3): 254–261

Carnes, M.A. and Vizniak, N.A. (2012) *Quick reference evidence-based conditions manual*. Professional Health Systems. Canada

Cejudo, A., Sainz de Baranda, P., Ayala, F. and Santonja, F. (2014) A simplified version of the weight-bearing ankle lunge test: Description and test-retest reliability. *Manual Therapy*. 19: 355–359

Clarkson, H.M. (2013) *Musculoskeletal assessment: Joint motion and muscle testing*, 3rd edition. Lippincott, Williams and Wilkins. Philadelphia, PA

Cole, C., Seto, C. and Gazewood, J. (2005) Plantar fasciitis: Evidence-based review of diagnosis and therapy. *American Family Physician*. 72 (11): 2237–2242

Cook, C.E. and Hegedus, E. (2013) *Orthopaedic physical examination tests*, 2nd edition. Prentice Hall. London, UK

Cook, J.L. and Purdam, C.R. (2009) Is tendon pathology a continuum? A pathology model to explain the clinical presentation of load-induced tendinopathy. *British Journal of Sports Medicine*. 43: 409–416

Cooke, M.W., Lamb, S.E., Marsh, J. and Dale, J. (2003) A survey of current consultant practice of treatment of severe ankle sprains in emergency departments in the United Kingdom. *Emergency Medicine Journal*. 20: 505–507

De Garceau, D., Dean, D., Requejo, S.M. and Thordarson, D.B. (2003) The association between diagnosis of plantar fasciitis and Windlass test results. *Foot and Ankle International*. 24 (3): 251–255

Den Hartog, B.D. (2009) Insertional Achilles tendinosis: Pathogenesis and treatment. *Foot and Ankle Clinics of North America*. 14: 639–650

Donahue, M., Simon, J. and Docherty, C.L. (2013) Reliability and validity of a new questionnaire created to establish the presence of functional ankle instability: The IdFAI. *Athletic Training and Sports Health Care*. 5 (1): 38–43

Dutton, M. (2008) *Orthopaedic examination, evaluation, and intervention*, 2nd edition. McGraw-Hill. New York

Ferber, R., Hreljac, A. and Kendall, K.D. (2009) Suspected mechanisms in the cause of overuse running injuries: A clinical review. *Sports Health: A Multidisciplinary Approach*. 1: 242

Ferran, N.A. and Maffulli, N. (2006) Epidemiology of sprains of the lateral ankle ligament complex. *Foot and Ankle Clinics*. 11 (3): 659–662

Fong, D.T., Hong, Y., Chan, L.K., Yung, P.S. and Chan, K.M. (2007) A systematic review on ankle injury and ankle sprain in sports. *Sports Medicine*. 37 (1): 73–94

Fong, D.T., Man, C., Yung, P.S., Cheng, S. and Chan, K.M. (2008) Sports-related ankle injuries attending accident and emergency department. *Injury (International Journal of the Care of the Injured)*. 39 (10): 1222–1227

Fuller, E.A. (2000). The windlass mechanism of the foot: A mechanical model to explain pathology. *Journal of the American Podiatric Medical Association*. 90: 35–46

Gaeta, M., Minutoli, F., Vinci, S., *et al.* (2006) High resolution CT grading of tibial stress reactions in distance runners. *American Journal of Radiology*. 187 (3): 789–793

Galbraith, R.M. and Lavallee, M.E. (2009) Medial tibial stress syndrome: Conservative treatment options. *Current Reviews in Musculoskeletal Medicine*. 2: 127–133

Gärdin, A., Movin, T., Svensson, L. and Shalabi, A. (2010) The long-term clinical and MRI results following eccentric calf muscle training in chronic Achilles tendinosis. *Skeletal Radiology*. 39: 435–442

Gefen, A., Megido-Ravid, M. and Itzchak, Y. (2001) In-vivo biomechanical behavior of the human heel pad during the stance phase of gait. *Journal of Biomechanics*. 34 (12): 1661–1665

Gill, L.H. (1997) Plantar fasciitis: Diagnosis and conservative management. *Journal of the American Academy of Orthopaedic Surgeons.* 5: 109–117

Gross, J.M., Fetto, J. and Rosen, E. (2009) *Musculoskeletal examination*, 3rd edition. Wiley-Blackwell. Chichester, UK

Hamill, J. and Knutzen, K.M. (2009). *Biomechanical basis of human movement*, 3rd edition. Lippincott, Williams and Wilkins. Philadelphia, PA

Hamilton, J.J. and Ziemer, L.K. (1981) Functional anatomy of the human ankle and foot. In Kiene, R.H. and Johnson, K.A. (eds) *Proceedings of the AAOS Symposium on the Foot and Ankle.* Mosby. St Louis, MO

Harradine, P. (2013) Medial tibial stress syndrome: A bone stress perspective to injury and treatment. *Running 2013 Conference Presentation.* Kettering, UK

Hassouna, H. and Singh, D. (2005). Morton's metatarsalgia: Pathogenesis, aetiology and current management. *Acta Orthopaedica Belgica.* 71 (6): 646

Hattam, P. and Smeatham, A. (2010) *Special tests in musculoskeletal examination: An evidence-based guide for clinicians.* Churchill Livingston. Edinburgh, UK

Helgeson, K. (2009) Examination and intervention for sinus tarsi syndrome. *North American Journal of Sports Physical Therapy.* 4 (1): 29–37

Hertel, J. (2002) Functional anatomy, pathomechanics and pathophysiology of lateral ankle instability. *Journal of Athletic Training.* 37 (4): 364–375

Hertel, J., Denegar, C.R., Monroe, M.M. and Stokes, W.L. (1999) Talocrural and subtalar joint instability after lateral ankle sprain. *Medicine and Science in Sports and Exercise.* 31 (11): 1501–1508

Hicks, J.H. (1954) The mechanics of the foot II: The plantar aponeurosis and the arch. *Journal of Anatomy.* 88: 25–31

Huang, C.K., Kitaoka, H.B., An, K.N. and Chao, E.Y. (1993) Biomechanical evaluation of longitudinal arch stability. *Foot and Ankle.* 14 (6): 353–357

Hunter, L.J. and Fortune, J. (2000) Foot and ankle biomechanics. *South African Journal of Physiotherapy.* 56 (1): 17–20

Jana, R. and Roy T.S. (2011) Variant insertion of the fibularis tertius muscle is an evidence of the progressive evolutionary adaptation for the bipedal gait. *Clinics and Practice.* 1 (4): e81

Jose, J., Fichter, B. and Clifford, P.D. (2011) Tibial stress injuries in athletes. *American Journal of Orthopaedics.* 40 (4): 202–203

Joseph, M.F., Taft, K., Moskwa, M. and Denegar, C.R. (2012) Deep friction massage to treat tendinopathy: A systematic review of a classic treatment in the face of a new paradigm of understanding. *Journal of Sport Rehabilitation.* 21 (4): 343–353

Joyce, D. (2010) Ankle complex injuries in sport. In Comfort, P. and Abrahamson, E. (eds) *Sports rehabilitation and injury prevention.* Wiley-Blackwell. Chichester, UK

Jungers, W.L., Meldrum, D.J. and Stern, J.T. (1993) The functional and evolutionary significance of the human peroneus tertius muscle. *Journal of Human Evolution.* 25: 377–386

Kakkar, R., Chambers, S. and Scott, M.M. (2011) Conservative management of bilateral tendoachilles (TA) rupture: A case report. *Surgical Science.* 2 (5): 224–227

Kaminski, T.W., Hertel, J., Amendola, N., *et al.* (2013) National Athletic Trainers' Association Position Statement: Conservative management and prevention of ankle sprains in athletes. *Journal of Athletic Training.* 48 (4): 528–545

Karlsson, J. (2006) Acute ankle injuries. In Brukner, P. and Khan, K. (eds) *Clinical sports medicine*, 3rd edition. McGraw-Hill. NSW, Australia

Kearney, R. and Costa, M.L. (2010) Insertional Achilles tendinopathy management: A systematic review. *Foot and Ankle International.* 31 (8): 689–694

Kelikian, A.S. and Sarrafian, S.K. (2011) *Sarrafian's anatomy of the foot and ankle: Descriptive, topographical, functional*, 3rd edition. Lippincott, Williams and Wilkins. Philadelphia, PA

Kendall, F.P., McCreary, E.K., Provance, P.G., Rodgers, M.M. and Romani, W.A. (2005) *Muscles, testing and function with posture and pain*, 5th edition. Lippincott, Williams and Wilkins. Baltimore, MD

Kerkhoffs, G.M, van den Bekerom, M., Elders, L.A.M., *et al.* (2013) Diagnosis, treatment and prevention of ankle sprains: An evidence-based clinical guideline. *British Journal of Sports Medicine.* 46: 854–860

Kim. W. and Voloshin, A.S. (1995) Role of plantar fascia in the load-bearing capacity of the human foot. *Journal of Biomechanics.* 28: 1025–1033

Knott, L. and Kenny, T. (2013) *Varicose veins.* www.patient.co.uk/health/varicose-veins-leaflet, accessed March 2014

Kohls-Gatzoulis, J., Angel, J.C., Singh, D., Haddad, F., Livingstone, J. and Berry, G. (2004) Tibialis posterior dysfunction: A common and treatable cause of adult acquired flatfoot. *British Medical Journal.* 329: 1328–1333

Konor, M.M., Morton, S., Eckerson, J.M. and Grindstaff, T.L. (2012) Reliability of three measures of ankle dorsiflexion range of motion. *International Journal of Sports Physical Therapy.* 7 (3): 279–287

Korpalainen, R., Orava, S., Karpakka, J., Siira, P. and Hulkko, A. (2001) Risk factors for recurrent stress fractures in athletes. *American Journal of Sports Medicine.* 29 (3): 304–310

Kortebein, P.M., Kaufman, K.R., Basford, J.R. and Stuart, M.J. (2000) Medial tibial stress syndrome. *Medicine and Science in Sports and Exercise.* 32 (3): S27–33

Kujala, U.M., Sarna, S. and Kaprio, J. (2005) Cumulative incidence of Achilles tendon rupture and tendinopathy in male former elite athletes. *Clinics in Sports Medicine.* 15: 133–135

Kwong, P.K., Kay, D., Voner, P.T. and White, M.W. (1988) Plantar fasciitis: Mechanics and pathomechanics of treatment. *Clinical Sports Medicine.* 7: 119–126

Landorf, K.B., Radford, J.A., Keenan, A.M., *et al.* (2005) Effectiveness of low-Dye taping for the short term management of plantar fasciitis. *Journal of American Podiatric Medical Association.* 95 (6): 525–530

Lemont, H., Ammirati, K.M. and Usen, N. (2003) Plantar fasciitis: A degenerative process (fasciosis) without inflammation. *Journal of the American Podiatric Medical Association.* 93 (3): 234–237

Leppilahti, J., Puranen, J. and Orava, S. (1996) Incidence of Achilles tendon rupture. *Acta Orthopaedica.* 67 (3): 277–279

Lombardi, C.M., Silhanek, A.D., Connolly, F.G. and Dennis, L.N. (2002) The effect of first metatarsophalangeal joint arthrodesis on the first ray and the medial longitudinal arch: A radiographic study. *Journal of Foot and Ankle Surgery.* 41: 96–103

Loudon, J., Swift, M. and Bell, S. (2008) *The clinical orthopedic assessment guide,* 2nd edition. Human Kinetics. Champaign, IL

Luttgens, K. and Hamilton, N. (1997) *Kinesiology: Scientific basis of human motion,* 9th edition. Brown and Benchmark. Madison, WI

Maffulli, N. (1999) Rupture of the Achilles tendon. *Journal of Bone and Joint Surgery (American Volume).* 81 (7): 1019–1036

Magee, D. (2008) *Orthopedic physical assessment,* 5th edition. Saunders. London, UK

Magnussen, R.A., Dunn, W.R. and Thomson, A.B. (2009) Nonoperative treatment of midportion Achilles tendinopathy: A systematic review. *Clinical Journal of Sports Medicine.* 19: 54–64

Mahadevan, V (2008a) Pelvic girdle and lower limb: Ankle and foot. In Standring, S. (ed.) *Gray's anatomy: The anatomical basis of clinical practice,* 40th edition. Elsevier, Churchill Livingstone. UK

Mahadevan, V (2008b) Pelvic girdle and lower limb: Overview and surface anatomy. In Standring, S. (ed.) *Gray's anatomy: The anatomical basis of clinical practice,* 40th edition. Elsevier, Churchill Livingstone. UK

Marieb, E.N. and Hoehn, K. (2009). *Human anatomy and physiology,* 8th edition. Benjamin Cummings. Redwood City, CA

McCaig, S. (2012) Chronic ankle instability: Rehabilitation to prevent long term problems. *From Pain to Performance.* Conference presentation. London, UK

McKeon, P.O. and Mattacola, C.G. (2008) Interventions for the prevention of first time and recurrent ankle sprains. *Clinics in Sports Medicine.* 27 (3): 371–382

Menton, D. (2000) The plantaris and the question of vestigial muscles in man. *Journal of Creation.* 14 (2): 50–53

Moen, M.H., Bongers, T., Bakker, E.W.P., *et al.* (2010) The additional value of a pneumatic leg brace in the treatment of recruits with medial tibial stress syndrome: A randomized study. *Journal of the Royal Army Medical Corps.* 156 (4): 236–240

Moen, M.H., Holtslag, L., Bakker, E., *et al.* (2012) The treatment of medial tibial stress syndrome in athletes: A randomized clinical trial. *Sports Science, Medicine and Rehabilitation.* 4 (1): 12

Molloy, S., Solan, M.C. and Bendall, S.P. (2003) Synovial impingement in the ankle: A new physical sign. *Journal of Bone and Joint Surgery.* 85: 330–333

Muller-Wohlfahrt, H.-W., Haensel, L., Ueblacker, P. and Binder, A. (2013) Conservative treatment of muscle injuries. In Muller-Wohlfahrt, H.-W., Ueblacker, P., Haensel, L. and Garrett, W.E. (eds) *Muscle injuries in sport.* Thieme. Stuttgart, Germany

Mulligan, E.P. (2012) Lower leg, ankle and foot rehabilitation. In Andrews, J.R., Harrelson, G.L. and Wilk, K.E. (eds) *Physical rehabilitation of the injured athlete,* 4th edition. Elsevier, Saunders. Philadelphia, PA

Muscolino, J. (2006) *Kinesiology: The skeletal system and function.* Mosby, Elsevier. Philadelphia, PA

Neeley, F.G. (1998) Biomechanical risk factors for exercise related lower limb injuries. *Sports Medicine*. 26 (6): 395–413

Norkin, C.C. and Levangie, P.K. (2001) *Joint structure and function: A comprehensive analysis*, 4th edition. FA Davis Company. Philadelphia, PA

Oatis, C.A. (2009) *Kinesiology: The mechanics and pathomechanics of human movement*, 2nd edition. Lippincott, Williams and Wilkins. Philadelphia, PA

Ohberg, L., Lorentzon, R. and Alfredson, H. (2004) Eccentric training in patients with chronic Achilles tendinosis: Normalised tendon structure and decreased thickness at follow up. *British Journal of Sports Medicine*. 4 (38): 8–11

Orchard, J.W., Alcott, E., James, T., Farhart, P., Portus, M. and Waugh, S.R. (2002) Exact moment of a gastrocnemius muscle strain captured on video. *British Journal of Sports Medicine*. 36 (3): 222–223

Palastanga, N., Soames, R. and Palastanga, D. (2008) *Anatomy and human movement pocketbook*. Churchill Livingstone, Elsevier. Philadelphia, PA

Palmer, M.L. and Epler, M.E. (1998) *Fundamentals of musculoskeletal assessment techniques*, 2nd edition. Lippincott-Raven. Philadelphia, PA

Pansky, B. and Gest, T.R. (2012) *Lippincott's concise illustrated anatomy: Back, upper limb and lower limb*. Lippincott, Williams and Wilkins. Philadelphia, PA

Park, J.S. (2014) Ankle and foot. In Miller, M.D., Chhabra, A.B., Konin, J. and Mistry, D. (eds) *Sports medicine conditions: Return to play – recognition, treatment, planning*. Lippincott, Williams and Wilkins. Philadelphia, PA

Petty, N. (2011) *Neuromusculoskeletal examination and assessment*, 4th edition. Churchill Livingstone, Elsevier. Edinburgh, UK

Prentice, W.E. (2009) *Arnheim's principles of athletic training: A competence-based approach*, 13th edition. McGraw-Hill. New York

Punam, G. and Chhaya, V. (2013) Study of the efficacy of the Mulligan's movement with mobilization and taping technique as an adjunct to the conventional therapy for lateral ankle sprain. *Indian Journal of Physiotherapy and Occupational Therapy*. 7 (3): 167–171

Ranson, C. (2013) Tendinopathy in runners and running sports. *Running 2013 Conference Presentation*. Kettering, UK

Rasmussen, S., Christensen, M., Mathiesen, I. and Simonson, O. (2008) Shockwave therapy for chronic Achilles tendinopathy: A double-blind, randomized clinical trial of efficacy. *Acta Orthopaedica*. 79 (2): 249–256

Rathleff, M.S., Samani, A., Olesen, C.G., Kersting, U.G. and Madeleine, P. (2011) Inverse relationship between the complexity of midfoot kinematics and muscle activation in patients with medial tibial stress syndrome. *Journal of Electromyography and Kinesiology*. 21 (4): 638–644

Rathleff, M.S., Mølgaard, C.M., Fredberg, U., *et al.* (2014) High-load strength training improves outcome in patients with plantar fasciitis: A randomized controlled trial with 12-month follow-up. *Scandinavian Journal of Medicine and Science in Sport*. doi: 10.1111/sms.12313 (published online first)

Rathur, S., Clifford, P.D. and Chapman, C.B. (2009) Posterior ankle impingement: Os trigonum syndrome. *American Journal of Orthopedics*. 38 (5): 252–253

Read, M.T.F. (2008) *Concise guide to sports injuries*, 2nd edition. Churchill Livingstone, Elsevier. Philadelphia, PA

Rees, J.D., Stride, M. and Scott, A. (2013) Tendons: Time to revisit inflammation. *British Journal of Sports Medicine*. http://dx.doi.org/10.1136/bjsports-2012-091957, accessed May 2013

Riddle, D.L. and Schappert, S.M. (2004) Volume of ambulatory care visits and patterns of care for patients diagnosed with plantar fasciitis: A national study of medical doctors. *Foot and Ankle International*. 25 (5): 303–310

Roass, A. and Andersson, G.B.R. (1982) Normal range of motion of the hip, knee and ankle joints in male subjects, 30–40 years of age. *Acta Orthopaedica Scandinavica*. 53: 205–208

Robinson, J.M., Cook, J.L., Purdam, C., *et al.* (2001) The VISA-A questionnaire: A valid and reliable index of the clinical severity of Achilles tendinopathy. *British Journal of Sports Medicine*. 35: 335–341

Rompe, J.D., Cacchio, A., Weil, L., *et al.* (2010) Plantar fascia-specific stretching versus radial shock-wave therapy as initial treatment of plantar fasciopathy. *Journal of Bone and Joint Surgery*. 92 (15): 2514–2522

Rowe, V., Hemmings, S., Barton, C., Malliaras, P., Maffulli, N. and Morrissey, D. (2012) Conservative management of midportion Achilles tendinopathy: A mixed methods study, integrating systematic review and clinical reasoning. *Sports Medicine*. 42 (11): 941–967

Rupp, R.E. (2008) Overcompression of the syndesmosis during ankle fracture fixation: A case report. *American Journal of Orthopedics*. 37 (5): 259–261

Sammarco, G.J. and Hockenbury, R.T. (2001). Biomechanics of the foot and ankle. In Nordin, M. and Frankel, V.H. (eds) *Basic biomechanics of the musculoskeletal system*, 3rd edition. Lippincott, Williams and Wilkins. Philadelphia, PA

Sarrafian, S.K. (1987) Functional characteristics of the foot and plantar aponeurosis under tibiotalar loading. *Foot and Ankle*. 8: 4–18

Sarrafian, S.K. (1993) Biomechanics of the subtalar joint complex. *Clinical Orthopaedics and Related Research*. 290: 17–26

Scholten, P.E., Breugem, S.J. and van Dijk, C.N. (2012) Tendoscopic treatment of recurrent peroneal tendon dislocation. *Knee Surgery, Sports Traumatology, Arthroscopy*. 21 (6): 1304–1306

Scott, A., Docking, S., Vicenzino, B., *et al.* (2013) Sports and exercise-related tendinopathies: A review of selected topical issues by participants of the second International Scientific Tendinopathy Symposium (ISTS), Vancouver, 2012. *British Journal of Sports Medicine*. 47: 536–544

Sewell, D., Watkins, P. and Griffin, M. (2013) *Sport and exercise science: An introduction*, 2nd edition. Routledge. Abingdon, UK

Sharma, P. and Maffulli, N. (2005) Tendon injury and tendinopathy: Healing and repair. *Journal of Bone and Joint Surgery*. 87: 187–202

Shultz, S., Houglum, P. and Perrin, D. (2000) *Assessment of athletic injuries*. Human Kinetics. Champaign, IL

Soderberg, G.L. (1986). *Kinesiology: Application to pathological motion*. Williams and Wilkins. Philadelphia, PA

Soutas-Little, R.W., Beavis, G.C., Verstraete, M.C. and Markus, T.L. (1987) Analysis of foot motion during running using a joint co-ordinate system. *Medicine and Science in Sports and Exercise*. 19 (3): 285–293

Stiell, I.G. (1996) Ottawa ankle rules. *Canadian Family Physician*. 42: 478–480

Stiell, I.G., McDowell, I., Nair, R.C., Aeta, H., Greenberg, G.H. and McKnight, R.D. (1992a) Use of radiography in acute ankle injuries: Physicians' attitudes and practice. *Canadian Medical Association Journal*. 147 (11): 1671–1678

Stiell, I.G., Greenberg, G.H., McKnight, R.D., Nair, R.C., McDowell, I. and Worthington, J.R. (1992b) A study to develop clinical decision rules for the use of radiography in acute ankle injuries. *Annals of Emergency Medicine*. 21 (4): 384–390

Stoita, R. and Walsh, M. (2010) Operative treatment of plantar fasciitis: Evaluation of a surgical technique that preserves the integrity of plantar aponeurosis. *Journal of Bone and Joint Surgery (British Volume)*. 92 (Suppl. I): 177

Tan, V., Lin, S.S. and Okereke, E. (2003) Superior peroneal retinaculoplasty: A surgical technique for peroneal subluxation. *Clinical Orthopaedics and Related Research*. 410: 320–325

Tidy, C. and Kenny, T. (2012) *Deep vein thrombosis*. www.patient.co.uk/health/deep-vein-thrombosis-leaflet, accessed June 2014

van Middelkoop, M., van Rijn, R.M., Verhaar, J.A.N., Koes, B.W. and Bierma-Zeinstra, S.M.A. (2012) Re-sprains during the first 3 months after initial ankle sprain are related to incomplete recovery: An observational study. *Journal of Physiotherapy*. 58: 181–188

Vega, J., Batista, J.P., Golanó, P., Dalmau, A. and Viladot, R. (2013) Tendoscopic groove deepening for chronic subluxation of the peroneal tendons. *Foot and Ankle International*. 34 (6): 832–840

Viel, E. and Esnault, M. (1989) The effect of increased tension in the plantar fascia: A biomechanical analysis. *Physiotherapy Practitioner*. 5: 69–73

Viladot, A., Lorenzo, J.C., Salazar, J. and Rodriguez, A. (1984) The subtalar joint: Embryology and morphology. *Foot and Ankle*. 5: 54–66

Volpi, P., Melegati, G., Tornese, D. and Bandi, M. (2004) Muscle strains in soccer: A five-year survey of an Italian major league team. *Knee Surgery, Sports Traumatology, Arthroscopy*. 12 (5): 482–485

Whiting, W.C. and Zernicke, R.F. (1998). *Biomechanics of musculoskeletal injury*. Human Kinetics. Champaign, IL

Willems, T.M., Witvrouw, E., Delbaere, K., Mahieu, N., De Bourdeaudhuij, I. and De Clercq, D. (2005) Intrinsic risk factors for inversion ankle sprains in male subjects: A prospective study. *American Journal of Sports Medicine*. 33 (3): 415–423

Willits, K., Amendola, A., Bryant, D., *et al.* (2010) Operative versus non-operative treatment of acute Achilles tendon ruptures: A multi-center randomized trial using accelerated functional rehabilitation. *Journal of Bone and Joint Surgery.* 92 (17): 2767–2775

Yates, B. and White, S. (2004) The incidence and risk factors in the development of medial tibial stress syndrome among naval patients. *American Journal of Sports Medicine.* 32 (3): 772–780

Yelland, M.J., Sweeting, K.R., Lyftogt, J.A., Ng, S.K., Scuffham, P.A. and Evans, K.A. (2011) Prolotherapy injections and eccentric loading exercises for painful Achilles tendinosis: A randomised trial. *British Journal of Sports Medicine.* 45 (5): 421–428

12

PROFESSIONALISM AND ETHICS IN SPORTS THERAPY

Paul Robertson, Keith Ward and Rob Di Leva

Over recent years, sports therapists have gained increased recognition as autonomous allied health care practitioners, and have a valid role to play in the increasingly multidisciplinary area of Sport and Exercise Medicine (SEM). While the process for establishing improved recognition has not been without its challenges, in the UK organizations and professional bodies such as the Society of Sports Therapists (SST), the British Association of Sports Rehabilitators and Trainers (BASRaT) and the Sports Therapy Organization (STO), among others, have sought to consolidate the position of sports therapists (or sports rehabilitators in the case of BASRaT). This chapter seeks to present an overview of the professional responsibilities that sports therapists are obliged to recognize and uphold. Additionally, ethical issues and challenges that practitioners may encounter in their daily practice are discussed.

Development of sports therapy

Zachazewski and Magee (2012) present an international perspective on 'sports therapy' and practitioners who work as 'sports therapists'. They correctly identify that *'The definition, number, type, background, educational preparation, expertise, and experience of these health care professionals vary broadly on an international basis.'* Zachazewski and Magee (2012) further identify a range of health care professionals who may practise sports therapy; these may include the sports physiotherapist, athletic trainer, coach or trainer, massage therapist, strength and conditioning coach, sports psychologist, sports nutritionist, osteopath or chiropractor. In the UK, while the field of sports therapy is open to a range of practitioners, the evolution of the occupational title 'Sports Therapist' formally defines specialized practitioners who are appropriately trained primarily to support physically active populations (i.e. sports performers, fitness enthusiasts, performance artists and those simply engaging in regular physical activity). However, sports therapists are also well-positioned to provide health care to a range of less active populations (O'Halloran et al., 2009; Seah et al., 2009).

At the time of writing, sports therapists are still under a voluntary regulation system in the UK – i.e. there is no protection of title and no mandatory requirement for practising sports therapists to belong to any particular professional association (PA) – and this remains a major concern to those seeking minimum and mandatory accredited standards of education and a clearly demarcated scope of practice commensurate with other autonomous allied health care professionals in order to effectively promote safe and reliable practice and ultimately protect the general public from harm. What constitutes ideal professional regulation of sports therapists (statutory or voluntary) in the UK is still to be confirmed. Ward (2012) has presented a detailed commentary on this process. Graduate Sports Therapists (GST) are trained in evidence-based prevention, assessment, treatment and rehabilitation of injuries, and the return of patients to optimal levels of physical performance. As the vast majority of injuries sustained while participating in physical activity are musculoskeletal in nature, the sports therapist is required to be a specialist in assessing and managing such injuries and conditions. The specificity of the sports therapist's remit, and their ability to provide injury prevention interventions, pitch-side trauma care and return patients/athletes to optimal levels of physical performance (including sports-specific regimes) is arguably what definitively differentiates sports therapists from other recognized allied health care professionals such as physiotherapists and osteopaths; this is in addition to the fact that sports therapists from the outset are educated – and must achieve competency – in such sports- and exercise-specific areas as sports and exercise physiology, strength and conditioning, sports massage, sports rehabilitation and fitness profiling. The recognition of SEM as a medical specialty by the UK government in 2005 (Batt and Tanji, 2011), and the drive to get an ageing general population more engaged with physical activity, furthers the need for the GST – a health care professional with a specific remit to work with and support those engaged in regular sport and exercise.

Practitioner Tip Box 12.1

What is a sports therapist?

A sports therapist is a health care professional who has the knowledge, skills and ability to:

- utilize sports and exercise principles to optimize performance, preparation and injury prevention programmes;
- provide the immediate care of injuries and basic life support in a recreational, training and competitive environment;
- assess, treat and, where appropriate, refer on for specialist advice and intervention;
- provide appropriate sport and remedial massage in a sport and exercise context;
- plan and implement appropriate rehabilitation programmes.

Source: adapted from the Society of Sports Therapists, 2013.

Although each of the PAs representing sports therapists will have in place specified criteria for membership, the five established competency areas for GSTs as specified by the SST (2012a) are:

1. The prevention of injury and illness risk.
2. The recognition and evaluation of injury and illness.
3. The management and treatment of injury in both exercise and clinical environments, and referral of patients where appropriate.
4. The rehabilitation and reconditioning of patients.
5. The provision of health care education and professional practice.

Table 12.1 Competencies of a Graduate Sports Therapist

Prevention	A GST must be able to: • identify injury and illness risk factors associated with participation in competitive and recreational sport and exercise; • design, plan and implement comprehensive fitness and exercise programmes; • plan and implement injury and illness prevention strategies and programmes that involve a comprehensive understanding of the components of sport and exercise science.
Recognition and evaluation	A GST must be able to: • conduct a thorough initial examination and assessment of injuries and identify illnesses common to competitive and recreational sport and exercise participants.
Management, treatment and referral	A GST must be able to: • administer appropriate emergency aid and manage trauma within the competitive and recreational sport and exercise environment; • plan and carry out an appropriate treatment programme; • determine when and where participants should be referred to other appropriate health care professionals; • maintain a comprehensive medical records system.
Rehabilitation	A GST must be able to: • plan and implement a comprehensive rehabilitation and reconditioning programme appropriate for the patient concerned.
Education and professional practice areas	A GST must be able to: • provide relevant health care information, appropriate to their scope of practice and promote sports therapy as a professional discipline.

Source: reproduced with permission from the Society of Sports Therapists (SST, 2012a).

Underpinning each of the specified professional competencies are a specified scope of practice and a stipulated set of learning objectives and practical skill applications. GSTs must also be able to demonstrate the integration of critical analysis and evaluation, and evidence-informed approaches into their work. Furthermore, practitioners are required to adhere to designated Standards of Proficiency and Standards of Conduct, Performance and Ethics (SST, 2012b).

Healthcare ethics in employment settings

Sports therapists practice in a variety of employment settings, including the clinical setting, the occupational setting, in amateur sport, elite sport, the performing arts and in general health and fitness settings. Consequently, sports therapists can find themselves practising privately, or independently, or as part of an interdisciplinary SEM or emergency medical team (EMT). Whether practising independently or as part of an interdisciplinary team, it is important that all health care professionals understand their responsibilities and operate within their professional scope of practice as specified by their professional body. Furthermore, the sports therapist must be aware of the variety of professional and ethical challenges that can accompany working in environments such as those in sport, and the level of communication required to work effectively as part of an interdisciplinary team that may comprise professionals from areas other than health care (such as sports coaches or choreographers).

Sports therapy practice, and health care practice in general, is typified by adherence to ethical tenets. Such adherence should be regardless of the practice environment, or the presence or otherwise of an interdisciplinary team. Confidentiality, autonomy, non-maleficence (do no harm), beneficence (do good) and justice are core and generic tenets that are highly esteemed in health care (Anderson, 2007; Orchard, 2002; Schlabach and Peer, 2008; Sim, 1993), and are typically reinforced in the codes of conduct put in place by professional organizations for their members to abide by (as in the SST Standards of Conduct, Performance and Ethics, 2012b). Codes of conduct are characteristic of established professions (Swisher and Page, 2005) and are a requirement of emerging health care professions. Codes of conduct provide practitioners with guidance for appropriate professional behaviour. However, they do not offer a specific course of action for a practitioner when faced with a challenging ethical situation (Schlabach and Peer, 2008), nor do they guarantee that practitioners will act in an ethical manner (Robertson, 2009). Therefore, an understanding of these key tenets and a highly internalized sense of personal responsibility (McNamee, 1998), in addition to familiarity with the relevant code of conduct, are necessary in order for practitioners to act in a suitable manner regardless of the practice situation. As autonomous health care professionals, sports therapists must recognize their responsibilities and accountability. The process begins during formal training; transition must occur as one qualifies for practice. Schlabach and Peer (2008) define this as 'professional enculturation': *'The process of transition from novice to professional … learning and internalizing the norms, values, beliefs and behaviours of that profession.'* Once qualified, the main source of professional information and support is derived from a designated PA. Hence, it is important to recognize the responsibilities of a reputable professional association and what they are expected to provide, efficiently, for their members.

Generic responsibilities of a professional association

- Maintenance and regulation of a register of members (which may incorporate full, associate and student membership categories).
- Provision of a detailed code of conduct and ethics for members to abide by.
- Provision of a set of detailed competencies and proficiencies (of which full members must be able to demonstrate evidence of achievement).
- Provision of detailed disciplinary and appeals procedures for members facing allegations of impaired fitness to practise (due to misconduct, negligence, conviction or caution for a criminal offence, or for physical or mental health reasons).
- Provision of a comprehensive and immediate source of educational, legal and employment advice and support to members.
- Development and validation of educational standards and qualifications.
- Provision of specific advice to the general public.
- Provision of advice for, and liaison with, external parties on all matters pertaining to sports therapy and sports therapists (i.e. educational organizations, sporting bodies, health associations, other national and international PAs and the media).
- To provide members with the facility to take out appropriate levels of professional indemnity and public liability insurance and other insurances where necessary (such as employer's liability or business contents insurance).

Having and maintaining up-to-date and appropriate levels of professional indemnity (malpractice) and public liability insurance is an absolute necessity for protection in practice, and is one of the fundamental responsibilities for all practising sports therapists.

Practitioner Tip Box 12.2

Recommended activities for professional success

- Undertake a recognized, accredited professional qualification.
- Join a reputable professional association (PA).
- Ensure that full professional indemnity and public liability insurance is in place.
- Fully understand your professional scope of practice and expected code of conduct.
- Fully recognize your professional responsibilities and aspire to achieve professional enculturalization.
- Undertake appropriate, varied and sufficient continued professional development (CPD).
- CPD can include attendance at conferences, workshops and courses; mentoring and being mentored; shadowing experienced practitioners; peer group discussion; reading and critically evaluating articles; writing articles; giving talks; teaching; undertaking research; and more. CPD needs to be effectively reflected upon and appropriately documented.
- Read and appraise current appropriate literature.
- Undertake research (i.e. literature reviews; clinical audits; case studies; interventional studies).
- Undertake advanced qualifications and/or adjunctive qualifications.
- Join a specialist interest group or society.
- Seek the support of your PA for any professionally challenging situation.
- Volunteer to gain experience and develop professional contacts.
- Recognize that you can learn from everyone – including yourself (i.e. learn from what you do well, as well as from your mistakes).
- Work to create your opportunities (i.e. networking; publishing; delivering presentations).
- Be organized in practice (i.e. maintain equipment; be punctual; be hygienic; maintain records; pay your bills).
- Appreciate that working as a sports therapist is likely to involve working long hours.
- Be prepared to sometimes put work first.
- Present a positive, professional image.
- Be welcoming, polite and respectful in all communications and situations.
- Proof-read all communications, including email, before sending.
- Use social media with care, and with professional responsibility.
- Remember that a therapist is a professional who is trained, qualified and expected to care.
- Develop a sense of humour and your ability to engage in small talk.
- Contribute to the team (i.e. do more than your basic role).
- Be wary of unprofessional subcultural activity (e.g. inappropriately discussing patients; binge-drinking; unsociable behaviour).
- Practise what you preach.
- Stay focused; be honest; be thorough; be ethical.
- Scrutinize carefully any job advert prior to application (i.e. job role; person specification).
- If you require a reference/referee for a job application, it is courteous to request their approval first.
- Do not be afraid to carefully express your opinion.
- Avoid being disparaging of other people and professionals.

- Appreciate the process for the attainment of expertise.
- Be reflective and perform periodic SWOT analysis of your performance (identifying your strengths; weaknesses; opportunities; and threats).
- Be flexible, forgiving, open to change and willing to take on challenges.
- Work hard, exercise regularly, eat well and rest effectively.
- Make sure you allow some time for yourself, and your family and friends.

Confidentiality

Confidentiality is deemed essential for those trusted with making medical decisions (Oriscello, 2005). The preservation of a patient's confidentiality is crucial if a practitioner is to develop trust in their relationship with the patient (Fabius and Frazee, 2008) and applies in all situations and with all patients (Oriscello, 2005). The security of patient information is paramount to maintaining confidentiality, and appropriate measures to ensure this must be taken (for example, the use of lockable filing cabinets and password protected computer files) (Mattacola and Mattacola, 1999).

Autonomy

Autonomy refers to an individual's right to determine and take what they deem the best course of action for their selves (Mathias, 2004). This contrasts with the concept of paternalism, which is to determine and advocate a course of action for another individual (Anderson, 2007). In health care, the principle of autonomy has now superseded that of paternalism (Mathias, 2004), and in order for a patient to make a wholly autonomous decision they must be fully informed of all available treatment options (Jonas, 2006) and of any associated risks to their health (Anderson, 2007). The concept of informed consent has been explained by Sim (1996). In coexistence with this is the issue of professional (practitioner) autonomy, whereby the appropriately qualified health care professional (i.e. the graduate sports therapist) has the right and must make it their responsibility to make their own informed decisions in practice. Being an autonomous health care professional requires qualification for such, and is underpinned by experience and confidence in practice, and a certain level of authority.

Non-maleficence

Non-maleficence (to do no harm) is often cited as the core principle of health care practice (Schlabach and Peer, 2008). Yet the administration of seemingly appropriate treatment interventions does have the potential to result in pain (such as with manual therapy, electrotherapy or exercise rehabilitation) or further damage to injured tissues (such as where reduced pain sensation due to analgesic medication may result in a patient not being aware that they are causing further damage). Additionally, not administering treatment, or failing to act when there is a risk to the patient, can also result in harm (Anderson, 2007; Schlabach and Peer, 2008; Sim, 1993). Therefore, the practitioner must consider the potential benefits of interventions against the potential risk for harm that they may cause (Karnani, 2008). Clearly, there is an element of risk with virtually any intervention; iatrogenic conditions are those resulting from medical or therapeutic care, whether expertly and correctly delivered or inappropriately delivered. Health care professionals must always act responsibly and set out to do no harm; by employing evidence-based practice and by always acting within the remit of their practice, sports therapists will be taking all precautions to cause no harm.

711

Beneficence

Beneficence (to do good) refers to the requirement for the practitioner to always act in the best interests of the patient (Schlabach and Peer, 2008). While non-maleficence could be said to be a constant duty, beneficence can be viewed as a limited duty (Karnani, 2008). For example, the practitioner is required to always act in the best interests of their patients, but this does not apply to those who are not patients of the practitioner. In contrast, the practitioner must not harm another individual, regardless of whether that individual is a patient or not.

Justice

For the practitioner, justice means that patients in similar situations (i.e. with similar conditions) should be treated in a similar manner (Karnani, 2008). However, the principle of justice has wider societal connotations. The provision of equal opportunities for all individuals to experience services and opportunities, and the fair distribution of resources across society, reflects a justice-oriented approach (Karnani, 2008; Lumpkin *et al.*, 2003). For the practitioner, the use of expensive modalities, or extended time allocation, for certain patients and not others must be considered in the context of justice on a societal level and in terms of fair access to resources (Schlabach and Peer, 2008). Essentially, practitioners must routinely exhibit non-discriminatory practice.

Application of key tenets in employment settings

Despite the requirement to adhere to the key ethical tenets of health care practice, regardless of the situation, the variety of environments that a sports therapist can practice in challenges the practitioner's ability to adhere to the tenets in all situations. While the clinical setting may be more conducive to sound ethical practice, performance-oriented environments (such as in sport or performing arts) have the potential to place the sports therapist in ethically challenging situations.

Clinical settings

Sports therapists are regularly employed within a clinical setting. While the sports therapist will work with sports people in a clinical setting, they will also work with the general population. As long as the sports therapist is working in and applying treatments and techniques in a sport and exercise context, they are working within their sports therapy scope of practice. Within the clinical setting the sports therapist will commonly use modalities such as soft tissue therapy, joint mobilizations, exercise therapy and other rehabilitation techniques. In the clinical environment, the establishment of practitioner–patient boundaries is arguably more achievable due to the setting and the structured, appointment-based contact that is likely to be in place. Additionally, as an autonomous practitioner in a clinical setting that is removed from the patient's occupational or sporting environment, there is a reduced likelihood of the goal of patient health being tempered by performance-oriented goals such as the desire of the athlete to compete regardless of the potential for further harm. The clinical setting therefore allows the practitioner to be able to adhere to the key health care tenets and their code of conduct with minimal interference from others, and from competitive pressures.

Despite the clinical setting providing an environment that appears to be more conducive to ethical practice, ethical dilemmas can still emerge. Ethical dilemmas occur when two or more key tenets come into opposition (Karnani, 2008), and as a result the final decision cannot satisfy all the key tenets. When such ethical dilemmas occur, the practitioner must be able to identify the principles in conflict and be able to justify why one principle should be given priority over another (Schlabach and Peer, 2008). Additionally, for sports therapists, the professional body's code of conduct plays an essential role in their decision-making, as it too must be adhered to if the practitioner is to fulfil the requirements of the professional body. Therefore, even in the absence of other professionals in the decision-making process, the sports therapist has to meet the conditions of both the key ethical tenets and their professional body's code of conduct. While the majority of health care professional bodies' codes of conduct encapsulate the key tenets, they do not resolve the satisfying of all the ethical and professional requirements. Indeed, codes of conduct, while necessary for the protection of the public, practitioner and profession, are not foolproof and can be contradictory in nature and open to interpretation.

The often deontological (rule-based) nature of codes of conduct necessitates that practitioners adhere to the code in all situations, often regardless of the outcome (i.e. where the means justify the end). However, it appears that some professional bodies are now recognizing the limitations of such a rule-based approach. Two such bodies involved in health care are the Chartered Society of Physiotherapy (CSP) in the UK and the National Athletic Trainer's Association (NATA) in the United States. The emphasis of the approach utilized by these bodies is to provide a framework that supports the decision-making of their members and recognizes the ability of practitioners to act in the best interests of their patients, rather than requiring practitioners to adhere to a set of rules that may, or may not, result in the best outcome for the patient. The focus upon achieving the most favourable health-oriented outcome for the patient suggests a move away from the deontological approach and towards a more teleological approach, where the appropriateness of the decision is assessed not by its adherence to the rules, but by the consequences of the decision-making process. Arguably, the practitioner should adopt an altruistic approach in that the health outcome should be favourable for the patient, with less concern paid to the consequences for the practitioner.

Performance-oriented settings

Settings where the goal of patient health co-exists alongside performance-oriented goals such as winning in sport or the need to achieve a certain aesthetic in dance choreography can arguably exacerbate the potential for professional and ethical dilemmas to arise. Furthermore, the patient who may not be motivated by performance, but who needs to return to paid employment as soon as possible, may also challenge the sports therapist as financial necessities may be placed ahead of health. For the sports therapist who is practising with the goal of achieving the best health-oriented outcomes for their patient, working with patients who potentially place health behind performance or financial needs can be challenging. This situation is perhaps best exemplified by the elite sport setting.

Injuries are a generally accepted hazard of sports participation, with elite athletes seemingly expected, and willing, to take risks with their health that are above those expected of other professions (Murphy and Waddington, 2007). Indeed, studies (such as those by Drawer and Fuller, 2002; and Gissane et al., 2003) have highlighted that the risk of injury in professional sport can exceed that of other so-called high-risk professions such as construction, mining and quarrying. Moreover, Drawer and Fuller (2002) identify that this risk is deemed unacceptable according to the work-based criteria utilized by the Health and Safety Executive (HSE) in the UK, therefore putting a duty upon the employers of professional athletes to reduce this risk (Gissane et al., 2003).

The impact of such a high level of injury risk is wide-ranging. Elite athletes can be in receipt of earnings from salaries and endorsement agreements that far exceed the national average, with some football players receiving as much as £100,000 per week (Murphy and Waddington,

2007). Injury thus restricts the athlete's earning potential and prevents their employer's utilization of an expensive asset. Additionally, previous injury appears to be a key risk factor for subsequent injury (Hagglund *et al.*, 2006), potentially further restricting the employer's use of their asset and the athlete's earning potential, thus making the reduction of initial injury risk very important. For the athlete, regardless of salary or competitive level, injury can have a negative psychological impact in the form of anxiety, loss of motivation, anger and self-pity (Heredia *et al.*, 2004; Udry, 1997; Walker *et al.*, 2008). Furthermore, injury can prevent individuals from obtaining the well-established physical and psychological health benefits that accrue from participation in physical activity (Biddle and Mutrie, 2001) and can have long-term implications for physical health, as illustrated by associations between previous injury and osteoarthritis in athletes (Golightly *et al.*, 2009; Thelin *et al.*, 2006).

Despite the apparent need for health care professionals in the sports environment, the removal of the practitioner and the patient from the clinical setting and into areas such as the changing room, team bus and sports club has the potential to blur practitioner–patient boundaries and alter relationships (Moore, 2003; Sim, 1993). Moreover, the disparate aims of health care and sport have the potential to put the practitioner in a position where they sacrifice health-oriented values in favour of those that emphasize results (Mathias, 2004) and serve the interests of the employer (i.e. the sports organization) rather than the interests of the patient (Waddington and Roderick, 2002). As a consequence, the key tenets of confidentiality, autonomy and non-maleficence are particularly challenged (Anderson, 2007; Collins *et al.*, 1999; Mathias, 2004).

The health care practitioner, as an employee of a sports organization, has an obligation to the employer, and this can lead to situations arising where the sports therapist may compromise outcomes for the patient by considering how decisions may affect their employment. Additionally, being a member of a multidisciplinary support team raises the concern that other members of the support team may not necessarily be bound by a code of conduct, or may be operating under a conflicting code. Consequently, problems may arise with regard to how information concerning an athlete's injury is used. Requests to both share information among the support team (Waddington and Roderick, 2002) and to withhold information from the athlete do occur (Murphy and Waddington, 2007) in what is an environment where coaches, managers and directors are under pressure to succeed. This compromising of key health care tenets, particularly in high-level sport (Collins *et al.*, 1999; Waddington and Roderick, 2002), has resulted in organizations and governing bodies reiterating the importance of practitioner adherence to their relevant professional code of conduct (such as with the British Olympic Association [BOA], 2000). Such documents call for those involved with interdisciplinary teams to be aware of the constraints imposed upon practitioners by their professional duties (BOA, 2000). Yet the presence of interdisciplinary team members whose primary role is to improve performance (such as with sport coaches, strength and conditioning coaches, exercise physiologists or psychologists), and the increasing integration of health care practitioners into a subculture where the goal is to continually push the boundaries of human performance, can see practitioners engaging in these result-oriented practices (Anderson, 2007; Mathias, 2004) despite the calls for adherence.

The integration of the health care practitioner into the sports environment, and in particular into the area of selection for competition, further compromises the practitioner's ability to serve the best interests of the patient and achieve health-oriented goals. If a patient is aware that the practitioner is asked for information regarding the patient's ability to perform by those whose role it is to select individuals for competition, then the patient may withhold information, seek another practitioner who is not involved with selection or avoid seeing a practitioner at all (Collins *et al.*, 1999). Accordingly, patients may not be fully informed of the risks to their health if they continue to compete, thus undermining their ability to make an autonomous decision and potentially resulting in harm. Yet it is arguable that, even with information regarding potential risks to health, athletes will opt not to compete. The presence of external pressures (such as sponsors), the expectation for athletes to compete while injured (Murphy and Waddington, 2007), the athlete's desire to retain their squad place and the need to compete to receive financial reward contribute to athletes often perceiving that they have little option but to compete while injured (Roderick *et al.*, 2000). Additionally, for those athletes who are unable to compete due to injury, internal pressures (for example, challenges to athletic identity and self-resentment) frequently exist and can drive an athlete to prematurely return to competition (Shrier *et al.*, 2010).

The existence of these pressures on athletes and the potential for athletes to further harm themselves by competing while injured or returning to competition too early suggests that a paternalistic approach on the part of the health care practitioner may be justified (Brown, 1985). The process of identifying if the principle of autonomy should be sacrificed is not a straightforward one. It involves the practitioner assessing, often in a time-constrained situation, the capacity of the individual to make informed decisions about their actions, the environment in which these decisions take place and the potential for harm (Anderson, 2007). Furthermore, the extent to which the athlete has surrendered their autonomy must also be assessed. By engaging in a professional relationship with a health care practitioner, an individual often views the practitioner as an expert and therefore allows decisions regarding their health to be made by the practitioner; although the extent that this occurs in sport is questionable due to athletes' typically greater awareness of their bodies (Thomas, 1991).

In situations where an athlete's capacity to make an informed decision is clearly compromised (such as when they are concussed), then it can be strongly argued that the practitioner is right to limit the athlete's participation (Anderson, 2007) for the beneficence of the athlete (Thomas, 1991). This soft, or weak, form of paternalism is often viewed as justifiable and the inability of the athlete to make an informed decision may additionally warrant the practitioner engaging in coercion to ensure the health of the athlete (Thomas, 1991). A coercive approach involves the utilization of a threat to present an individual with no other option but to take the course of action deemed desirable by another (Anderson, 2007). For the practitioner, such threats may involve informing competition officials that the athlete is not medically fit to continue, therefore leaving the athlete with no option but to withdraw from competition.

If an injury does not obviously compromise an athlete's ability to make an informed decision (such as with a lateral ankle sprain), the practitioner must be aware of how truly voluntary an athlete's decision making is if they express a desire to continue playing or a return to competition. The explanation of risks to health by the practitioner does not necessarily mean that the athlete is then going to make a voluntary decision (Anderson, 2007), as they typically operate in a pressurized, win-at-all-costs environment (Volkwein, 1995). Thus, while athletes are not necessarily coerced, the presence of offers (such as financial rewards for a certain number of appearances) and the expectations of others (i.e. coaches, fans and teammates) can reduce the voluntariness of an athlete's decision (Anderson, 2007). If the practitioner does deem that an athlete's decision making is coerced, then a soft paternalistic approach may be warranted in such situations. Yet caution is necessary, as while the practitioner may perceive the athlete's decision to risk their health to be the result of coercion, there is a possibility that such risk-taking behaviours are the norm to the athlete and the decision is therefore wholly voluntary (Anderson, 2007). Any interference with actions that are wholly voluntary is termed hard, or strong, paternalism and is extremely hard to justify. Cases where both the severity and likelihood of harm to the individual, or to others, are high are perhaps the only time hard paternalism is warranted (Anderson, 2007).

The issues identified above highlight the difficulties for health practitioners working in the sports environment. The seemingly disparate aims of healthcare and sport, the presence of other professionals, financial implications and the overriding win-at-all-costs subculture of sport challenges the practitioner's loyalties and gives rise to ethical dilemmas. The re-emphasis of adherence to a professional code of conduct alone does not appear to be sufficient in such a multifaceted and pressurized environment; therefore, the practitioner must have both an awareness of the relevant code of conduct and of all factors that influence athletes being withdrawn from, or returned to, competition. An attempt to conceptualize this process with specific regard to return-to-competition decisions has been made (Creighton *et al.*, 2010). This three-step process recognizes the multifaceted nature of decision making in the sports environment and involves, first, evaluating the health status of the athlete through analysis of relevant medical factors (for example, clinical examination and functional tests). Second, an evaluation of the participation risk is made; this involves looking at factors that can modify the risk involved with participation (such as permitted protection, type of sport or competitive level). Finally, the practitioner must investigate the factors that could modify a decision to return to competition. For example, external pressures, the use of analgesics and pressure from the athlete should all be considered in light of the key tenets discussed previously (Creighton *et al.*, 2010).

Such models, while useful for the practitioner, only reflect a preliminary attempt to clarify what is a complex sociological process (Shrier *et al.*, 2010). However, it is arguable that despite such attempts to clarify the decision-making process, the practitioner will remain unable to achieve the necessary critical distance from the process in order to be wholly objective (Thomas, 1991). Furthermore, the values of the practitioner, as shaped by their exposure to various environments (Lumpkin *et al.*, 2003), will potentially motivate practitioners to behave in a certain way (Loisel *et al.*, 2005). That these values may conflict with what is considered desirable for the health of the athlete and the values of other members of the support team requires the practitioner to not just be aware of their relevant code of conduct or decision-making models, but to also be aware of their own values, the influence they can have on the practitioner's behaviour, the effect on other members of the support team and ultimately the effect on the health of the athlete (Schlabach and Peer, 2008). Engagement in activities that raise awareness of the values held by members of the support team can serve to create openness (Schlabach and Peer, 2008) and potentially aid the decision-making process when considering permitting athletes to continue to compete or return to competition.

Summary

Aspects of sports therapy have been in existence for many years; however, it is only recently that sports therapists have emerged as independent and autonomous health care practitioners. Several organizations and professional bodies have a vested interest in the development of sports therapy in the UK, yet coherence among these groups has been challenged for a number of political and processual reasons. Such issues are, however, not insurmountable and must be seen as being simply part of the evolutionary process for improved regulation and recognition. Despite its regulatory challenges, the sports therapy profession is experiencing significant progress and reputation as a viable and definitively different health care profession, with the capability to contribute effectively in a variety of settings and with a number of populations.

Working in different settings and with different populations requires the sports therapist to be aware of the professional and ethical challenges that they may face. Health care practice, regardless of setting or population, is characterized by several key tenets. However, for the sports therapist working in environments such as sport, adhering to the fundamental tenets can be challenging. The presence of external pressures on athletes and other members of the interdisciplinary support team, the varying values and codes that are present among other support team members, the win-at-all-costs subculture evident in sport and the desire to push the boundaries of human performance all contribute to the challenges the practitioner will face and make adherence to a code of conduct difficult. Moreover, the practitioner's own values will influence their motivation and ultimately their behaviour. Therefore, practitioners must have clear knowledge of their professional code of conduct, recognition of their own values, appreciation of the values of others and the understanding of pressures that exist in the sports environment in order to engage in effective decision making – all of which contribute to the characteristic hallmarks of an autonomous professional.

Useful websites

- Association of Chartered Physiotherapists in Sports and Exercise Medicine (ACPSEM): www.physiosinsport.org
- British Association of Sport and Exercise Medicine (BASEM): www.basem.co.uk
- British Association of Sport Rehabilitators and Trainers (BASRaT): www.basrat.org
- Chartered Society of Physiotherapy (CSP): www.csp.org.uk
- Complementary and Natural Healthcare Council (CNHC): www.cnhc.org.uk
- Federation of Holistic Therapists (FHT): www.fht.org.uk
- Health and Care Professions Council (HCPC): www.hpc-uk.org
- National Athletic Trainer's Association (NATA): www.nata.org
- Professional Standards Authority for Health and Social Care (PSA): www.chre.org.uk
- Society of Sports Therapists (SST): www.society-of-sports-therapists.org
- Sports Massage Association (SMA): www.thesma.org
- Sports Therapy Organisation (STO): www.uksportstherapy.org.uk
- World Federation of Athletic Training and Therapy (WFATT): www.wfatt.org

References

Anderson, L. (2007) Doctoring risk: Responding to risk-taking in athletes. *Sport, Ethics and Philosophy*. 1 (2): 119–134

Batt, M.E. and Tanji, J.L. (2011) The future of chronic disease management and the role of sport and exercise medicine physicians. *Clinical Journal of Sports Medicine*. 21: 1

Biddle, S.J. and Mutrie, N.M. (2001) *Psychology of physical activity: Determinants, well-being and health.* Routledge. London, UK

British Olympic Association (2000) The British Olympic Association's position statement on athlete confidentiality. *Journal of Sports Sciences*. 18: 133–135

Brown, W.M. (1985) Paternalism, drugs and the nature of sports. *Journal of the Philosophy of Sport*. 11: 14–22

Collins, D., Moore, P., Mitchell, D. and Alpress, F. (1999) Role conflict and confidentiality in multidisciplinary athlete support programmes. *British Journal of Sports Medicine*. 33: 208–211

Creighton, D.W., Shrier, I., Shultz, R., Meeuwisse, W.H. and Matheson, G.O. (2010) Return-to-play in sport: A decision-based model. *Clinical Journal of Sport Medicine*. 20 (5): 379–385

Drawer, S. and Fuller, C.W. (2002) Evaluating the level of injury in English professional football using a risk based assessment process. *British Journal of Sports Medicine*. 36: 446–451

Fabius, R. and Frazee, S.G. (2008) The 'trusted clinician': An alternative approach to worksite health promotion? *American Journal of Health Promotion*. 22 (3): supplement, 1–7

Gissane, C., White, J., Kerr, K., Jennings, S. and Jennings, D. (2003) Health and safety implications on injury in professional rugby league football. *Occupational Medicine*. 53: 512–517

Golightly, Y., Marshall, S.W. and Guskiewicz, K.M. (2009) Early-onset arthritis in retired National Football League players. *Journal of Physical Activity and Health.* 6 (5): 638–643

Hagglund, M., Walden, M. and Ekstrand, J. (2006) Previous injury as a risk factor for injury in elite football: A prospective study over two consecutive seasons. *British Journal of Sports Medicine.* 40: 767–772

Heredia, R.A., Munoz, A. and Artaza, J.L. (2004) The effect of psychological response on recovery of sport injury. *Research in Sports Medicine.* 12 (1): 15–31

Jonas, J. (2006) Ethics in injury management. *Athletic Therapy Today.* 11 (1): 28–30

Karnani, N. (2008) Bioethics: Applying the basic principles to resolve an ethical dilemma. *Northeast Florida Medical Supplement.* 59: 3–5

Loisel, P., Falardeau, M., Baril, R., *et al.* (2005) The values underlying team decision-making in work rehabilitation for musculoskeletal disorders. *Disability and Rehabilitation.* 27 (10): 561–569

Lumpkin, A., Stoll, S.K. and Beller, J.M. (2003) *Sport ethics: Applications for fair play,* 3rd edition. McGraw-Hill. New York

Mathias, M.B. (2004) The competing demands of sport and health: An essay on the history of ethics in sports medicine. *Clinical Sports Medicine.* 23: 195–214

Mattacola, C.G. and Mattacola, G.A. (1999) Confidentiality in athletic therapy: The legal perspective. *Athletic Therapy Today.* 4 (2): 13–14

McNamee, M. (1998) Celebrating trust: Virtues and rules in the ethical conduct of sports coaches. In McNamee, M.J. and Parry, S.J. (eds). *Ethics and sport.* E. and F.N. Spon. London, UK

Moore, Z.M. (2003) Ethical dilemmas in sport psychology: Discussion and recommendations for practice. *Professional Psychology: Research and Practice.* 34: 601–610

Murphy, P. and Waddington, I. (2007) Are elite athletes exploited? *Sport in Society.* 10 (2): 239–255

O'Halloran, P., Brown, V.T. and Morgan, K. (2009) The role of the sports and exercise medicine physician in the National Health Service: Questionnaire-based survey. *British Journal of Sports Medicine.* 43: 1143–1148

Orchard, J. (2002) Who owns the information? *British Journal of Sports Medicine.* 36 (1): 16–18

Oriscello, R.G. (2005) Ethical considerations in sports medicine. In O'Connor, F.G., Sallis, R.E., Wilder, R.P. and St. Pierre, P (eds). *Sports medicine: Just the facts.* McGraw-Hill. New York

Robertson, P. (2009) Ethical challenges in the sports environment: Implications for sports therapy. *Journal of Sports Therapy.* 2 (1): 1–2

Roderick, M., Waddington, I. and Parker, G. (2000) Playing hurt: Managing injuries in English professional football. *International Review for the Sociology of Sport.* 35 (2): 165–180

Schlabach, G.A. and Peer, K.S. (2008) *Professional ethics in athletic training.* Mosby, Elsevier. St. Louis, MO

Seah, R., Radford, D., Tillett, E. and Creaney, L. (2009) *NHS consultants in sport and exercise medicine: A new medical specialty to facilitate a physically active population, job plans and service description.* Faculty of Sport and Exercise Medicine UK. www.fsem.co.uk/DesktopModules/Documents, accessed May 2011

Shrier, I., Charland, L., Mohtadi, N.G.H., Meeuwisse, W.H. and Matheson, G.O. (2010) The sociology of return-to-play decision-making: A clinical perspective. *Clinical Journal of Sport Medicine.* 20 (5): 333–335

Sim, J. (1993) Sports medicine: Some ethical issues. *British Journal of Sports Medicine.* 27: 95–100

Sim, J. (1996) The elements of informed consent. *Manual Therapy.* 1 (2): 104–106

SST (Society of Sports Therapists) (2012a) *Standards of education and training: Competencies of a Graduate Sports Therapist.* Society of Sports Therapists. Glasgow, UK

SST (Society of Sports Therapists) (2012b) *Standards of conduct, performance and ethics.* www.society-of-sports-therapists.org/flipbooks/Standards%20of%20conduct%20performance%20and%20ethics/index.html, accessed January 2014

SST (Society of Sports Therapists) (2013) *What is sports therapy?* www.society-of-sports-therapists.org/index.php/public_information/what-is-sports-therapy, accessed December 2013

Swisher, L.L. and Page, C.G. (2005) *Professionalism in physical therapy.* Elsevier. St. Louis, MO

Thelin, N., Holmberg, S. and Thelin, A. (2006) Knee injuries account for the sports-related increase risk of increased osteoarthritis. *Scandinavian Journal of Medicine and Science in Sports.* 16 (5): 329–333

Thomas, C.E. (1991) Locus of authority, coercion, and critical distance in the decision to play an injured player. *Quest.* 43: 352–362

Udry, E. (1997) Coping and social support amongst injured athletes following surgery. *Journal of Sport and Exercise Psychology.* 19: 71–90

Volkwein, K.A.E. (1995) Ethics and top-level sport: A paradox? *International Review for the Sociology of Sport*. 30: 311–320

Waddington, I. and Roderick, M. (2002) Management of medical confidentiality in English professional clubs: Some ethical problems and issues. *British Journal of Sports Medicine*. 36: 118–123

Walker, N., Thatcher, J. and Lavallee, D. (2008) Psychological responses to injury in competitive sport: A critical review. *Perspectives in Public Health*. 127 (4): 174–180

Ward, K. (2012) The United States of sports therapy: A commentary on current progress and challenges of the profession. *Journal of Sports Therapy*. 5 (2): 2–13

Zachazewski, J.E. and Magee, D.J. (2012) Sports therapy: Who? What? When? Where? Why? and How? In Zachazewski, J.E. and Magee, D.J. (eds) *Sports therapy services: Organization and operations*. Wiley-Blackwell. Chichester, UK

Appendix

SPORTS THERAPY CLINIC   **Date:** _____

CONFIDENTIAL PATIENT RECORD FORM

Patient name: DoB: Age:	Address: Email: Tel. (mobile): Tel. (home / work):
GP details (name; address):	Consent for Assessment and Treatment: Y / N
Occupation(s):	ADL / Exercise / Sport:

| **Previous Medical History/General Health**
System   **Comment**
Skin
Musculoskeletal
Neurological
Gastrointestinal
Endocrine
Cardiovascular
Respiratory
Renal
Reproductive
Visual
Ear, nose and throat
Mental | **Recent visits to any of the following?**
(circle):

GP / consultant / physiotherapist / osteopath / chiropractor / podiatrist / sports therapist / sports massage practitioner / complementary therapist / other

Details (i.e. dates; diagnoses; treatments; advice): |
| **Medication History**
Current prescription medications and
dosage:

Non-prescription medications:

Other (homeopathic / supplements): | **History of Major Illness:**

History of Major Surgery (type / date):

Investigations (X-ray / MRI / CT / US / DEXA / blood tests / nerve conduction / arthroscopy / other): |

Any other conditions not mentioned above (e.g. allergies; general malaise; headache; dizziness; stress):

- *I, the undersigned, agree to undertake assessment and treatment, as advised by my sports therapist.*
- *I am aware I have the right to see my assessment and treatment records and these will not be released to any other party without my written consent.*
- *I have been informed that I may be accompanied during all treatment sessions.*
- *I declare that the information I have provided is correct and I will notify the therapist of any change in my medical condition as soon as I am aware of it.*

Patient signature:		Date:
Guardian signature (U 18s):	Guardian name:	Date:
Sports therapist signature:	Sports therapist name:	Date:

SPORTS THERAPY CLINIC   Date: _____

CONFIDENTIAL PATIENT RECORD FORM

PPW:

HPC (MoI; Onset; SIN; VAS; AF; RF):

Body charts:

CI / DDx:

Observations (skin; contours; posture):

Cleared joints:

Joint movements (ARoM; PRoM; Acc. mvts; RRoM):

721

SPORTS THERAPY CLINIC   Date: _____

CONFIDENTIAL PATIENT RECORD FORM

Special tests:

Functional tests:

Palpation:

Neurological assessment completed? Yes / No (see additional form)

Red / Yellow Flags / Referral (details):

Working Dx:

Problem list:	**Goals** (short / long term; SMART):	**Tx plan:**

Sports therapist signature: **Sports therapist name:**   **Date:**

SPORTS THERAPY CLINIC   **Date:** _____

CONFIDENTIAL PATIENT RECORD FORM

Tx / Ex / Advice provided	Sports therapist signature

CONTINUATION NOTES   Patient name:_____

Date / Tx no.	SOAP / Tx / Ex / Advice provided	Sports therapist signature

SPORTS THERAPY CLINIC   Date: _____

CONFIDENTIAL PATIENT RECORD FORM

NEUROLOGICAL ASSESSMENT Patient name: _____

Reflexes	Nerve Root	Reflexes	Comments:
Biceps / brachioradialis	C5 / C6		
Triceps	C7 / C8		
Patella	L3 / L4		
Achilles	S1 / S2		
Myotomes			
Shoulder elevation	C4		
Shoulder abduction	C5		
Elbow flexion/wrist extension	C6		
Elbow extension	C7		
Thumb extension	C8		
Finger abduction / adduction	T1		
Hip flexion	L2		
Knee extension	L3		
Ankle dorsiflexion	L4		
Hallux extension	L5		
Foot eversion	S1		
Gluteal contraction	S1 / S2		
Knee flexion	S1 / S2		
Plantarflexion	S1 / S2		

Dermatomes		Nerve Root	
		C4	
		C5	
		C6	
		C7	
		L2	
		L3	
		L4	
		L5	
		S1	
		S2	
		Comments:	

Appendix

SPORTS THERAPY CLINIC Date: _____
CONFIDENTIAL PATIENT RECORD FORM

NEUROLOGICAL ASSESSMENT Patient name: _____

Neural tests	Comments
Spurling's test R/L:	
Cervical compression / distraction test:	
ULNT 1 R/L (brachial plexus / median nv / anterior interosseous nv / C5 / C6 / C7):	
ULNT 2a R/L (median nv / musculocutaneous nv / axillary nv):	
ULNT 2b R/L (radial nv):	
ULNT 3 R/L (ulnar nv / C8 / T1):	
SLR test R/L:	
Slump test R/L:	
Femoral nv test R/L:	
UMN tests R/L (Babinski; clonus; Romberg's test; other):	
Comments:	
Sports therapist signature:	**Sports therapist name:** **Date:**

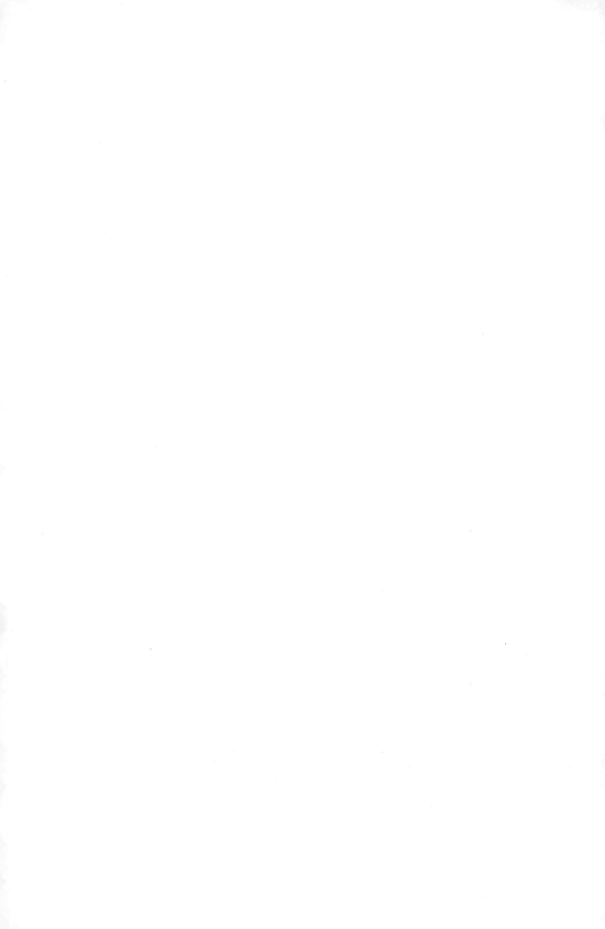

INDEX